"十三五"国家重点出版物出版规划项目

总 主 编　刘树伟

副总主编　赵　斌　柳　澄　李振平　徐以发

Color Atlas of Digital Human Cross Sectional Anatomy
Abdomen

数字人连续横断层解剖学彩色图谱
腹部分册

主编　汤煜春　于德新　任福欣

山东科学技术出版社

图书在版编目（CIP）数据

数字人连续横断层解剖学彩色图谱. 腹部分册 / 汤煜春, 于德新, 任福欣主编. -- 济南：山东科学技术出版社, 2020.12
ISBN 978-7-5723-0677-8

Ⅰ. ①数… Ⅱ. ①汤… ②于… ③任… Ⅲ. ①腹—计算机X线扫描体层摄影—断面解剖学—图谱 Ⅳ. ①R814.42-64

中国版本图书馆CIP数据核字(2020)第166507号

数字人连续横断层解剖学彩色图谱·腹部分册
SHUZIREN LIANXU HENGDUANCENG JIEPOUXUE CAISE TUPU · FUBU FENCE

责任编辑：徐日强　孙小杰
装帧设计：侯　宇　李晨溪

主管单位：山东出版传媒股份有限公司
出 版 者：山东科学技术出版社
　　　　　地址：济南市市中区英雄山路189号
　　　　　邮编：250002　电话：（0531）82098088
　　　　　网址：www.lkj.com.cn
　　　　　电子邮件：sdkj@sdcbcm.com
发 行 者：山东科学技术出版社
　　　　　地址：济南市市中区英雄山路189号
　　　　　邮编：250002　电话：（0531）82098071
印 刷 者：济南新先锋彩印有限公司
　　　　　地址：济南市工业北路188-6号
　　　　　邮编：250101　电话：（0531）88615699

规格：8开（285mm×420mm）
印张：34.75　字数：271千　印数：1~2000
版次：2020年12月第1版　2020年12月第1次印刷
定价：420.00元

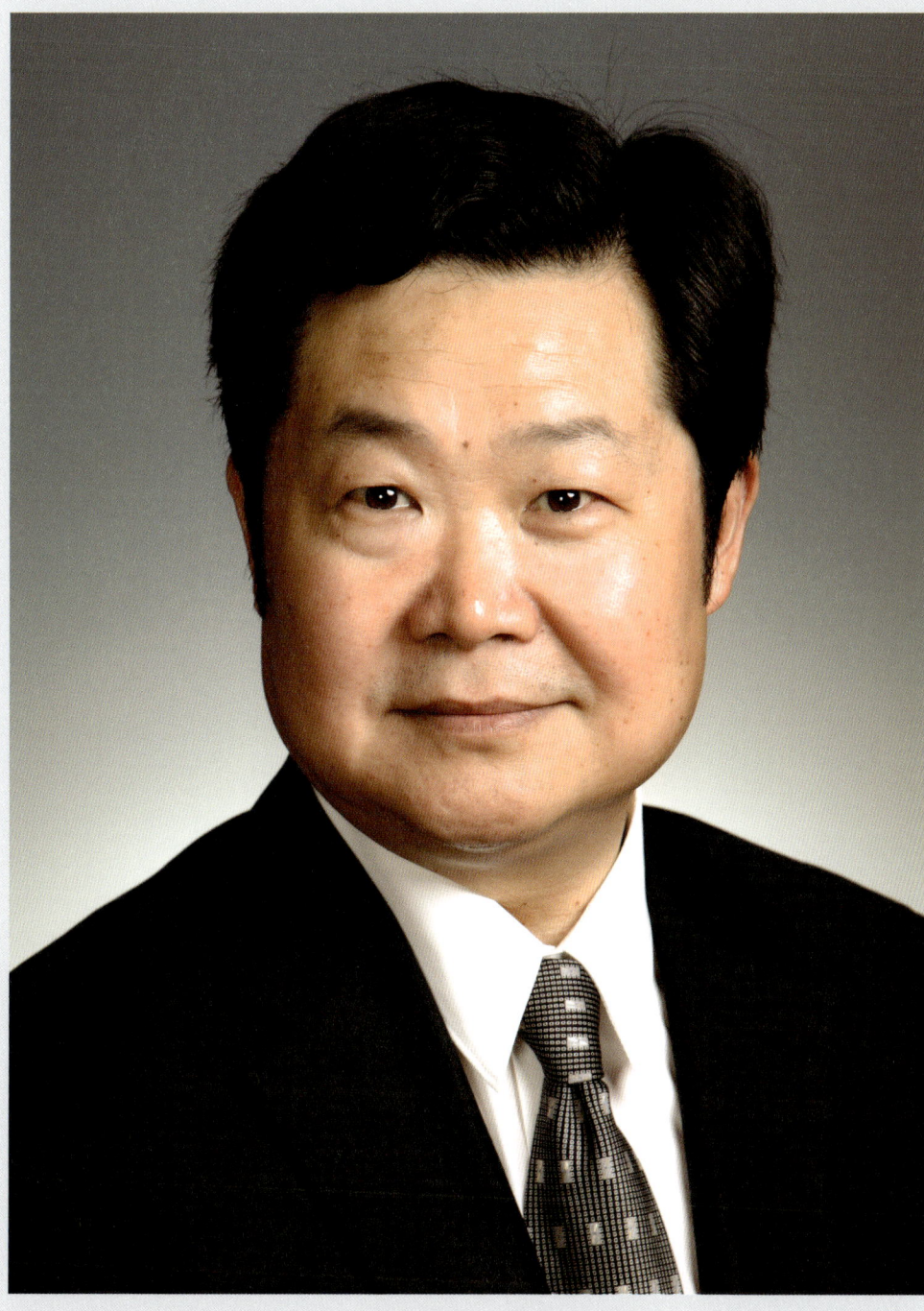

总主编 刘树伟

刘树伟，医学博士，山东大学基础医学院解剖学与神经生物学系教授、博士生导师，山东大学断层影像解剖学研究中心主任，山东大学数字人研究院院长，山东大学脑与类脑科学研究院副院长。曾任山东大学研究生院常务副院长、医学院副院长、人体解剖与组织胚胎学系主任等职，兼任亚洲临床解剖学会副主席、中国解剖学会副理事长和断层影像解剖学分会主任委员、中华医学会数字医学分会常务委员等职。获"卫生部有突出贡献的中青年专家"和"山东省教学名师"称号，享受国务院政府特殊津贴。潜心断层影像解剖学、数字人体和计算神经科学研究，承担国家及省部级课题20余项，在 *Radiology*、*NeuroImage* 和 *Cerebral Cortex* 等杂志发表论文320余篇（其中SCI收录70余篇），主编《人体断层解剖学》《临床中枢神经解剖学》和《功能神经影像学》等著作40余部，获省部级科技进步奖4项（其中一等奖1项）。长期从事人体解剖学教学，主持的"顺应现代影像学发展，创建断层解剖学课程"教学改革项目于1997年获山东省教学成果奖一等奖和国家级教学成果奖二等奖，主持完成的"我国数字解剖学教学体系创建与推广"教学研究项目于2018年获山东省教学成果奖特等奖和国家级教学成果奖二等奖。

主要学术著作、论文如下：

1. 刘树伟. 断层解剖学. 北京：人民卫生出版社, 1998.
2. 刘树伟. 人体断层解剖学图谱. 济南：山东科学技术出版社, 2003.
3. 刘树伟. 人体断层解剖学. 北京：高等教育出版社, 2006.
4. 刘树伟, 柳澄, 胡三元. 腹部外科临床解剖学图谱. 济南：山东科学技术出版社, 2006.
5. 刘树伟, 王怀经. 应用解剖学（全六册）. 北京：高等教育出版社, 2007.
6. 刘树伟, 尹岭, 唐一源. 功能神经影像学. 济南：山东科学技术出版社, 2011.
7. 刘树伟, 李瑞锡. 局部解剖学. 8版. 北京：人民卫生出版社, 2013.
8. 刘树伟, 杨晓飞, 邓雪飞. 临床解剖学·腹盆部分册. 2版. 北京：人民卫生出版社, 2014.
9. 刘树伟. 断层解剖学. 3版. 北京：高等教育出版社, 2017.
10. 刘树伟, 林祥涛. 影像解剖学系列图谱（全六册）. 济南：山东科学技术出版社, 2020.
11. Tang Y, Hojatkashani C, Dinov ID, Sun B, Fan L, Lin X, Qi H, Hua X, Liu S*, Toga AW*. The construction of a Chinese MRI brain atlas: a morphometric comparison study between Chinese and Caucasian cohorts. NeuroImage, 2010, 51(1): 33-41.
12. Liu F, Zhang Z, Lin X, Teng G, Meng H, Yu T, Fang F, Zang F, Li Z, Liu S*. Development of the human fetal cerebellum in the second trimester: a post mortem magnetic resonance imaging evaluation. J Anat, 2011, 219: 582–588.
13. Zuo Y, Liu C, Liu S*. Pulmonary intersegmental planes: imaging appearance and possible reasons leading to their visualization. Radiology, 2013, 267(1): 267-275.
14. Yin X, Han Y, Ge H, Xu W, Huang R, Zhang D, Xu J, Fan L, Pang Z, Liu S*. Inferior frontal white matter asymmetry correlates with executive control of attention. Hum Brain Mapp, 2013, 34(4): 796-813.
15. Zhan J, Dinov ID, Li J, Zhang Z, Hobel S, Shi Y, Lin X, Zamanyan A, Lei F, Teng G, Fang F, Tang Y, Zang F, Toga AW*, Liu S*. Spatial-temporal atlas of fetal brain development during the early second trimester. NeuroImage, 2013, 82:115-126.
16. Ge X, Shi Y, Li J, Zhang Z, Lin X, Zhan J, Ge H, Xu J, Yu Q, Leng Y, Teng G, Feng L, Meng H, Tang Y, Zang F, Toga AW*, Liu S*. Development of the human fetal hippocampal formation during early second trimester. NeuroImage, 2015, 119: 33-43.
17. Xu J, Yin X, Ge H, Han Y, Pang Z, Liu B*, Liu S*, Friston K. Heritability of the effective connectivity in the resting-state default mode network. Cerebral Cortex, 2017, 27(12): 5626-5634.
18. Tang Y, Zhao L, Lou Y, Shi Y, Fang R, Lin X, Liu S*, Toga AW. Brain structure differences between Chinese and Caucasian cohorts: A comprehensive morphometry study. Hum Brain Mapp, 2018, 39(5): 2147-2155.
19. Li Z, Xu F, Zhang Z, Lin X, Teng G, Zang F, Liu S*. Morphologic evolution and coordinated development of the fetal lateral ventricles in the second and third trimesters. Am J Neuroradiol, 2019, 40(4): 718-725.
20. Xu F, Ge X, Shi Y, Zhang Z, Tang Y, Lin X, Teng G, Zang F, Gao N, Liu H, Toga AW*, Liu S*. Morphometric development of the human fetal cerebellum during the early second trimester. NeuroImage, 2020, 207: 116372.

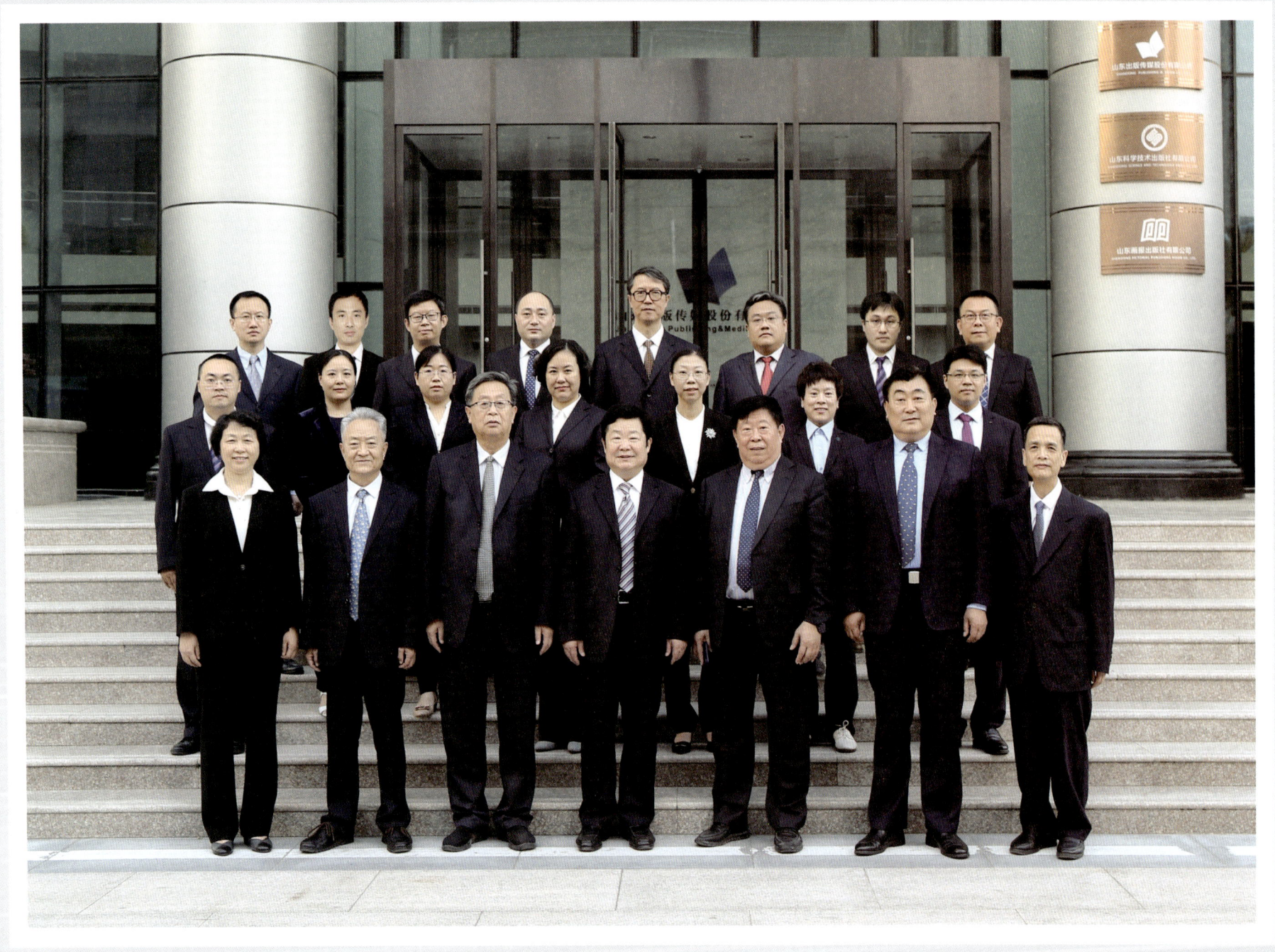

编委会全体人员合影

前排（从左至右）：王 青 李振平 柳 澄 刘树伟 赵 斌 徐以发 林祥涛
中排（从左至右）：孙 博 孟海伟 冯 蕾 张 杨 吴凤霞 王韶玉 任福欣
后排（从左至右）：侯中煜 左一智 于德新 汤煜春 于台飞 张忠和 于乔文 王增涛

《数字人连续横断层解剖学彩色图谱》编委会

总 主 编 刘树伟

副总主编 赵 斌　柳 澄　李振平　徐以发

编　　委（以姓氏笔画为序）

于台飞（山东省医学影像学研究所）　　　　汤煜春（山东大学齐鲁医学院）
于乔文（山东省立医院）　　　　　　　　　吴凤霞（山东大学齐鲁医学院）
于德新（山东大学齐鲁医院）　　　　　　　张　杨（山东大学齐鲁医院）
王　青（山东大学齐鲁医院）　　　　　　　张忠和（山东省立医院）
王韶玉（山东大学齐鲁医院）　　　　　　　李振平（山东大学齐鲁医学院）
王增涛（山东大学齐鲁医学院，山东省立医院）　孟海伟（山东大学齐鲁医学院）
刘树伟（山东大学齐鲁医学院）　　　　　　林祥涛（山东大学齐鲁医学院，山东省立医院）
冯　蕾（山东大学齐鲁医学院）　　　　　　赵　斌（山东省医学影像学研究所）
左一智（南京医科大学）　　　　　　　　　柳　澄（山东省医学影像学研究所）
孙　博（山东省医学影像学研究所）　　　　侯中煜（山东省立医院）
任福欣（山东省医学影像学研究所）　　　　徐以发（山东省数字人工程技术研究中心）

腹部分册

主　　编　汤煜春　于德新　任福欣

编　　者　（以姓氏笔画为序）

于德新（山东大学齐鲁医院）　　　　　　　刘宇宁（山东大学齐鲁医学院）

王　宝（山东大学齐鲁医院）　　　　　　　齐亚飞（山东大学齐鲁医院）

王　红（山东大学齐鲁医学院）　　　　　　胡旻琦（山东大学齐鲁医学院）

汤煜春（山东大学齐鲁医学院）　　　　　　龚　鑫（皖南医学院）

任福欣（山东省医学影像学研究所）　　　　缪化春（皖南医学院）

标本图像处理

魏　昱（山东省数字人工程技术研究中心）

李照群（山东省数字人工程技术研究中心）

任晓雪（山东省数字人工程技术研究中心）

序 一

我在人体解剖学园地里已耕耘七十余年了，对这个园地里新出现的每一朵鲜花和每一颗小草，都备感欣慰和鼓舞。今天，当看到山东大学刘树伟教授寄来的《数字人连续横断层解剖学彩色图谱》的书稿时，我眼前一亮，心情十分振奋。这将是一部巨著，是人体解剖学园地里一朵引人注目的鲜花。第一，它的人体标本数字断层彩色图像国际领先。"剖开顽石方知玉，淘尽泥沙始见金。"外形适中、结构正常、色泽鲜艳的人体断层标本相当难得。刘树伟教授团队历时5年，共铣削了6具人体标本，选择其中2具的断层图像来制成这部图谱，十分难能可贵。这套断层图像的分辨率高达16 000像素×26 000像素，为当今国际上人体标本断层图像的最高分辨率。更令人感到欣喜的是，动脉和静脉均灌注颜料，使小血管得以展示，更有益于疾病的影像诊断和微创外科手术参考，大大增加了这套图谱的临床适用性。第二，书中标本断层与活体薄层CT、MR图像匹配得当。"天机云锦用在我，裁剪妙处非刀尺。"由于非同一个体，人体标本断层与活体CT、MR图像的匹配十分困难，在毫米级的层厚上二者间的匹配更是难上加难。同时，在国内外同类图谱中往往不配CT、MR图像。刘树伟教授团队"明知山有虎，偏向虎山行"，动员了十几名志愿者参与CT、MR配图，终获成功，使这部图谱的科学性、临床实用价值大为提高。第三，这部图谱是"医工结合""解剖与影像结合"的典范。"几番磨砺方成器，十载耕耘自见功。"刘树伟教授在山东大学先后创建了山东大学断层影像解剖学研究中心、数字人研究院，形成了一支"医工结合""解剖与影像结合"的科研团队，承担了一批国家级科研项目，在国内外杂志上发表了400余篇论文，获得10余项省部级科技进步奖和国家级教学成果奖，开发了教学软件"中国数字人解剖系统"，为我国断层影像解剖学和数字医学的发展做出了突出贡献。这部图谱是这种合作的杰出代表，我十分赞赏。

总之，刘树伟教授总主编的这部《数字人连续横断层解剖学彩色图谱》具有极强的创新性、科学性和实用性，出版价值重大。我真诚地希望不远的将来有数字人连续矢状断层和冠状断层的解剖学图谱出版。若如斯，解剖与影像皆幸莫大焉！

中国工程院院士 钟世镇

2020年10月

序 二

进入21世纪以来，医学影像技术发展迅速，扫描层厚越来越薄，图像分辨率不断提高，所显示的解剖细节也越来越丰富，亟需与之相适应的断层解剖学图谱为其提供形态学基础。正值此时，山东大学刘树伟教授团队利用数控冷冻铣削技术获得了0.1 mm层厚的人体标本连续断层数据集，并编写成《数字人连续横断层解剖学彩色图谱》。我有幸先于广大读者看到书稿，感到此部图谱有以下特色：

特色之一，断层薄，精度高。人体连续断层标本彩色图像0.1 mm层厚，每隔20层选1层，分辨率高达16 000像素×26 000像素，达到了同类图谱的国际领先水平。CT、MR图像均为2 mm层厚，能做到与断层标本较好地契合。

特色之二，标注细，结构全。全书对5 000多个解剖结构进行了中英文标注，脑部结构标注到了大脑沟回、神经核团，肺、肝等均标注到了亚段级结构，对心包腔、胸膜腔、腹膜腔等均进行了连续追踪观察。

特色之三，注重将具体知识总结提升为解剖学理论。每一断层均有概要性文字，不仅描述了断层结构的整体配布规律，还讨论了关键结构的断面形态变化类型、大小、变异及其影像学特征等。

特色之四，努力做到理论联系实际。关键结构的选择以临床需要为原则，具体内容强调结合临床诊疗技术进展讨论解剖结构在疾病影像学诊断、介入治疗和外科手术中的应用。

总之，这是一部优秀的大型人体断层解剖学专著。它的公开出版，不仅在解剖学上有着重要的意义，而且对疾病影像诊断水平的提高也将大有裨益。因之为序，并郑重地向广大临床工作者推荐。

中国工程院院士 张运

2020年10月

序 三

山东大学刘树伟教授是我国著名的断层影像解剖学专家，目前担任中国解剖学会副理事长兼断层影像解剖学分会主任委员。他不仅在 Radiology 和 NeuroImage 等国际著名杂志上发表了一系列研究论文，而且在断层解剖学和数字解剖学教学方面 2 次获得国家级教学成果奖。最近，刘树伟教授团队用数控冷冻铣削技术获取了 6 套中国人连续横断层解剖数据，计划出版一部《数字人连续横断层解剖学彩色图谱》。我仔细阅读了他寄来的书稿，感到这是一部人体断层解剖学的巨著，拥有以下创新：

（1）人体标本连续断层彩色图像来源于数字人研究，分辨率高，达到了同类图谱的国际领先水平。刘树伟教授团队改进了数控冷冻铣削技术，使用了大型龙门刨床，革新了切削刀具和切削工艺，使用 LED 光源和线阵扫描式相机摄影，获得了 0.1 mm 层厚的真彩色人体标本断层图像，分辨率达到了 16 000 像素 ×26 000 像素，而且较好地保留了标本原始色彩。

（2）使用 2 mm 间距选择标本和活体 CT、MR 图像制作图谱，8 开本印刷，是国内外同类图谱中绝无仅有的。使用数字人断面制作断层解剖学图谱在美国和中国已有先例，但断面间距均在 10 mm 以上，且无活体 CT、MR 图像相匹配，因此已不能满足当今数字人研究和疾病 CT、MR 图像诊断的需求，亟需薄层断层解剖学图谱的出版。

（3）标注细致和断面特点总结是该部图谱的又一显著特点。该部图谱使用《中国解剖学名词》对 5 000 多个解剖结构进行了中英文标注，每幅图像的标注结构大多超过 40 个，每隔 10 mm 增加了重要结构断层解剖的特点总结、断面数值和临床应用意义介绍，使这部图谱不仅科学理论价值巨增，也提高了其临床实用性，受众面大大增加。

我相信这部图谱代表了当今断层影像解剖学的发展前沿，将使该学科又上了一个新台阶，不仅将促进我国断层解剖学学科水平的整体提高，也将推动疾病 CT、MR 诊断水平的进一步改善，从而产生巨大的社会效益。因此，我很高兴为之作序，并向广大读者推荐。

中国工程院院士

2020 年 11 月

总前言

"图谱是表达断层解剖的最好形式。"这是我的导师四川大学王永贵教授34年前的谆谆教诲,当时只是一名硕士研究生的我并未完全理解。随着岁月的磨炼,我逐渐认识到这真是一句至理名言。时间进入21世纪,尤其是近10年间,人体断层解剖学发展迅速。在断层数据的获取方面,数控冷冻铣削技术使标本断层层厚达到了亚毫米水平,以CT和MRI为代表的医学影像设备的扫描速度更快、层厚更薄、分辨力更高;在断层图像的处理方面,多平面重组、三维重建、多模态影像融合、虚拟现实、增强现实和生物学计量等技术的发展更加深入、应用更趋广泛;在研究内容方面,对人体局部断层解剖信息的要求更加精细,形态与功能的结合更加密切,临床应用的针对性更强。在这种学术背景下,无论是人体解剖学工作者,还是临床医师,均呼唤着层厚在毫米级的薄层连续人体断层解剖彩色图谱的出版。"好雨知时节,当春乃发生。"这部《数字人连续横断层解剖学彩色图谱》应运而生,既是人体解剖学领域最重要的前沿进展之一,又迎合了临床医师尤其是医学影像学医师的祈盼,还实现了本人的终生夙愿。

《数字人连续横断层解剖学彩色图谱》共包括头颈部、胸部、腹部、盆部与会阴、上肢和下肢6个分册,图像共4 519幅(含断层标本彩色图像917幅、螺旋CT图像1 753幅、3T MR图像1 841幅、其他图像8幅),文字约170万字。从图像采集到全书定稿,主要由山东大学数字人研究院完成。我们的目标是把本套图谱打造成断层解剖学的传世经典、解剖学工作者案头必备的工具书、临床工作者爱不释手的阅片指南。努力追求做到以下四个突出。第一,突出薄层断层解剖。以往的厚片断层解剖切片多在厘米级,许多解剖结构难以显示。本图谱标本断层层厚为0.1 mm,每隔20层选用1层,因此可充分展示一些细小的解剖结构。在标注和文字描述中,重点突出那些以往厚片无法展示的解剖细节,使断层解剖学为之一新。第二,突出解剖与影像的融合。标本断层和影像断层是断层解剖学两大支柱内容,在以往的研究中往往强调相互对照,而融合不够。本图谱不但强调二者之间的相互匹配,而且更强调二者的融合,旨在给出关键结构影像学表现的精准解剖学阐释。第三,突出断层解剖学规律的总结。以往的许多图谱,只注重断层结构的标注,而忽略了解剖结构在连续断层中的变化规律。本图谱每一断层均有300～500字的总结性短文,以讨论关键结构的断层形态变化规律、类型、大小、位置、毗邻、分区、发育、变异、影像学特征、生理功能、诊断和治疗意义等,以期将具体知识总结升华为断层解剖学理论。第四,突出基础理论与临床应用的结合。伟大导师恩格斯说过:"没有解剖学就没有医学。"因此,解剖学知识只有应用于临床才能显示出其巨大实用意义和社会价值。书中关键结构的选择以临床需要为标准,在写作中强调精选内容,重点讨论关键结构在疾病诊断、介入治疗和外科手术中的应用价值。

"雄关漫道真如铁,而今迈步从头越。"在全书即将付梓之际,心中百感交集,思绪万千。我要衷心感谢国家自然科学基金委员会和山东省科技厅,是其立项的科研项目使本图谱使用的原始数据得以成功获取;我要衷心感谢我的同事们和研究生们,是大家齐心协力、忘我无私的工作,才使本书得以完成;我要衷心感谢中国工程院钟世镇院士、张运院士、顾晓松院士及西安交通大学刘军教授,是他们的推荐意见和序,照亮了我前进的道路;我要衷心感谢我的解剖学、影像学和外科学同仁,他们富有建设性的意见和建议使得本书内容在解剖学与临床的结合上更加紧密;我要衷心感谢山东科学技术出版社,是其领导和编辑们的视野、耐心和意志使得本图谱历尽千辛万苦而得以出版并入选"十三五"国家重点出版物出版规划项目。书是在使用中日臻完善的。最后,我衷心希望和感谢广大读者,不断提出您的意见和需求,以使本书更具理论价值和临床适用性。

2020年是中国解剖学会成立100周年。特将本部图谱献给中国解剖学会,以隆重纪念其百年华诞。

总主编 刘树伟

2020年10月15日

前 言

《数字人连续横断层解剖学彩色图谱·腹部分册》共有 640 幅图像（含断层标本彩色图像 128 幅，螺旋 CT 图像 256 幅，3.0 T MR 图像 256 幅），文字约 27 万字。从图像采集到结构标注，从文字撰写到全书定稿，主要由山东大学数字人研究院完成。人体连续横断层解剖图像来源于一名腹部无异常的女性尸体标本，以膈右穹窿平面为上界，经 L5-S1 椎间盘平面为下界，总共获取 2 560 个断面，层厚为 0.1 mm，每隔 20 层选 1 层，共选取 128 幅断层彩色图像用于本图谱。匹配良好的 CT 和 MR 图像源自一名腹部无异常的女性志愿者，均为 2 mm 层厚，包括螺旋 CT 常规扫描和增强扫描的图像各 128 幅，3T 磁共振扫描 T1 加权和 T2 加权图像各 128 幅，以便读者能够各取所需。

这 128 层腹部横断层结构的配布，由上而下大致可分为 6 段。

第 1 段（断层 1～6）：从膈右穹窿出现平面至膈左穹窿出现平面，该段腹部结构相对简单，主要为膈右穹窿、肝右叶、膈腔静脉孔和下腔静脉。

第 2 段（断层 7～32）：从第二肝门出现平面至第一肝门出现平面，由右向左依次为肝、胃和脾。肝的断面从上至下逐渐增大，占据上腹部的大部分，其内从上到下肝静脉逐渐变细、肝门静脉逐渐变粗。膈食管裂孔出现，食管腹段连至胃贲门。大、小网膜次第出现，肝镰状韧带、冠状韧带明显，肝周围的腹膜腔为肝周间隙，脾周围的腹膜腔为脾周间隙。此例标本横结肠与降结肠位置高，出现于胃左前方。

第 3 段（断层 33～56）：从肝门静脉分叉平面至肝门静脉合成平面，腹部结构渐趋复杂，从上到下出现肝蒂、肾上腺、肾、胰、胆囊、升降结肠、横结肠、胃体部与幽门部、十二指肠。肝断面逐渐变小，肝内管道明显变细。胰头、颈、体、尾出现，门腔间隙位于此段。大网膜、小网膜、镰状韧带、肝圆韧带明显，网膜囊居胃与胰体之间，肝肾隐窝介于肝与肾之间。胆外胆道出现于此段。双肾明显，肾门、肾盂内结构易于辨认。膈主动脉裂孔出现，腹主动脉向前依次发出腹腔干和肠系膜上动脉，脾动脉、脾静脉出现。空肠显露于左上腹。可仔细寻找腹腔神经节、交感干、淋巴结等。

第 4 段（断层 57～86）：从肝门静脉合成至胰头消失平面，从前向后大致可将腹部结构分为三层，前层由右向左为升结肠、大网膜与胃体、横结肠、空肠和降结肠，中层由右向左为肝右叶、十二指肠降部、胰头、肠系膜上动静脉、十二指肠升部，后层由右向左为右肾、下腔静脉与左肾静脉、主动腹部与肾动脉、左肾等。淋巴结散在于上述结构之间。

第 5 段（断层 87～107）：从胰头消失平面至腹主动脉分叉平面，主要为肠道和肠系膜，右侧为升结肠，中间为横结肠及其系膜，左侧为降结肠、小肠及肠系膜，脊柱前方为下腔静脉和腹主动脉。腹壁结构明显，可于此段观察。

第 6 段（断层 108～128）：从腹主动脉分叉平面至 L5-S1 椎间盘平面，主要为肠道，如升结肠、回肠、空肠、降结肠，髂骨翼出现，髂总动脉、静脉逐渐分向两侧。腹前外侧壁结构清晰，可见白线、腹直肌与腹直肌鞘、腹外斜肌及其腱膜、腹内斜肌与腹横肌。腹后壁肌可见腰大肌与腰方肌。此段亦适于观察输尿管、腹壁浅筋膜、淋巴结等。

呕心沥血终成卷，千呼万唤始出来。回顾整个编写历程，真是感慨万千。衷心感谢著名解剖学家、本书的总主编刘树伟教授的信任和委托，让我们成为《数字人连续横断层解剖彩色图谱》这套传世经典之作的参与者和见证者；衷心感谢我们的解剖学同事和影像学同仁们，在大家的共同努力下，本图谱终于付梓。尽管我们反复校阅，书中难免会有错误和不足之处，衷心希望读者多多提出需求和建议，以使本书在使用中不断完善。

汤煜春　于德新　任福欣

2020 年 11 月 16 日

目 录

腹部连续横断层解剖

腹部连续横断层 1（FH.11910）..2
腹部连续横断层 2（FH.11890）..4
腹部连续横断层 3（FH.11870）..6
腹部连续横断层 4（FH.11850）..8
腹部连续横断层 5（FH.11830）...10
腹部连续横断层 6（FH.11810）...12
腹部连续横断层 7（FH.11790）...14
腹部连续横断层 8（FH.11770）...16
腹部连续横断层 9（FH.11750）...18
腹部连续横断层 10（FH.11730）...20
腹部连续横断层 11（FH.11710）...22
腹部连续横断层 12（FH.11690）...24
腹部连续横断层 13（FH.11670）...26
腹部连续横断层 14（FH.11650）...28
腹部连续横断层 15（FH.11630）...30
腹部连续横断层 16（FH.11610）...32
腹部连续横断层 17（FH.11590）...34
腹部连续横断层 18（FH.11570）...36
腹部连续横断层 19（FH.11550）...38
腹部连续横断层 20（FH.11530）...40
腹部连续横断层 21（FH.11510）...42
腹部连续横断层 22（FH.11490）...44
腹部连续横断层 23（FH.11470）...46
腹部连续横断层 24（FH.11450）...48
腹部连续横断层 25（FH.11430）...50
腹部连续横断层 26（FH.11410）...52
腹部连续横断层 27（FH.11390）...54
腹部连续横断层 28（FH.11370）...56
腹部连续横断层 29（FH.11350）...58
腹部连续横断层 30（FH.11330）...60
腹部连续横断层 31（FH.11310）...62
腹部连续横断层 32（FH.11290）...64
腹部连续横断层 33（FH.11270）...66
腹部连续横断层 34（FH.11250）...68
腹部连续横断层 35（FH.11230）...70
腹部连续横断层 36（FH.11210）...72
腹部连续横断层 37（FH.11190）...74
腹部连续横断层 38（FH.11170）...76
腹部连续横断层 39（FH.11150）...78
腹部连续横断层 40（FH.11130）...80
腹部连续横断层 41（FH.11110）...82
腹部连续横断层 42（FH.11090）...84
腹部连续横断层 43（FH.11070）...86
腹部连续横断层 44（FH.11050）...88
腹部连续横断层 45（FH.11030）...90
腹部连续横断层 46（FH.11010）...92
腹部连续横断层 47（FH.10990）...94
腹部连续横断层 48（FH.10970）...96
腹部连续横断层 49（FH.10950）...98
腹部连续横断层 50（FH.10930）...100
腹部连续横断层 51（FH.10910）...102
腹部连续横断层 52（FH.10890）...104
腹部连续横断层 53（FH.10870）...106
腹部连续横断层 54（FH.10850）...108
腹部连续横断层 55（FH.10830）...110

腹部连续横断层 56（FH.10810）..........112	腹部连续横断层 94（FH.10050）..........188
腹部连续横断层 57（FH.10790）..........114	腹部连续横断层 95（FH.10030）..........190
腹部连续横断层 58（FH.10770）..........116	腹部连续横断层 96（FH.10010）..........192
腹部连续横断层 59（FH.10750）..........118	腹部连续横断层 97（FH.9990）..........194
腹部连续横断层 60（FH.10730）..........120	腹部连续横断层 98（FH.9970）..........196
腹部连续横断层 61（FH.10710）..........122	腹部连续横断层 99（FH.9950）..........198
腹部连续横断层 62（FH.10690）..........124	腹部连续横断层 100（FH.9930）..........200
腹部连续横断层 63（FH.10670）..........126	腹部连续横断层 101（FH.9910）..........202
腹部连续横断层 64（FH.10650）..........128	腹部连续横断层 102（FH.9890）..........204
腹部连续横断层 65（FH.10630）..........130	腹部连续横断层 103（FH.9870）..........206
腹部连续横断层 66（FH.10610）..........132	腹部连续横断层 104（FH.9850）..........208
腹部连续横断层 67（FH.10590）..........134	腹部连续横断层 105（FH.9830）..........210
腹部连续横断层 68（FH.10570）..........136	腹部连续横断层 106（FH.9810）..........212
腹部连续横断层 69（FH.10550）..........138	腹部连续横断层 107（FH.9790）..........214
腹部连续横断层 70（FH.10530）..........140	腹部连续横断层 108（FH.9770）..........216
腹部连续横断层 71（FH.10510）..........142	腹部连续横断层 109（FH.9750）..........218
腹部连续横断层 72（FH.10490）..........144	腹部连续横断层 110（FH.9730）..........220
腹部连续横断层 73（FH.10470）..........146	腹部连续横断层 111（FH.9710）..........222
腹部连续横断层 74（FH.10450）..........148	腹部连续横断层 112（FH.9690）..........224
腹部连续横断层 75（FH.10430）..........150	腹部连续横断层 113（FH.9670）..........226
腹部连续横断层 76（FH.10410）..........152	腹部连续横断层 114（FH.9650）..........228
腹部连续横断层 77（FH.10390）..........154	腹部连续横断层 115（FH.9630）..........230
腹部连续横断层 78（FH.10370）..........156	腹部连续横断层 116（FH.9610）..........232
腹部连续横断层 79（FH.10350）..........158	腹部连续横断层 117（FH.9590）..........234
腹部连续横断层 80（FH.10330）..........160	腹部连续横断层 118（FH.9570）..........236
腹部连续横断层 81（FH.10310）..........162	腹部连续横断层 119（FH.9550）..........238
腹部连续横断层 82（FH.10290）..........164	腹部连续横断层 120（FH.9530）..........240
腹部连续横断层 83（FH.10270）..........166	腹部连续横断层 121（FH.9510）..........242
腹部连续横断层 84（FH.10250）..........168	腹部连续横断层 122（FH.9490）..........244
腹部连续横断层 85（FH.10230）..........170	腹部连续横断层 123（FH.9470）..........246
腹部连续横断层 86（FH.10210）..........172	腹部连续横断层 124（FH.9450）..........248
腹部连续横断层 87（FH.10190）..........174	腹部连续横断层 125（FH.9430）..........250
腹部连续横断层 88（FH.10170）..........176	腹部连续横断层 126（FH.9410）..........252
腹部连续横断层 89（FH.10150）..........178	腹部连续横断层 127（FH.9390）..........254
腹部连续横断层 90（FH.10130）..........180	腹部连续横断层 128（FH.9370）..........256
腹部连续横断层 91（FH.10110）..........182	
腹部连续横断层 92（FH.10090）..........184	**参考文献**..........258
腹部连续横断层 93（FH.10070）..........186	**索　引**..........261

腹部分册
腹部连续横断层解剖

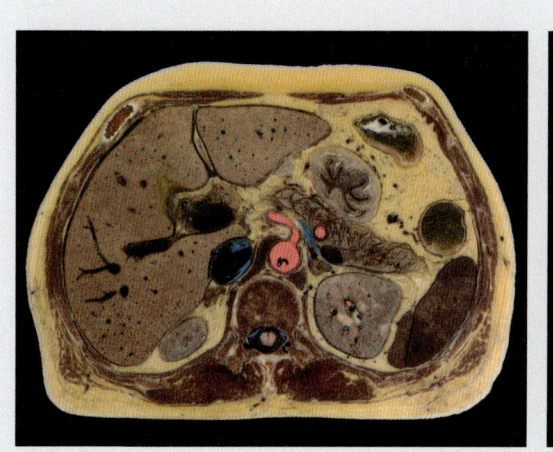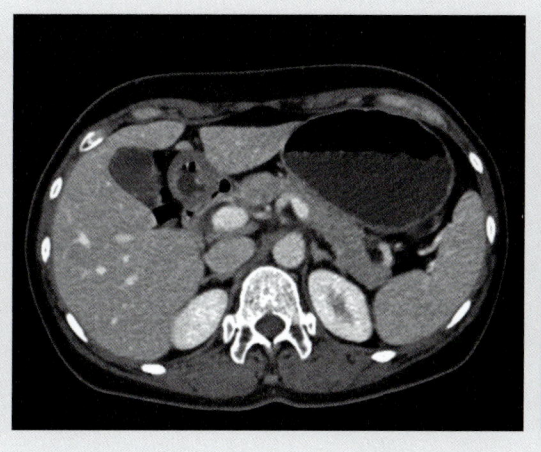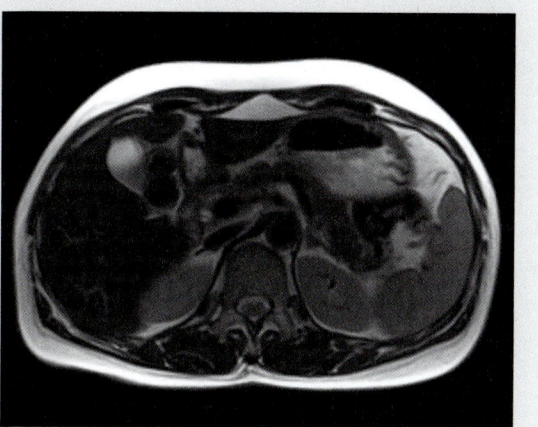

腹部连续横断层 1（FH.11910）

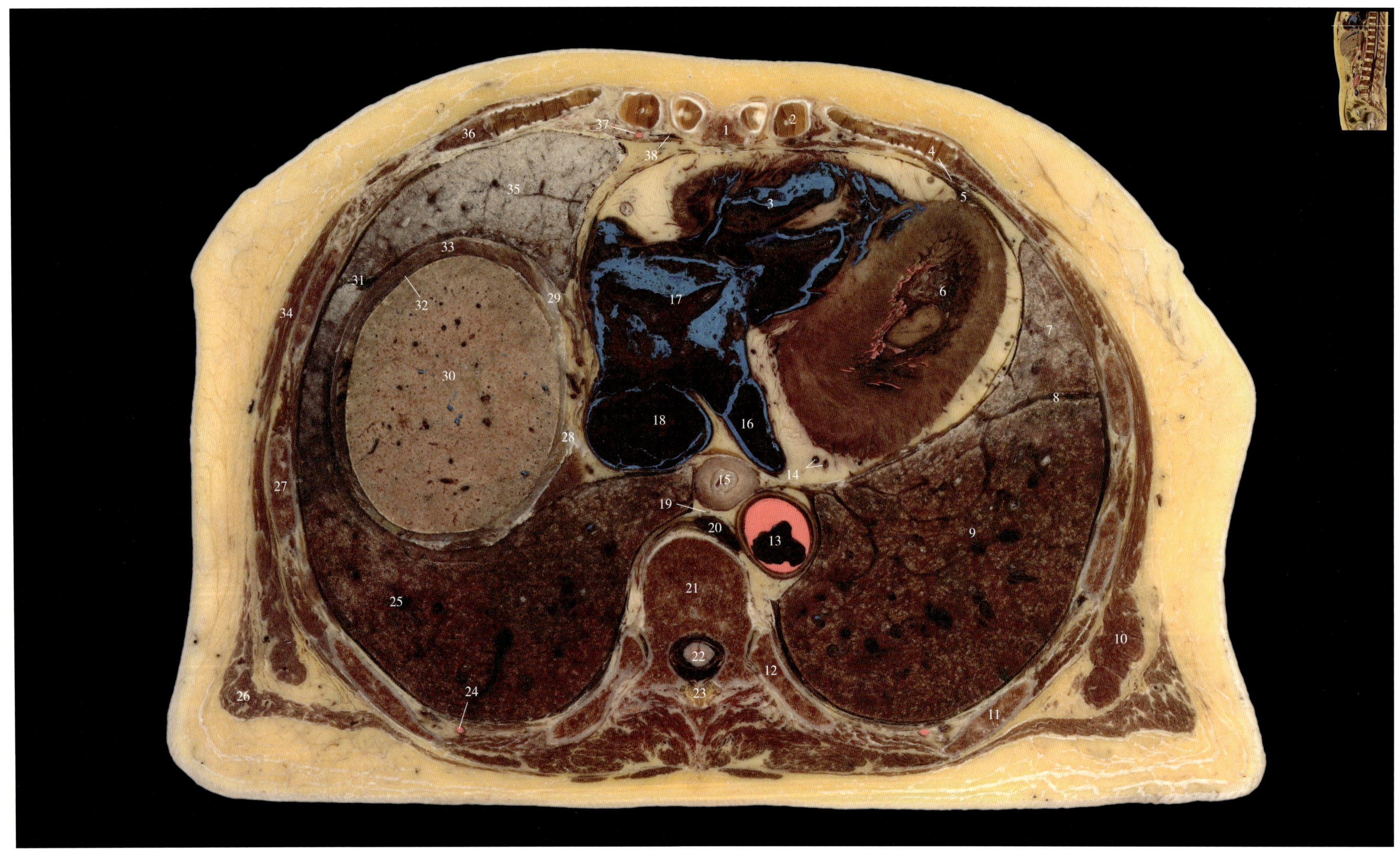

A. 断层标本图像

1. 胸骨体 body of sternum
2. 第 5 肋软骨 5th costal cartilage
3. 右心室 right ventricle
4. 肋纵隔隐窝 costomediastinal recess
5. 心包腔 pericardial cavity
6. 左心室 left ventricle
7. 左肺上叶 superior lobe of left lung
8. 左肺斜裂 oblique fissure of left lung
9. 左肺下叶 inferior lobe of left lung
10. 前锯肌 serratus anterior
11. 第 8 肋骨 8th costal bone
12. 第 9 肋骨 9th costal bone
13. 胸主动脉 thoracic aorta
14. 左冠状动脉左缘支 left marginal branch of left coronary artery
15. 食管 esophagus
16. 冠状窦 coronary sinus
17. 右心房 right atrium
18. 下腔静脉 inferior vena cava
19. 胸导管 thoracic duct
20. 奇静脉 azygos vein
21. 第 9 胸椎椎体 body of 9th thoracic vertebra
22. 脊髓 spinal cord
23. 黄韧带 ligamenta flava
24. 肋间后动脉 posterior intercostal artery
25. 右肺下叶 inferior lobe of right lung
26. 背阔肌 latissimus dorsi
27. 第 7 肋骨 7th costal bone
28. 冠状韧带上层 superior layer of coronary ligament
29. 冠状韧带下层 inferior layer of coronary ligament
30. 肝右叶 right lobe of liver
31. 右肺斜裂 oblique fissure of right lung
32. 右肝上间隙 right suprahepatic space
33. 膈 diaphragm
34. 腹外斜肌 obliquus externus abdominis
35. 右肺中叶 middle lobe of right lung
36. 第 5 肋骨 5th costal bone
37. 腹壁上动脉 superior epigastric artery
38. 胸廓内静脉 internal thoracic vein

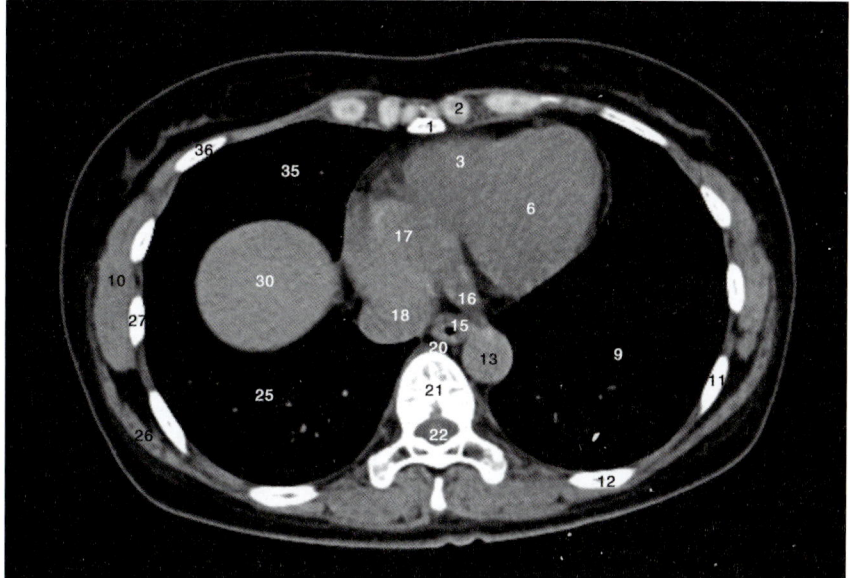

B. CT 平扫图像

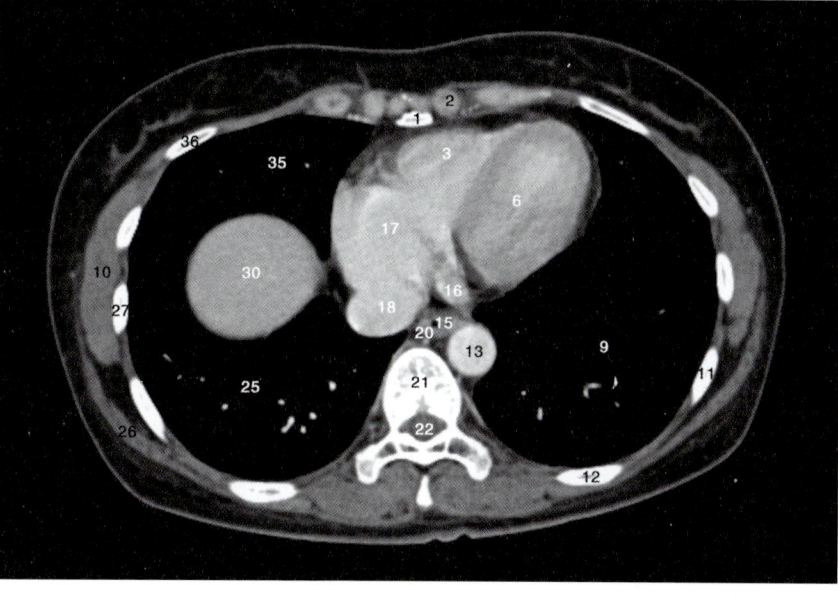

C. CT 增强图像

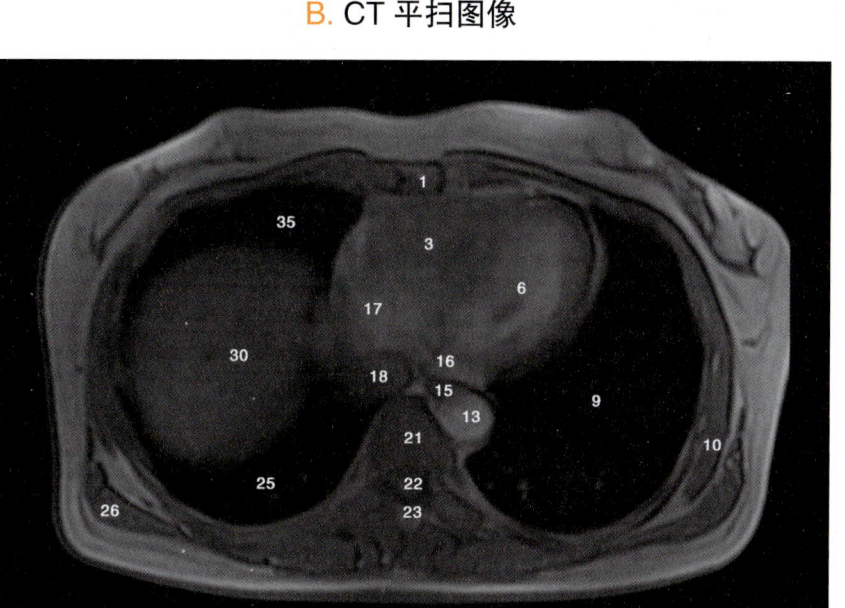

D. MR T1WI

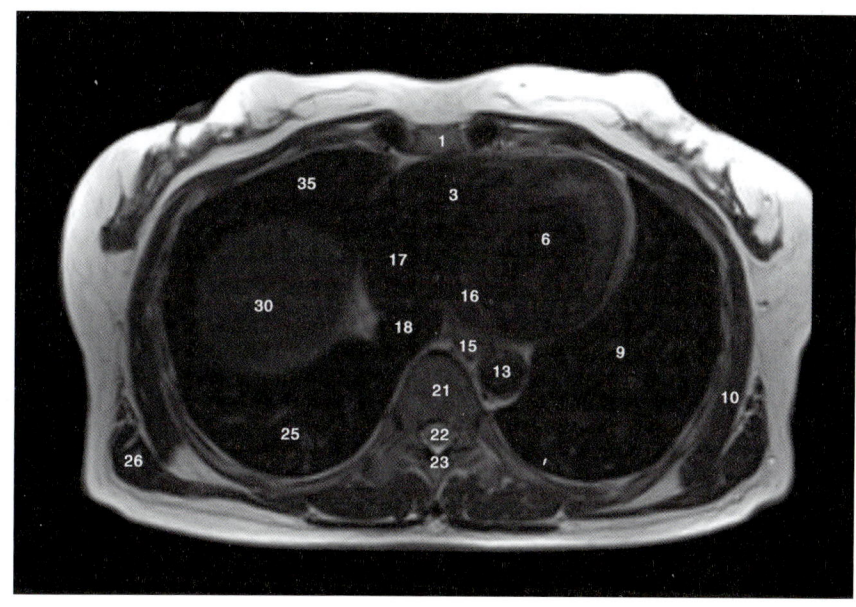

E. MR T2WI

关键结构：膈右穹窿，心，肺。

此断面经第 9 胸椎椎体下份。

心与左、右肺占据此断面的绝大部分，可见右心房、左、右心室和冠状窦等结构，其右侧为膈右穹窿和肝右叶。冠状韧带由膈下及肝上面的腹膜移行而成，由上、下两层腹膜构成。下腔静脉穿过膈的腔静脉孔，注入右心房。食管逐渐左移，走向膈的食管裂孔。胸主动脉位于食管左后方，贴椎体向下走行。膈右穹窿和肝右叶的出现 85% 集中于第 9~10 胸椎水平，其最高点居第 5 胸肋关节的高处[1]。膈肌收缩时下降 1~3 cm，使胸腔扩大，帮助吸气。在进行腹部 CT 等影像学检查时，为减少呼吸动度误差，大约 1/4 的胸部会保留在扫描野内，应注意充分利用这些影像信息（如 CT 可调整为肺窗以便观察更多的肺信息）来对肺、胸膜等病变进行筛查式诊断，如发现肺的炎症、肿瘤等。如腹部检查阴性的腹疼患者可通过观察扫描野内胸膜是否增厚、有无胸腔积液等来判断是否为胸膜炎所致的放射性腹痛。

3

腹部连续横断层 2（FH.11890）

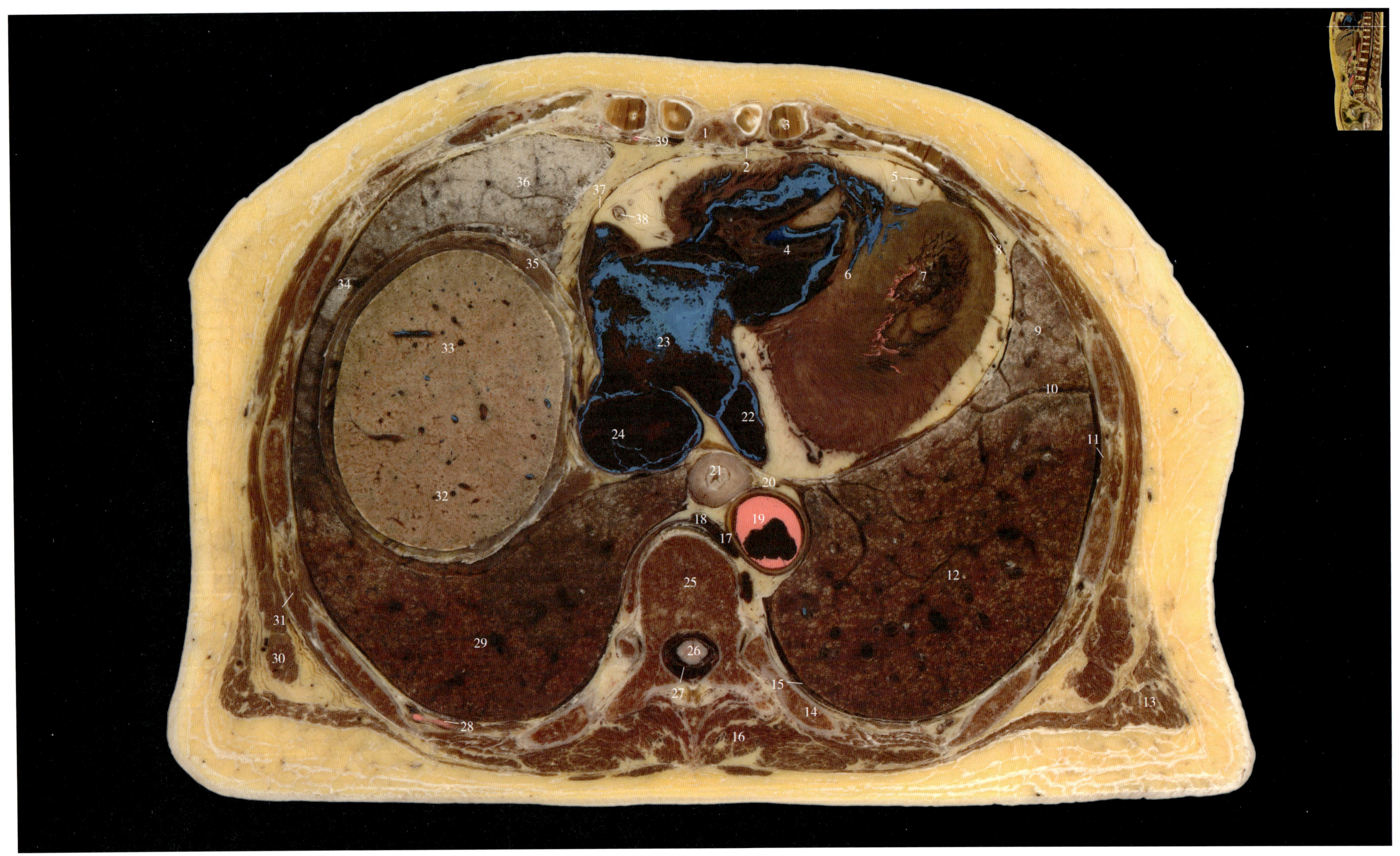

A. 断层标本图像

1. 胸骨体 body of sternum
2. 胸廓内静脉 internal thoracic vein
3. 第5肋软骨 5th costal cartilage
4. 右心室 right ventricle
5. 左冠状动脉前室间支 anterior interventricular branch of left coronary artery
6. 室间隔 interventricular septum
7. 左心室 left ventricle
8. 心包前下窦 anterior inferior sinus of pericardium
9. 左肺上叶 superior lobe of left lung
10. 左肺斜裂 oblique fissure of left lung
11. 肋间内肌 intercostale interni
12. 左肺下叶 inferior lobe of left lung
13. 背阔肌 latissimus dorsi
14. 第9肋骨 9th costal bone
15. 胸膜腔 pleural cavity
16. 竖脊肌 erector spinae
17. 半奇静脉 hemiazygos vein
18. 奇静脉 azygos vein
19. 胸主动脉 thoracic aorta
20. 左肺韧带 left pulmonary ligament
21. 食管 esophagus
22. 冠状窦 coronary sinus
23. 右心房 right atrium
24. 下腔静脉 inferior vena cava
25. 第9胸椎椎体 body of 9th thoracic vertebra
26. 脊髓 spinal cord
27. 硬脊膜 spinal dura mater
28. 肋间后动脉 posterior intercostal artery
29. 右肺下叶 inferior lobe of right lung
30. 后锯肌 serratus posterior
31. 肋间外肌 intercostale externi
32. 肝右后叶上段 superior segment of right posterior lobe of liver
33. 肝右前叶上段 superior segment of right anterior lobe of liver
34. 右肺斜裂 oblique fissure of right lung
35. 膈 diaphragm
36. 右肺中叶 middle lobe of right lung
37. 心包腔 pericardial cavity
38. 右冠状动脉 right coronary artery
39. 腹壁上动脉 superior epigastric artery

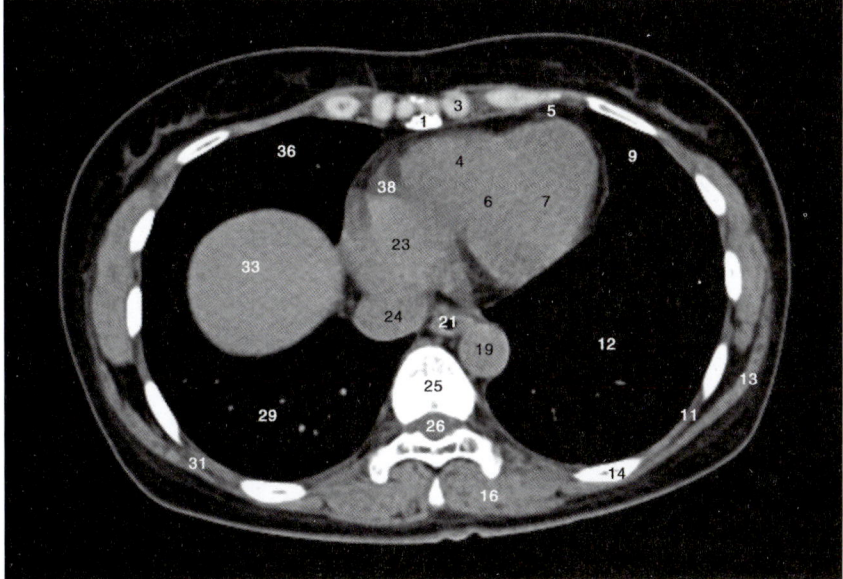

B. CT 平扫图像

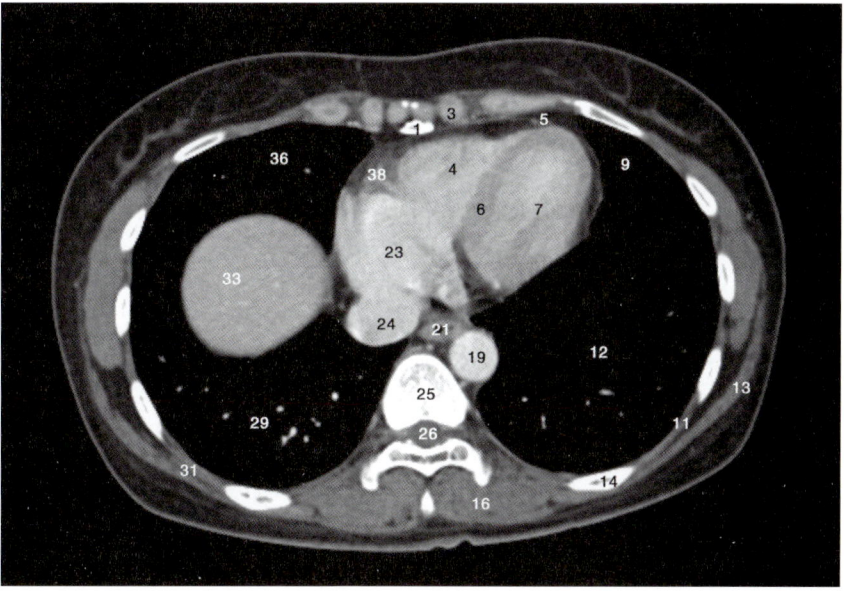

C. CT 增强图像

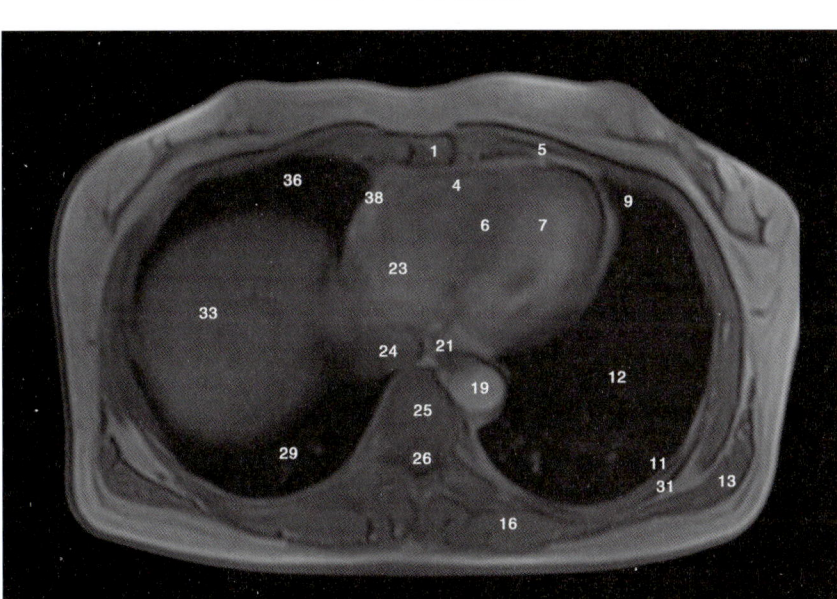

D. MR T1WI

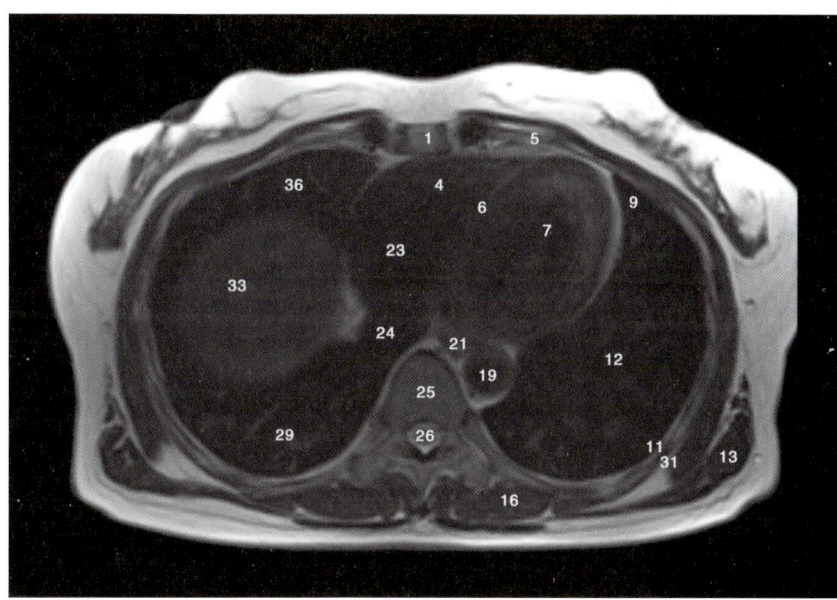

E. MR T2WI

关键结构：腔静脉孔，下腔静脉，右心房。

此断面经第9胸椎椎体下份。

下腔静脉穿过膈的腔静脉孔，向上注入右心房，腔静脉孔平约T8-9椎间盘水平，略呈四边形，位于膈中心腱的右侧与腱中心部交界处。下腔静脉由左、右髂总静脉汇合而成，沿腹主动脉右侧上行。在下腔静脉开口于右心房的左前方，有肌性（占53.20%±5.30%）、膜性（占27.20%±4.60%）或半肌半膜性（占19.60%±4.10%）的瓣膜，即下腔静脉瓣。此瓣胚胎时期较明显，成人已不显著，有时可阙如（8.0%）。下腔静脉全程可分为5段，由膈至右心房为第5段，又称膈上段，其长度平均为1.80cm，超过2.0cm者占31.40%，最长者可达3.0cm，下腔静脉穿膈处管径为3.40cm±0.40cm[2]。部分肿瘤可通过下腔静脉蔓延或脱落而进入右心房，常见的既有原发性又有继发性肿瘤，如下腔静脉平滑肌瘤、平滑肌肉瘤、肝癌等，甚至可来源于子宫[3]。另外，来自下腔静脉的血栓栓子（主要来源于下肢静脉，长期卧床患者突然起床行走等为主因），也可经过右心房、右心室进入肺动脉，造成肺动脉栓塞，严重者可危及生命。

腹部连续横断层 3（FH.11870）

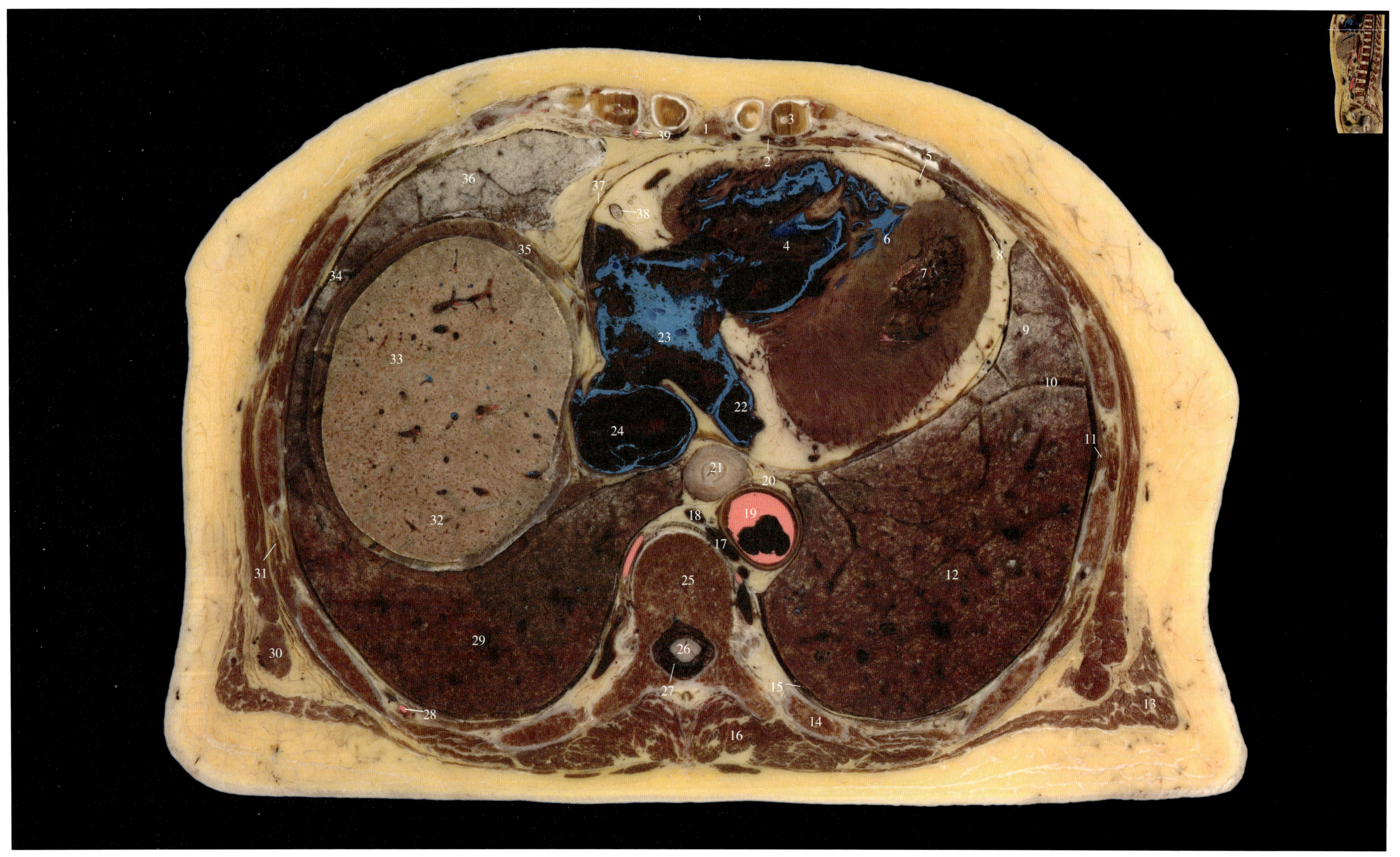

A. 断层标本图像

1. 胸骨体 body of sternum
2. 胸廓内静脉 internal thoracic vein
3. 第5肋软骨 5th costal cartilage
4. 右心室 right ventricle
5. 左冠状动脉前室间支 anterior interventricular branch of left coronary artery
6. 室间隔 interventricular septum
7. 左心室 left ventricle
8. 心包前下窦 anterior inferior sinus of pericardium
9. 左肺上叶 superior lobe of left lung
10. 左肺斜裂 oblique fissure of left lung
11. 肋间内肌 intercostale interni
12. 左肺下叶 inferior lobe of left lung
13. 背阔肌 latissimus dorsi
14. 第9肋骨 9th costal bone
15. 胸膜腔 pleural cavity
16. 竖脊肌 erector spinae
17. 半奇静脉 hemiazygos vein
18. 奇静脉 azygos vein
19. 胸主动脉 thoracic aorta
20. 左肺韧带 left pulmonary ligament
21. 食管 esophagus
22. 冠状窦 coronary sinus
23. 右心房 right atrium
24. 下腔静脉 inferior vena cava
25. 第9胸椎椎体 body of 9th thoracic vertebra
26. 脊髓 spinal cord
27. 硬脊膜 spinal dura mater
28. 肋间后动脉 posterior intercostal artery
29. 右肺下叶 inferior lobe of right lung
30. 后锯肌 serratus posterior
31. 肋间外肌 intercostale externi
32. 肝右后叶上段 superior segment of right posterior lobe of liver
33. 肝右前叶上段 superior segment of right anterior lobe of liver
34. 右肺斜裂 oblique fissure of right lung
35. 膈 diaphragm
36. 右肺中叶 middle lobe of right lung
37. 心包腔 pericardial cavity
38. 右冠状动脉 right coronary artery
39. 腹壁上动脉 superior epigastric artery

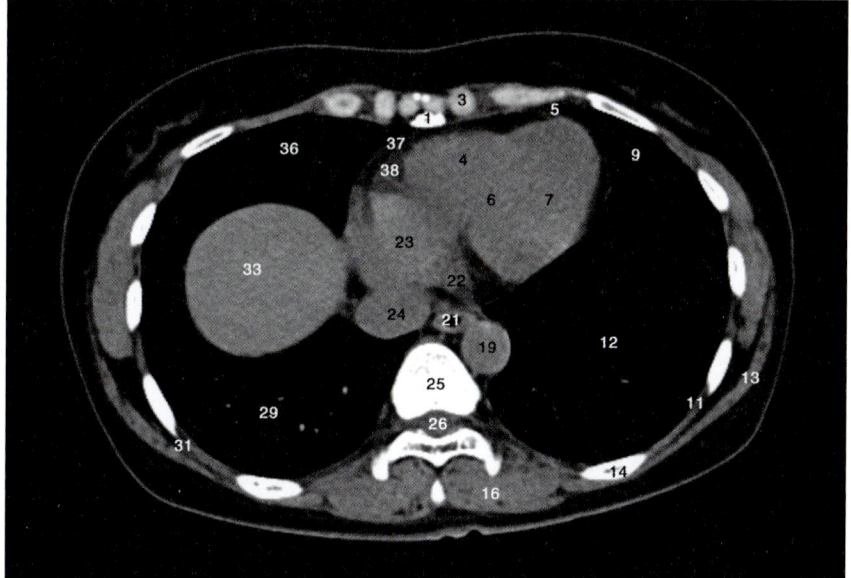

B. CT 平扫图像

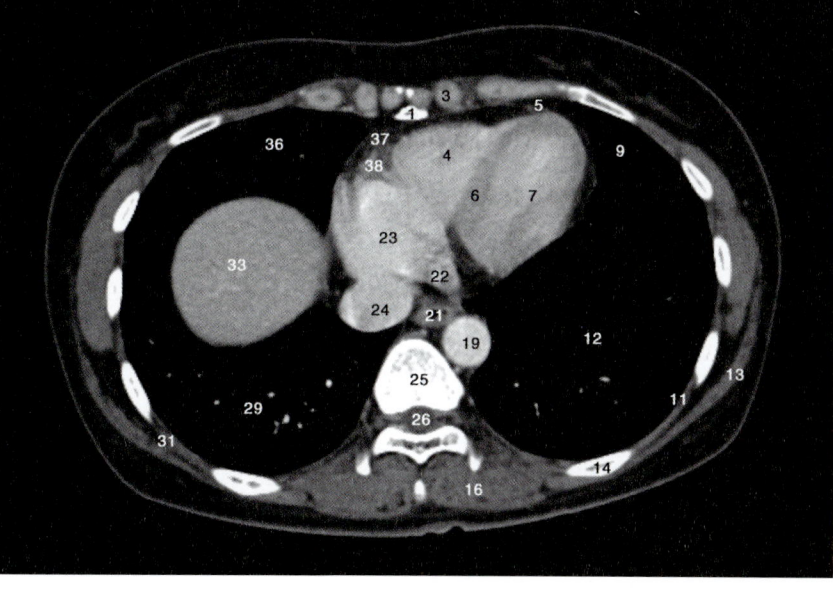

C. CT 增强图像

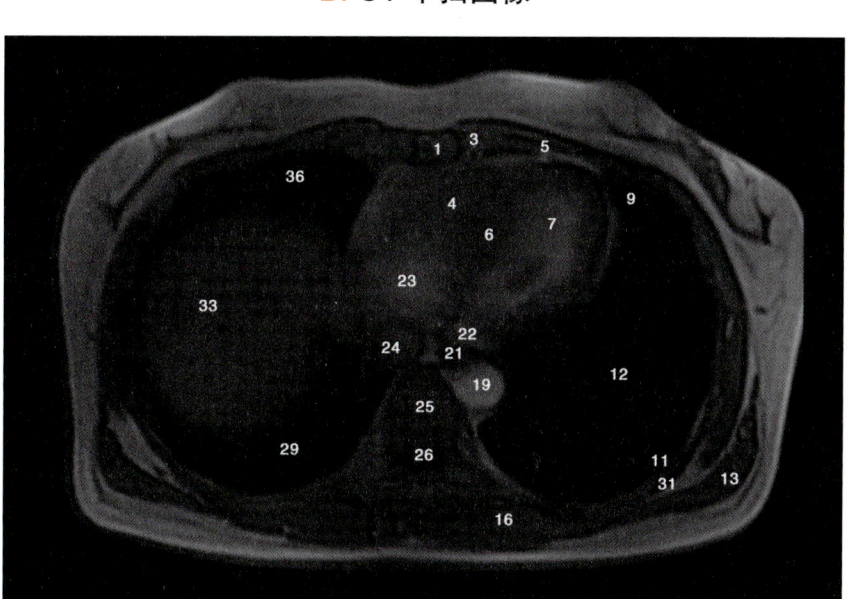

D. MR T1WI

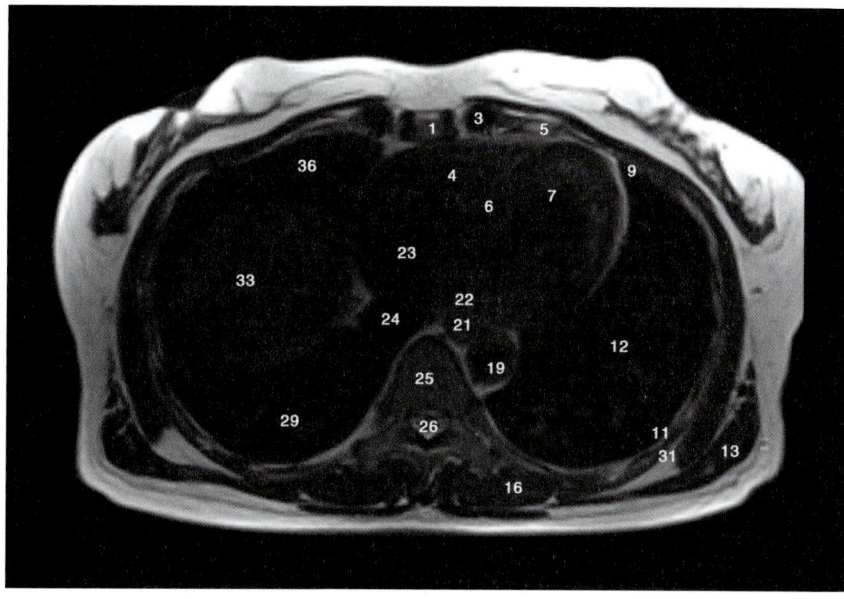

E. MR T2WI

关键结构：肝右叶，膈。

此断面经第9胸椎椎体下份。

肝的断面逐渐增大，主要为肝右叶，被右肺中叶、右肺下叶和右心房、下腔静脉包绕。肝右叶大而厚，呈楔子形，约占全肝的3/4。膈呈穹隆状，覆盖于肝的上方，位于胸、腹腔之间，上面与胸膜腔、肺和心包腔相邻，下面与肝、胃和脾相邻，封闭胸廓下口。由于膈穹隆是由下向上突，故膈的下方和内侧为腹腔，而胸腔则居其上方和外侧。膈的周边是肌性部，中央为腱膜，称中心腱。肌束起自胸廓下口的周缘和腰椎前面，可分为3部：胸骨部起自剑突后面；肋部起自下6对肋骨和肋软骨；腰部以左、右2个膈脚起自上2~3个腰椎及内、外侧弓状韧带。各部肌束均止于中心腱[4]。CT等横轴位图像上，膈附近胸、腹水的鉴别可通过"横膈征"来鉴别：即当腹水或胸腹水存在时，膈可显示为弧形线状影，该线状影前内侧的液体为腹水，后外侧的为胸腔积液。

腹部连续横断层 4（FH.11850）

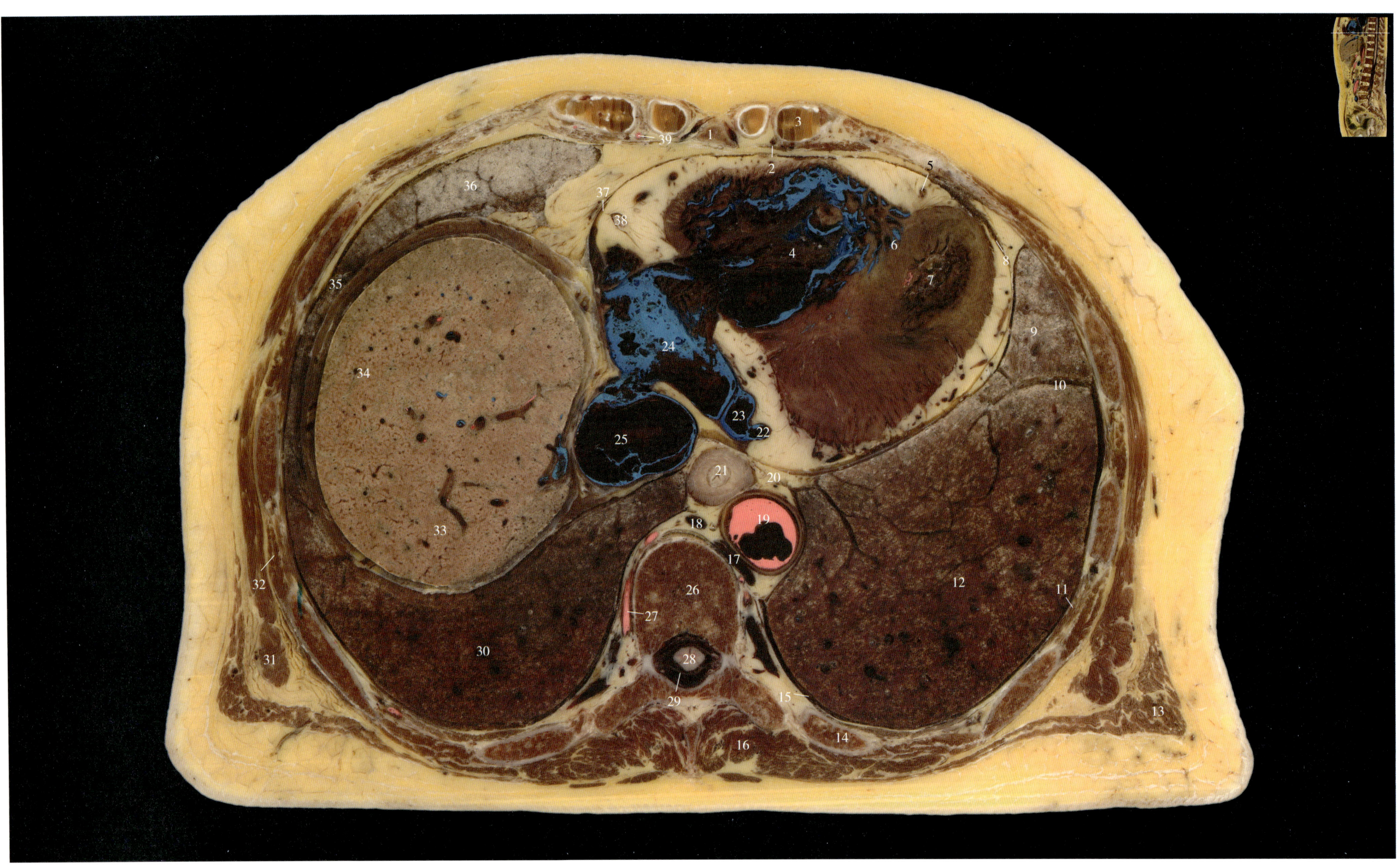

A. 断层标本图像

1. 胸骨体 body of sternum
2. 胸廓内静脉 internal thoracic vein
3. 第 5 肋软骨 5th costal cartilage
4. 右心室 right ventricle
5. 左冠状动脉前室间支 anterior interventricular branch of left coronary artery
6. 室间隔 interventricular septum
7. 左心室 left ventricle
8. 心包前下窦 anterior inferior sinus of pericardium
9. 左肺上叶 superior lobe of left lung
10. 左肺斜裂 oblique fissure of left lung
11. 肋间内肌 intercostale interni
12. 左肺下叶 inferior lobe of left lung
13. 背阔肌 latissimus dorsi
14. 第 9 肋骨 9th costal bone
15. 胸膜腔 pleural cavity
16. 竖脊肌 erector spinae
17. 半奇静脉 hemiazygos vein
18. 奇静脉 azygos vein
19. 胸主动脉 thoracic aorta
20. 左肺韧带 left pulmonary ligament
21. 食管 esophagus
22. 心大静脉 great cardiac vein
23. 冠状窦 coronary sinus
24. 右心房 right atrium
25. 下腔静脉 inferior vena cava
26. 第 9 胸椎椎体 body of 9th thoracic vertebra
27. 肋间后动脉 posterior intercostal artery
28. 脊髓 spinal cord
29. 硬脊膜 spinal dura mater
30. 右肺下叶 inferior lobe of right lung
31. 后锯肌 serratus posterior
32. 肋间外肌 intercostale externi
33. 肝右后叶上段 superior segment of right posterior lobe of liver
34. 肝右前叶上段 superior segment of right anterior lobe of liver
35. 右肺斜裂 oblique fissure of right lung
36. 右肺中叶 middle lobe of right lung
37. 心包腔 pericardial cavity
38. 右冠状动脉 right coronary artery
39. 腹壁上动脉 superior epigastric artery

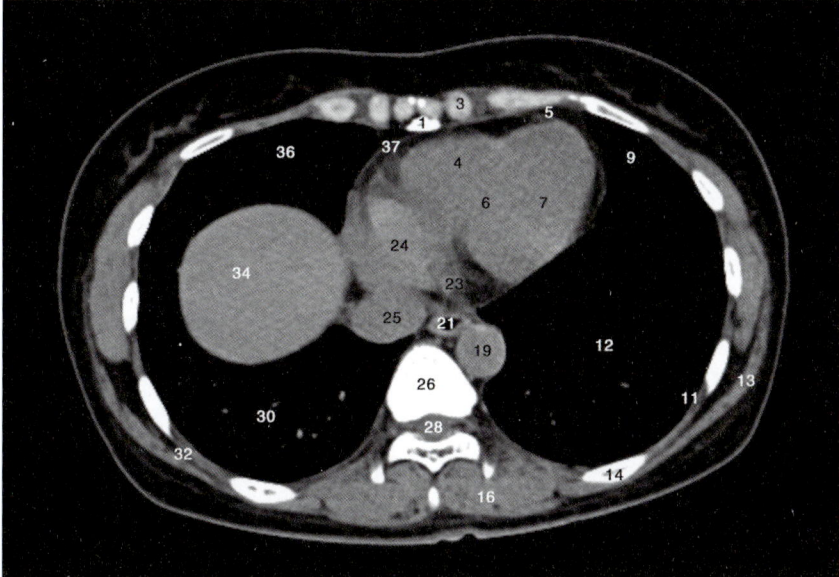

B. CT 平扫图像

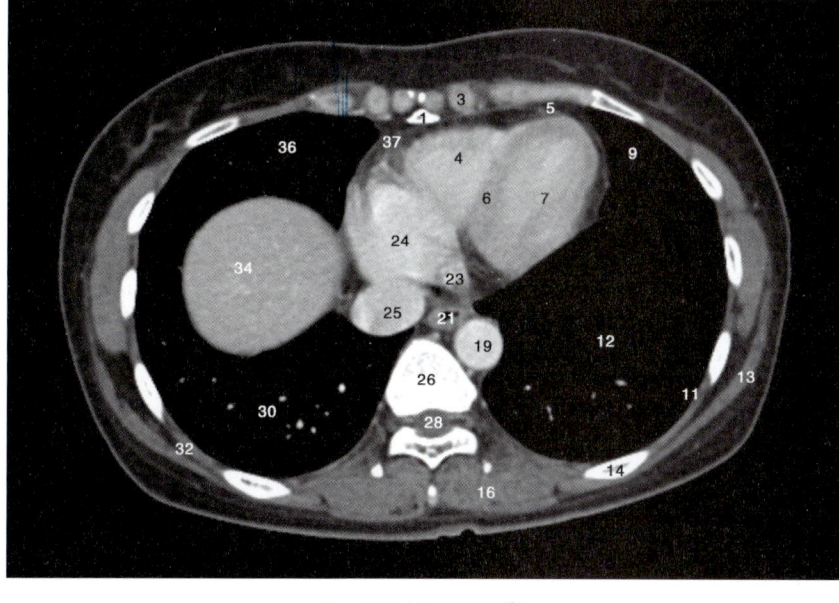

C. CT 增强图像

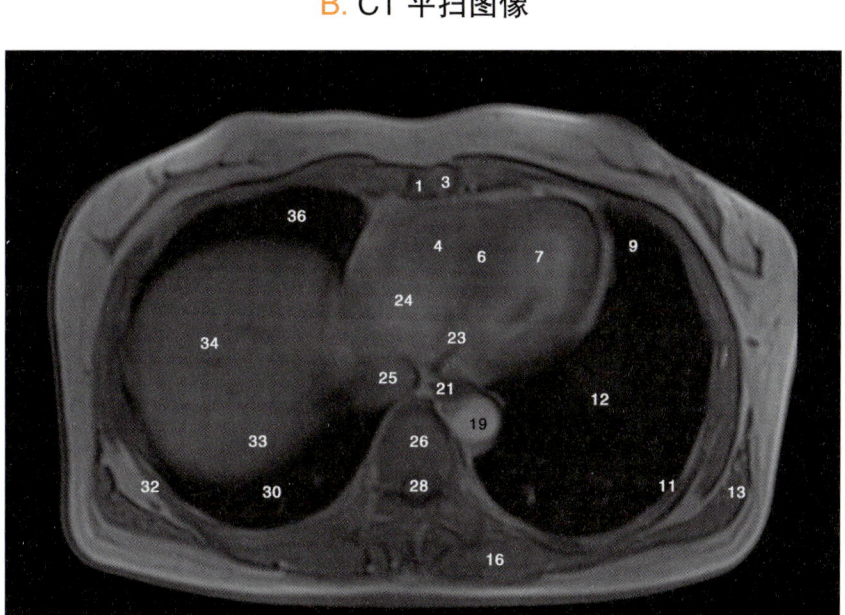

D. MR T1WI

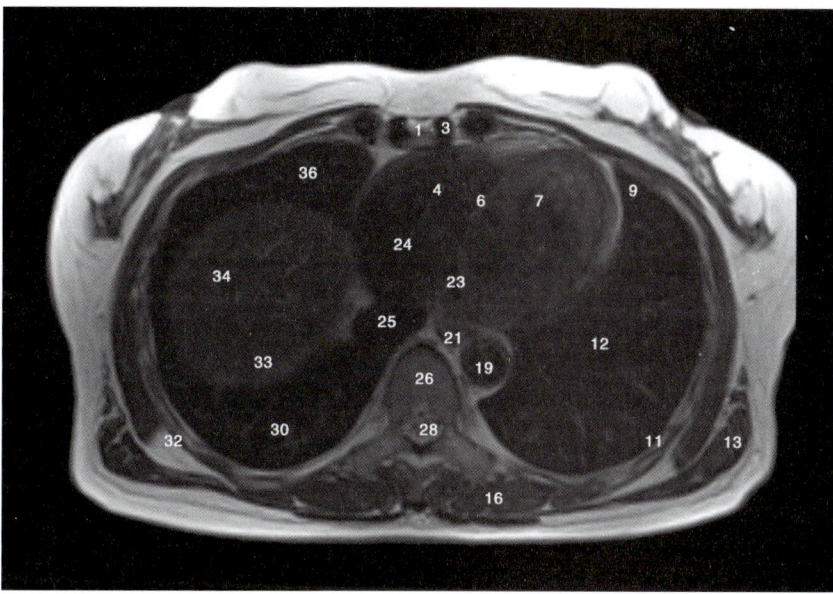

E. MR T2WI

关键结构：冠状窦，第 9 胸椎椎体。

此断面经第 9 胸椎椎体下份。

胸椎椎体前凸后凹，矢径略大于横径；胸椎管近似圆形，矢径为 1.4~1.5 cm，横径与矢径大致相等，内含硬脊膜和脊髓。此断面切及心大静脉汇入冠状窦的部位。冠状窦位于心后面的冠状沟内，左心房和左心室之间，向右以冠状窦口通向右心房。冠状窦口位于下腔静脉口和右房室口之间，其开口处有瓣膜，即冠状窦瓣，亦称 Thebesius 瓣，其作用是防止血液倒流。冠状窦长为 2.34 cm ± 0.13 cm，起始段直径为 0.82 cm ± 0.27 cm，中段直径为 0.92 cm ± 0.24 cm，末段直径为 1.05 cm ± 0.28 cm。冠状窦瓣多数呈嵴状或镰刀状，瓣膜出现率为 70.00% ± 6.48%[2]。冠状窦及其属支是心脏静脉系统的重要组成部分，也是许多心脏疾患诊断、治疗的重要标志和通道，如左心室起搏和部分消融手术等都需要冠状窦置管这一重要环节。

腹部连续横断层 5（FH.11830）

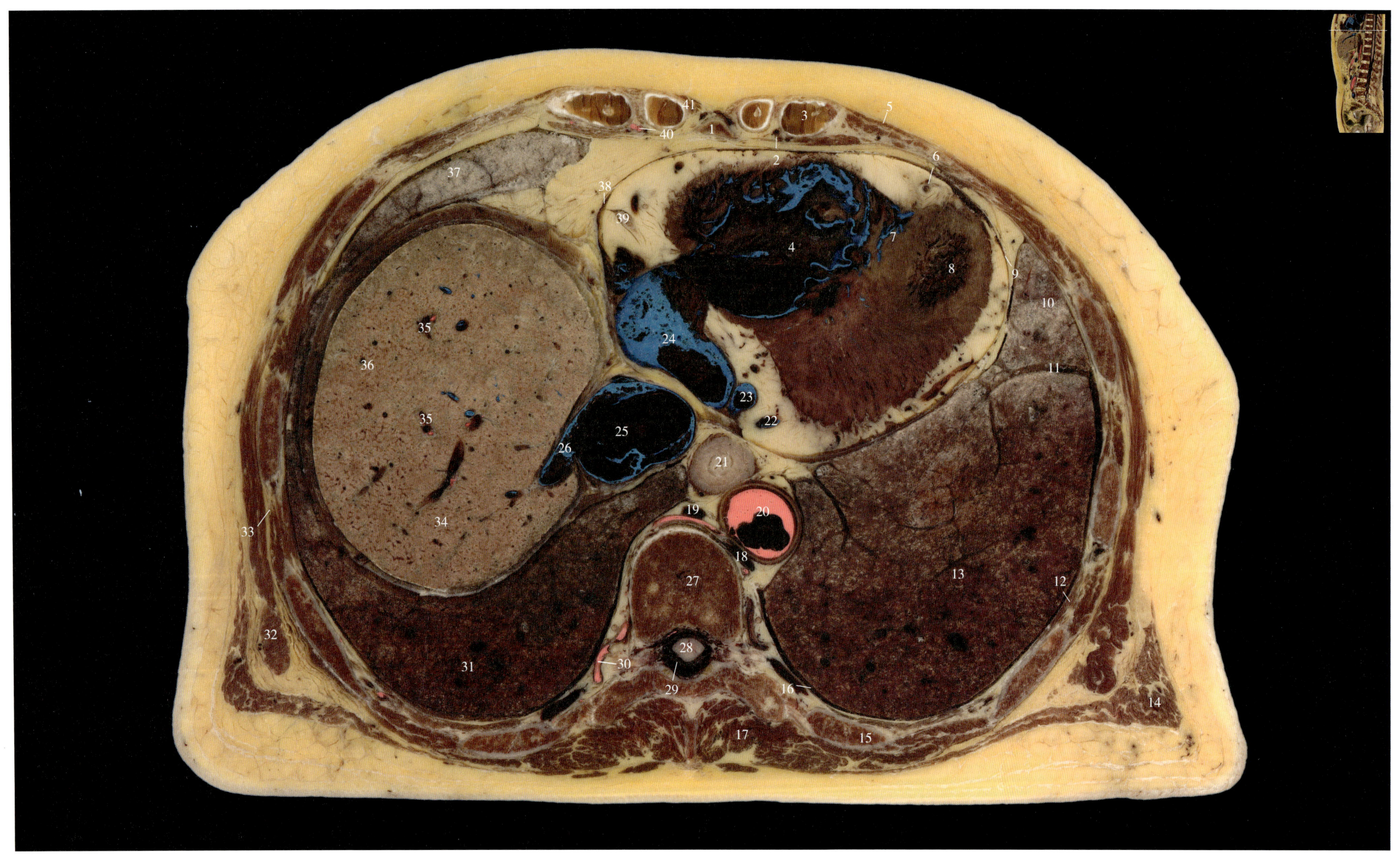

A. 断层标本图像

1. 胸骨体 body of sternum
2. 胸廓内静脉 internal thoracic vein
3. 第5肋软骨 5th costal cartilage
4. 右心室 right ventricle
5. 腹外斜肌 obliquus externus abdominis
6. 左冠状动脉前室间支 anterior interventricular branch of left coronary artery
7. 室间隔 interventricular septum
8. 左心室 left ventricle
9. 心包前下窦 anterior inferior sinus of pericardium
10. 左肺上叶 superior lobe of left lung
11. 左肺斜裂 oblique fissure of left lung
12. 肋间内肌 intercostale interni
13. 左肺下叶 inferior lobe of left lung
14. 背阔肌 latissimus dorsi
15. 第9肋骨 9th costal bone
16. 胸膜腔 pleural cavity
17. 竖脊肌 erector spinae
18. 半奇静脉 hemiazygos vein
19. 奇静脉 azygos vein
20. 胸主动脉 thoracic aorta
21. 食管 esophagus
22. 心大静脉 great cardiac vein
23. 冠状窦 coronary sinus
24. 右心房 right atrium
25. 下腔静脉 inferior vena cava
26. 肝右静脉 right hepatic vein
27. 第9胸椎椎体 body of 9th thoracic vertebra
28. 脊髓 spinal cord
29. 硬脊膜 spinal dura mater
30. 肋间后动脉 posterior intercostal artery
31. 右肺下叶 inferior lobe of right lung
32. 后锯肌 serratus posterior
33. 肋间外肌 intercostale externi
34. 肝右后叶上段 superior segment of right posterior lobe of liver
35. 肝门静脉右前上支 right anterosuperior branch of hepatic portal vein
36. 肝右前叶上段 superior segment of right anterior lobe of liver
37. 右肺中叶 middle lobe of right lung
38. 心包腔 pericardial cavity
39. 右冠状动脉 right coronary artery
40. 腹壁上动脉 superior epigastric artery
41. 腹直肌 rectus abdominis

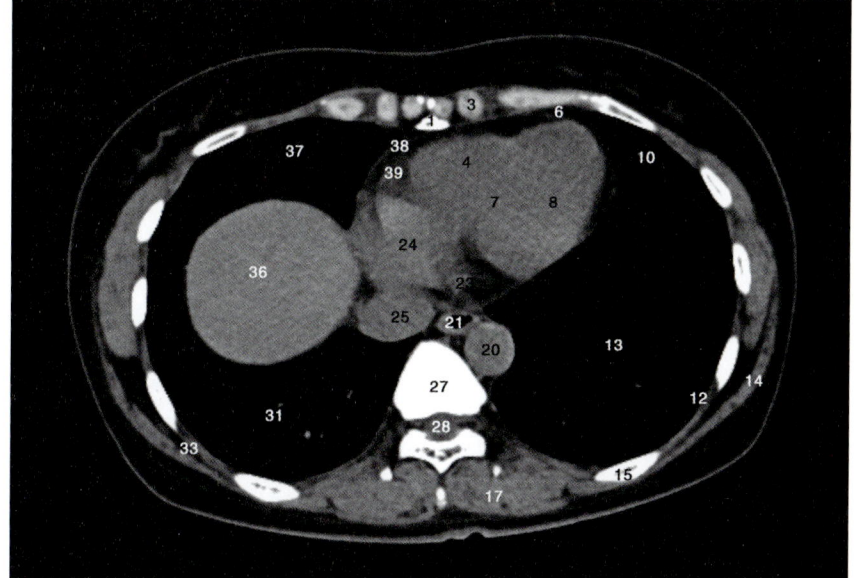

B. CT 平扫图像

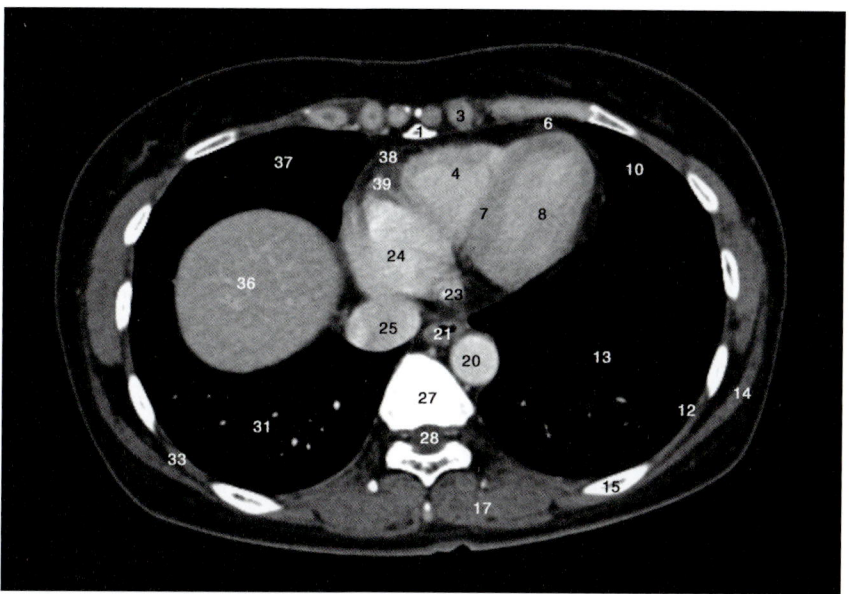

C. CT 增强图像

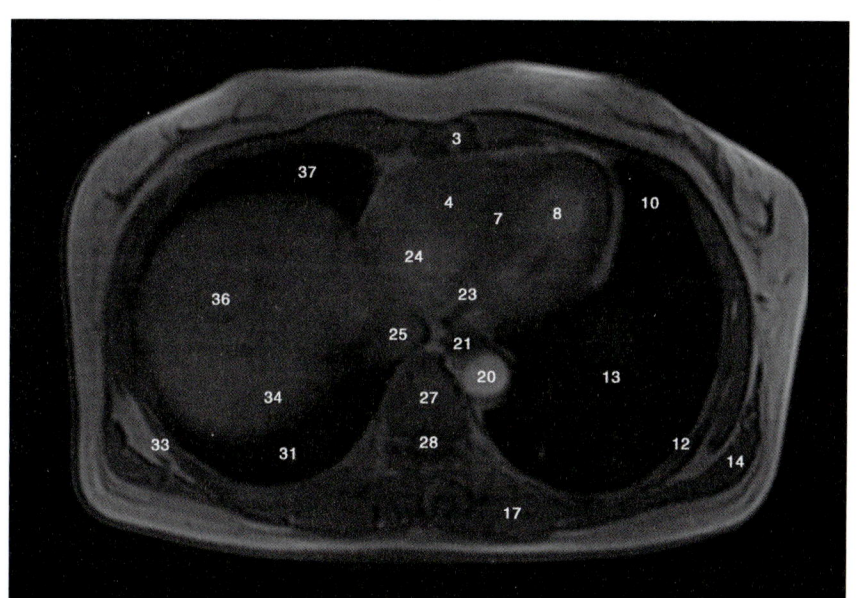

D. MR T1WI

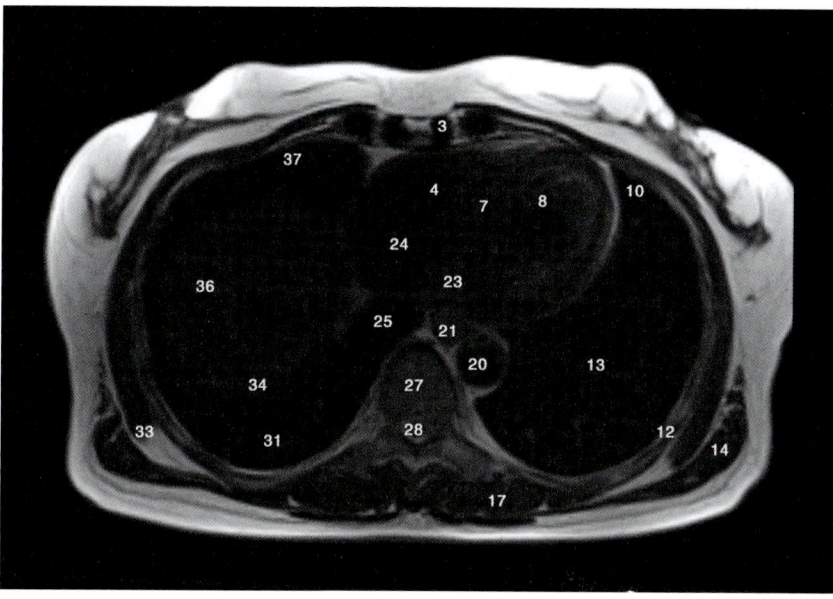

E. MR T2WI

关键结构：肝右静脉，肝右后上段。

此断面经第9胸椎体下份。

肝右静脉汇入下腔静脉右壁。肝右静脉为最长、最粗的肝静脉属支，位于肝右叶间裂内，通常仅有1支，但偶见2支，可作为右叶间裂的标志。肝右静脉收集肝右后叶和肝右前叶上部的静脉血，其主要属支有右后上缘静脉，出现率为48.8%。据国人解剖数值资料：肝右静脉的内径为 0.84 cm ± 0.14 cm，另据文献报道为 1.18 cm ± 0.86 cm。肝右静脉注入处外径为 1.56 cm ± 0.41 cm，分叉处为 1.14 cm ± 0.28 cm。肝右静脉主干长为 2.28 cm ± 0.95 cm，由前、后2支合成者占96.94%，由3支汇合而成者占3.1%。肝右静脉后根长为 2.94 cm ± 0.73 cm，前根长为 2.79 cm ± 0.81 cm[2]。右叶间裂将右肝分为右前叶和右后叶，右段间裂又将右后叶分为右后叶上段和右后叶下段，此断层切及肝右后叶上段。肝右叶占据肝脏总体积的大部分，约占3/4；肝左叶约占1/4。但肝硬化患者随着病情严重程度的发展，会出现肝左叶所占比例有所增加（以左外叶为著），肝右叶所占比例有所减少（以右前叶为著）的情况[5]。

腹部连续横断层 6 (FH.11810)

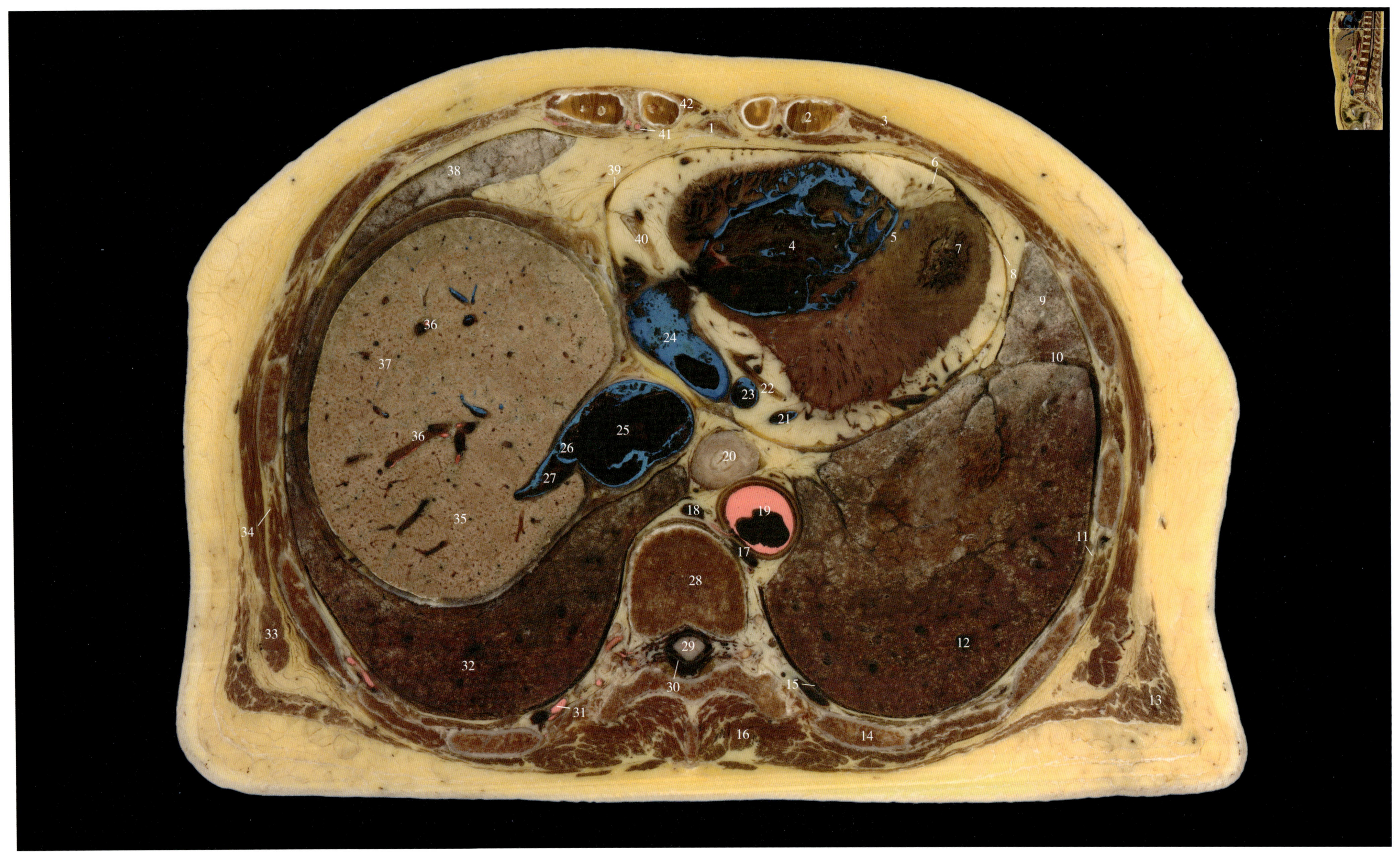

A. 断层标本图像

1. 胸骨体 body of sternum
2. 第5肋软骨 5th costal cartilage
3. 腹外斜肌 obliquus externus abdominis
4. 右心室 right ventricle
5. 室间隔 interventricular septum
6. 左冠状动脉前室间支 anterior interventricular branch of left coronary artery
7. 左心室 left ventricle
8. 心包前下窦 anterior inferior sinus of pericardium
9. 左肺上叶 superior lobe of left lung
10. 左肺斜裂 oblique fissure of left lung
11. 肋间内肌 intercostale interni
12. 左肺下叶 inferior lobe of left lung
13. 背阔肌 latissimus dorsi
14. 第9肋骨 9th costal bone
15. 胸膜腔 pleural cavity
16. 竖脊肌 erector spinae
17. 半奇静脉 hemiazygos vein
18. 奇静脉 azygos vein
19. 胸主动脉 thoracic aorta
20. 食管 esophagus
21. 心大静脉 great cardiac vein
22. 左冠状动脉 left coronary artery
23. 冠状窦 coronary sinus
24. 右心房 right atrium
25. 下腔静脉 inferior vena cava
26. 肝右静脉 right hepatic vein
27. 肝右后上缘静脉 right posterosuperior marginal vein of liver
28. 第9胸椎椎体 body of 9th thoracic vertebra
29. 脊髓 spinal cord
30. 硬脊膜 spinal dura mater
31. 肋间后动脉 posterior intercostal artery
32. 右肺下叶 inferior lobe of right lung
33. 后锯肌 serratus posterior
34. 肋间外肌 intercostale externi
35. 肝右后叶上段 superior segment of right posterior lobe of liver
36. 肝门静脉右前上支 right anterosuperior branch of hepatic portal vein
37. 肝右前叶上段 superior segment of right anterior lobe of liver
38. 右肺中叶 middle lobe of right lung
39. 心包腔 pericardial cavity
40. 右冠状动脉 right coronary artery
41. 腹壁上动脉 superior epigastric artery
42. 腹直肌 rectus abdominis

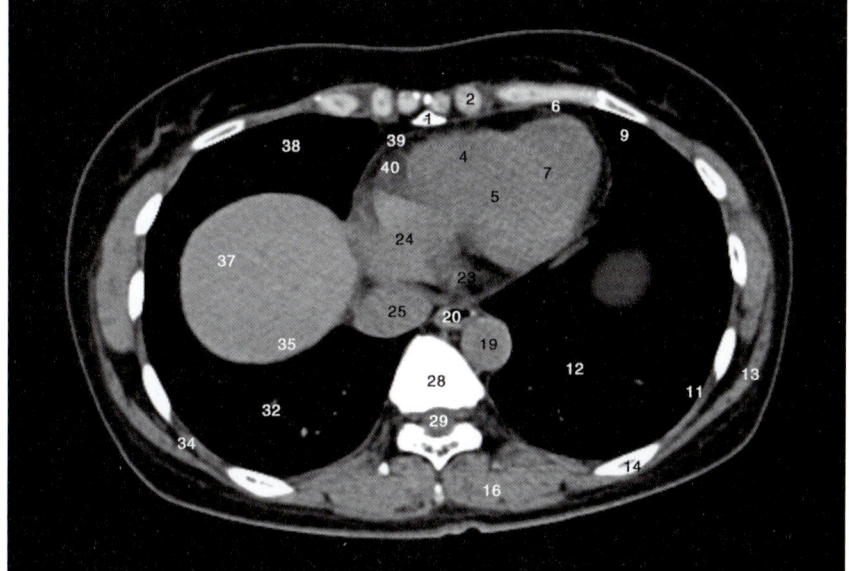

B. CT 平扫图像

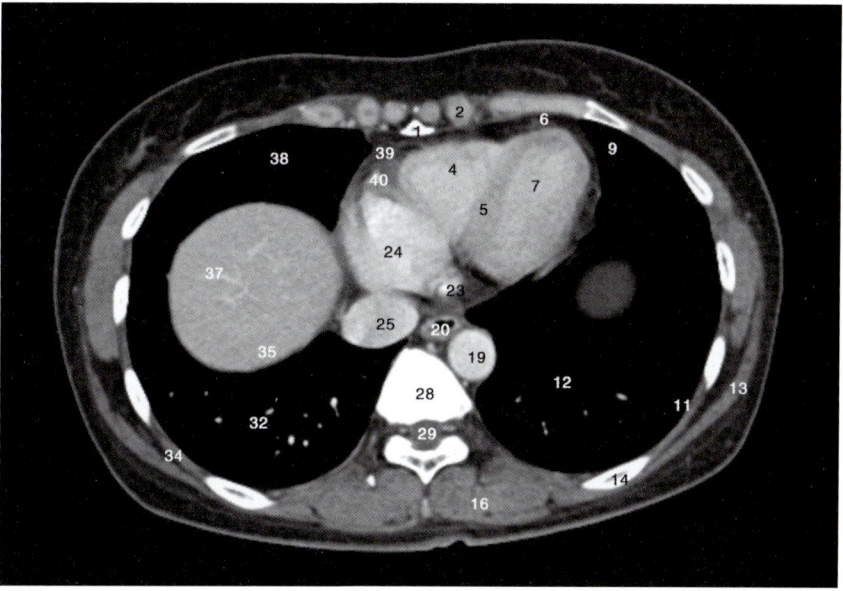

C. CT 增强图像

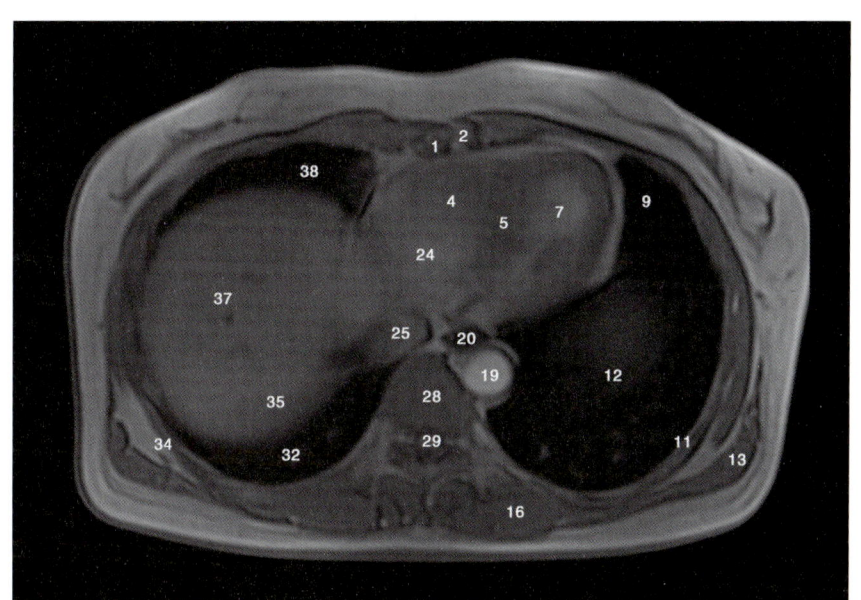

D. MR T1WI

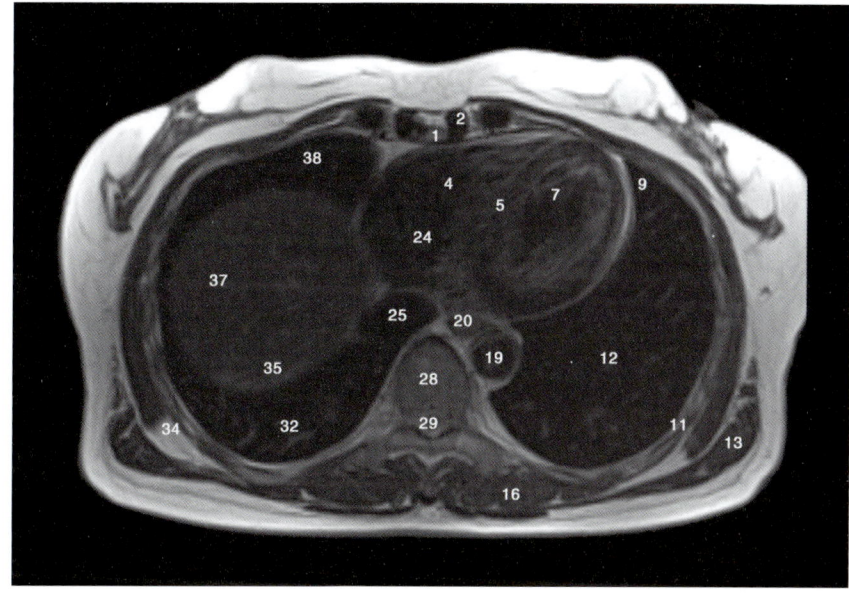

E. MR T2WI

关键结构：腹直肌，右肺中叶。

此断面经第9胸椎椎体下份。

腹直肌出现，位于腹前壁正中线的两侧，居腹直肌鞘内，上宽下窄。两侧腹直肌内侧缘以白线相隔，因白线在脐以上呈带状，脐以下为线形，故两侧腹直肌上部距离较远（>1 cm），而下方几乎相贴。起自第5~7肋软骨的前面和剑突，肌纤维直向下方，止于耻骨上缘（耻骨结节与耻骨联合之间）及耻骨联合的前面。肌纤维被数个锯齿状的腱划分隔。人类通常有3个腱划：最上方的一个在胸骨剑突的稍下方，最下方的一个居脐的水平线上，中间的一个位于二者之间[2]。腱划与腹直肌鞘前层紧密愈合，与腹直肌鞘后层无愈合，可自由移动。手术时，切开腹直肌鞘前层后可向外侧牵拉腹直肌，暴露腹直肌鞘后层，但尽量不要向内侧牵拉，以防损伤胸神经前支[4]。此断面中，在膈的前上方，肺仅留右肺中叶内侧段和左肺上叶下舌段，且此两段最靠近心脏，在CT图像上因受心脏搏动的影响，部分肺组织萎陷，常可观察到条索状的纤维灶，边缘多较清晰，部分模糊者应首先考虑心脏搏动所致的运动伪影，不能轻易给出肺炎的诊断。

腹部连续横断层 7 (FH.11790)

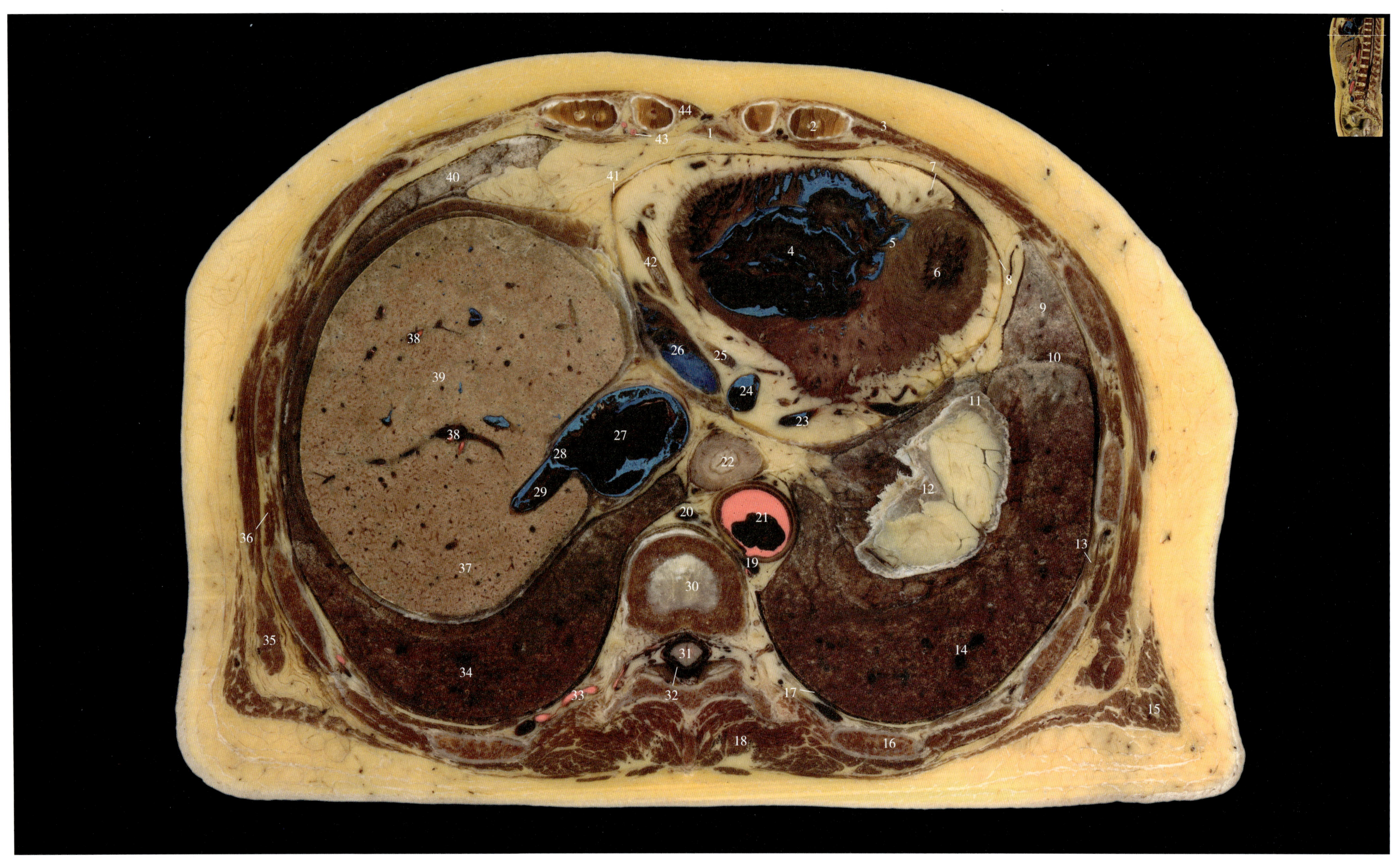

A. 断层标本图像

1. 胸骨体 body of sternum
2. 第5肋软骨 5th costal cartilage
3. 腹外斜肌 obliquus externus abdominis
4. 右心室 right ventricle
5. 室间隔 interventricular septum
6. 左心室 left ventricle
7. 左冠状动脉前室间支 anterior interventricular branch of left coronary artery
8. 心包前下窦 anterior inferior sinus of pericardium
9. 左肺上叶 superior lobe of left lung
10. 左肺斜裂 oblique fissure of left lung
11. 膈 diaphragm
12. 胃底 fundus of stomach
13. 肋间内肌 intercostale interni
14. 左肺下叶 inferior lobe of left lung
15. 背阔肌 latissimus dorsi
16. 第9肋骨 9th costal bone
17. 胸膜腔 pleural cavity
18. 竖脊肌 erector spinae
19. 半奇静脉 hemiazygos vein
20. 奇静脉 azygos vein
21. 胸主动脉 thoracic aorta
22. 食管 esophagus
23. 心大静脉 great cardiac vein
24. 冠状窦 coronary sinus
25. 左冠状动脉 left coronary artery
26. 右心房 right atrium
27. 下腔静脉 inferior vena cava
28. 肝右静脉 right hepatic vein
29. 肝右后上缘静脉 right posterosuperior marginal vein of liver
30. T9-10椎间盘 T9-10 intervertebral disc
31. 脊髓 spinal cord
32. 硬脊膜 spinal dura mater
33. 肋间后动脉 posterior intercostal artery
34. 右肺下叶 inferior lobe of right lung
35. 后锯肌 serratus posterior
36. 肋间外肌 intercostale externi
37. 肝右后叶上段 superior segment of right posterior lobe of liver
38. 肝门静脉右前上支 right anterosuperior branch of hepatic portal vein
39. 肝右前叶上段 superior segment of right anterior lobe of liver
40. 右肺中叶 middle lobe of right lung
41. 心包腔 pericardial cavity
42. 右冠状动脉 right coronary artery
43. 腹壁上动脉 superior epigastric artery
44. 腹直肌 rectus abdominis

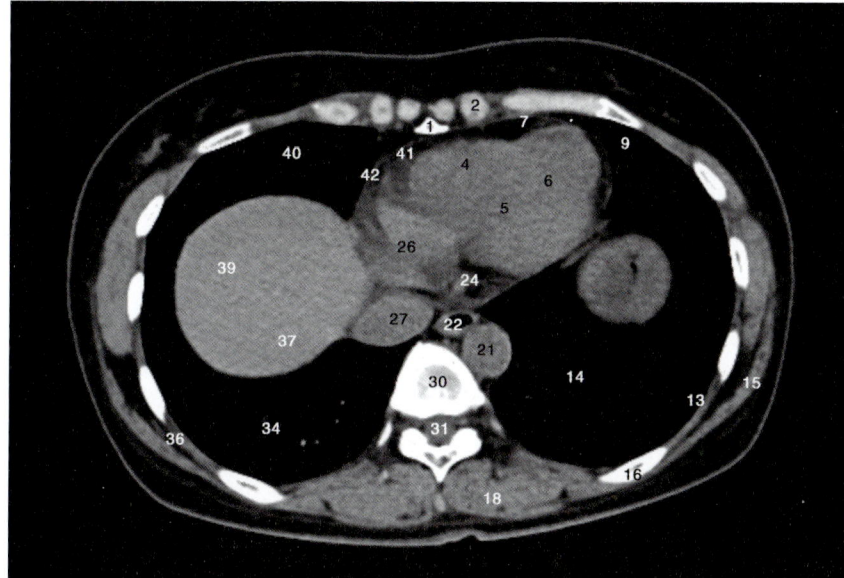

B. CT 平扫图像

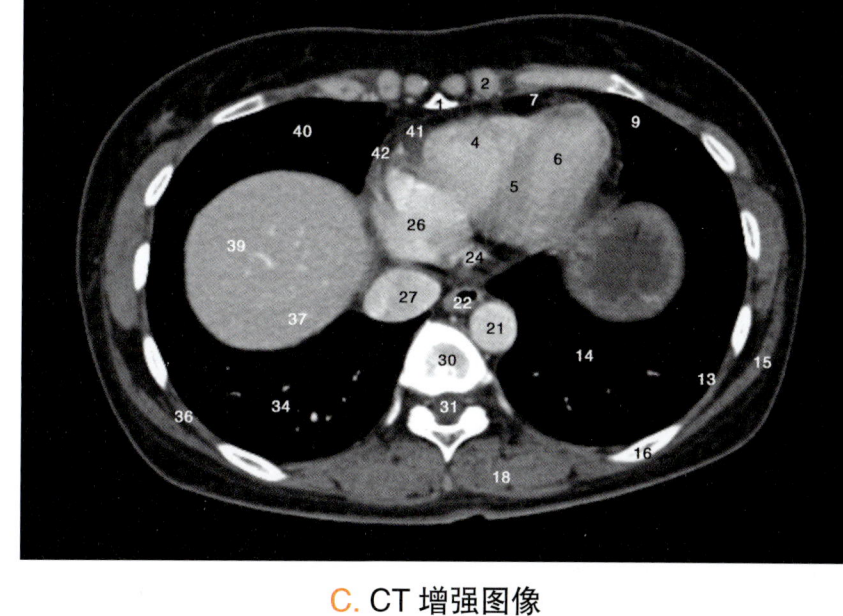

C. CT 增强图像

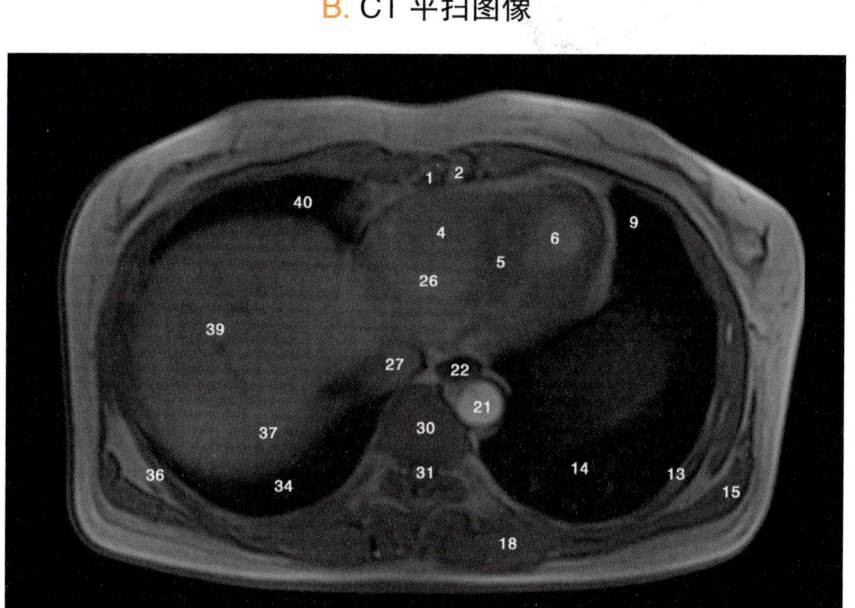

D. MR T1WI

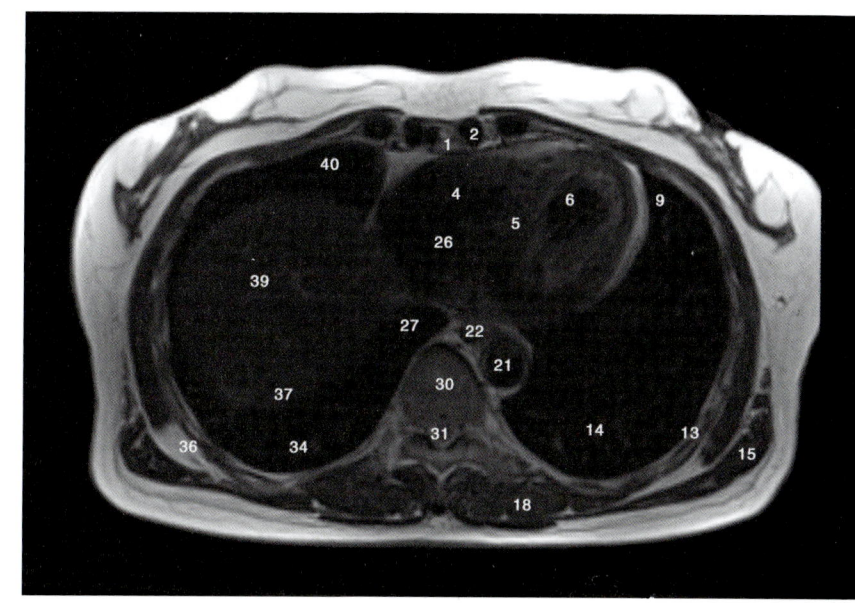

E. MR T2WI

关键结构：膈左穹窿，T9-10 椎间盘。

此断面经第9胸椎椎体下份及T9-10椎间盘。

心脏结构为右心房及左、右心室。膈右穹窿和肝右叶的占比较上一断面增大，膈左穹窿首次出现，膈左穹窿低于右穹窿，其最高点位于第5肋间隙的高处，因受胃、结肠含气量的影响，其变化范围较右侧大[1]。左右肺逐渐缩小，围绕在膈左、右穹窿外侧。显示第9胸椎椎体及其椎板和棘突的断面，从后向前左右两侧的第9、8、7、6肋骨及第5、6肋软骨依次排列，围成胸廓。贴近前正中线的两侧可见腹直肌，腹壁前外侧、外侧和后外侧分别见前锯肌、后锯肌和背阔肌。背部可见竖脊肌，依照肌纤维的位置和起始点，竖脊肌分为外侧的髂肋肌、中间的最长肌和内侧的棘肌。膈穹窿的上移称为膈膨升，系膈发育异常或因膈神经损伤麻痹而引起膈部分或全部抬高，而膈形态完整无缺损。膈膨升按病因可分为先天性和获得性（如创伤性、医源性）两种，可单独存在，也可能是全身疾病的一部分[6]。

15

腹部连续横断层 8（FH.11770）

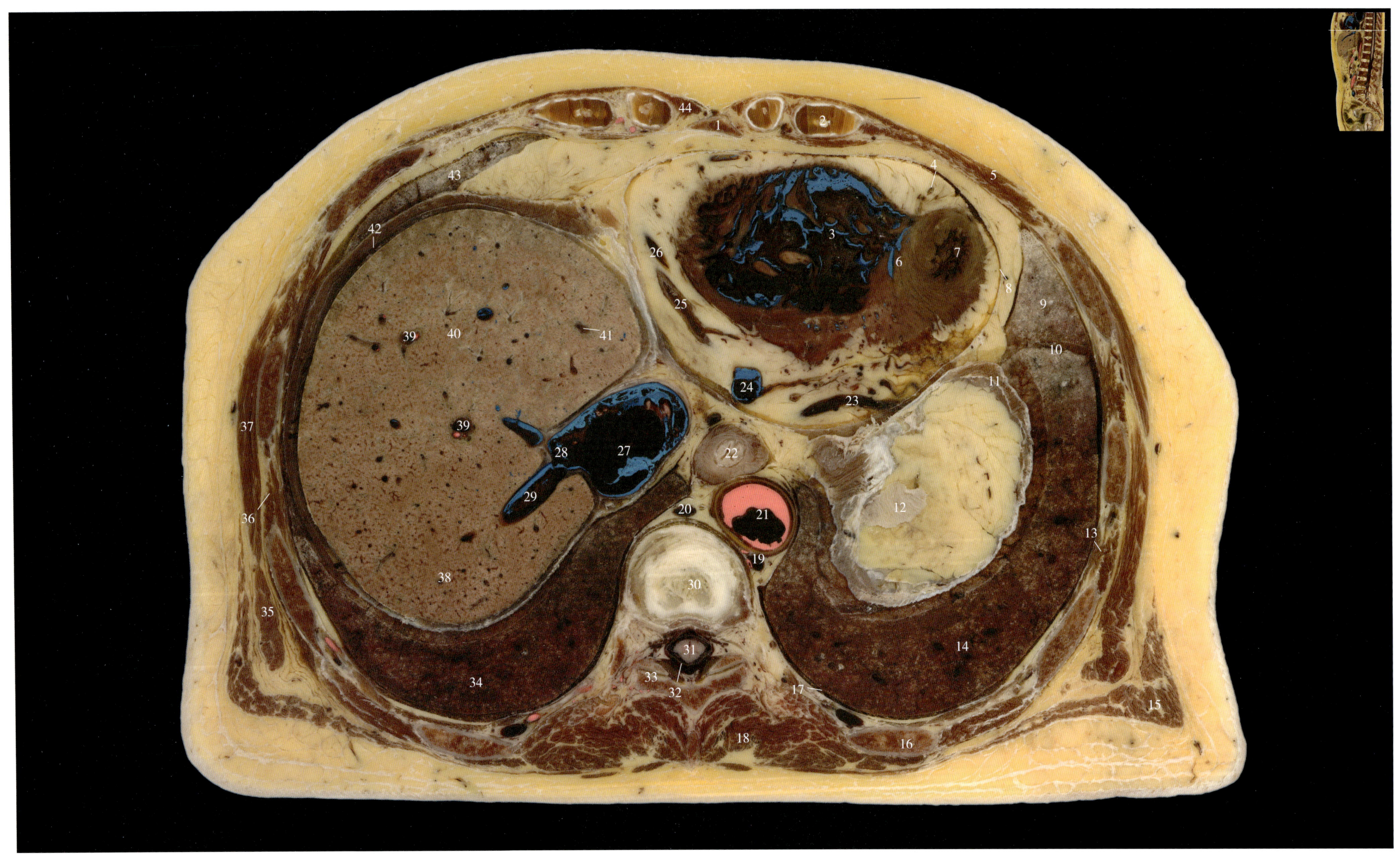

A. 断层标本图像

1. 胸骨体 body of sternum
2. 第5肋软骨 5th costal cartilage
3. 右心室 right ventricle
4. 左冠状动脉前室间支 anterior interventricular branch of left coronary artery
5. 腹外斜肌 obliquus externus abdominis
6. 室间隔 interventricular septum
7. 左心室 left ventricle
8. 心包前下窦 anterior inferior sinus of pericardium
9. 左肺上叶 superior lobe of left lung
10. 左肺斜裂 oblique fissure of left lung
11. 膈 diaphragm
12. 胃底 fundus of stomach
13. 肋间内肌 intercostale interni
14. 左肺下叶 inferior lobe of left lung
15. 背阔肌 latissimus dorsi
16. 第9肋骨 9th costal bone
17. 胸膜腔 pleural cavity
18. 竖脊肌 erector spinae
19. 半奇静脉 hemiazygos vein
20. 奇静脉 azygos vein
21. 胸主动脉 thoracic aorta
22. 食管 esophagus
23. 心大静脉 great cardiac vein
24. 冠状窦 coronary sinus
25. 右冠状动脉 right coronary artery
26. 心小静脉 small cardiac vein
27. 下腔静脉 inferior vena cava
28. 肝右静脉 right hepatic vein
29. 肝右后上缘静脉 right posterosuperior marginal vein of liver
30. T9-10椎间盘 T9-10 intervertebral disc
31. 脊髓 spinal cord
32. 硬脊膜 spinal dura mater
33. 关节突关节 zygapophysial joints
34. 右肺下叶 inferior lobe of right lung
35. 后锯肌 serratus posterior
36. 肋间外肌 intercostale externi
37. 前锯肌 serratus anterior
38. 肝右后叶上段 superior segment of right posterior lobe of liver
39. 肝门静脉右前上支 right anterosuperior branch of hepatic portal vein
40. 肝右前叶上段 superior segment of right anterior lobe of liver
41. 肝门静脉左外上支 left laterosuperior branch of hepatic portal vein
42. 右肝上间隙 right suprahepatic space
43. 右肺中叶 middle lobe of right lung
44. 腹直肌 rectus abdominis

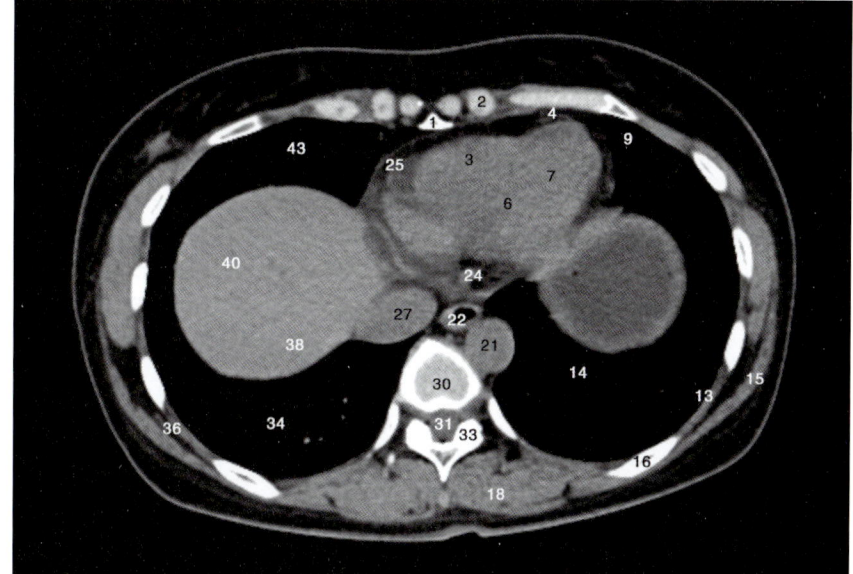

B. CT平扫图像

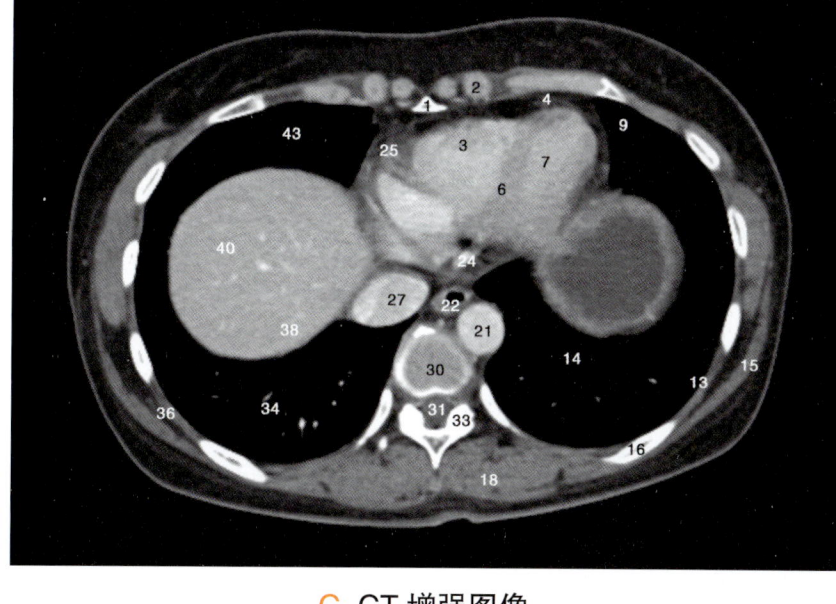

C. CT增强图像

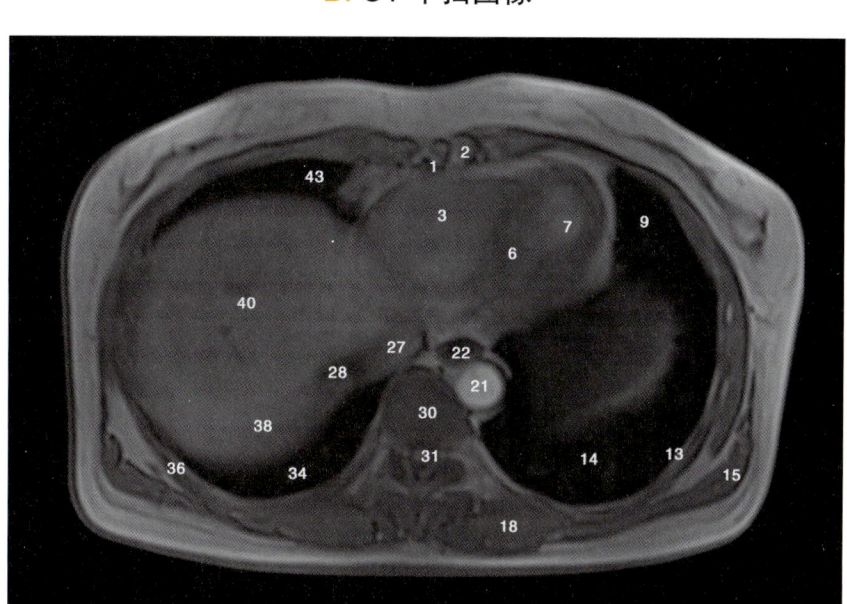

D. MR T1WI

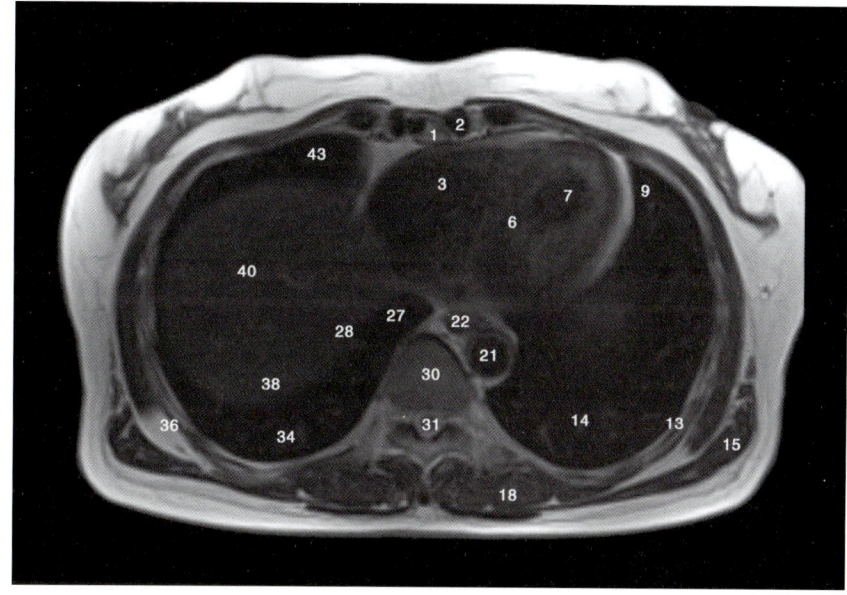

E. MR T2WI

关键结构：食管，胸主动脉。

此断面经T9-10椎间盘。

右心房消失，心脏仅存左、右心室。左肺上叶和右肺中叶仅余小部分，左、右肺下叶呈"C"字形分别围绕在膈左、右穹窿后部。食管继续左移，位于胸主动脉左前方，走向膈食管裂孔。此处为消化管最狭窄的部分。依照食管所占据的位置可将其分为颈部、胸部和腹部三部分。食管腹部甚短，仅为1~2 cm，向左下方行，经肝左叶后缘的食管切迹，末端与胃贲门相续。

胸主动脉是降主动脉的一部分，上接主动脉弓，下至第12胸椎下缘处，穿过膈的主动脉裂孔移行为腹主动脉。食管最常见的恶性肿瘤为食管癌，CT在食管癌的术前评估中有重要作用，在CT-TNM分期中，食管壁的厚度改变、是否突破管壁浆膜层等，是T分期的关键，如CT图像上食管与胸主动脉间脂肪间隙模糊或消失，甚至肿瘤包绕主动脉生长，则提示手术困难或无法手术，预后不良。

腹部连续横断层 9（FH.11750）

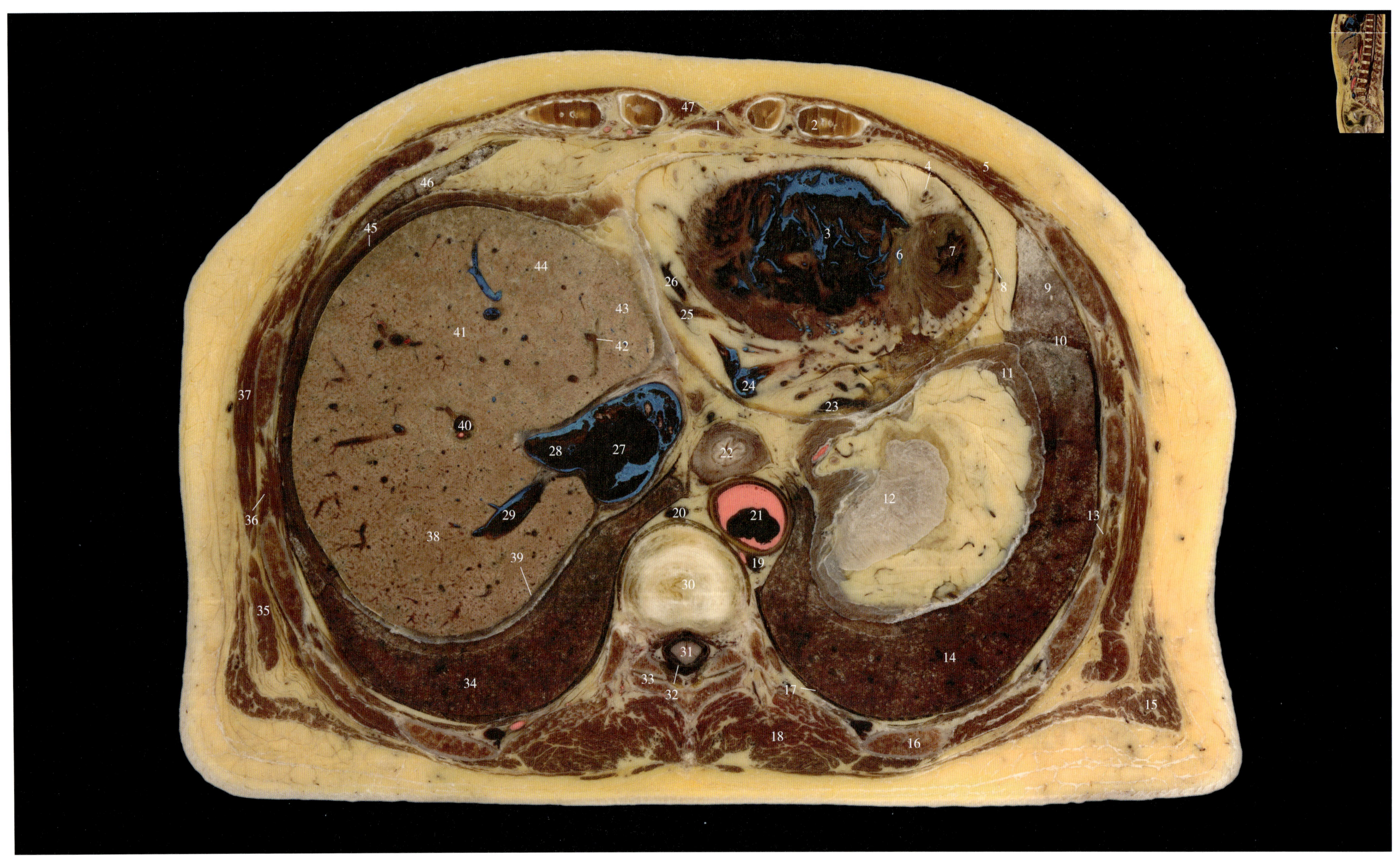

A. 断层标本图像

1. 胸骨体 body of sternum
2. 第 5 肋软骨 5th costal cartilage
3. 右心室 right ventricle
4. 左冠状动脉前室间支 anterior interventricular branch of left coronary artery
5. 腹外斜肌 obliquus externus abdominis
6. 室间隔 interventricular septum
7. 左心室 left ventricle
8. 心包前下窦 anterior inferior sinus of pericardium
9. 左肺上叶 superior lobe of left lung
10. 左肺斜裂 oblique fissure of left lung
11. 膈 diaphragm
12. 胃底 fundus of stomach
13. 肋间内肌 intercostale interni
14. 左肺下叶 inferior lobe of left lung
15. 背阔肌 latissimus dorsi
16. 第 9 肋骨 9th costal bone
17. 胸膜腔 pleural cavity
18. 竖脊肌 erector spinae
19. 半奇静脉 hemiazygos vein
20. 奇静脉 azygos vein
21. 胸主动脉 thoracic aorta
22. 食管 esophagus
23. 心大静脉 great cardiac vein
24. 冠状窦 coronary sinus
25. 右冠状动脉 right coronary artery
26. 心小静脉 small cardiac vein
27. 下腔静脉 inferior vena cava
28. 肝右静脉 right hepatic vein
29. 肝右后上缘静脉 right posterosuperior marginal vein of liver
30. T9-10 椎间盘 T9-10 intervertebral disc
31. 脊髓 spinal cord
32. 硬脊膜 spinal dura mater
33. 关节突关节 zygapophysial joints
34. 右肺下叶 inferior lobe of right lung
35. 后锯肌 serratus posterior
36. 肋间外肌 intercostale externi
37. 前锯肌 serratus anterior
38. 肝右后叶上段 superior segment of right posterior lobe of liver
39. 肝裸区 bare area of liver
40. 肝门静脉右前上支 right anterosuperior branch of hepatic portal vein
41. 肝右前叶上段 superior segment of right anterior lobe of liver
42. 肝门静脉左外上支 left laterosuperior branch of hepatic portal vein
43. 肝左外叶上段 superior segment of left lateral lobe of liver
44. 肝左内叶段 left medial lobe of liver
45. 右肝上间隙 right suprahepatic space
46. 右肺中叶 middle lobe of right lung
47. 腹直肌 rectus abdominis

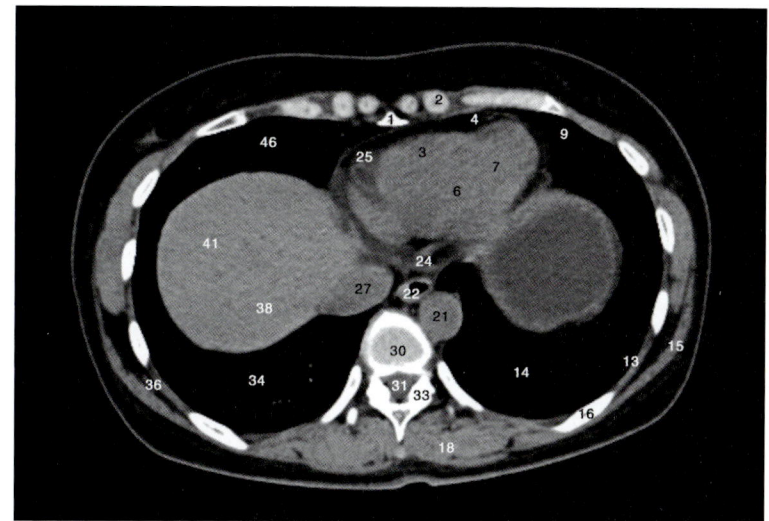

B. CT 平扫图像

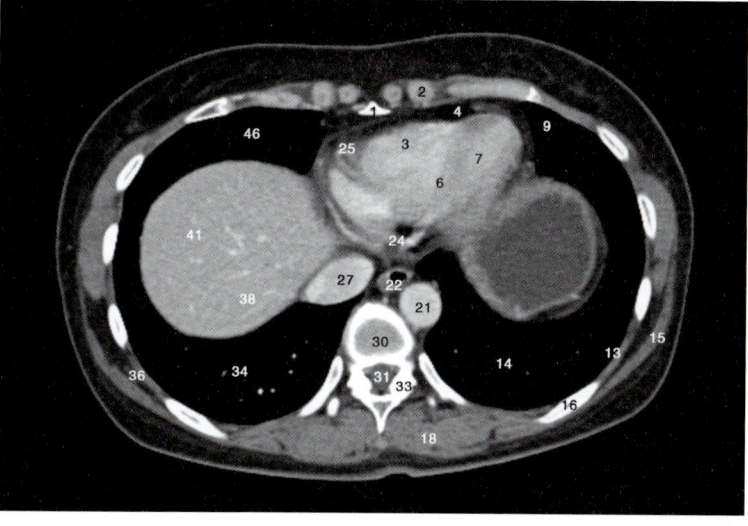

C. CT 增强图像

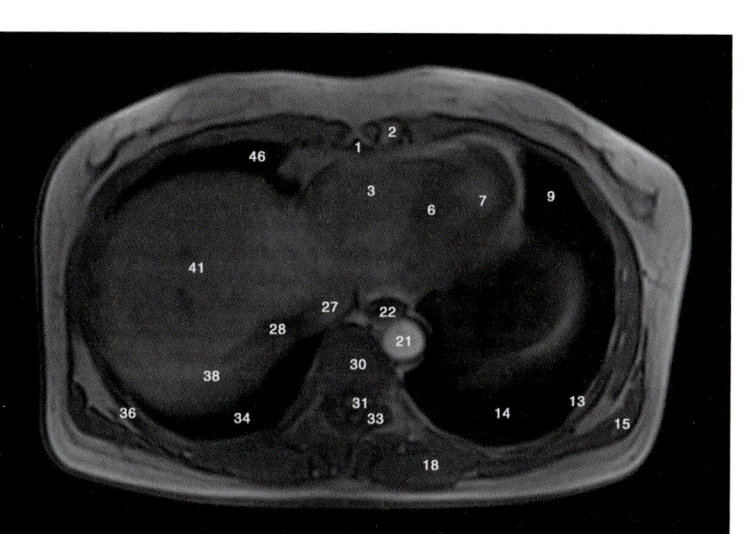

D. MR T1WI

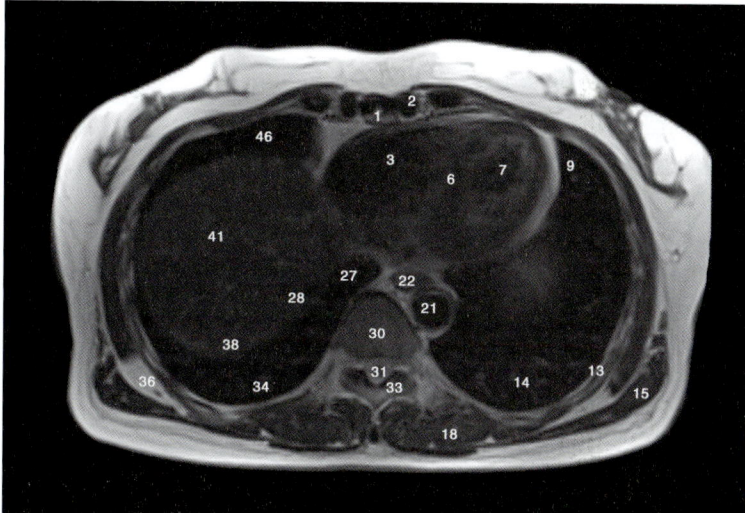

E. MR T2WI

关键结构：奇静脉，半奇静脉。

此断面经 T9-10 椎间盘。

在椎体前方，胸主动脉后方可见奇静脉和半奇静脉。奇静脉由右腰升静脉和右肋下静脉在第 12 肋头的下方互相汇合而成，大部分位于腰大肌深面。奇静脉于胸主动脉和胸导管的右侧上行，右肋间后动脉经行于奇静脉的背侧，食管则位于其腹侧。奇静脉全长与右侧纵隔胸膜接触，至第 3~5 胸椎高度（约 40% 位于第 4 胸椎高度），儿童在第 2~4 胸椎高度，奇静脉向前方构成奇静脉弓，跨过右肺根，注入上腔静脉。半奇静脉为奇静脉属支，走行于胸主动脉左侧和左侧内脏大神经的右侧、食管的背侧、左侧肋后动脉的腹侧[2]。在 CT、MR 平扫或增强图像上，由于有周围脂肪间隙的衬托，尽管奇静脉和半奇静脉较细，但依然可能较清晰地显示，但应注意与邻近的胸导管的鉴别；在增强 CT 静脉期图像上，奇静脉和半奇静脉强化，密度高于胸导管。

腹部连续横断层 10（FH.11730）

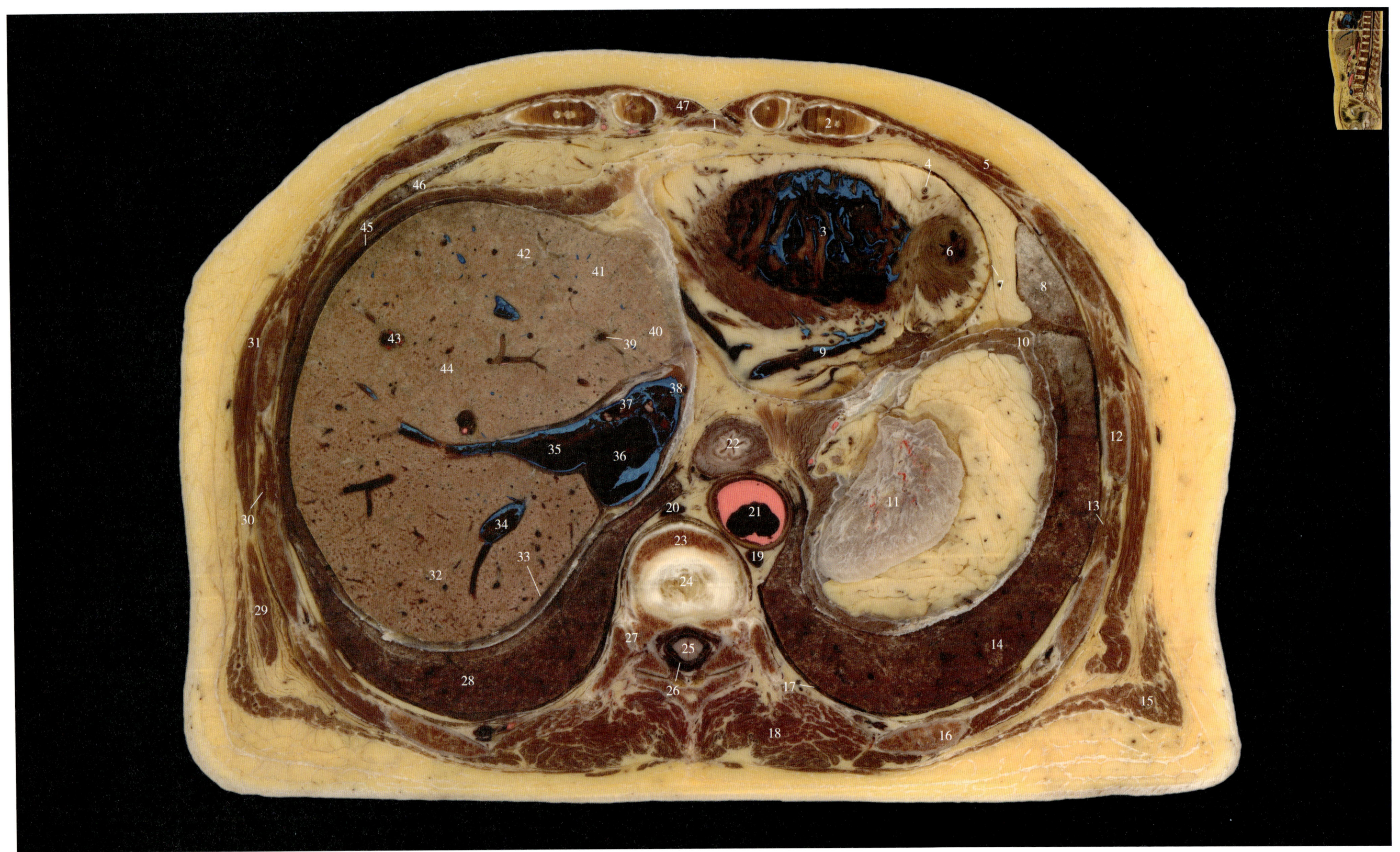

A. 断层标本图像

1. 胸骨体 body of sternum
2. 第 5 肋软骨 5th costal cartilage
3. 右心室 right ventricle
4. 左冠状动脉前室间支 anterior interventricular branch of left coronary artery
5. 腹外斜肌 obliquus externus abdominis
6. 左心室 left ventricle
7. 心包前下窦 anterior inferior sinus of pericardium
8. 左肺上叶 superior lobe of left lung
9. 心中静脉 middle cardiac vein
10. 膈 diaphragm
11. 胃底 fundus of stomach
12. 第 7 肋骨 7th costal bone
13. 肋间内肌 intercostale interni
14. 左肺下叶 inferior lobe of left lung
15. 背阔肌 latissimus dorsi
16. 第 9 肋骨 9th costal bone
17. 胸膜腔 pleural cavity
18. 竖脊肌 erector spinae
19. 半奇静脉 hemiazygos vein
20. 奇静脉 azygos vein
21. 胸主动脉 thoracic aorta
22. 食管 esophagus
23. 第 10 胸椎椎体 body of 10th thoracic vertebra
24. T9-10 椎间盘 T9-10 intervertebral disc
25. 脊髓 spinal cord
26. 硬脊膜 spinal dura mater
27. 肋头关节 joint of costal head
28. 右肺下叶 inferior lobe of right lung
29. 后锯肌 serratus posterior
30. 肋间外肌 intercostale externi
31. 前锯肌 serratus anterior
32. 肝右后叶上段 superior segment of right posterior lobe of liver
33. 肝裸区 bare area of liver
34. 肝右后上缘静脉 right posterosuperior marginal vein of liver
35. 肝右静脉 right hepatic vein
36. 下腔静脉 inferior vena cava
37. 肝中静脉 middle hepatic vein
38. 肝左静脉 left hepatic vein
39. 肝门静脉左外上支 left laterosuperior branch of hepatic portal vein
40. 肝左外叶上段 superior segment of left lateral lobe of liver
41. 肝左外叶下段 inferior segment of left lateral lobe of liver
42. 肝左内叶段 left medial lobe of liver
43. 肝门静脉右前上支 right anterosuperior branch of hepatic portal vein
44. 肝右前叶上段 superior segment of right anterior lobe of liver
45. 右肝上间隙 right suprahepatic space
46. 右肺中叶 middle lobe of right lung
47. 腹直肌 rectus abdominis

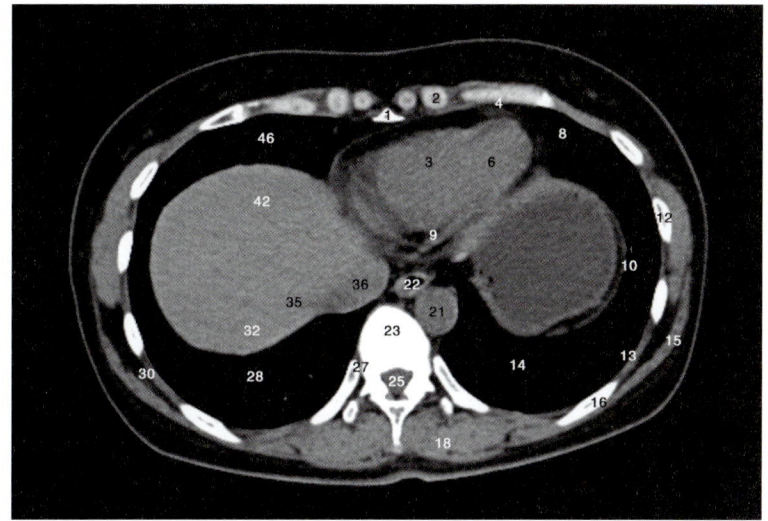

B. CT 平扫图像

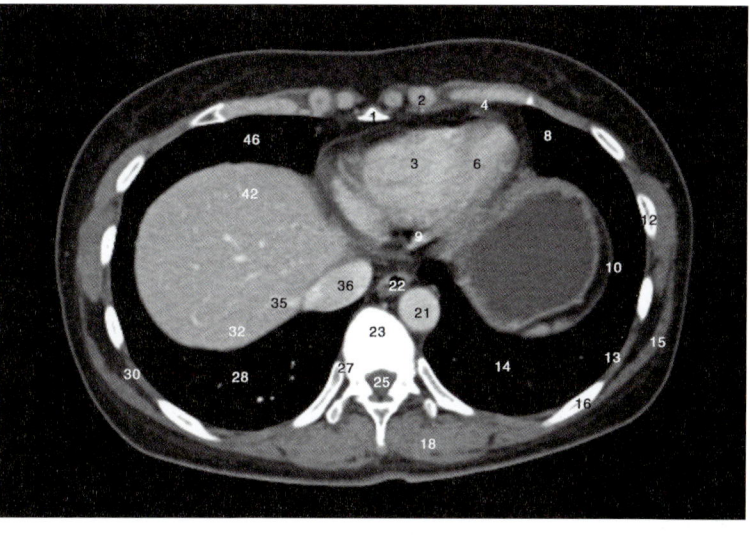

C. CT 增强图像

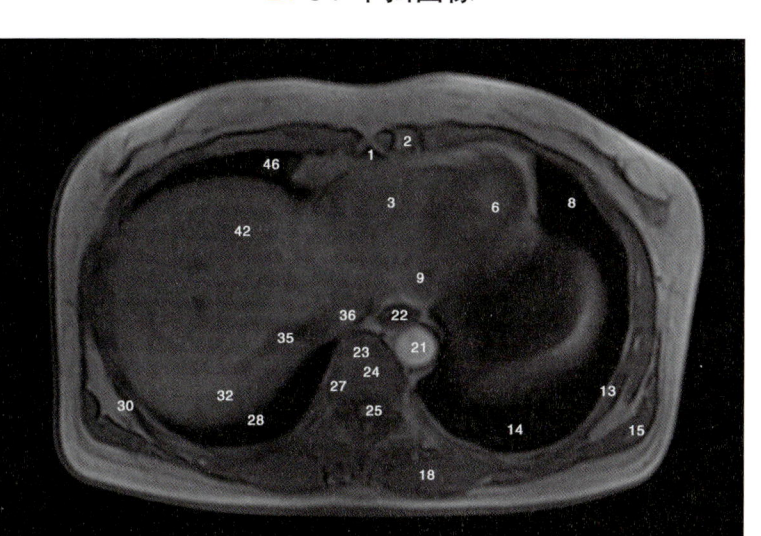

D. MR T1WI

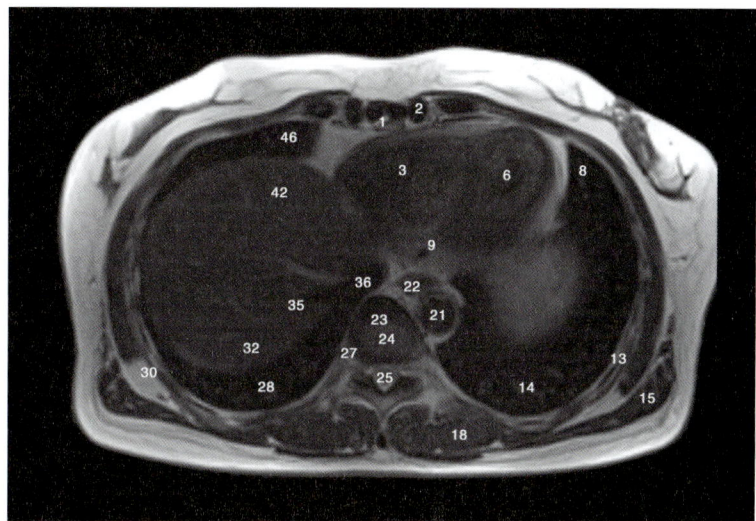

E. MR T2WI

关键结构：肝左静脉，肝右后上缘静脉。

此断面经 T9-10 椎间盘和第 10 胸椎椎体上份。

肝中静脉和肝左静脉在此断面汇入下腔静脉。肝左静脉位于左段间裂内，由上、下 2 根合成，收集左外叶上段和左外叶下段的静脉血。国人解剖数值显示肝左静脉内径为 0.58 cm ± 0.07 cm，肝左静脉注入处外径为 1.07 cm ± 0.29 cm，分叉处为 1.04 cm ± 0.25 cm。肝左静脉主干长为 2.28 cm ± 0.88 cm，肝左静脉与下腔静脉的夹角为 76.88° ± 11.93°[2]。肝右后上缘静脉位于右后叶，是肝右静脉最高位的属支，出现率约为 50%。由于该支平行于肝右后上缘，因此超声横位较难显示，但在右肋缘下向第二肝门扫描，则容易发现[7]。该断面上，肺的面积进一步减小，CT 纵隔窗上显示的膈前上方低密度区并不一定都是肺组织，对于中老年较肥胖者，两侧心膈角处经常有较大的三角形脂肪堆积，在 X 线胸片上有时可造成诊断上的困惑，CT 经过测量 CT 值或调整窗宽窗位可以清晰地显示为脂肪密度，MRI 的 T1WI 和 T2WI 均表现为高信号，可明确为脂肪组织。

腹部连续横断层 11（FH.11710）

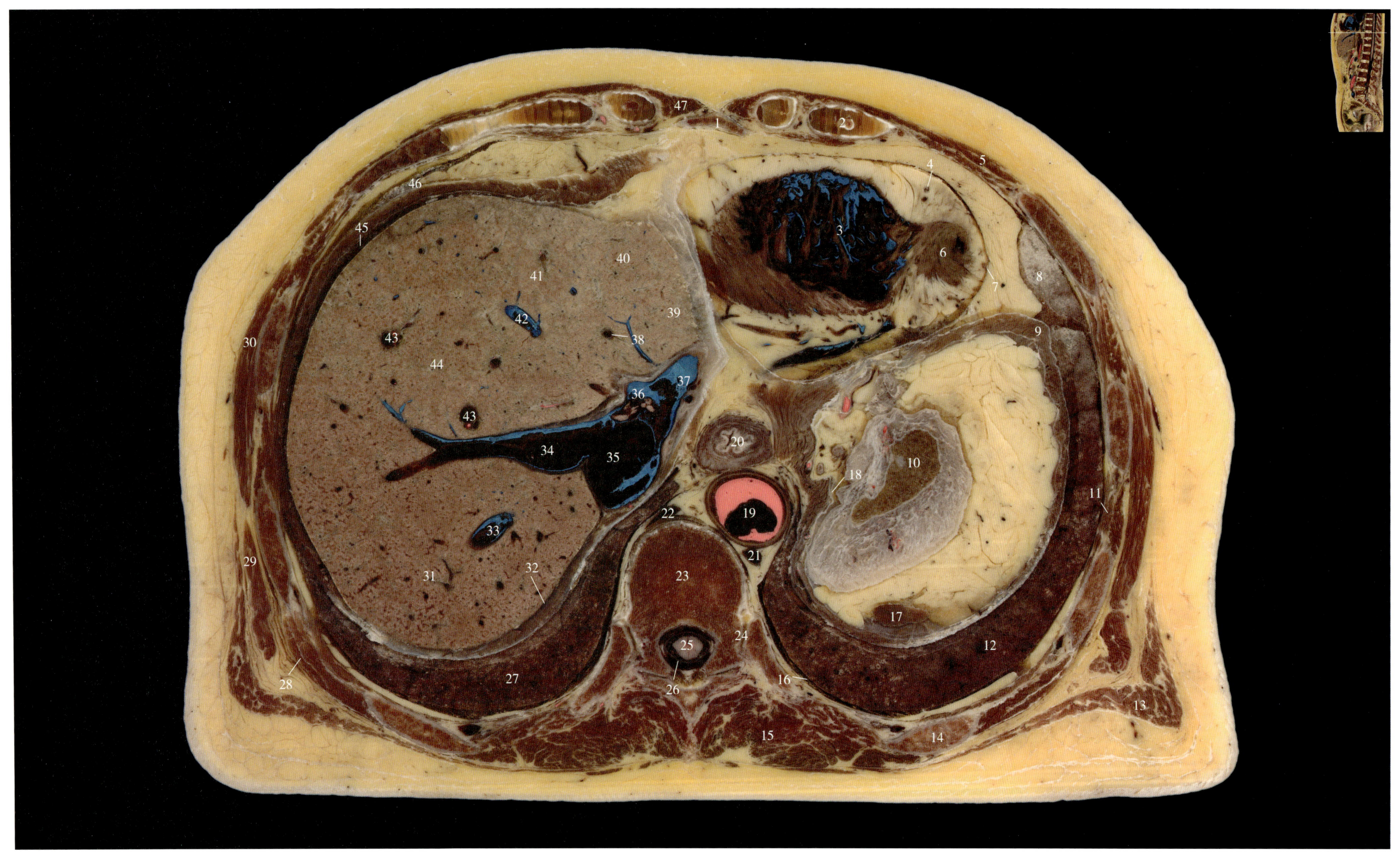

A. 断层标本图像

1. 胸骨体 body of sternum
2. 第 5 肋软骨 5th costal cartilage
3. 右心室 right ventricle
4. 左冠状动脉前室间支 anterior interventricular branch of left coronary artery
5. 腹外斜肌 obliquus externus abdominis
6. 左心室 left ventricle
7. 心包前下窦 anterior inferior sinus of pericardium
8. 左肺上叶 superior lobe of left lung
9. 膈 diaphragm
10. 胃底 fundus of stomach
11. 肋间内肌 intercostale interni
12. 左肺下叶 inferior lobe of left lung
13. 背阔肌 latissimus dorsi
14. 第 9 肋骨 9th costal bone
15. 竖脊肌 erector spinae
16. 胸膜腔 pleural cavity
17. 脾 spleen
18. 胃裸区 bara area of stomach
19. 胸主动脉 thoracic aorta
20. 食管 esophagus
21. 半奇静脉 hemiazygos vein
22. 奇静脉 azygos vein
23. 第 10 胸椎椎体 body of 10th thoracic vertebra
24. 肋头关节 joint of costal head
25. 脊髓 spinal cord
26. 硬脊膜 spinal dura mater
27. 右肺下叶 inferior lobe of right lung
28. 肋间外肌 intercostale externi
29. 下后锯肌 serratus posterior inferior
30. 前锯肌 serratus anterior
31. 肝右后叶上段 superior segment of right posterior lobe of liver
32. 肝裸区 bare area of liver
33. 肝右后上缘静脉 right posterosuperior marginal vein of liver
34. 肝右静脉 right hepatic vein
35. 下腔静脉 inferior vena cava
36. 肝中静脉 middle hepatic vein
37. 肝左静脉 left hepatic vein
38. 肝门静脉左外上支 left laterosuperior branch of hepatic portal vein
39. 肝左外叶上段 superior segment of left lateral lobe of liver
40. 肝左外叶下段 inferior segment of left lateral lobe of liver
41. 肝左内叶 left medial lobe of liver
42. 肝中静脉属支 tributary of middle hepatic vein
43. 肝门静脉右前上支 right anterosuperior branch of hepatic portal vein
44. 肝右前叶上段 superior segment of right anterior lobe of liver
45. 右肝上间隙 right suprahepatic space
46. 右肺中叶 middle lobe of right lung
47. 腹直肌 rectus abdominis

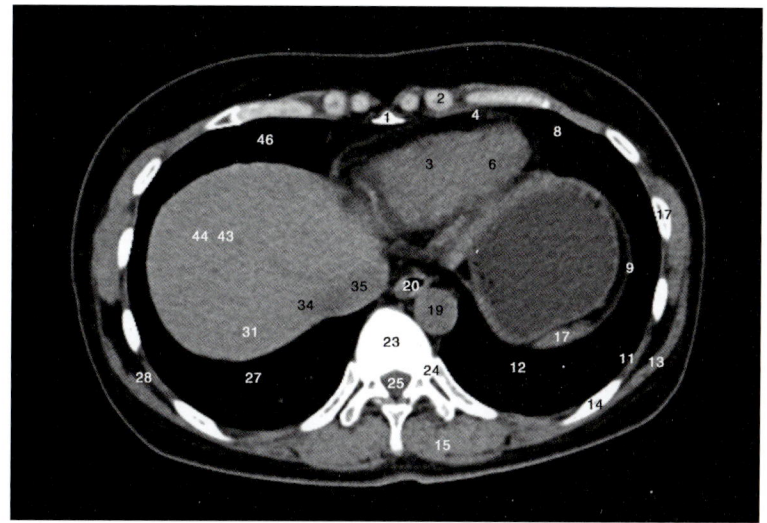

B. CT 平扫图像　　　　　　　　C. CT 增强图像

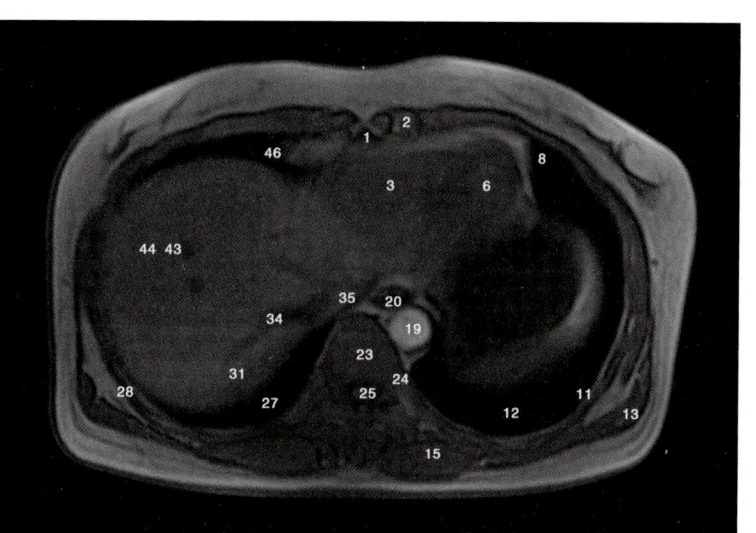 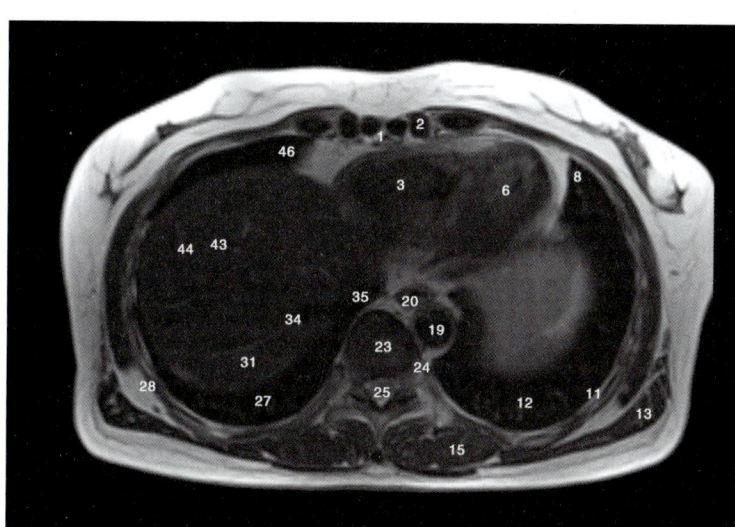

D. MR T1WI　　　　　　　　E. MR T2WI

关键结构：食管裂孔，胃底。

此断面经第 10 胸椎椎体上份。

胃、脾出现在膈左穹窿内。胃分为贲门部、胃底、胃体和幽门部四部分，最上方为胃底。食管左移至胸主动脉前方，穿膈食管裂孔。食管裂孔是膈的 3 个较大的裂孔之一，有食管、迷走神经及食管的血管和淋巴管通过，是 1 个呈矢状位的椭圆形孔，位于膈主动脉裂孔的左前上方，高度约平对第 10 胸椎。其肌纤维主要来自膈的左、右内侧脚。特别是右内侧脚的纤维，分裂成浅、深 2 个肌束，浅层者绕行于食管右侧，形成食管裂孔的右缘，深层者绕行于食管左侧，形成食管裂孔的左缘，深、浅两肌束在裂孔前缘相交，形成食管裂孔。而左膈脚内侧肌纤维尽管也绕行于食管左侧，但未参与食管裂孔的形成，此类型被称为标准型。据刘正津观察，国人以Ⅰ型（标准型）食管裂孔居多，约占 75.8%；食管裂孔完全由左膈脚内侧肌纤维形成者属Ⅱ型，约占 3.2%；Ⅰ、Ⅱ型结构兼有者为Ⅲ型，约占 15.4%；其余各型则更少见。食管裂孔各径为外径为 18.53 mm ± 2.71 mm，内径为 11.68 mm ± 3.14 mm，前后径为 9.76 mm ± 0.27 mm[2]。膈食管裂孔对防止胃食管反流及胃向胸腔内疝入具有重要作用。若食管腹段、食管胃连接部和部分胃组织等通过膈食管裂孔进入胸腔，则称为食管裂孔疝，多见于中老年患者，多无明显症状，部分患者表现为胸痛、咽下疼痛伴吞咽困难，可伴有反流和胸骨后及背部烧灼感等，治疗上可利用腹腔镜进行手术修补。

腹部连续横断层 12（FH.11690）

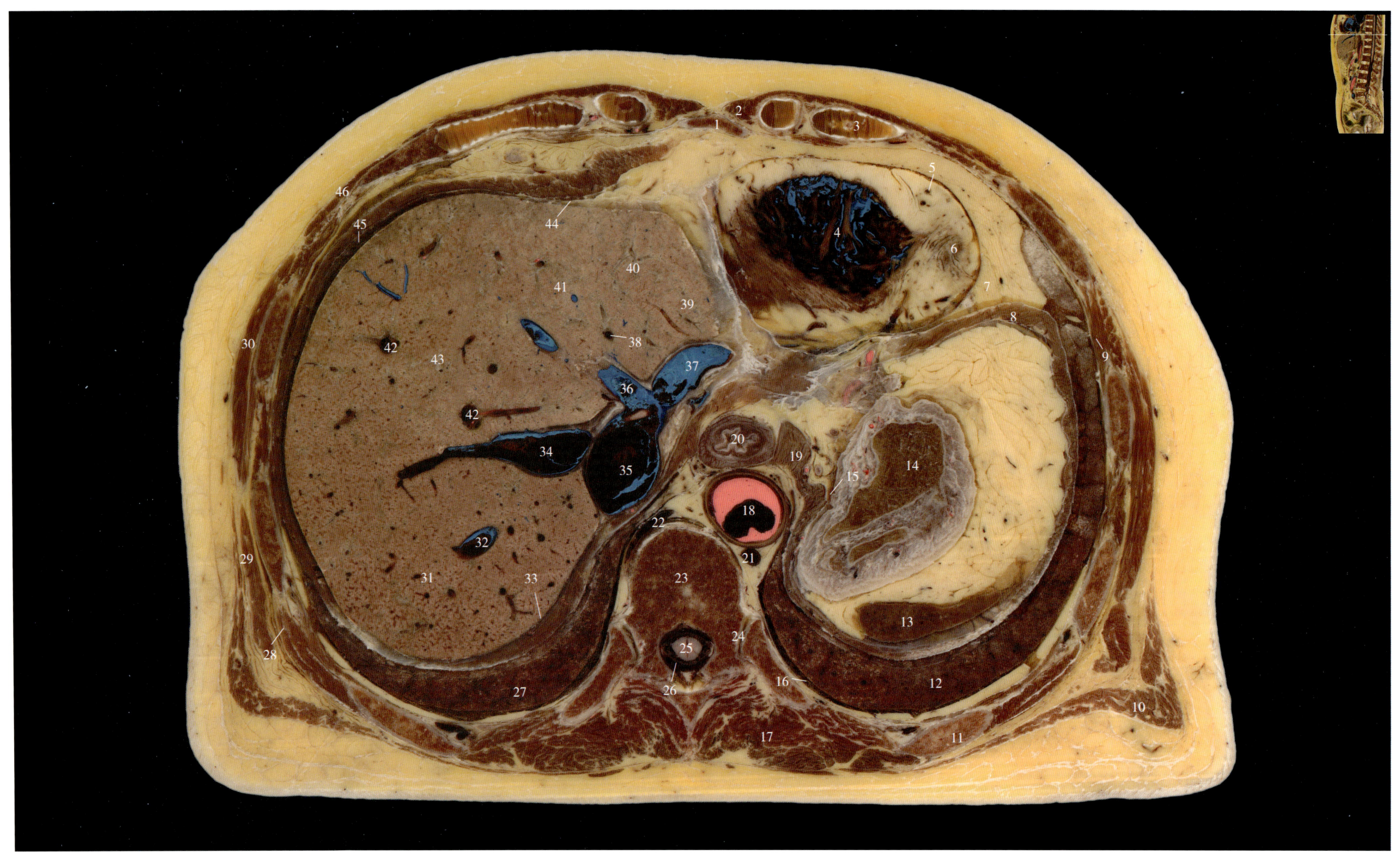

A. 断层标本图像

1. 胸骨体 body of sternum
2. 腹直肌 rectus abdominis
3. 第5肋软骨 5th costal cartilage
4. 右心室 right ventricle
5. 左冠状动脉前室间支 anterior interventricular branch of left coronary artery
6. 左心室 left ventricle
7. 心包前下窦 anterior inferior sinus of pericardium
8. 膈 diaphragm
9. 肋间内肌 intercostale interni
10. 背阔肌 latissimus dorsi
11. 第9肋骨 9th costal bone
12. 左肺下叶 inferior lobe of left lung
13. 脾 spleen
14. 胃底 fundus of stomach
15. 胃裸区 bara area of stomach
16. 胸膜腔 pleural cavity
17. 竖脊肌 erector spinae
18. 胸主动脉 thoracic aorta
19. 左膈脚 left crus of diaphragm
20. 食管腹部 abdominal part of esophagus
21. 半奇静脉 hemiazygos vein
22. 奇静脉 azygos vein
23. 第10胸椎椎体 body of 10th thoracic vertebra
24. 肋头关节 joint of costal head
25. 脊髓 spinal cord
26. 硬脊膜 spinal dura mater
27. 右肺下叶 inferior lobe of right lung
28. 肋间外肌 intercostale externi
29. 下后锯肌 serratus posterior inferior
30. 前锯肌 serratus anterior
31. 肝右后叶上段 superior segment of right posterior lobe of liver
32. 肝右后上缘静脉 right posterosuperior marginal vein of liver
33. 肝裸区 bare area of liver
34. 肝右静脉 right hepatic vein
35. 下腔静脉 inferior vena cava
36. 肝中静脉 middle hepatic vein
37. 肝左静脉 left hepatic vein
38. 肝门静脉左外上支 left laterosuperior branch of hepatic portal vein
39. 肝左外叶上段 superior segment of left lateral lobe of liver
40. 肝左外叶下段 inferior segment of left lateral lobe of liver
41. 肝左内叶 left medial lobe of liver
42. 肝门静脉右前上支 right anterosuperior branch of hepatic portal vein
43. 肝右前叶上段 superior segment of right anterior lobe of liver
44. 肝镰状韧带 falciform ligament of liver
45. 右肝上间隙 right suprahepatic space
46. 腹外斜肌 obliquus externus abdominis

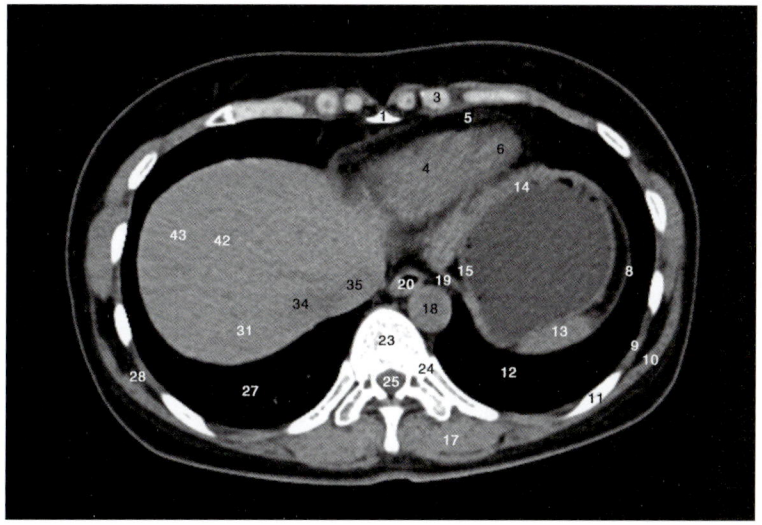

B. CT 平扫图像

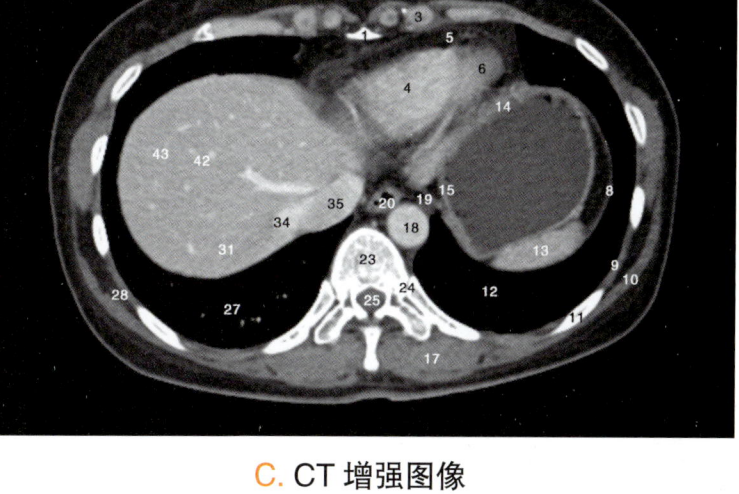

C. CT 增强图像

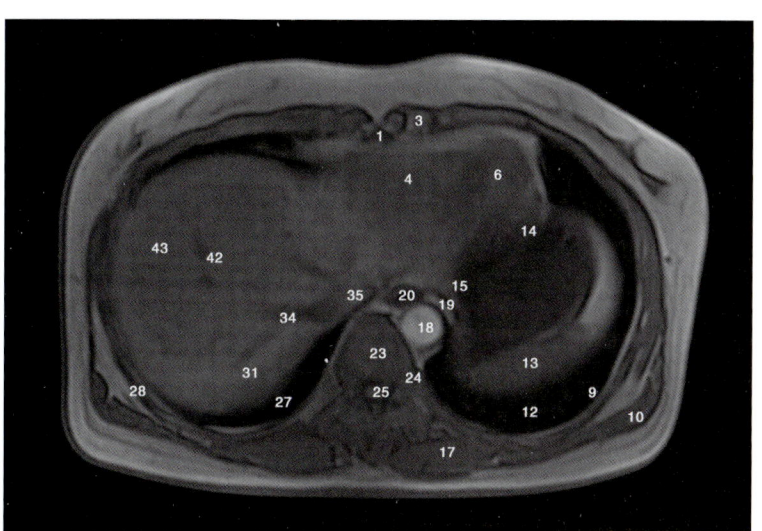

D. MR T1WI

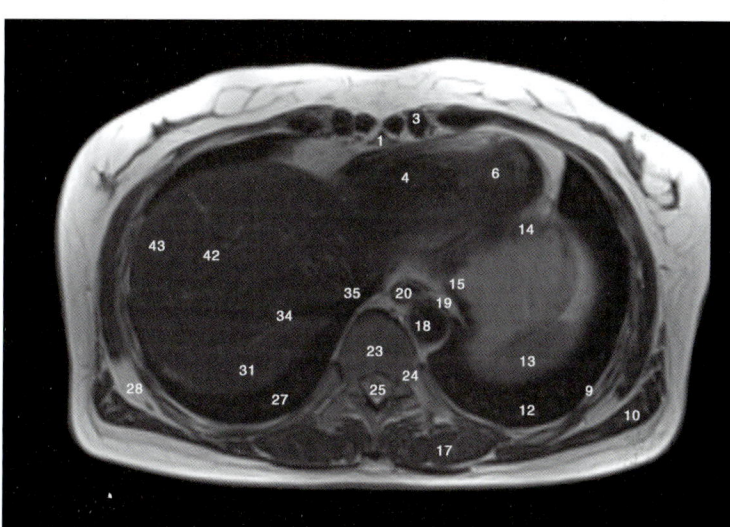

E. MR T2WI

关键结构：第二肝门，肝左、中、右静脉。

此断面经第10胸椎椎体上份。

第二肝门是指肝左、中、右静脉出肝并汇入下腔静脉处，多位于第10胸椎椎体上份水平（56.67%）。于此断面上，可见肝右静脉出肝后开口于下腔静脉右壁，肝中静脉和肝左静脉共同开口于下腔静脉左前壁。据国人446例的观察资料，65.7%的肝左静脉与肝中静脉同干汇入下腔静脉，33.2%的单独汇至下腔静脉的左前壁或左壁。肝左、中、右静脉排列于下腔静脉的左前、前和右后侧。据韩景茹等对30例腹部横断层标本的观测，肝左、中、右静脉长轴与经下腔静脉中点所做左右水平线的夹角分别为69°、57°和14°[1]。当肝静脉因各种原因阻塞导致肝静脉回流障碍，肝脏淤血而产生门静脉高压临床症候群，称之为布加综合征。布加综合征的广义定义为肝静脉和/或其开口以上的下腔静脉阻塞所导致的门静脉和/或下腔静脉高压临床症候群，病理生理学定义为从肝小静脉到下腔静脉和右心房汇合处的任何部位的肝静脉流出道阻塞[7]，主要临床表现为腹痛、肝脾肿大、腹水及下肢水肿等，急性期CT平扫可见肝脏弥漫性肿大、密度减低，伴大量腹水；增强CT静脉期显示下腔静脉肝后段及肝静脉内出现充盈缺损为特异性表现。MR除了能发现充盈缺损等直接征象，对肝间接信号改变更敏感。平扫可见肝信号不均匀，急性期者周边区域可见稍长T1和稍长T2异常信号，且周边强化程度弱于中心区域。布加综合征一般需要介入等手术治疗。

25

腹部连续横断层 13（FH.11670）

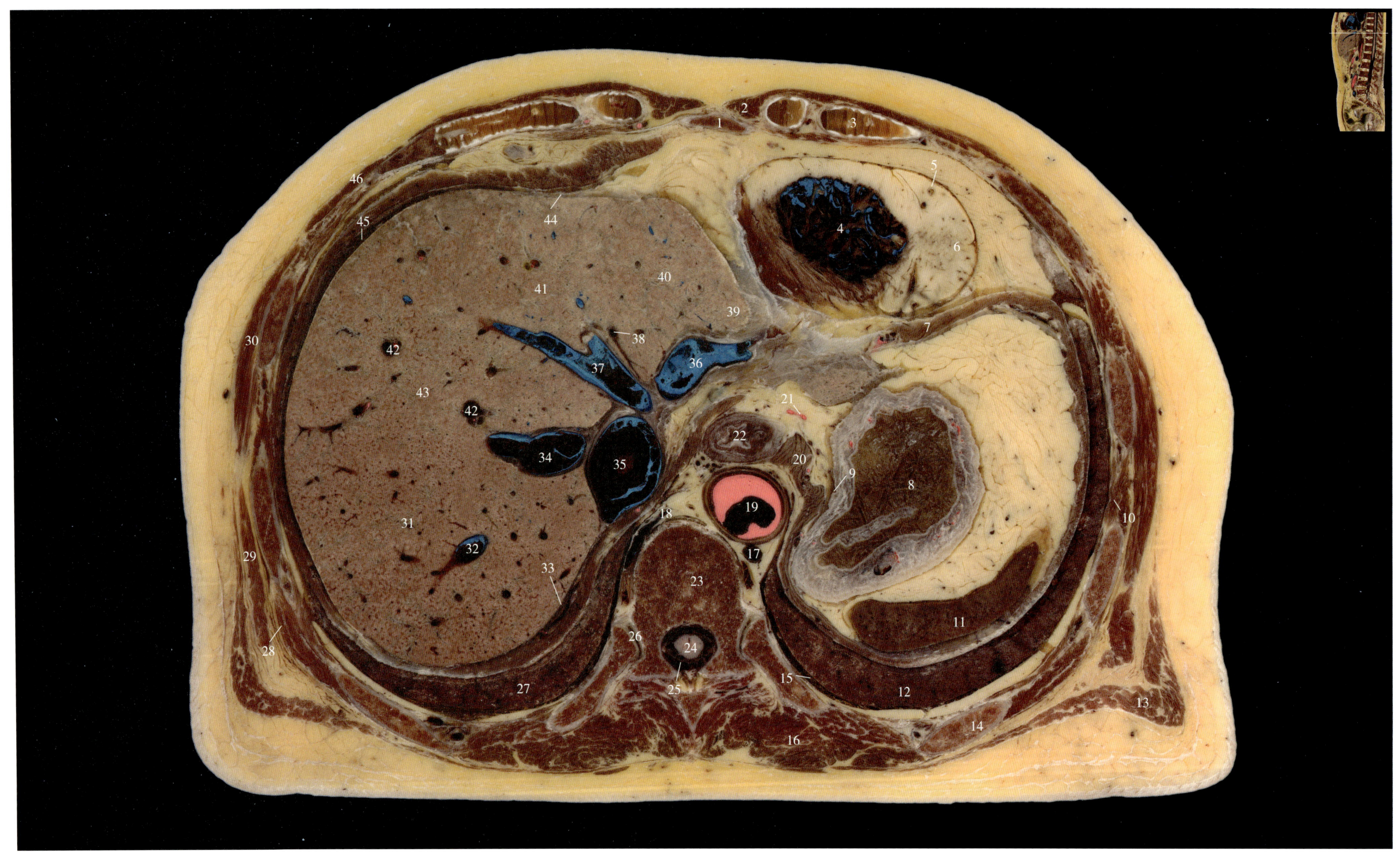

A. 断层标本图像

1. 胸骨体 body of sternum
2. 腹直肌 rectus abdominis
3. 第5肋软骨 5th costal cartilage
4. 右心室 right ventricle
5. 左冠状动脉前室间支 anterior interventricular branch of left coronary artery
6. 心包脂肪垫 pericardial fat pad
7. 膈 diaphragm
8. 胃底 fundus of stomach
9. 胃裸区 bara area of stomach
10. 肋间内肌 intercostale interni
11. 脾 spleen
12. 左肺下叶 inferior lobe of left lung
13. 背阔肌 latissimus dorsi
14. 第9肋骨 9th costal bone
15. 胸膜腔 pleural cavity
16. 竖脊肌 erector spinae
17. 半奇静脉 hemiazygos vein
18. 奇静脉 azygos vein
19. 胸主动脉 thoracic aorta
20. 左膈脚 left crus of diaphragm
21. 胃左动脉 left gastric artery
22. 食管腹部 abdominal part of esophagus
23. 第10胸椎椎体 body of 10th thoracic vertebra
24. 脊髓 spinal cord
25. 硬脊膜 spinal dura mater
26. 肋头关节 joint of costal head
27. 右肺下叶 inferior lobe of right lung
28. 肋间外肌 intercostale externi
29. 下后锯肌 serratus posterior inferior
30. 前锯肌 serratus anterior
31. 肝右后叶上段 superior segment of right posterior lobe of liver
32. 肝右后上缘静脉 right posterosuperior marginal vein of liver
33. 肝裸区 bare area of liver
34. 肝右静脉 right hepatic vein
35. 下腔静脉 inferior vena cava
36. 肝左静脉 left hepatic vein
37. 肝中静脉 middle hepatic vein
38. 肝门静脉左外下支 left lateroinferior branch of hepatic portal vein
39. 肝左外叶上段 superior segment of left lateral lobe of liver
40. 肝左外叶下段 inferior segment of left lateral lobe of liver
41. 肝左内叶 left medial lobe of liver
42. 肝门静脉右前上支 right anterosuperior branch of hepatic portal vein
43. 肝右前叶上段 superior segment of right anterior lobe of liver
44. 肝镰状韧带 falciform ligament of liver
45. 右肝上间隙 right suprahepatic space
46. 腹外斜肌 obliquus externus abdominis

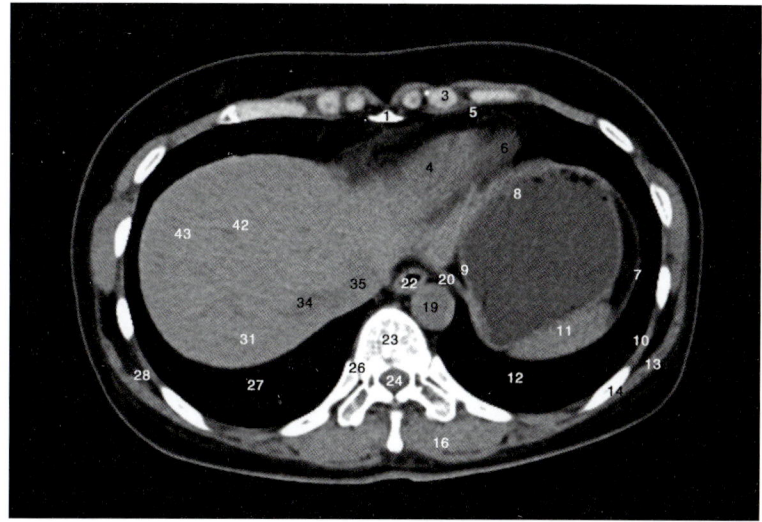

B. CT 平扫图像

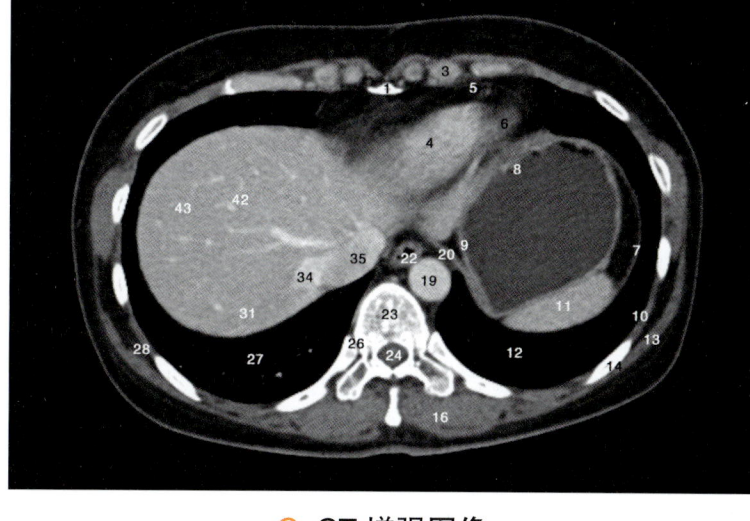

C. CT 增强图像

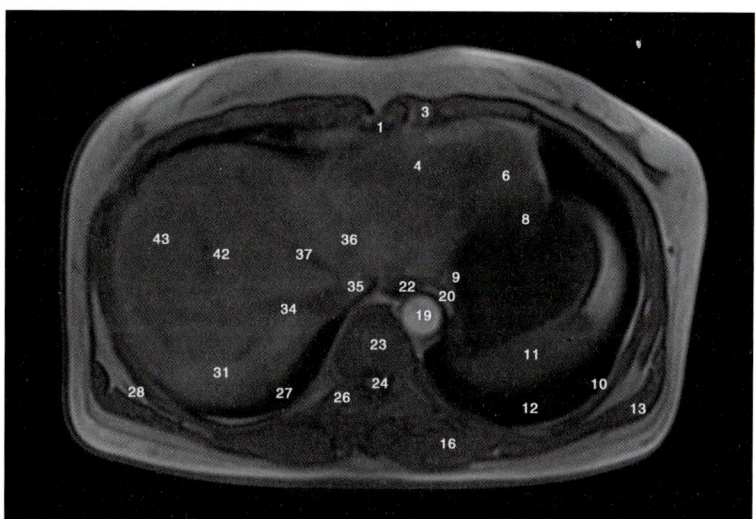

D. MR T1WI

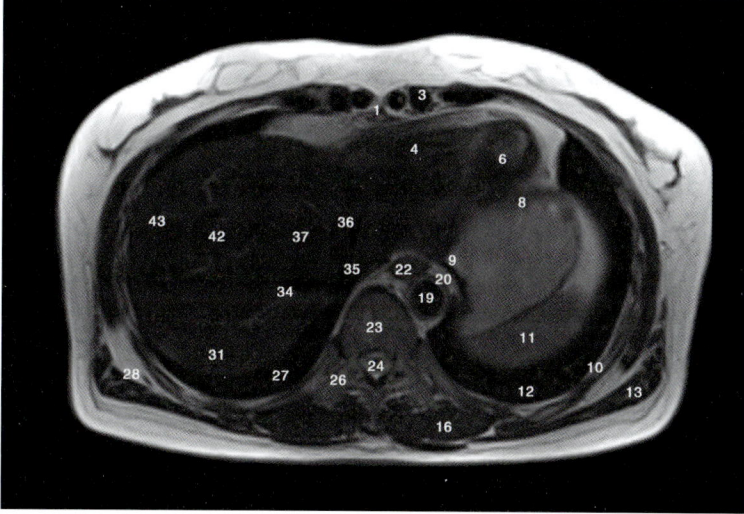

E. MR T2WI

关键结构：右肝上间隙，胃壁。

此断面经第10胸椎椎体上份。

在腹腔内，肝占据右侧，肝左外叶首次出现于膈左穹窿的下内侧。膈与肝左叶之间为右肝上间隙，肝上间隙借镰状韧带和左三角韧带分为右肝上间隙、左肝上前间隙和左肝上后间隙，右肝上间隙左界为镰状韧带，后方达冠状韧带上层，右侧向下与右结肠旁沟交通。胃底居腹腔左侧，胃壁由黏膜、黏膜下层、肌层、外膜4层结构组成，并有血管、淋巴管和神经分布。其中，胃黏膜厚 0.3~1.5 mm，以幽门附近最厚，贲门附近相对较薄。黏膜表面可见皱襞，皱襞由黏膜和黏膜下层共同形成，高低不一，排列不甚规则，但在贲门和幽门处，皱襞多呈放射状。黏膜下层由疏松结缔组织构成，含较大的血管、神经和淋巴管。肌层较厚，由内斜性、中环形和外纵行3层平滑肌构成[2]。胃最常见恶性肿瘤是胃癌，也是消化系统最常见的恶性肿瘤，按形态学分期可分为早期胃癌和进展期胃癌。早期胃癌是指癌组织局限于黏膜或黏膜下层的浸润性胃癌，不论是否有区域淋巴结转移的证据。当癌组织侵犯胃壁肌层或以上时称为进展期胃癌。Borrman 分型根据大体形态将进展期胃癌分为4种类型：Ⅰ型，结节隆起型；Ⅱ型，局限溃疡型；Ⅲ型，浸润溃疡型；Ⅳ型，弥漫浸润性（局部 Bor.Ⅳ，革囊胃）。

腹部连续横断层 14（FH.11650）

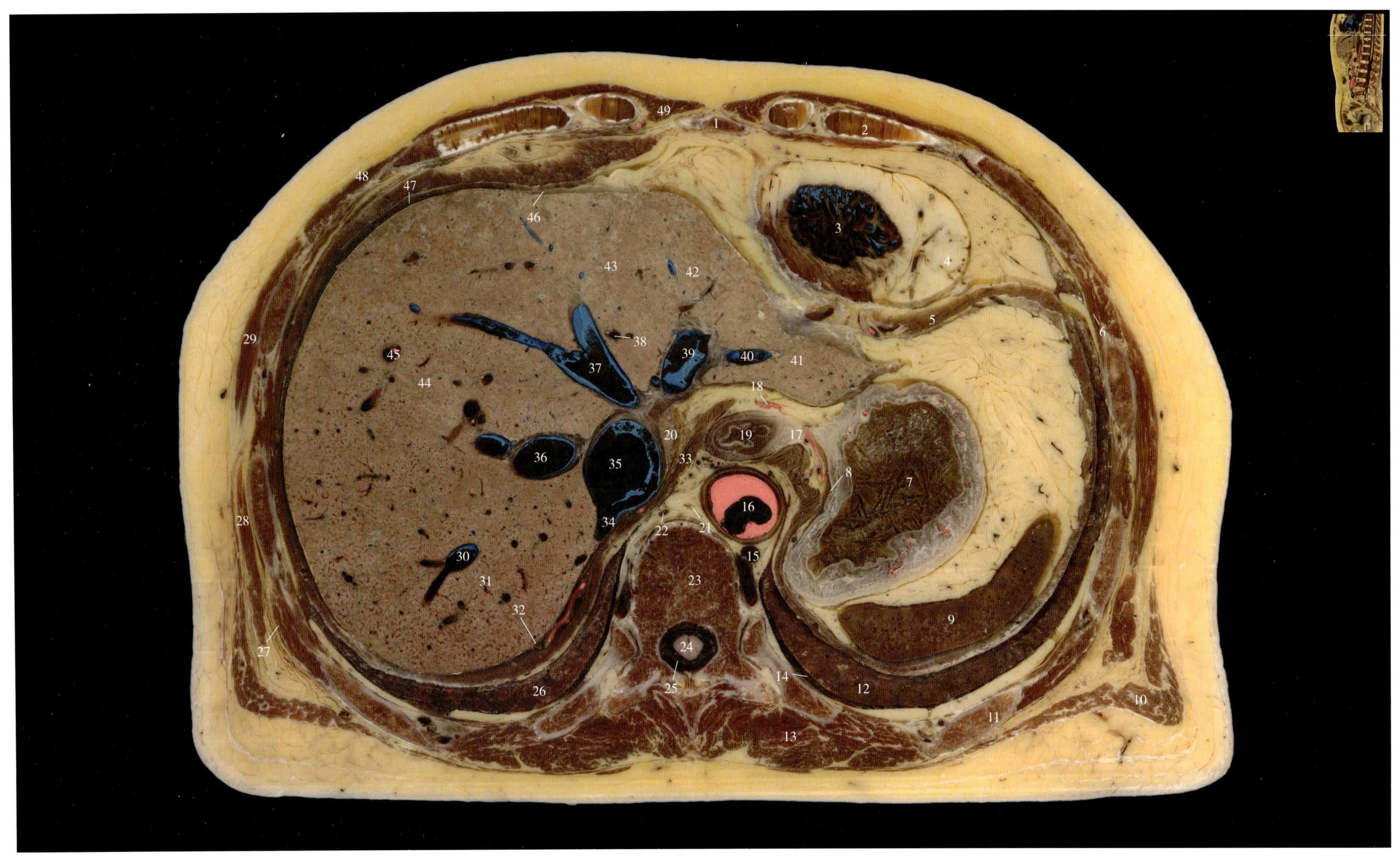

A. 断层标本图像

1. 胸骨体 body of sternum
2. 第 5 肋软骨 5th costal cartilage
3. 右心室 right ventricle
4. 心包脂肪垫 pericardial fat pad
5. 膈 diaphragm
6. 肋间内肌 intercostale interni
7. 胃底 fundus of stomach
8. 胃裸区 bara area of stomach
9. 脾 spleen
10. 背阔肌 latissimus dorsi
11. 第 9 肋骨 9th costal bone
12. 左肺下叶 inferior lobe of left lung
13. 竖脊肌 erector spinae
14. 胸膜腔 pleural cavity
15. 半奇静脉 hemiazygos vein
16. 胸主动脉 thoracic aorta
17. 胃贲门 cardia of stomach
18. 胃左动脉 left gastric artery
19. 食管腹部 abdominal part of esophagus
20. 肝尾状叶 caudate lobe of liver
21. 胸导管 thoracic duct
22. 奇静脉 azygos vein
23. 第 10 胸椎椎体 body of 10th thoracic vertebra
24. 脊髓 spinal cord
25. 硬脊膜 spinal dura mater
26. 右肺下叶 inferior lobe of right lung
27. 肋间外肌 intercostale externi
28. 下后锯肌 serratus posterior inferior
29. 前锯肌 serratus anterior
30. 肝右后上缘静脉 right posterosuperior marginal vein of liver
31. 肝右后叶上段 superior segment of right posterior lobe of liver
32. 肝裸区 bare area of liver
33. 右膈脚 right crus of diaphragm
34. 副肝静脉 accessory hepatic veins
35. 下腔静脉 inferior vena cava
36. 肝右静脉 right hepatic vein
37. 肝中静脉 middle hepatic vein
38. 肝门静脉左外下支 left lateroinferior branch of hepatic portal vein
39. 肝左静脉 left hepatic vein
40. 肝左后上缘静脉 left posterosuperior marginal vein of liver
41. 肝左外叶上段 superior segment of left lateral lobe of liver
42. 肝左外叶下段 inferior segment of left lateral lobe of liver
43. 肝左内叶 left medial lobe of liver
44. 肝右前叶上段 superior segment of right anterior lobe of liver
45. 肝门静脉右前上支 right anterosuperior branch of hepatic portal vein
46. 肝镰状韧带 falciform ligament of liver
47. 右肝上间隙 right suprahepatic space
48. 腹外斜肌 obliquus externus abdominis
49. 腹直肌 rectus abdominis

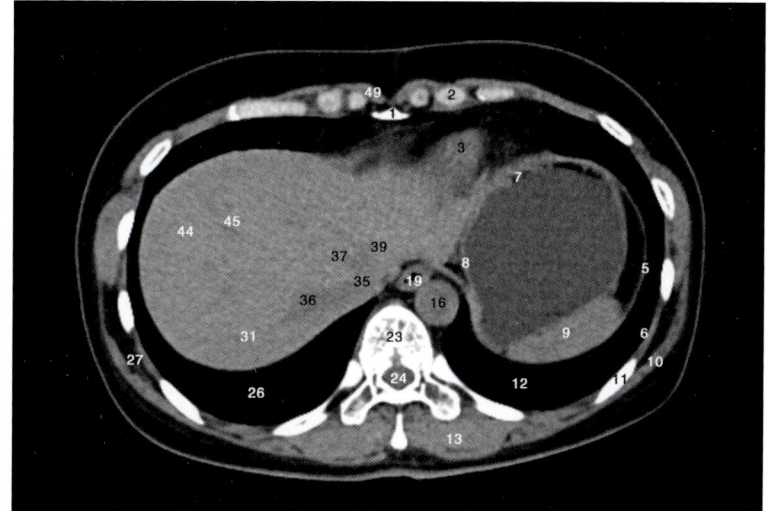

B. CT 平扫图像

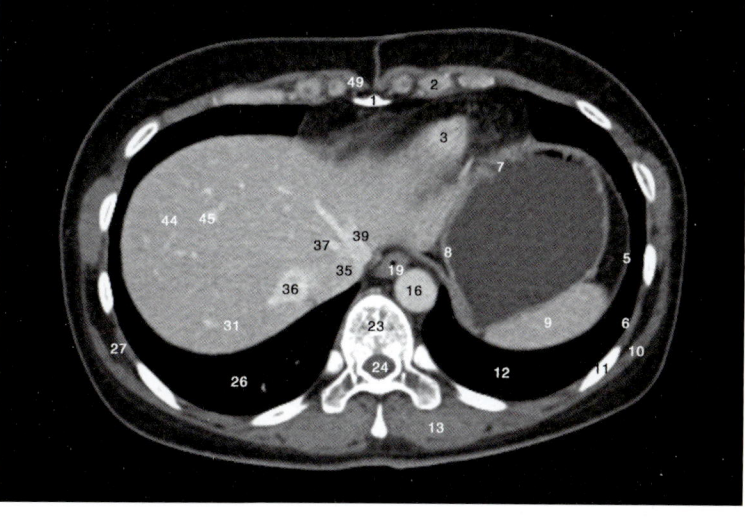

C. CT 增强图像

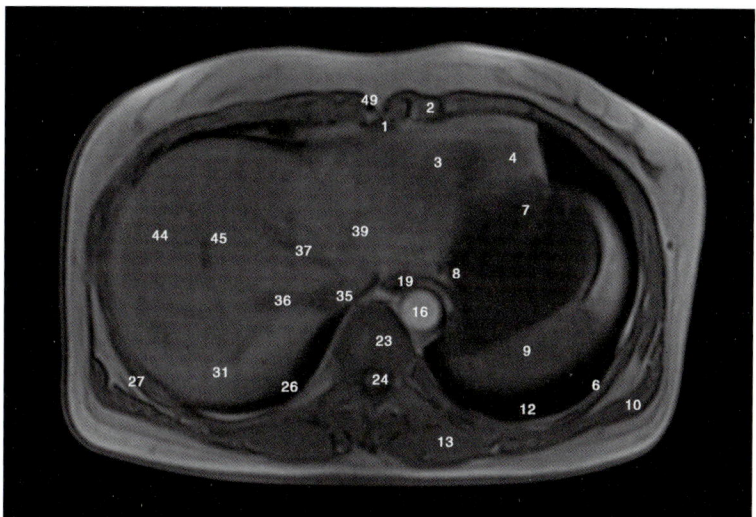

D. MR T1WI

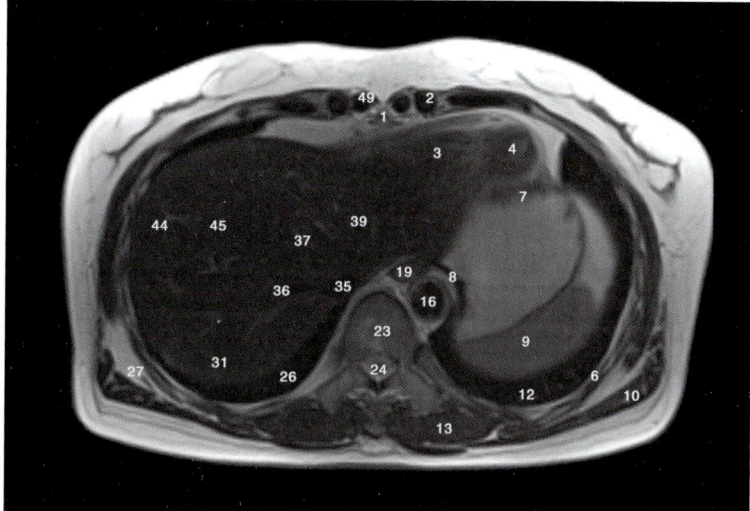

E. MR T2WI

关键结构：肝裸区，胃裸区。

此断面经第 10 胸椎椎体上份。

心脏结构仅余右心室，双肺仅余下叶的小部分。肝较上一断层进一步增大，并越过脊柱伸向左季肋区，肝尾状叶首次出现于下腔静脉左前方，并向左突入网膜囊上隐窝。肝冠状韧带下层位于下腔静脉后方、肝尾状叶右缘，与上层之间为肝裸区。右肝上间隙向左后方仅能延伸至冠状韧带上层处，难以达到肝裸区。而膈肌外侧的右肋膈下隐窝向左均越过肝裸区而延伸至脊柱的右前方。因此，在 CT、MR 等图像上，若液体能延伸至脊柱右前方则为胸腔积液，反之为腹腔积液。肝裸区的阻断范围是有限的，裸区以上和以下腹水仍可自由移动。胃底借胃膈韧带固定于膈，胃膈韧带右层向右续于食管前方的腹膜，左层连系于膈。胃膈韧带左、右层之间的胃面无腹膜覆盖，称胃裸区，出现率为 100%，面积在成人平均为 6.1 cm^2，儿童平均为 1.8 cm^2。胃裸区与膈之间为左膈下腹膜外间隙。在横断面上，胃裸区于食管腹段平面较小，向下逐渐增大，至第 12 胸椎平面达到最大，向下胃膈韧带两层相互靠拢而延续为胃胰韧带[1]。

腹部连续横断层 15（FH.11630）

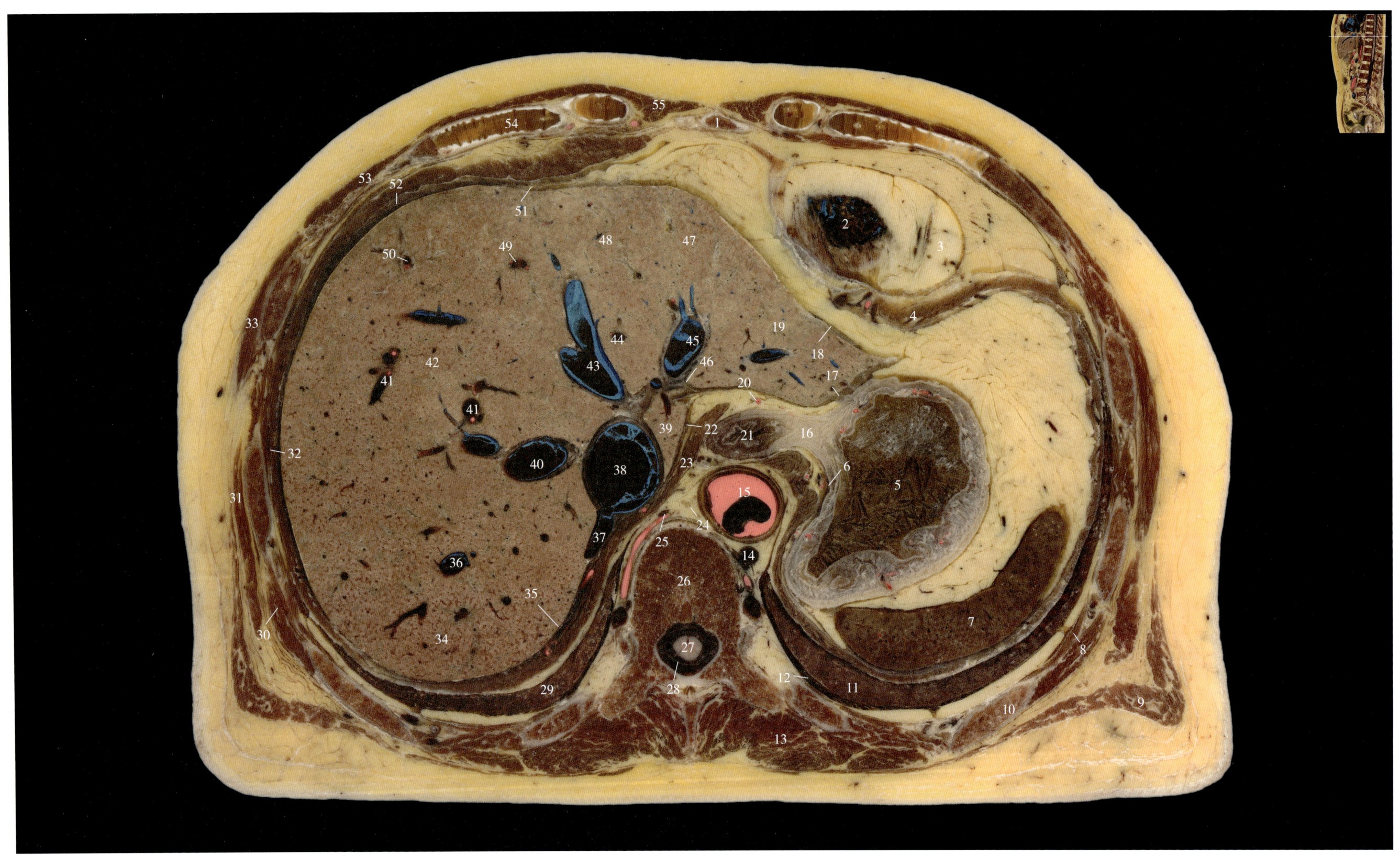

A. 断层标本图像

1. 胸骨体 body of sternum
2. 右心室 right ventricle
3. 心包脂肪垫 pericardial fat pad
4. 膈 diaphragm
5. 胃底 fundus of stomach
6. 胃裸区 bara area of stomach
7. 脾 spleen
8. 肋间内肌 intercostale interni
9. 背阔肌 latissimus dorsi
10. 第 9 肋骨 9th costal bone
11. 左肺下叶 inferior lobe of left lung
12. 胸膜腔 pleural cavity
13. 竖脊肌 erector spinae
14. 半奇静脉 hemiazygos vein
15. 胸主动脉 thoracic aorta
16. 胃贲门 cardia of stomach
17. 左肝下前间隙 anterior left subrahepatic space
18. 左肝上前间隙 anterior left suprahepatic space
19. 肝左外叶上段 superior segment of left lateral lobe of liver
20. 胃左动脉 left gastric artery
21. 食管腹部 abdominal part of esophagus
22. 网膜囊上隐窝 superior omental recess
23. 右膈脚 right crus of diaphragm
24. 胸导管 thoracic duct
25. 奇静脉 azygos vein
26. 第 10 胸椎椎体 body of 10th thoracic vertebra
27. 脊髓 spinal cord
28. 硬脊膜 spinal dura mater
29. 右肺下叶 inferior lobe of right lung
30. 肋间外肌 intercostale externi
31. 下后锯肌 serratus posterior inferior
32. 肋膈隐窝 costodiaphragmatic recess
33. 前锯肌 serratus anterior
34. 肝右后叶上段 superior segment of right posterior lobe of liver
35. 肝裸区 bare area of liver
36. 肝右后上缘静脉 right posterosuperior marginal vein of liver
37. 副肝静脉 accessory hepatic veins
38. 下腔静脉 inferior vena cava
39. 肝尾状叶 caudate lobe of liver
40. 肝右静脉 right hepatic vein
41. 肝门静脉右前上支 right anterosuperior branch of hepatic portal vein
42. 肝右前叶上段 superior segment of right anterior lobe of liver
43. 肝中静脉 middle hepatic vein
44. 肝门静脉左外下支 left lateroinferior branch of hepatic portal vein
45. 肝左静脉 left hepatic vein
46. 静脉韧带裂和肝胃韧带 fissure for ligamentum venosum and hepatogastric ligament
47. 肝左外叶下段 inferior segment of left lateral lobe of liver
48. 肝左内叶 left medial lobe of liver
49. 肝门静脉左内支 left medial branch of hepatic portal vein
50. 肝门静脉右前支 right anterior branch of hepatic portal vein
51. 肝镰状韧带 falciform ligament of liver
52. 右肝上间隙 right suprahepatic space
53. 腹外斜肌 obliquus externus abdominis
54. 第 5 肋软骨 5th costal cartilage
55. 腹直肌 rectus abdominis

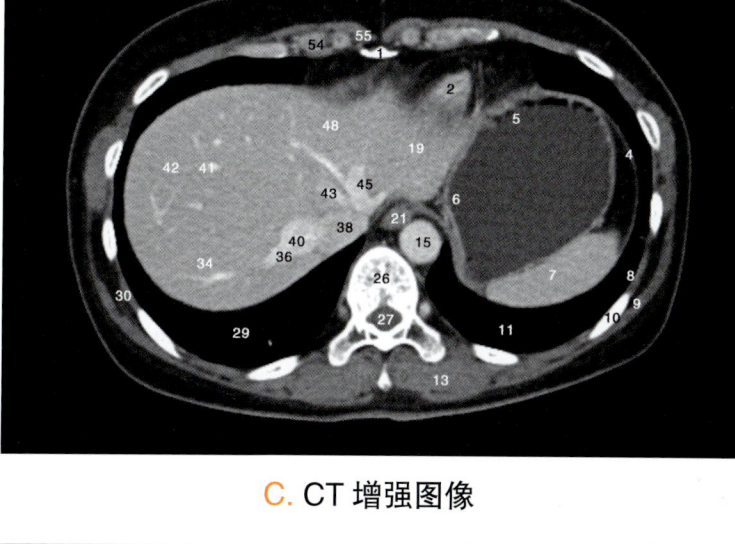

B. CT 平扫图像

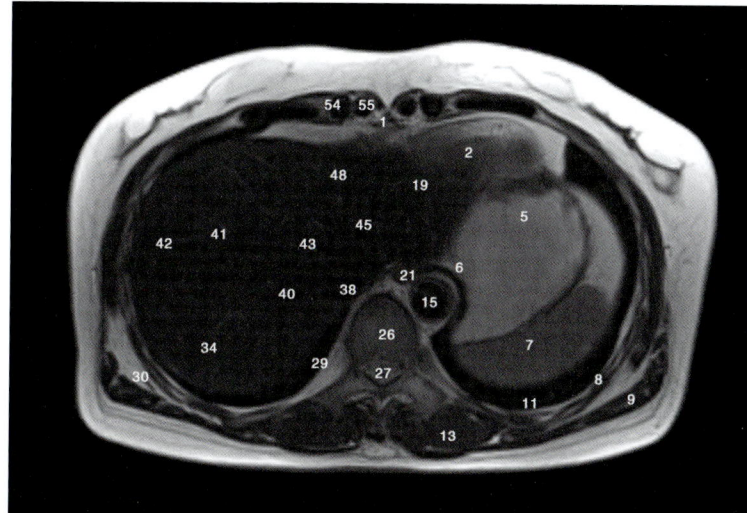

C. CT 增强图像

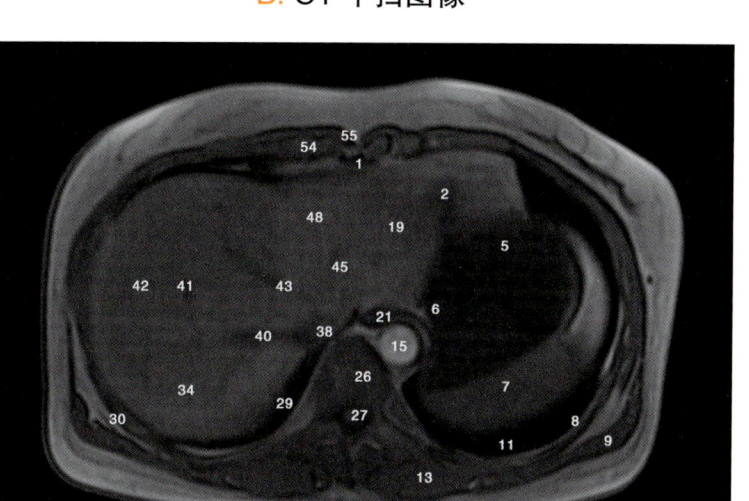

D. MR T1WI

E. MR T2WI

关键结构：肝段，肝裂。

此断面经第 10 胸椎椎体下份。

肝段是依据 Glisson 系统的分支与分布和肝静脉的走行进行的功能性区域划分，因解剖学上肝段之间并没有天然的界线，目前多依赖一些人为的连线或肝裂等解剖标记来划分为 8 个段（Couinaud 分段法）。肝裂为各肝段之间的分界线，包括：正中裂、背裂、左叶间裂、左段间裂、右叶间裂、右段间裂。本层是在肝左、中、右静脉分隔肝叶、段的典型断面。从下腔静脉左前壁引虚线，经肝中静脉长轴向前外延伸为正中裂，分隔右前叶和左内叶。从下腔静脉右侧壁，经肝右静脉长轴向外引虚线为右叶间裂，将右前叶和右后叶分开。由于左叶间裂内未见有标志性血管，因此，可从静脉韧带裂右端这一天然标志向前偏 10° 引虚线表示左叶间裂，将左内叶和左外叶分开。沿肝左静脉长轴引虚线，将左外叶分为后方的上段和前方的下段。下腔静脉右前壁与静脉韧带裂右端之间的弧形线为背裂，该裂后方为尾状叶，前方分别为右前叶和左内叶[7]。然而，肝段是根据 Glisson 管道系统分布呈不规则状的，边界不可能是直线，早在 1998 年 Fasel 等就应用门静脉塑化标本研究证实了传统划线分段法与真实的解剖分段相差较大[8]，后来又提出了一些观点，如 "1-2-20 概念" 等[9,10]。目前，借助计算机技术，一些 CT 工作站提供了一些可能更接近真实的肝段分析工具，利用 CT 增强门脉期图像，根据肝门静脉各支的实际分布范围，分析和展示相应的肝段范围，以期对手术等起到更好的指导作用。

腹部连续横断层 16（FH.11610）

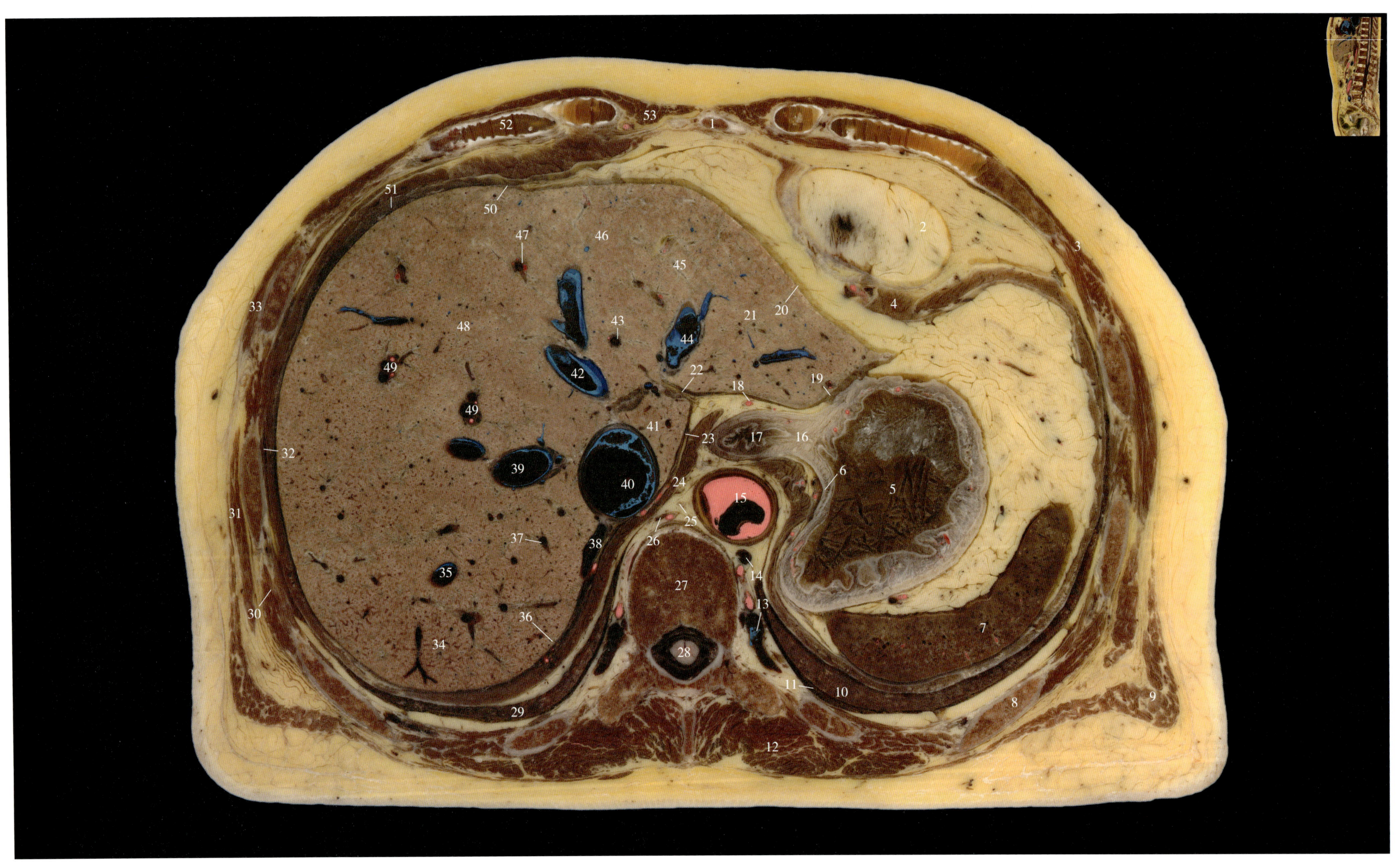

A. 断层标本图像

1. 胸骨体 body of sternum
2. 心包脂肪垫 pericardial fat pad
3. 腹外斜肌 obliquus externus abdominis
4. 膈 diaphragm
5. 胃底 fundus of stomach
6. 胃裸区 bara area of stomach
7. 脾 spleen
8. 第 9 肋骨 9th costal bone
9. 背阔肌 latissimus dorsi
10. 左肺下叶 inferior lobe of left lung
11. 胸膜腔 pleural cavity
12. 竖脊肌 erector spinae
13. 椎外静脉丛 external vertebral venous plexus
14. 半奇静脉 hemiazygos vein
15. 胸主动脉 thoracic aorta
16. 胃贲门 cardia of stomach
17. 食管腹部 abdominal part of esophagus
18. 胃左动脉 left gastric artery
19. 左肝下前间隙 anterior left subrahepatic space
20. 左肝上前间隙 anterior left suprahepatic space
21. 肝左外叶上段 superior segment of left lateral lobe of liver
22. 静脉韧带裂和肝胃韧带 fissure for ligamentum venosum and hepatogastric ligament
23. 网膜囊上隐窝 superior omental recess
24. 右膈脚 right crus of diaphragm
25. 胸导管 thoracic duct
26. 奇静脉 azygos vein
27. 第 10 胸椎椎体 body of 10th thoracic vertebra
28. 脊髓 spinal cord
29. 右肺下叶 inferior lobe of right lung
30. 肋间外肌 intercostale externi
31. 下后锯肌 serratus posterior inferior
32. 肋膈隐窝 costodiaphragmatic recess
33. 前锯肌 serratus anterior
34. 肝右后叶上段 superior segment of right posterior lobe of liver
35. 肝右后上缘静脉 right posterosuperior marginal vein of liver
36. 肝裸区 bare area of liver
37. 肝门静脉右后上支 right posterosuperior branch of hepatic portal vein
38. 副肝静脉 accessory hepatic veins
39. 肝右静脉 right hepatic vein
40. 下腔静脉 inferior vena cava
41. 肝尾状叶 caudate lobe of liver
42. 肝中静脉 middle hepatic vein
43. 肝门静脉左外下支 left lateroinferior branch of hepatic portal vein
44. 肝左静脉 left hepatic vein
45. 肝左外叶下段 inferior segment of left lateral lobe of liver
46. 肝左内叶 left medial lobe of liver
47. 肝门静脉左内支 left medial branch of hepatic portal vein
48. 肝右前叶上段 superior segment of right anterior lobe of liver
49. 肝门静脉右前上支 right anterosuperior branch of hepatic portal vein
50. 肝镰状韧带 falciform ligament of liver
51. 右肝上间隙 right suprahepatic space
52. 第 5 肋软骨 5th costal cartilage
53. 腹直肌 rectus abdominis

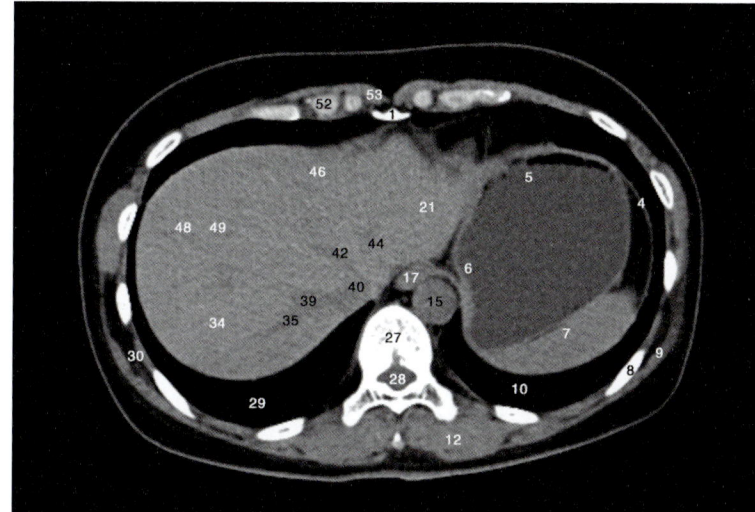

B. CT 平扫图像

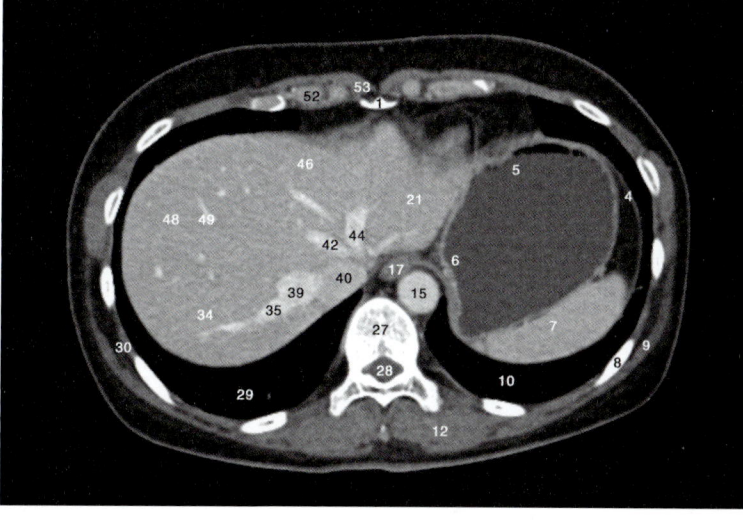

C. CT 增强图像

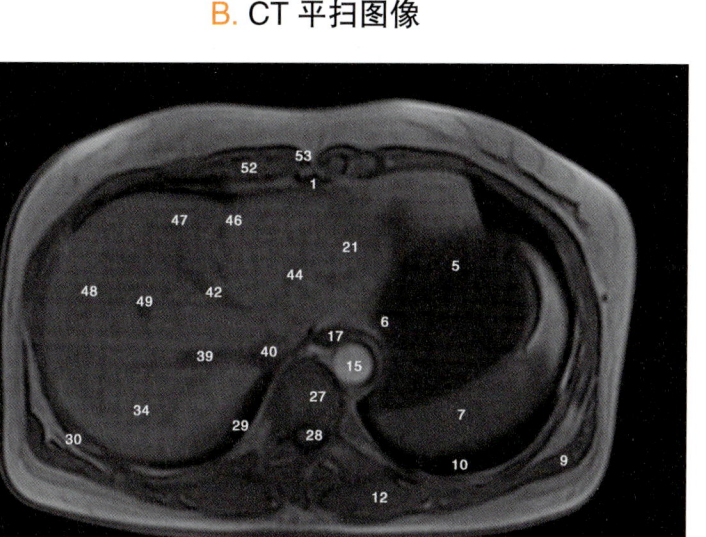

D. MR T1WI

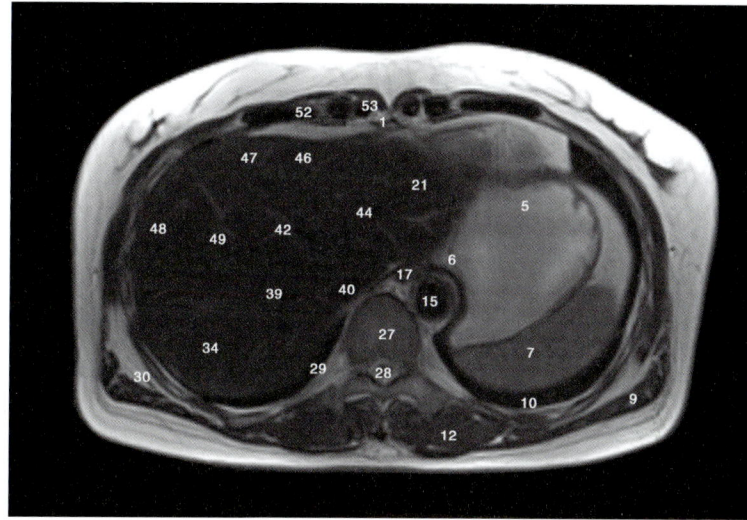

E. MR T2WI

关键结构：肝尾状叶，副肝静脉，肝左叶间静脉。

此断面经第 10 胸椎椎体下份。

肋膈隐窝出现于胸壁上的肋胸膜与膈胸膜之间。肝脏占据腹腔的右前方，呈楔形，下腔静脉左前方可见肝尾状叶，且向左突入网膜囊上隐窝。尾状叶居背裂后方，左界为静脉韧带裂。下方断面上可见此叶的左前角向前下方呈圆形突起，称乳头突，右前角向右延伸形成与右叶实质相连的隆起，称尾状突，此突介于胆囊窝与腔静脉沟之间。肝的血液回流除了三大肝静脉外，尚有数支直接汇入下腔静脉的细小肝静脉，统称为副肝静脉或肝短静脉，其数目较多，形态和分布变异较大。如本例中，此断面及 FH.11190 断面均显示有较清晰的副肝静脉，分别引流了肝尾状叶及肝右后叶的静脉血。有研究显示副肝静脉有 3~32 支，其内径为 0.10~3.43 cm，内径 > 0.5 cm 的静脉占 9.6%~40.7%，内径 > 1.0 cm 的静脉占 2.6%~25.4%。副肝静脉在布加综合征三大主肝静脉阻塞时起到代偿作用[11,12]。左叶间静脉是肝左静脉的属支，位于左叶间裂内，肝门静脉左支矢状部的前方，可作为左内叶和左外叶分界的标志，出现率为 85.4%，一般较细小[7]。

33

腹部连续横断层 17（FH.11590）

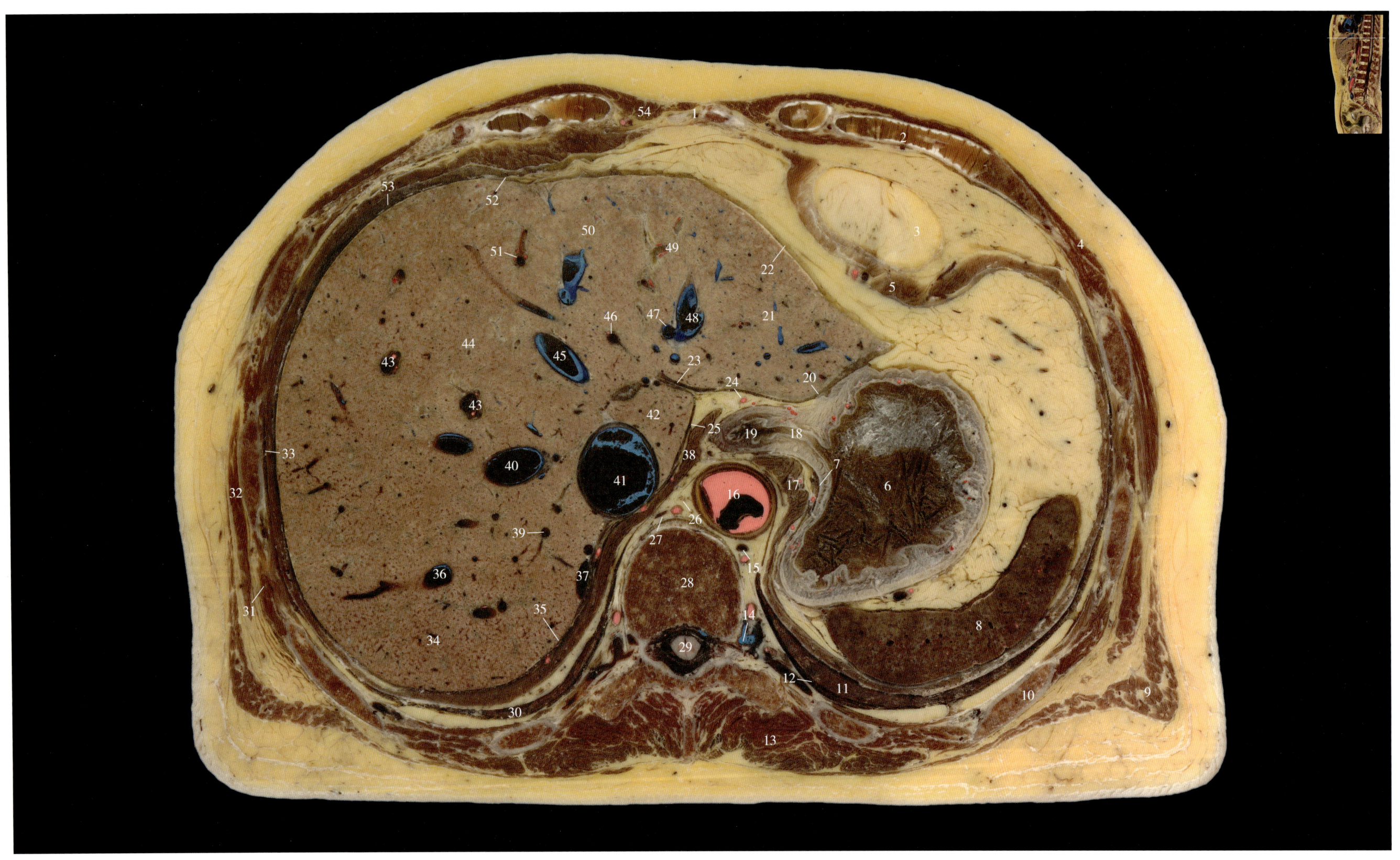

A. 断层标本图像

1. 剑突 xiphoid process
2. 第5肋软骨 5th costal cartilage
3. 心包脂肪垫 pericardial fat pad
4. 腹外斜肌 obliquus externus abdominis
5. 膈 diaphragm
6. 胃底 fundus of stomach
7. 胃裸区 bara area of stomach
8. 脾 spleen
9. 背阔肌 latissimus dorsi
10. 第9肋骨 9th costal bone
11. 左肺下叶 inferior lobe of left lung
12. 胸膜腔 pleural cavity
13. 竖脊肌 erector spinae
14. 椎外静脉丛 external vertebral venous plexus
15. 半奇静脉 hemiazygos vein
16. 胸主动脉 thoracic aorta
17. 左膈脚 left crus of diaphragm
18. 胃贲门 cardia of stomach
19. 食管腹部 abdominal part of esophagus
20. 左肝下前间隙 anterior left subrahepatic space
21. 肝左外叶上段 superior segment of left lateral lobe of liver
22. 左肝上前间隙 anterior left suprahepatic space
23. 静脉韧带裂和肝胃韧带 fissure for ligamentum venosum and hepatogastric ligament
24. 胃左动脉 left gastric artery
25. 网膜囊上隐窝 superior omental recess
26. 胸导管 thoracic duct
27. 奇静脉 azygos vein
28. 第10胸椎椎体 body of 10th thoracic vertebra
29. 脊髓 spinal cord
30. 右肺下叶 inferior lobe of right lung
31. 肋间外肌 intercostale externi
32. 下后锯肌 serratus posterior inferior
33. 肋膈隐窝 costodiaphragmatic recess
34. 肝右后叶上段 superior segment of right posterior lobe of liver
35. 肝裸区 bare area of liver
36. 肝右后上缘静脉 right posterosuperior marginal vein of liver
37. 副肝静脉 accessory hepatic veins
38. 右膈脚 right crus of diaphragm
39. 肝门静脉右后上支 right posterosuperior branch of hepatic portal vein
40. 肝右静脉 right hepatic vein
41. 下腔静脉 inferior vena cava
42. 肝尾状叶 caudate lobe of liver
43. 肝门静脉右前上支 right anterosuperior branch of hepatic portal vein
44. 肝右前叶上段 superior segment of right anterior lobe of liver
45. 肝中静脉 middle hepatic vein
46. 肝门静脉左外下支 lateroinferior branch of hepatic portal vein
47. 左叶间静脉 left interlobar vein
48. 肝左静脉 left hepatic vein
49. 肝左外叶下段 inferior segment of left lateral lobe of liver
50. 肝左内叶 left medial lobe of liver
51. 肝门静脉左内支 left medial branch of hepatic portal vein
52. 肝镰状韧带 falciform ligament of liver
53. 右肝上间隙 right suprahepatic space
54. 腹直肌 rectus abdominis

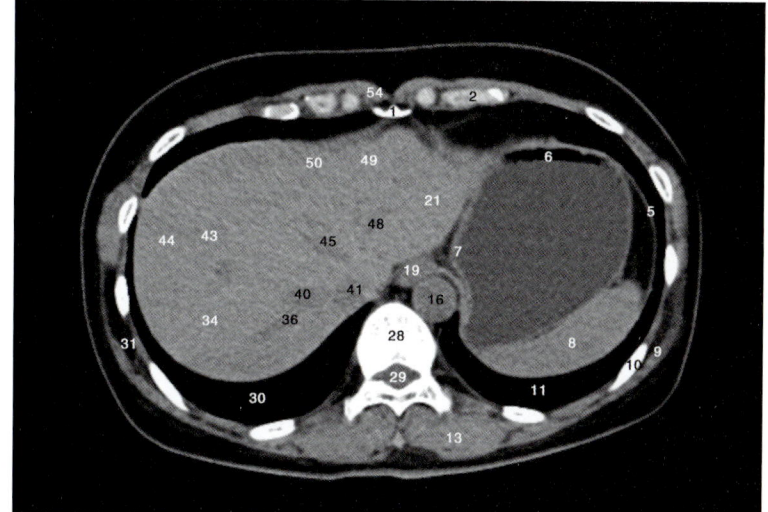

B. CT 平扫图像

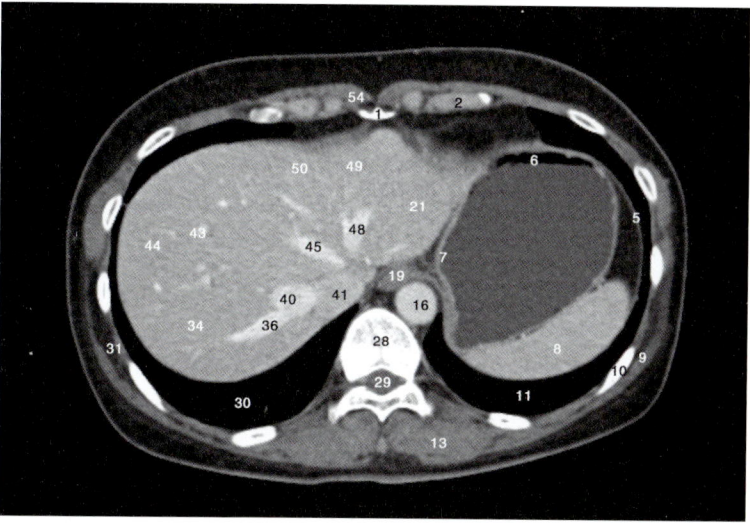

C. CT 增强图像

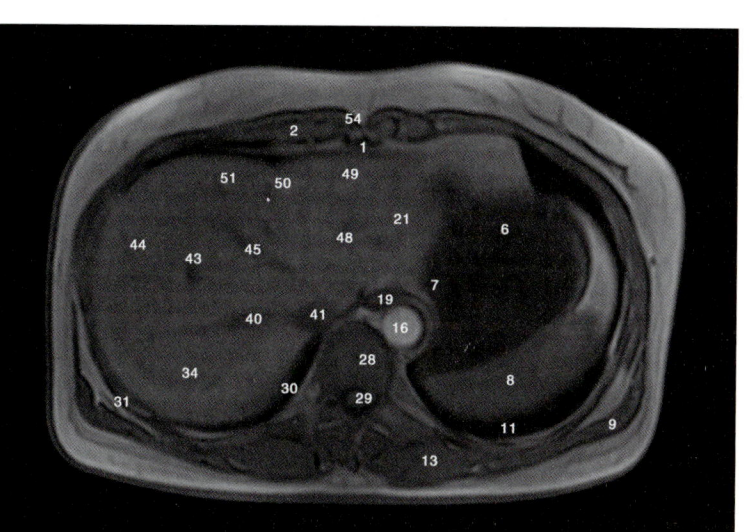

D. MR T1WI

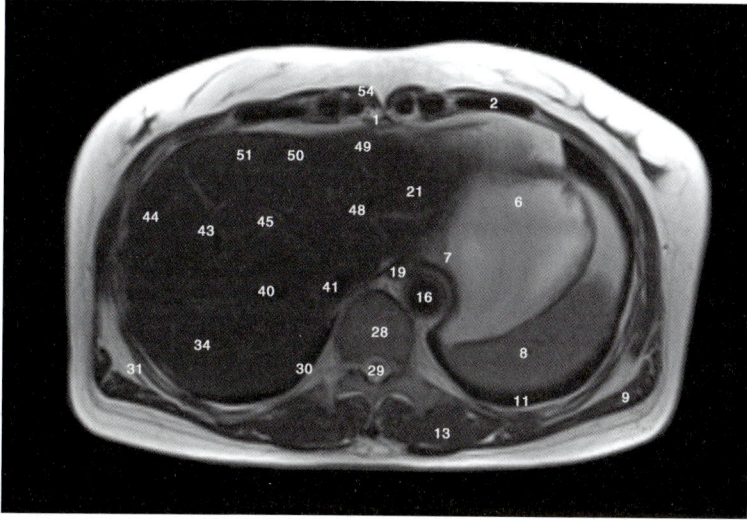

E. MR T2WI

关键结构：肝中静脉，副肝中静脉。

此断面经第10胸椎椎体下份。

肝中静脉位于肝正中裂内，由左、右2根合成。收纳左内叶和右前叶的静脉血，常与肝左静脉汇合共同注入下腔静脉。肝中静脉有如下特征：①管径和长度，内径为 0.71 cm ± 0.14 cm，另有文献报道为 0.57 cm ± 0.10 cm。肝中静脉注入处管径为 0.95 cm ± 0.38 cm，分叉处管径为 0.78 cm ± 0.22 cm。肝中静脉主干长为 5.10 cm ± 2.39 cm，左根长为 2.18 cm ± 0.89 cm，右根长为 2.76 cm ± 1.37 cm；②合成类型，左下支和右下支合成者占 83.6% ± 5.0%，单干型组成者占 16.4% ± 5.0%。另据文献报道肝中静脉由左、右2根合成者占 93.8%，3根汇合而成者占 3.1%，4根汇合而成者占 3.1%；③合成部位，在肝门静脉分叉处下方合成者占 71.7% ± 6.6%；平肝门静脉分叉处者占 17.4% ± 5.6%；在肝门静脉分叉处上方者占 10.9% ± 4.6%；④与下腔静脉的夹角为 73.75° ± 19.72°；⑤属支，肝中静脉右上支的出现率为 90.9% ± 3.9%，副肝中静脉（直接注入下腔静脉的右上支）的出现率为 1.82% ± 1.89%[2]。如本例第12层（FH.11690）对应的CT和MR图像中，就有一较粗大的副肝中静脉。

腹部连续横断层 18（FH.11570）

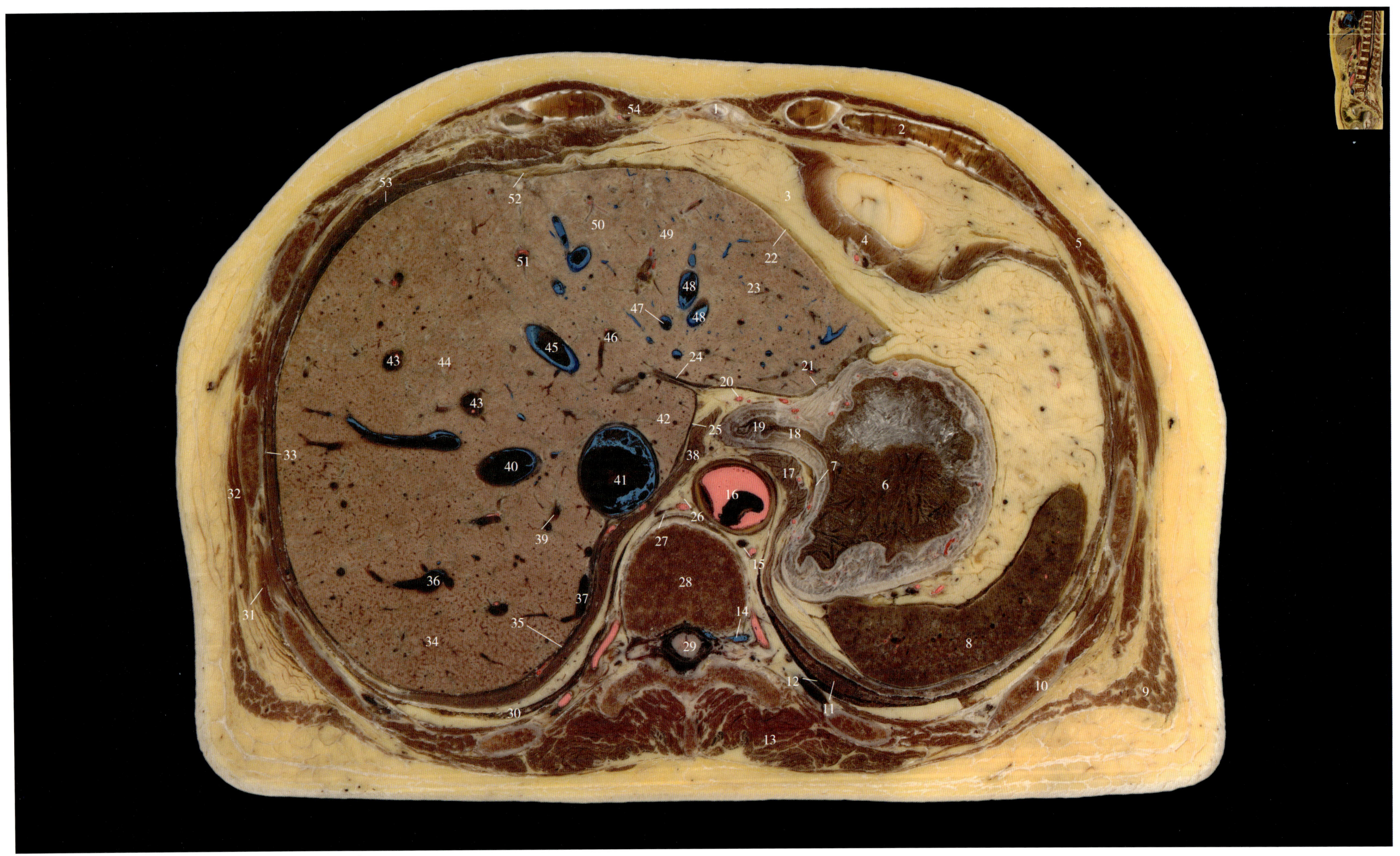

A. 断层标本图像

1. 剑突 xiphoid process
2. 第5肋软骨 5th costal cartilage
3. 大网膜 greater omentum
4. 膈 diaphragm
5. 腹外斜肌 obliquus externus abdominis
6. 胃底 fundus of stomach
7. 胃裸区 bara area of stomach
8. 脾 spleen
9. 背阔肌 latissimus dorsi
10. 第9肋骨 9th costal bone
11. 左肺下叶 inferior lobe of left lung
12. 胸膜腔 pleural cavity
13. 竖脊肌 erector spinae
14. 椎外静脉丛 external vertebral venous plexus
15. 半奇静脉 hemiazygos vein
16. 胸主动脉 thoracic aorta
17. 左膈脚 left crus of diaphragm
18. 胃贲门 cardia of stomach
19. 食管腹部 abdominal part of esophagus
20. 胃左动脉 left gastric artery
21. 左肝下前间隙 anterior left subrahepatic space
22. 左肝上前间隙 anterior left suprahepatic space
23. 肝左外叶上段 superior segment of left lateral lobe of liver
24. 静脉韧带裂和肝胃韧带 fissure for ligamentum venosum and hepatogastric ligament
25. 网膜囊上隐窝 superior omental recess
26. 胸导管 thoracic duct
27. 奇静脉 azygos vein
28. 第10胸椎椎体 body of 10th thoracic vertebra
29. 脊髓 spinal cord
30. 右肺下叶 inferior lobe of right lung
31. 肋间外肌 intercostale externi
32. 下后锯肌 serratus posterior inferior
33. 肋膈隐窝 costodiaphragmatic recess
34. 肝右后叶上段 superior segment of right posterior lobe of liver
35. 肝裸区 bare area of liver
36. 肝右后上缘静脉 right posterosuperior marginal vein of liver
37. 副肝静脉 accessory hepatic veins
38. 右膈脚 right crus of diaphragm
39. 肝门静脉右后上支 right posterosuperior branch of hepatic portal vein
40. 肝右静脉 right hepatic vein
41. 下腔静脉 inferior vena cava
42. 肝尾状叶 caudate lobe of liver
43. 肝门静脉右前上支 right anterosuperior branch of hepatic portal vein
44. 肝右前叶上段 superior segment of right anterior lobe of liver
45. 肝中静脉 middle hepatic vein
46. 肝门静脉左外下支 left lateroinferior branch of hepatic portal vein
47. 左叶间静脉 left interlobar vein
48. 肝左静脉 left hepatic vein
49. 肝左外叶下段 inferior segment of left lateral lobe of liver
50. 肝左内叶 left medial lobe of liver
51. 肝门静脉左内支 left medial branch of hepatic portal vein
52. 肝镰状韧带 falciform ligament of liver
53. 右肝上间隙 right suprahepatic space
54. 腹直肌 rectus abdominis

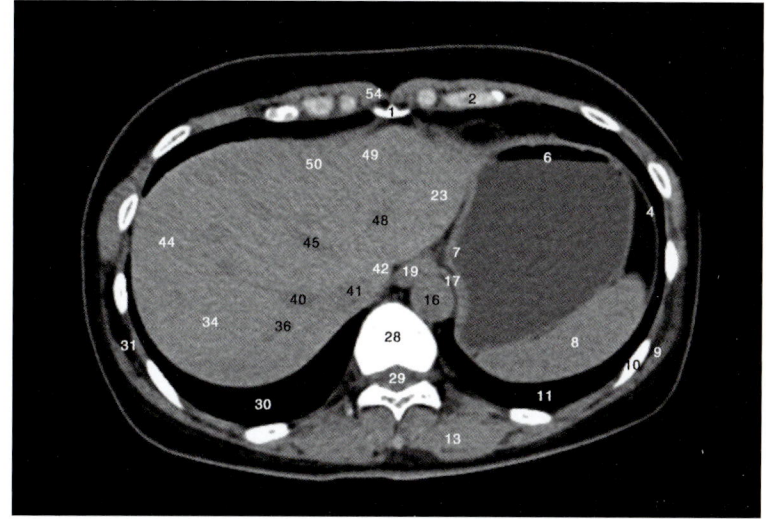

B. CT 平扫图像

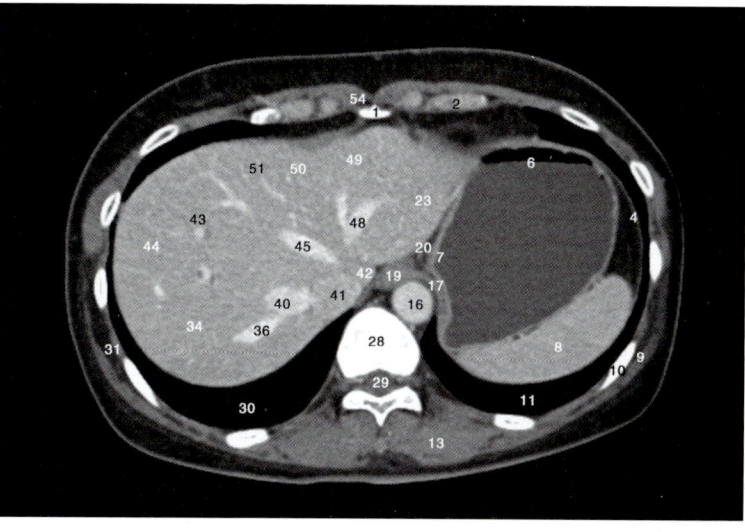

C. CT 增强图像

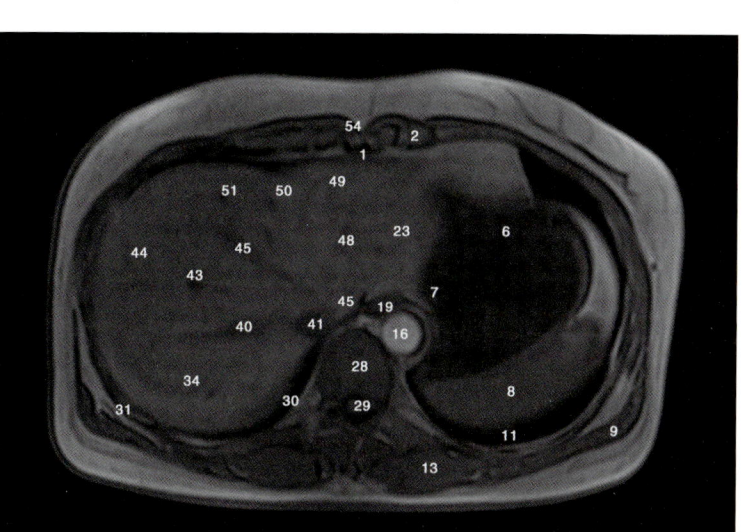

D. MR T1WI

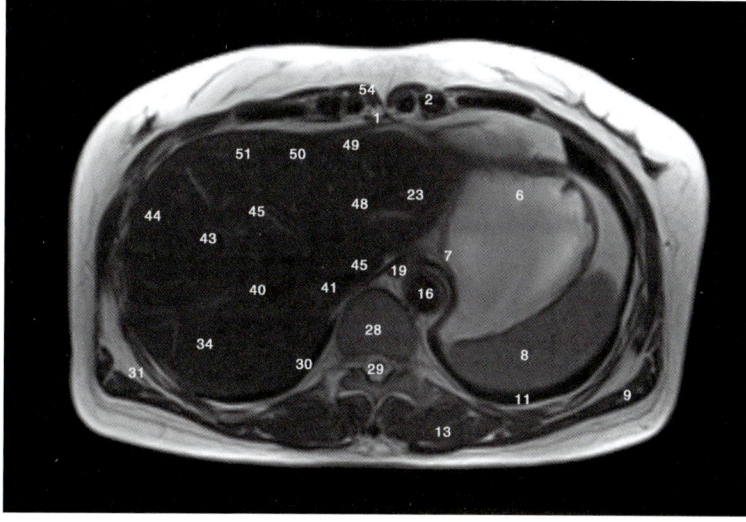

E. MR T2WI

关键结构：肝镰状韧带，肝静脉。

此断面经第10胸椎椎体下份。

肝脏断面逐渐增大，占据腹腔右前方，切及肝右后上段、右前上段、左内叶、左外下段和尾状叶。白线位于腹前壁正中线上，是由两侧腹直肌鞘的纤维彼此交织形成的腱性结构，上自剑突，下至耻骨联合。白线上宽下窄，坚韧而缺少血管，约在中点处有疏松的瘢痕组织区即脐环，为脐带附着处[13]。白线呈褐白色，孕妇颜色会变深，但不同于妊娠纹。妊娠纹一般呈紫红色，形似西瓜纹，产后妊娠纹会逐渐减退甚至消失，而腹白线从出生就存在。另外，部分过度肥胖者腹部皮肤纤维断裂，在突然消瘦后腹部也会出现白纹。镰状韧带位于肝的前面与腹白线后方之间，其肝附着点多数位于正中矢状面右侧，将肝连于腹前壁，其左侧1cm处与下腔静脉左前壁的连线可作为左叶间裂的标志。镰状韧带起源于胚胎时期胃背系膜腹侧部，为双层结构，起自正中线上的腹前壁后面与膈的下表面，向后连于肝的前面与上面，其行程略偏右。

腹部连续横断层 19（FH.11550）

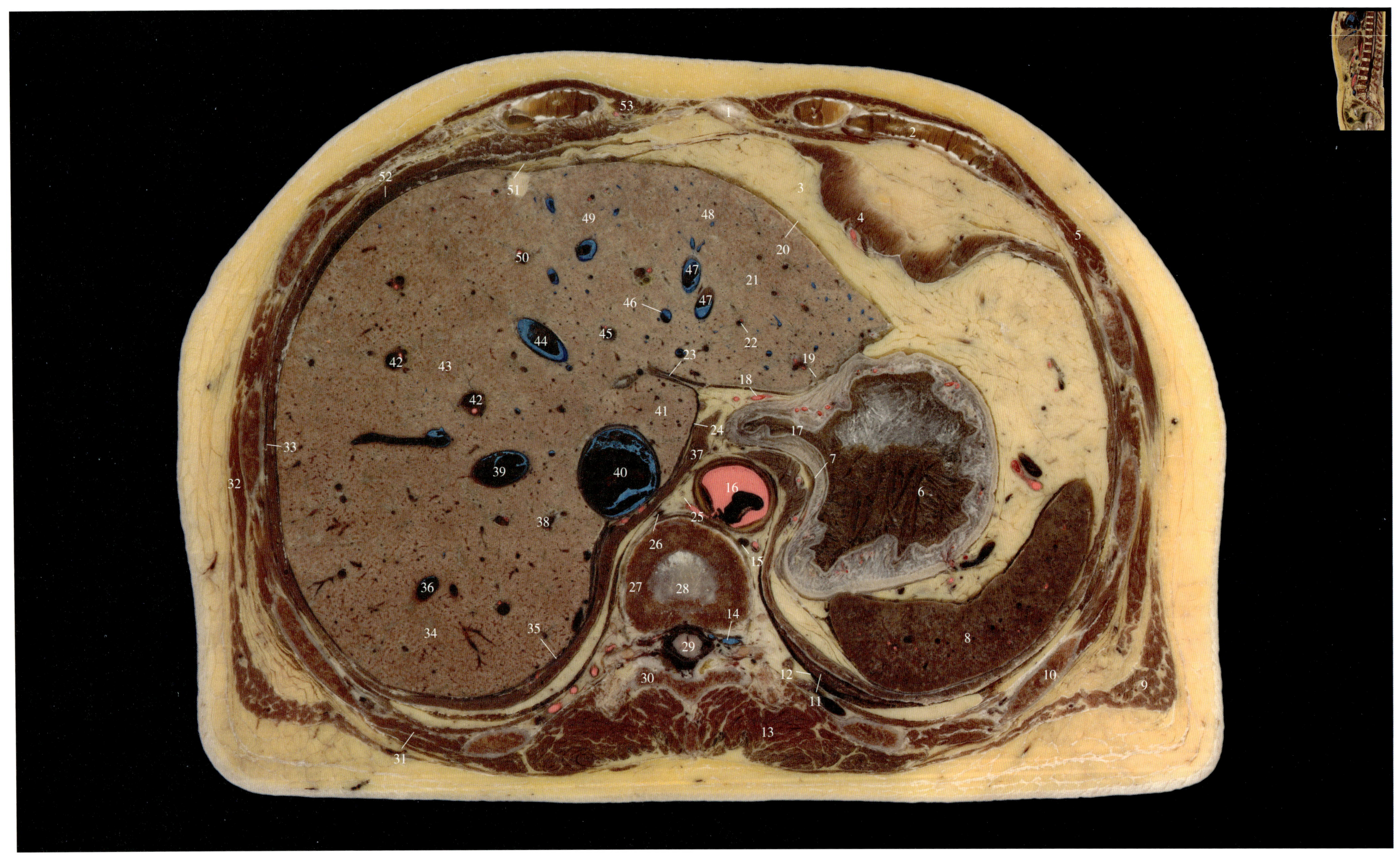

A. 断层标本图像

1. 剑突 xiphoid process
2. 第5肋软骨 5th costal cartilage
3. 大网膜 greater omentum
4. 膈 diaphragm
5. 腹外斜肌 obliquus externus abdominis
6. 胃 stomach
7. 胃裸区 bara area of stomach
8. 脾 spleen
9. 背阔肌 latissimus dorsi
10. 第9肋骨 9th costal bone
11. 左肺下叶 inferior lobe of left lung
12. 胸膜腔 pleural cavity
13. 竖脊肌 erector spinae
14. 椎外静脉丛 external vertebral venous plexus
15. 半奇静脉 hemiazygos vein
16. 胸主动脉 thoracic aorta
17. 胃贲门 cardia of stomach
18. 胃左动脉 left gastric artery
19. 左肝下前间隙 anterior left subhepatic space
20. 左肝上前间隙 anterior left suprahepatic space
21. 肝左外叶上段 superior segment of left lateral lobe of liver
22. 肝门静脉左外上支 left laterosuperior branch of hepatic portal vein
23. 静脉韧带裂和肝胃韧带 fissure for ligamentum venosum and hepatogastric ligament
24. 网膜囊上隐窝 superior omental recess
25. 胸导管 thoracic duct
26. 奇静脉 azygos vein
27. 第10胸椎椎体 body of 10th thoracic vertebra
28. T10-11椎间盘 T10-11 intervertebral disc
29. 脊髓 spinal cord
30. 第10胸椎横突 transverse process of 10th thoracic vertebra
31. 肋间外肌 intercostale externi
32. 下后锯肌 serratus posterior inferior
33. 肋膈隐窝 costodiaphragmatic recess
34. 肝右后叶上段 superior segment of right posterior lobe of liver
35. 肝裸区 bare area of liver
36. 肝右后上缘静脉 right posterosuperior marginal vein of liver
37. 右膈脚 right crus of diaphragm
38. 肝门静脉右后上支 right posterosuperior branch of hepatic portal vein
39. 肝右静脉 right hepatic vein
40. 下腔静脉 inferior vena cava
41. 肝尾状叶 caudate lobe of liver
42. 肝门静脉右前上支 right anterosuperior branch of hepatic portal vein
43. 肝右前叶上段 superior segment of right anterior lobe of liver
44. 肝中静脉 middle hepatic vein
45. 肝门静脉左外下支 left lateroinferior branch of hepatic portal vein
46. 左叶间静脉 left interlobar vein
47. 肝左静脉 left hepatic vein
48. 肝左外叶下段 inferior segment of left lateral lobe of liver
49. 肝左内叶 left medial lobe of liver
50. 肝门静脉左内支 left medial branch of hepatic portal vein
51. 肝镰状韧带 falciform ligament of liver
52. 右肝上间隙 right suprahepatic space
53. 腹直肌 rectus abdominis

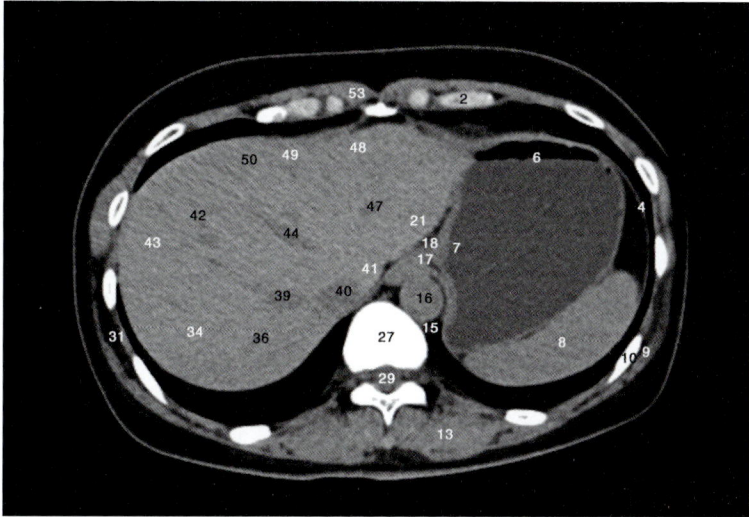

B. CT平扫图像

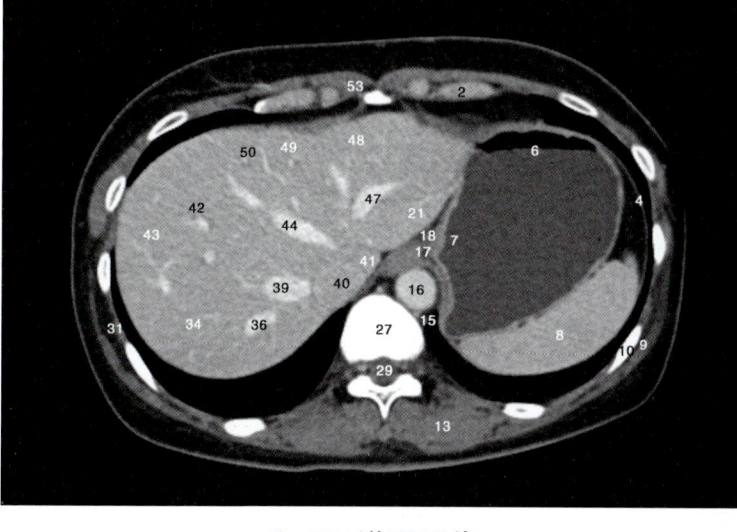

C. CT增强图像

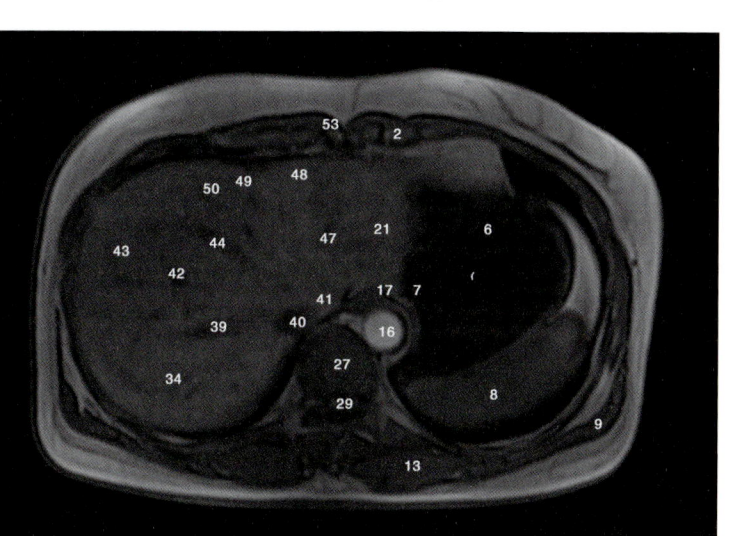

D. MR T1WI

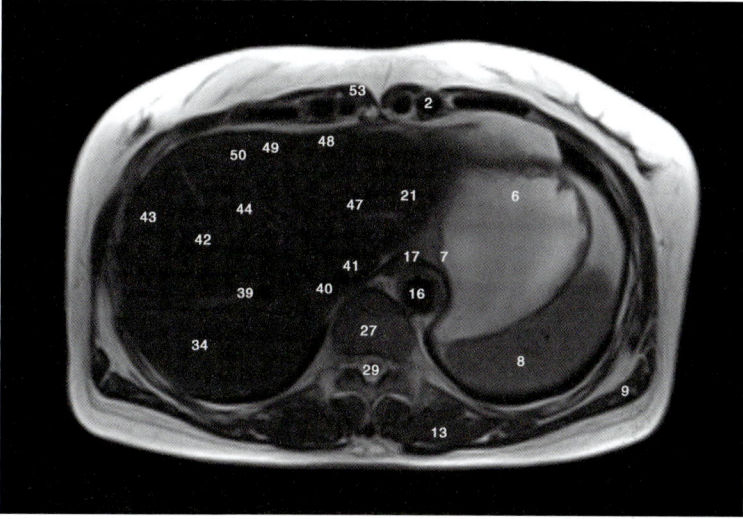

E. MR T2WI

关键结构：胃贲门，剑突。

此断面经第10胸椎椎体下份及T10-11椎间盘。

贲门位于胸主动脉和肝左叶之间，是胃的入口，新生儿贲门相对较大，括约肌不发达，是婴儿易于溢乳的主要原因。贲门癌为发生于贲门的上皮类恶性肿瘤，2000年WHO将其称为胃食管交界部（gastroesophageal junction，GEJ）癌。2018年，在美国癌症联合会（American Joint Committee on Cancer，AJCC）和国际抗癌联盟（Union for International Cancer Control，UICC）联合发布的第8版胃癌和食管癌/胃食管交界部癌TNM分期对该区域的肿瘤分期标准做出了明确的定义：对于GEJ癌，若肿瘤侵及GEJ且肿瘤中心位于胃食管交界线以下≤2 cm的范围内，采用食管癌分期标准；若累及GEJ但肿瘤中心位于胃食管交界线以下2 cm以外的，以及未累及胃食管交界线的所有胃内肿瘤，采用胃癌分期标准。因此，准确判断胃食管交界线的位置及其是否受到肿瘤侵犯对于评估这一区域肿瘤至关重要。值得注意的是，该版分期所采用的数据中国人群的占比很小，可能会产生一定的偏倚，还需要通过国内大样本研究验证和完善[14]。幽门螺杆菌感染与该区域的肿瘤发生有密切关系，饮酒和吸烟也是其重要因素。剑突是位于胸骨下端的薄骨片，幼年时为软骨，老年后完全骨化。

腹部连续横断层 20（FH.11530）

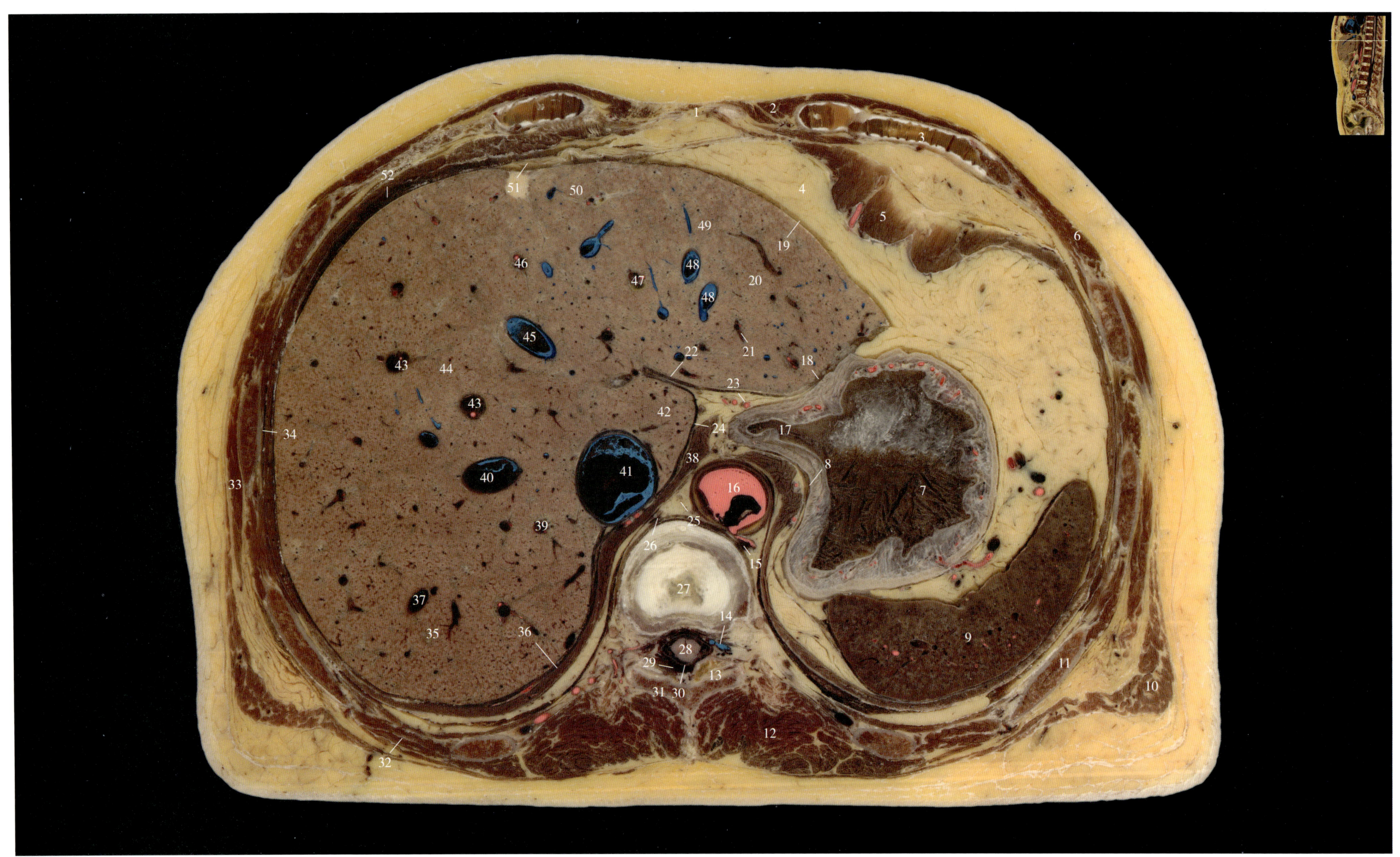

A. 断层标本图像

1. 腹白线 linea alba
2. 腹直肌 rectus abdominis
3. 第5肋软骨 5th costal cartilage
4. 大网膜 greater omentum
5. 膈 diaphragm
6. 腹外斜肌 obliquus externus abdominis
7. 胃 stomach
8. 胃裸区 bara area of stomach
9. 脾 spleen
10. 背阔肌 latissimus dorsi
11. 第9肋骨 9th costal bone
12. 竖脊肌 erector spinae
13. 关节突关节 zygophysial joints
14. 椎内静脉丛 internal vertebral venous plexus
15. 半奇静脉 hemiazygos vein
16. 胸主动脉 thoracic aorta
17. 胃贲门 cardia of stomach
18. 左肝下前间隙 anterior left subrahepatic space
19. 左肝上前间隙 anterior left suprahepatic space
20. 肝左外叶上段 superior segment of left lateral lobe of liver
21. 肝门静脉左外上支 left laterosuperior branch of hepatic portal vein
22. 静脉韧带裂和肝胃韧带 fissure for ligamentum venosum and hepatogastric ligament
23. 胃左动脉 left gastric artery
24. 网膜囊上隐窝 superior omental recess
25. 胸导管 thoracic duct
26. 奇静脉 azygos vein
27. T10-11椎间盘 T10-11 intervertebral disc
28. 脊髓 spinal cord
29. 硬膜外隙 epidural space
30. 硬脊膜 spinal dura matter
31. 第10胸椎横突 transverse process of 10th thoracic vertebra
32. 肋间外肌 intercostale externi
33. 下后锯肌 serratus posterior inferior
34. 肋膈隐窝 costodiaphragmatic recess
35. 肝右后叶上段 superior segment of right posterior lobe of liver
36. 肝裸区 bare area of liver
37. 肝右后上缘静脉 right posterosuperior marginal vein of liver
38. 右膈脚 right crus of diaphragm
39. 肝门静脉右后上支 right posterosuperior branch of hepatic portal vein
40. 肝右静脉 right hepatic vein
41. 下腔静脉 inferior vena cava
42. 肝尾状叶 caudate lobe of liver
43. 肝门静脉右前上支 right anterosuperior branch of hepatic portal vein
44. 肝右前叶上段 superior segment of right anterior lobe of liver
45. 肝中静脉 middle hepatic vein
46. 肝门静脉左内支 left medial branch of hepatic portal vein
47. 肝门静脉左外下支 left lateroinferior branch of hepatic portal vein
48. 肝左静脉 left hepatic vein
49. 肝左外叶下段 inferior segment of left lateral lobe of liver
50. 肝左内叶 left medial lobe of liver
51. 肝镰状韧带 falciform ligament of liver
52. 右肝上间隙 right suprahepatic space

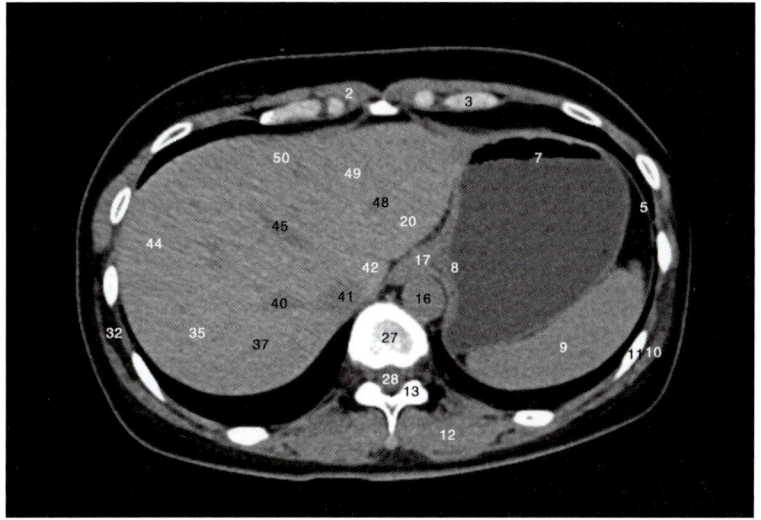

B. CT 平扫图像

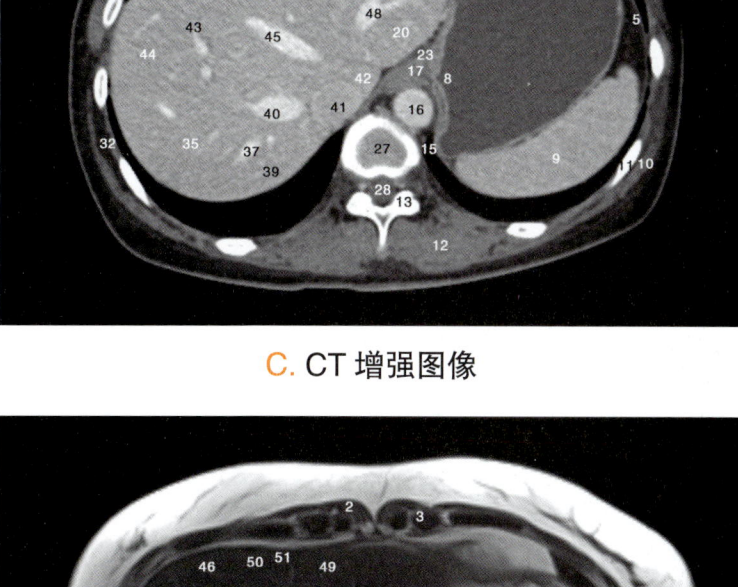

C. CT 增强图像

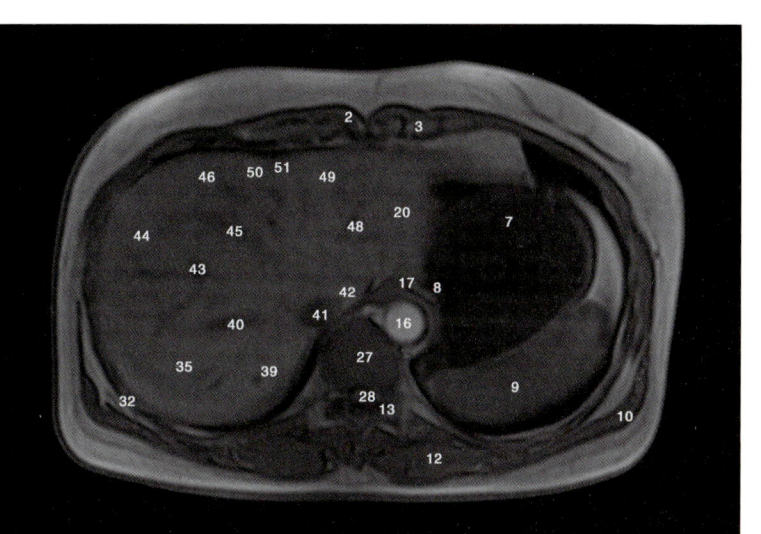

D. MR T1WI

E. MR T2WI

关键结构：静脉韧带裂，肝胃韧带，网膜囊上隐窝。

此断面经 T10-11 椎间盘。

肝尾状叶与左外叶之间为静脉韧带裂。小网膜的肝胃韧带部分起始于其右端，并分其为前、后两部。静脉韧带裂前部向左通胃肝隐窝，二者合称左肝下前间隙。肝尾状叶左侧与胃之间为小网膜。小网膜是连于膈、肝静脉韧带裂和肝门与胃小弯和十二指肠上部之间的双层腹膜，其左侧部从肝门连于胃小弯，称肝胃韧带，右侧部从肝门连至十二指肠上部，称肝十二指肠韧带。肝韧带内含有胃左动、静脉，淋巴结和脂肪组织，有时迷走肝左动脉亦居其中。网膜囊前壁自上而下依次为小网膜两层腹膜的后层、覆盖胃后壁及十二指肠起始2 cm段后面的腹膜和胃结肠韧带的后层腹膜或大网膜的第二层腹膜；网膜囊后壁由下而上依次是大网膜后两层腹膜的前层、横结肠、横结肠系膜的上层及覆于胰、左肾及左肾上腺前面的腹膜壁层；上壁为肝尾状叶和膈下面的腹膜；下壁为大网膜二、三层的愈着部；左界为脾及胃脾韧带和脾肾韧带。网膜囊按部位可分为网膜囊前庭及数个隐窝，自网膜孔进入网膜囊即为网膜囊前庭，自前庭向上移行于肝尾状叶和膈腰部之间称为网膜囊上隐窝[2]。静脉韧带裂后部为网膜囊上隐窝的一部分，此隐窝呈">"形间隙围绕肝尾状叶。CT可显示91%的肝胃韧带，略呈三角形或半月形，其内的结构一般为4~6 mm，若>6 mm，可能是变异结构，如胰体、横结肠、迂曲的脾动脉或腹腔干，亦可能是上腹部疾病引起的腹腔淋巴结或胃左淋巴结肿大、淋巴瘤或胃左静脉曲张[1]。

腹部连续横断层 21（FH.11510）

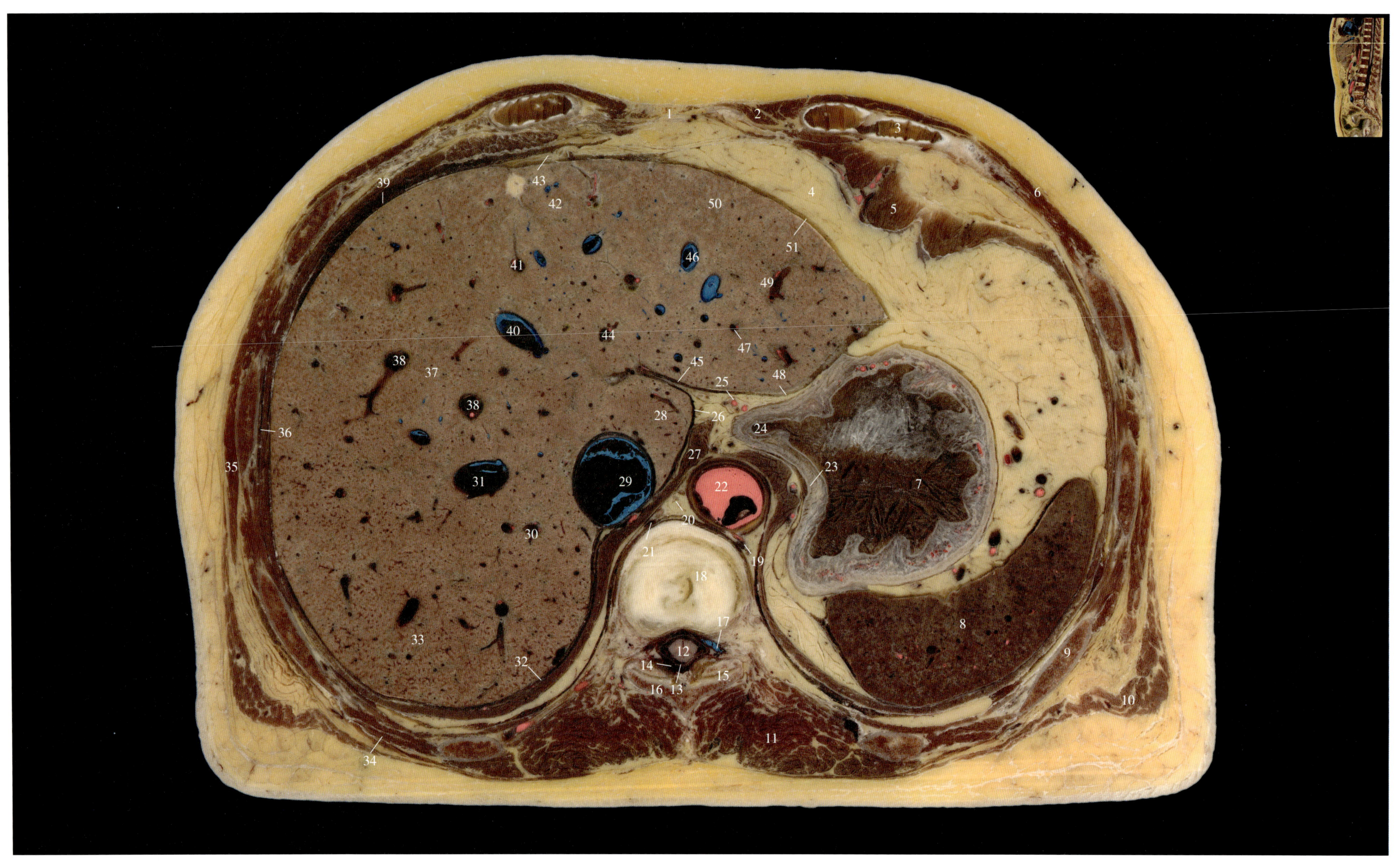

A. 断层标本图像

1. 腹白线 linea alba
2. 腹直肌 rectus abdominis
3. 第 5 肋软骨 5th costal cartilage
4. 大网膜 greater omentum
5. 膈 diaphragm
6. 腹外斜肌 obliquus externus abdominis
7. 胃 stomach
8. 脾 spleen
9. 第 9 肋骨 9th costal bone
10. 背阔肌 latissimus dorsi
11. 竖脊肌 erector spinae
12. 脊髓 spinal cord
13. 硬脊膜 spinal dura matter
14. 硬膜外隙 epidural space
15. 关节突关节 zygapophysial joints
16. 第 10 胸椎横突 transverse process of 10th thoracic vertebra
17. 椎内静脉丛 internal vertebral venous plexus
18. T10-11 椎间盘 T10-11 intervertebral disc
19. 半奇静脉 hemiazygos vein
20. 胸导管 thoracic duct
21. 奇静脉 azygos vein
22. 胸主动脉 thoracic aorta
23. 胃裸区 bara area of stomach
24. 胃贲门 cardia of stomach
25. 胃左动脉 left gastric artery
26. 网膜囊上隐窝 superior omental recess
27. 右膈脚 right crus of diaphragm
28. 肝尾状叶 caudate lobe of liver
29. 下腔静脉 inferior vena cava
30. 肝门静脉右后上支 right posterosuperior branch of hepatic portal vein
31. 肝右静脉 right hepatic vein
32. 肝裸区 bare area of liver
33. 肝右后叶上段 superior segment of right posterior lobe of liver
34. 肋间外肌 intercostale externi
35. 下后锯肌 serratus posterior inferior
36. 肋膈隐窝 costodiaphragmatic recess
37. 肝右前叶上段 superior segment of right anterior lobe of liver
38. 肝门静脉右前上支 right anterosuperior branch of hepatic portal vein
39. 右肝上间隙 right suprahepatic space
40. 肝中静脉 middle hepatic vein
41. 肝门静脉左内支 left medial branch of hepatic portal vein
42. 肝左内叶 left medial lobe of liver
43. 肝镰状韧带 falciform ligament of liver
44. 肝门静脉左外下支 left lateroinferior branch of hepatic portal vein
45. 静脉韧带裂和肝胃韧带 fissure for ligamentum venosum and hepatogastric ligament
46. 肝左静脉 left hepatic vein
47. 肝门静脉左外上支 left laterosuperior branch of hepatic portal vein
48. 左肝下前间隙 anterior left subrahepatic space
49. 肝左外叶上段 superior segment of left lateral lobe of liver
50. 肝左外叶下段 inferior segment of left lateral lobe of liver
51. 左肝上前间隙 anterior left suprahepatic space

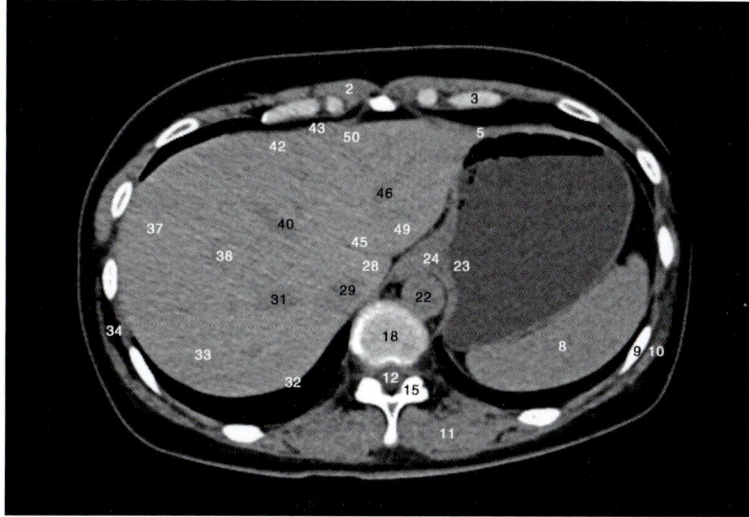

B. CT 平扫图像

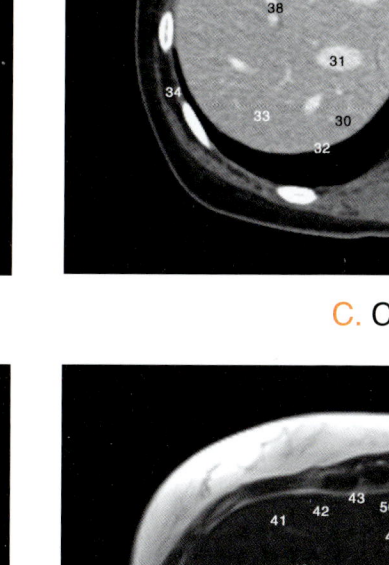

C. CT 增强图像

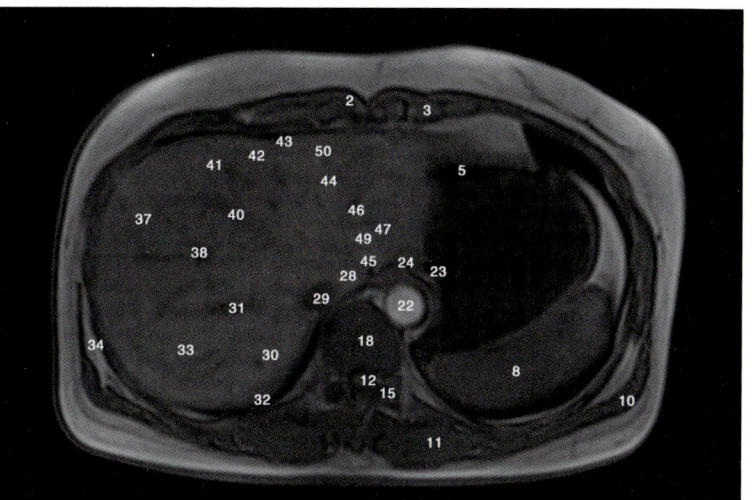

D. MR T1WI

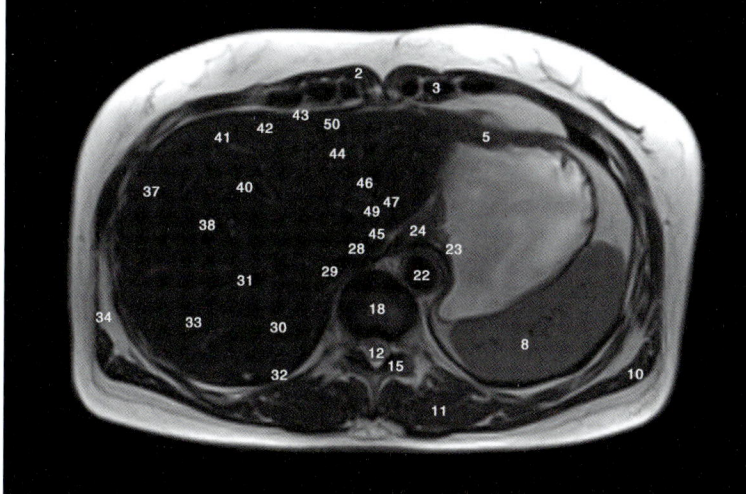

E. MR T2WI

关键结构：左、右膈脚，胸导管。

此断面经 T10-11 椎间盘。

胸腔内肺已完全消失，仅剩下肋膈隐窝。膈脚以肌腱起始，其纤维与脊柱前纵韧带融合，右膈脚较左膈脚宽而长，起于上 3 节腰椎椎体及椎间盘的前外侧面。左膈脚起于上 2 个腰椎的相应部位。左、右膈脚内侧缘于腰椎间盘水平在中线汇合，在主动脉前方形成一跨越主动脉的纤维弓，即正中弓状韧带。在 CT 或 MR 图像上，有时可通过观察膈脚移位征来鉴别脊柱附近的胸腹水；当胸腔积液积聚在膈脚与脊柱间，可使膈脚向前外侧移位；当腹水积聚在膈脚的前外侧，可将膈脚推向后内侧。脊柱区显示 T10-11 椎间盘，左、右膈脚后方和椎体前方之间为膈后间隙，内可见奇静脉、半奇静脉和胸导管。胸导管是全身最粗大的淋巴管，全长 30~40 cm，通常在第 12 胸椎下缘高度起自膨大的乳糜池，沿脊柱前面上行，经胸腔至颈根部左侧，注入左静脉角。

腹部连续横断层 22（FH.11490）

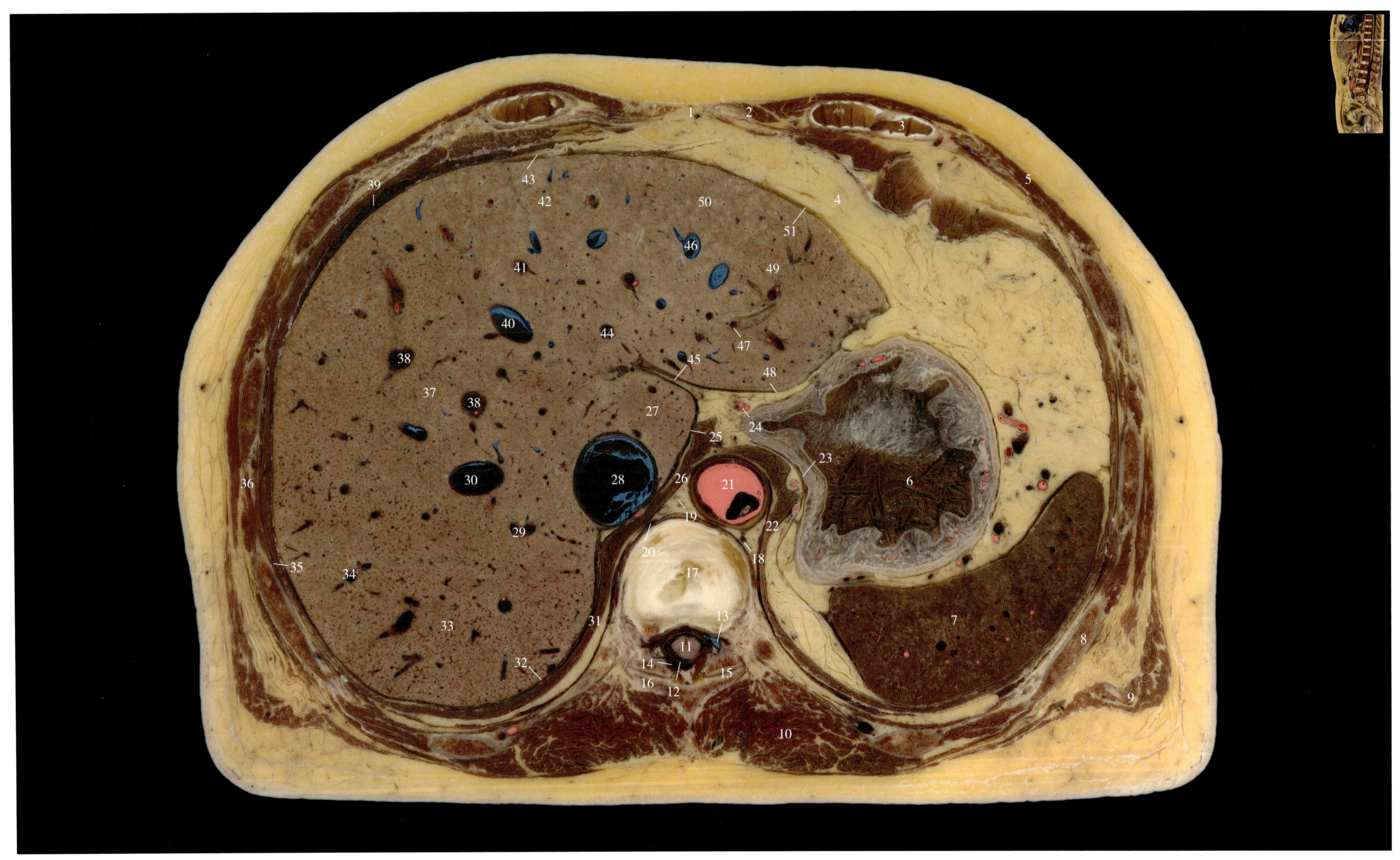

A. 断层标本图像

1. 腹白线 linea alba
2. 腹直肌 rectus abdominis
3. 第5肋软骨 5th costal cartilage
4. 大网膜 greater omentum
5. 腹外斜肌 obliquus externus abdominis
6. 胃 stomach
7. 脾 spleen
8. 第9肋骨 9th costal bone
9. 背阔肌 latissimus dorsi
10. 竖脊肌 erector spinae
11. 脊髓 spinal cord
12. 硬脊膜 spinal dura matter
13. 椎内静脉丛 internal vertebral venous plexus
14. 硬膜外隙 epidural space
15. 关节突关节 zygapophysial joints
16. 第10胸椎横突 transverse process of 10th thoracic vertebra
17. T10-11 椎间盘 T10-11 intervertebral disc
18. 半奇静脉 hemiazygos vein
19. 胸导管 thoracic duct
20. 奇静脉 azygos vein
21. 胸主动脉 thoracic aorta
22. 左膈脚 left crus of diaphragm
23. 胃裸区 bara area of stomach
24. 胃左动脉 left gastric artery
25. 网膜囊上隐窝 superior omental recess
26. 右膈脚 right crus of diaphragm
27. 肝尾状叶 caudate lobe of liver
28. 下腔静脉 inferior vena cava
29. 肝门静脉右后上支 right posterosuperior branch of hepatic portal vein
30. 肝右静脉 right hepatic vein
31. 膈 diaphragm
32. 肝裸区 bare area of liver
33. 肝右后叶上段 superior segment of right posterior lobe of liver
34. 肝门静脉右后上支及肝动脉 right posterosuperior branch of hepatic portal vein and corresponding hepatic artery
35. 肋膈隐窝 costodiaphragmatic recess
36. 肋间外肌 intercostale externi
37. 肝右前叶上段 superior segment of right anterior lobe of liver
38. 肝门静脉右前上支 right anterosuperior branch of hepatic portal vein
39. 右肝上间隙 right suprahepatic space
40. 肝中静脉 middle hepatic vein
41. 肝门静脉左内支 left medial branch of hepatic portal vein
42. 肝左内叶 left medial lobe of liver
43. 肝镰状韧带 falciform ligament of liver
44. 肝门静脉左外下支 left lateroinferior branch of hepatic portal vein
45. 静脉韧带裂和肝胃韧带 fissure for ligamentum venosum and hepatogastric ligament
46. 肝左静脉 left hepatic vein
47. 肝门静脉左外上支 left laterosuperior branch of hepatic portal vein
48. 左肝下前间隙 anterior left subrahepatic space
49. 肝左外叶上段 superior segment of left lateral lobe of liver
50. 肝左外叶下段 inferior segment of left lateral lobe of liver
51. 左肝上前间隙 anterior left suprahepatic space

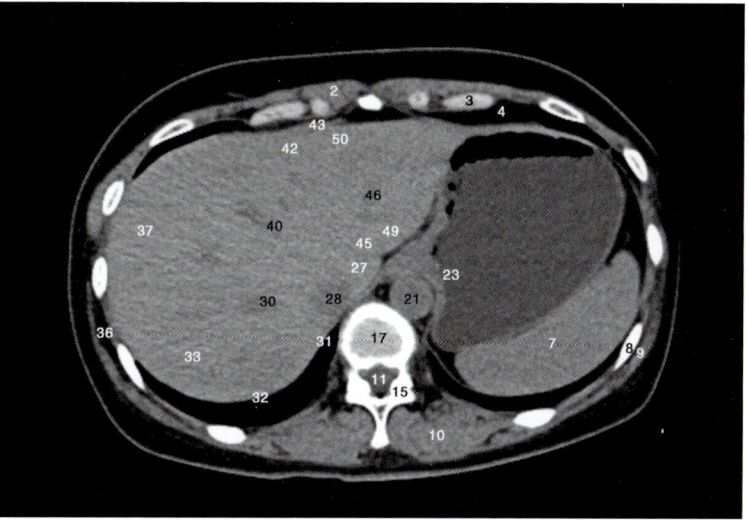

B. CT 平扫图像

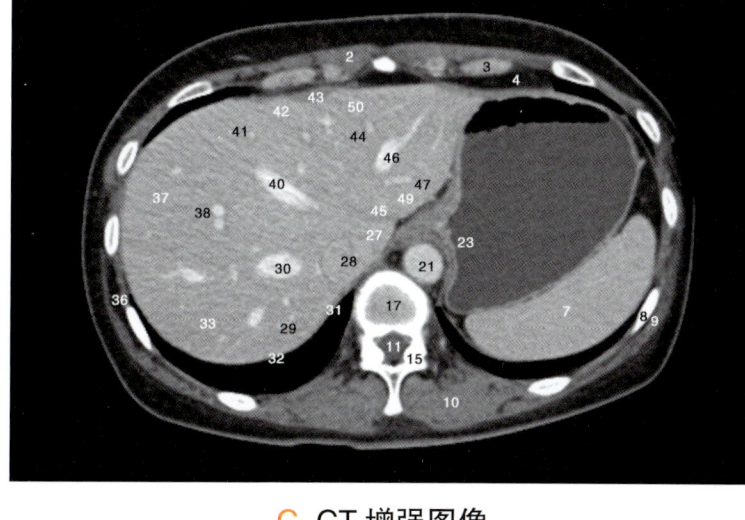

C. CT 增强图像

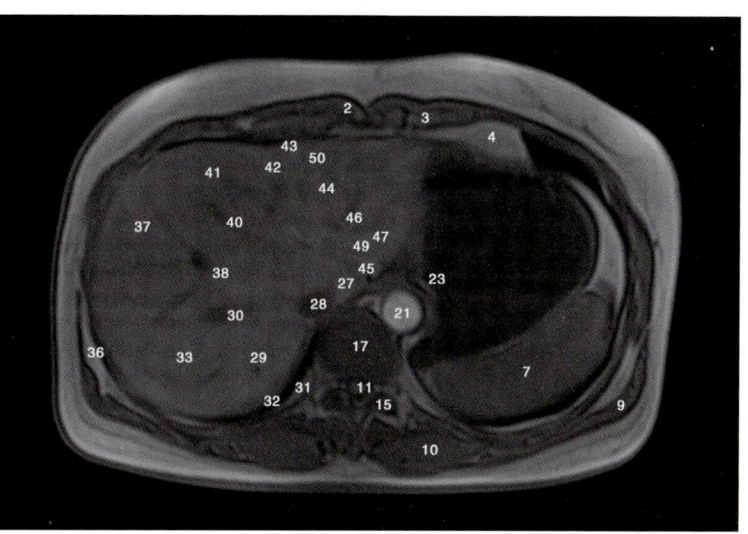

D. MR T1WI

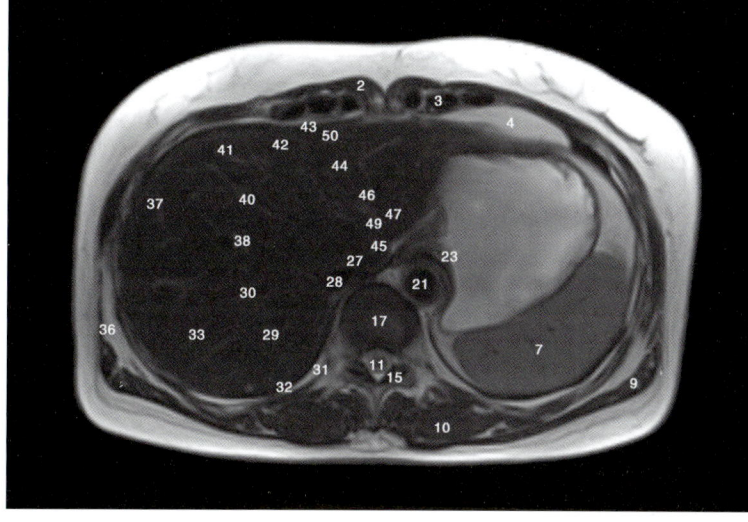

E. MR T2WI

关键结构：T10-11 椎间盘，椎内静脉丛。

此断面经 T10-11 椎间盘。

肋膈隐窝依然可见，腹腔内的结构由右至左表现为肝、胃底和脾。断面上肝占据腹腔的大部分，肝左、中、右静脉进一步远离下腔静脉，肝左静脉的两大属支向左侧延伸。椎内静脉丛位于椎管内，分布于椎骨骨膜与硬脊膜之间，收集脊髓、椎骨和韧带的静脉血，向上与颅内的枕窦、乙状窦、基底丛等有吻合，并与椎外静脉丛有广泛的交通。这些静脉丛沟通了上、下腔静脉系统，并且与颅内有直接交通，因此某些盆腔、胸腔、腹腔的感染、肿瘤或寄生虫卵等，可不经过肺循环而直接通过椎静脉丛侵入颅内。在增强 CT 或 MR 静脉期图像上有时可见椎管内较粗的椎内静脉丛属支沿脊髓两侧上行。

腹部连续横断层 23（FH.11470）

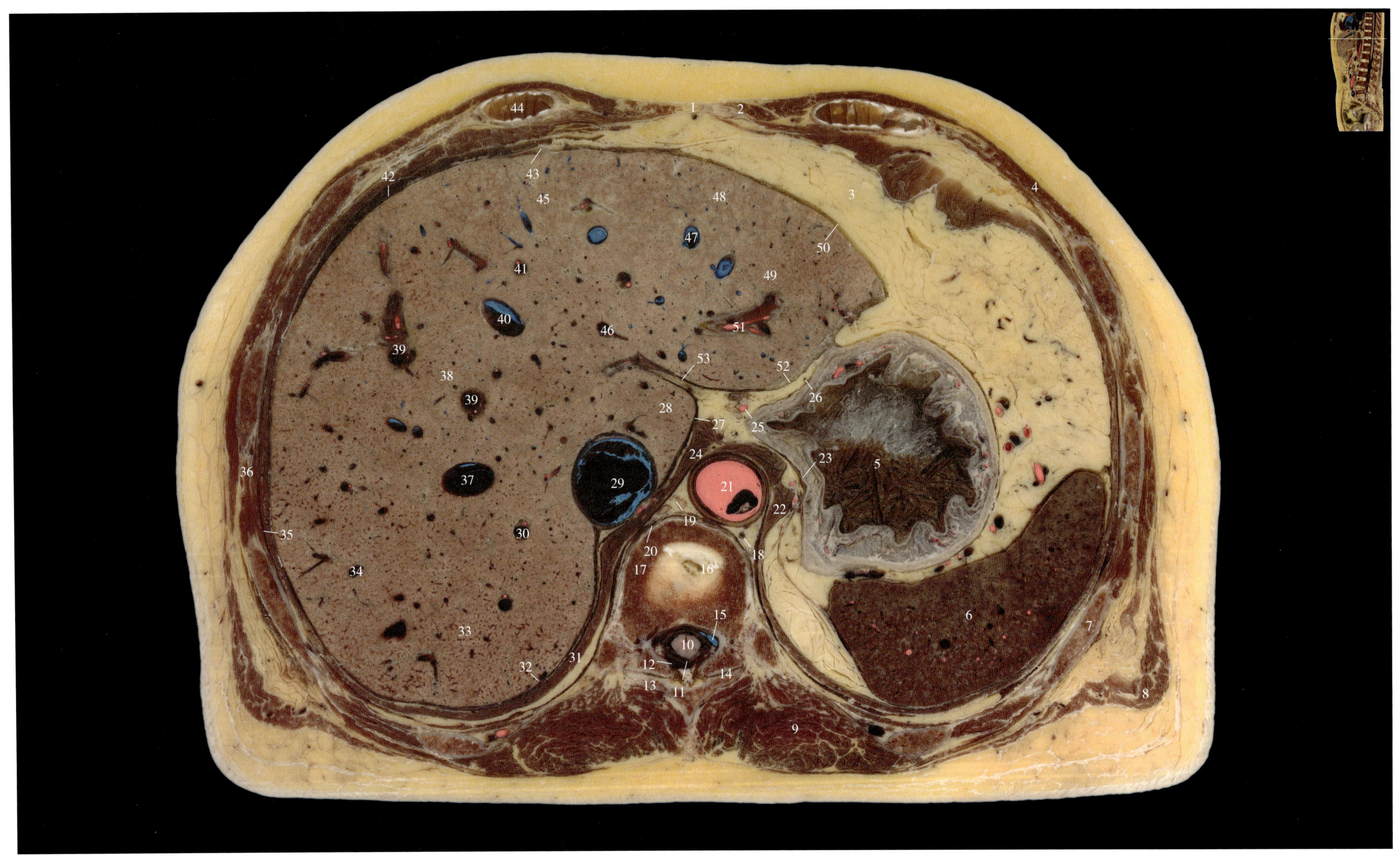

A. 断层标本图像

1. 腹白线 linea alba
2. 腹直肌 rectus abdominis
3. 大网膜 greater omentum
4. 腹外斜肌 obliquus externus abdominis
5. 胃 stomach
6. 脾 spleen
7. 第9肋骨 9th costal bone
8. 背阔肌 latissimus dorsi
9. 竖脊肌 erector spinae
10. 脊髓 spinal cord
11. 硬脊膜 spinal dura matter
12. 硬膜外隙 epidural space
13. 第11胸椎横突 transverse process of 11th thoracic vertebra
14. 关节突关节 zygapophysial joints
15. 椎内静脉丛 internal vertebral venous plexus
16. T10-11椎间盘 T10-11 intervertebral disc
17. 第11胸椎椎体 body of 11th thoracic vertebra
18. 半奇静脉 hemiazygos vein
19. 胸导管 thoracic duct
20. 奇静脉 azygos vein
21. 胸主动脉 thoracic aorta
22. 左膈脚 left crus of diaphragm
23. 胃裸区 bara area of stomach
24. 右膈脚 right crus of diaphragm
25. 胃左动脉 left gastric artery
26. 胃左静脉 left gastric vein
27. 网膜囊上隐窝 superior omental recess
28. 肝尾状叶 caudate lobe of liver
29. 下腔静脉 inferior vena cava
30. 肝门静脉右后上支 right posterosuperior branch of hepatic portal vein
31. 膈 diaphragm
32. 肝裸区 bare area of liver
33. 肝右后叶上段 superior segment of right posterior lobe of liver
34. 肝门静脉右后上支及肝动脉 right posterosuperior branch of hepatic portal vein and corresponding hepatic artery
35. 肋膈隐窝 costodiaphragmatic recess
36. 肋间外肌 intercostale externi
37. 肝右静脉 right hepatic vein
38. 肝右前叶上段 superior segment of right anterior lobe of liver
39. 肝门静脉右前上支 right anterosuperior branch of hepatic portal vein
40. 肝中静脉 middle hepatic vein
41. 肝门静脉左内支 left medial branch of hepatic portal vein
42. 右肝上间隙 right suprahepatic space
43. 肝镰状韧带 falciform ligament of liver
44. 第6肋软骨 6th costal cartilage
45. 肝左内叶 left medial lobe of liver
46. 肝门静脉左外下支 left lateroinferior branch of hepatic portal vein
47. 肝左静脉 left hepatic vein
48. 肝左外叶下段 inferior segment of left lateral lobe of liver
49. 肝左外叶上段 superior segment of left lateral lobe of liver
50. 左肝上前间隙 anterior left suprahepatic space
51. 肝门静脉左外上支及肝动脉 left laterosuperior branch of hepatic portal vein and corresponding hepatic artery
52. 左肝下前间隙 anterior left subrahepatic space
53. 静脉韧带裂和肝胃韧带 fissure for ligamentum venosum and hepatogastric ligament

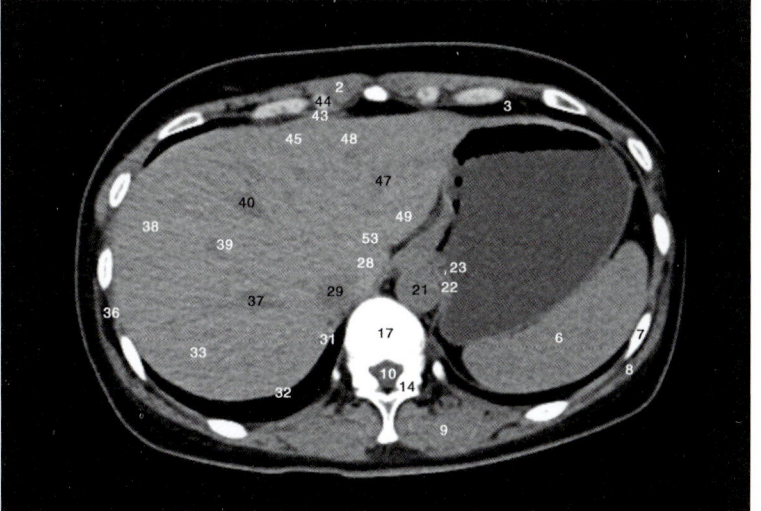

B. CT 平扫图像

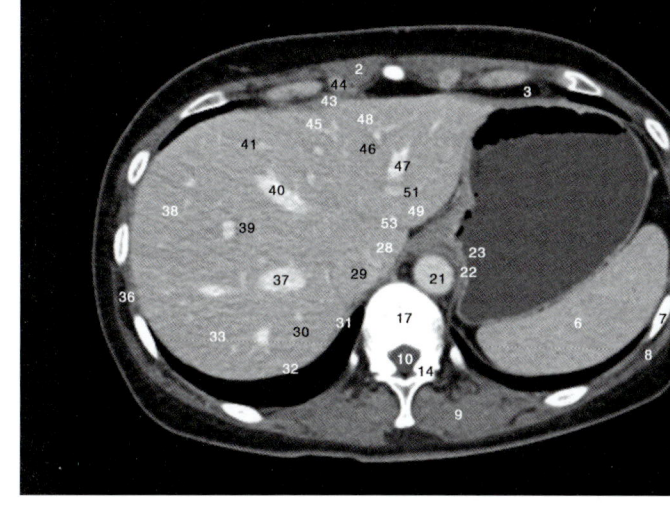

C. CT 增强图像

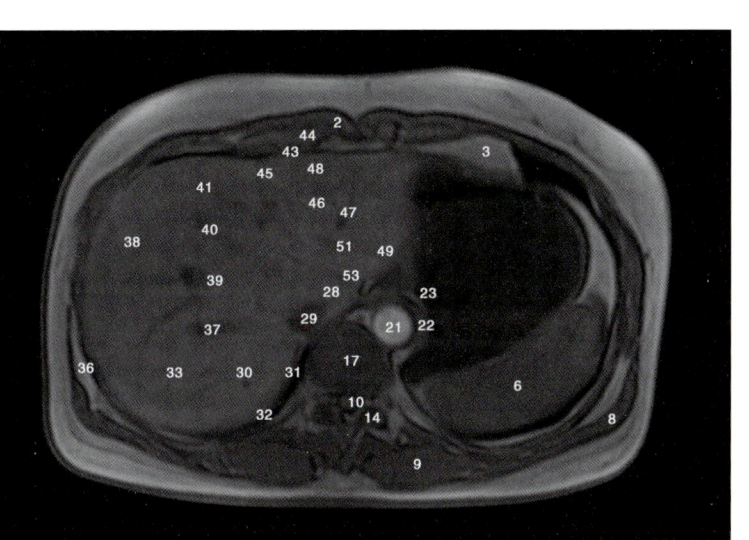

D. MR T1WI

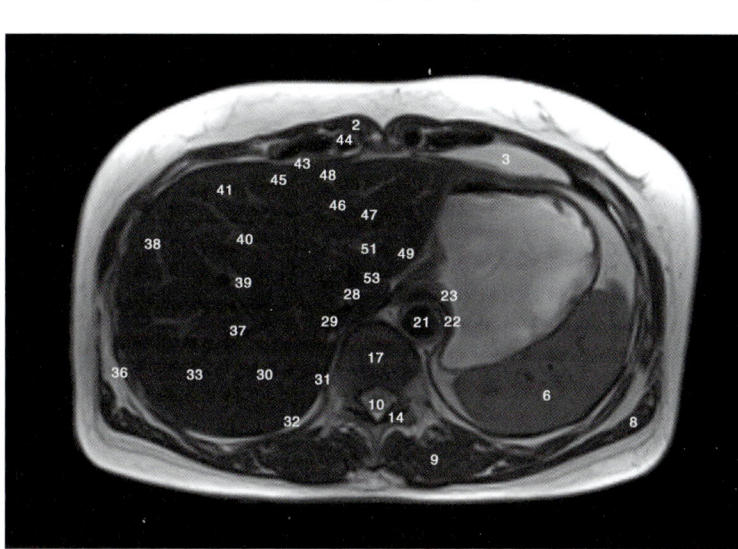

E. MR T2WI

关键结构：肝门静脉属支，胃左动、静脉。

此断面经第11胸椎椎体上份。

肝上间隙被镰状韧带分为右肝上间隙、左肝上间隙（被左冠状韧带和左三角韧带分为左肝上前间隙和左肝上后间隙）和腹膜外间隙。胃左动脉起于腹腔干，向左上方走行至贲门附近，然后转向前下，在肝胃韧带两层之间沿胃小弯向右下行走。终支多与胃右动脉吻合，沿途在贲门附近分出食管支；经胃小弯分出5~6支至胃。胃大部切除术常在第1、2壁分支间切断胃小弯。偶尔肝固有动脉左支或副肝左动脉（临床上称之为"迷走肝左动脉"）起于胃左动脉，故胃手术时切忌盲目结扎[15]。胃左静脉又称胃冠状静脉，沿胃小弯左行再转向右下，汇入肝门静脉或脾静脉。胃周血管是胃癌区域淋巴结分组的重要参考结构，在术前CT、MR等图像上应予仔细识别并进行描述，有助于手术清扫、判断分期、评估预后等。如胃左动脉周围淋巴结为第7组淋巴结，有别于同在胃小弯的第3组淋巴结。对于不同位置的胃癌，淋巴结的转移情况也不尽相同。一般来说贲门附近的肿瘤多见贲门右淋巴结（第1组）、贲门左淋巴结（第2组）转移，胃体或胃小弯的肿瘤多见胃小弯淋巴结（第3组）、胃左动脉淋巴结（第7组）转移，而胃窦癌多见幽门上淋巴结（第5组）、幽门下淋巴结（第6组）转移，其次才是为胃小弯侧及大弯侧的淋巴结转移。胃大弯侧的淋巴结（第4组），根据胃周血管分为4sa-胃短血管淋巴结、4sb-胃网膜左血管淋巴结、4d-胃网膜右血管淋巴结[14]。

腹部连续横断层 24（FH.11450）

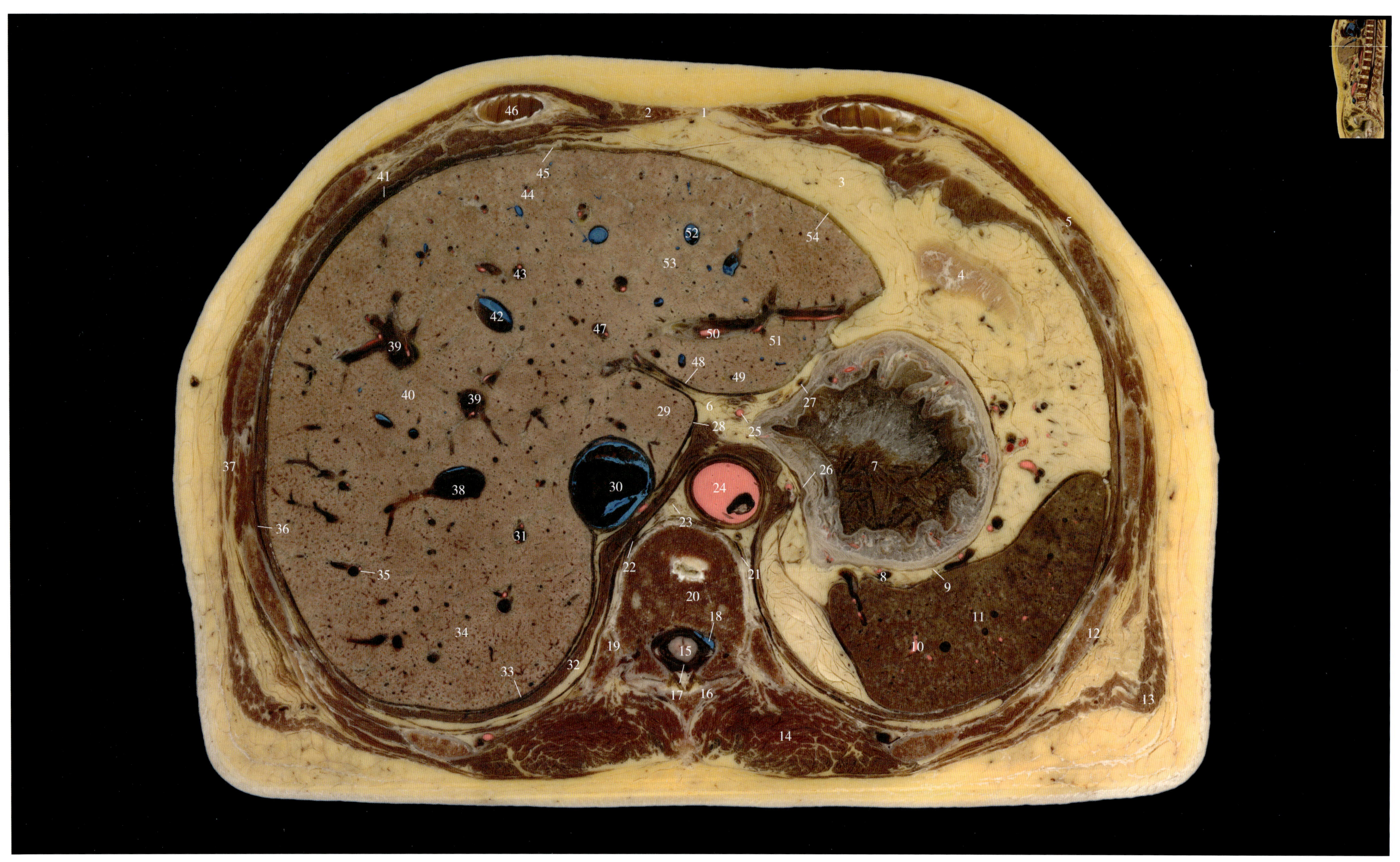

A. 断层标本图像

1. 腹白线 linea alba
2. 腹直肌 rectus abdominis
3. 大网膜 greater omentum
4. 横结肠 transverse colon
5. 腹外斜肌 obliquus externus abdominis
6. 小网膜 lesser omentum
7. 胃 stomach
8. 脾静脉 splenic vein
9. 网膜囊脾隐窝 splenic recess omental bursa
10. 脾动脉 splenic artery
11. 脾 spleen
12. 第 9 肋骨 9th costal bone
13. 背阔肌 latissimus dorsi
14. 竖脊肌 erector spinae
15. 脊髓 spinal cord
16. 第 11 胸椎横突 transverse process of 11th thoracic vertebra
17. 硬脊膜 spinal dura matter
18. 椎内静脉丛 internal vertebral venous plexus
19. 肋头关节 joint of costal head
20. 第 11 胸椎椎体 body of 11th thoracic vertebra
21. 肋间后静脉 posterior intercostal vein
22. 奇静脉 azygos vein
23. 胸导管 thoracic duct
24. 胸主动脉 thoracic aorta
25. 胃左动脉 left gastric artery
26. 胃裸区 bara area of stomach
27. 胃左静脉 left gastric vein
28. 网膜囊上隐窝 superior omental recess
29. 肝尾状叶 caudate lobe of liver
30. 下腔静脉 inferior vena cava
31. 肝门静脉右后上支 right posterosuperior branch of hepatic portal vein
32. 膈 diaphragm
33. 肝裸区 bare area of liver
34. 肝右后叶上段 superior segment of right posterior lobe of liver
35. 肝门静脉右后上支及肝动脉 right posterosuperior branch of hepatic portal vein and corresponding hepatic artery
36. 肋膈隐窝 costodiaphragmatic recess
37. 肋间外肌 intercostale externi
38. 肝右静脉 right hepatic vein
39. 肝门静脉右前上支 right anterosuperior branch of hepatic portal vein
40. 肝右前叶上段 superior segment of right anterior lobe of liver
41. 右肝上间隙 right suprahepatic space
42. 肝中静脉 middle hepatic vein
43. 肝门静脉左内支 left medial branch of hepatic portal vein
44. 肝左内叶 left medial lobe of liver
45. 肝镰状韧带 falciform ligament of liver
46. 第 6 肋软骨 6th costal cartilage
47. 肝门静脉左外下支 left lateroinferior branch of hepatic portal vein
48. 静脉韧带裂 fissure for ligamentum venosum
49. 左肝下前间隙 anterior left subrahepatic space
50. 肝门静脉左外上支及肝动脉 left laterosuperior branch of hepatic portal vein and corresponding hepatic artery
51. 肝左外叶上段 superior segment of left lateral lobe of liver
52. 肝左静脉 left hepatic vein
53. 肝左外叶下段 inferior segment of left lateral lobe of liver
54. 左肝上前间隙 anterior left suprahepatic space

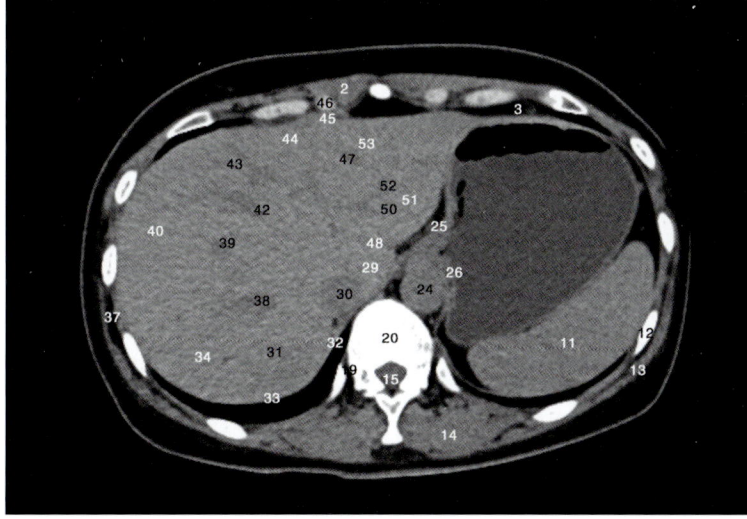

B. CT 平扫图像

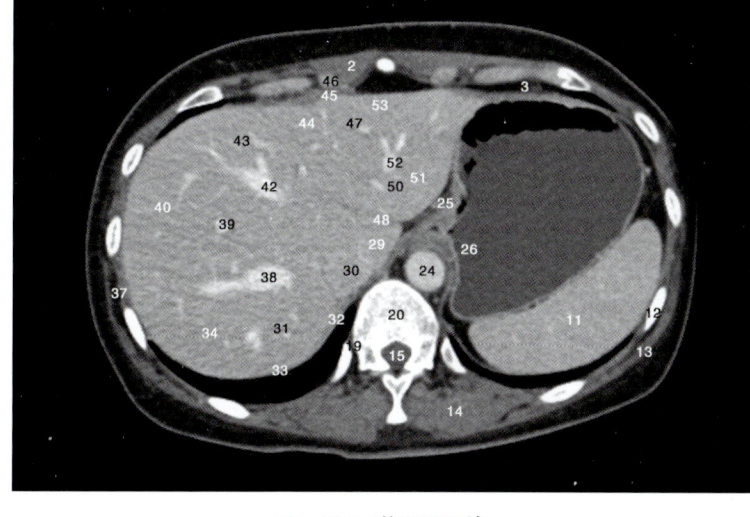

C. CT 增强图像

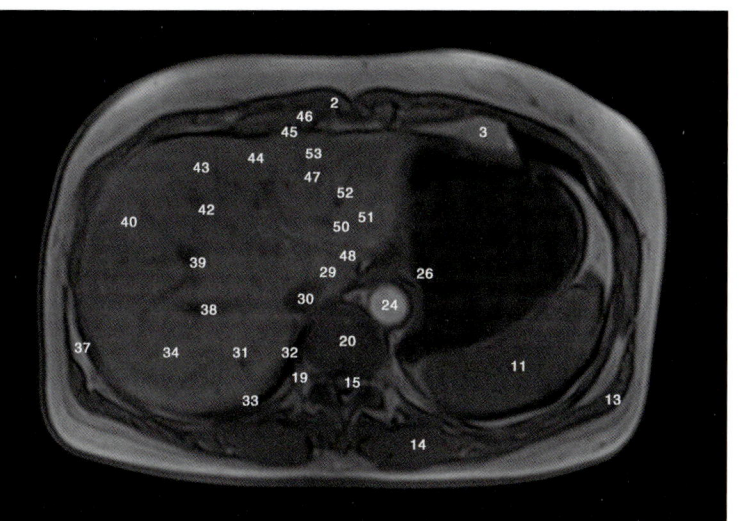

D. MR T1WI

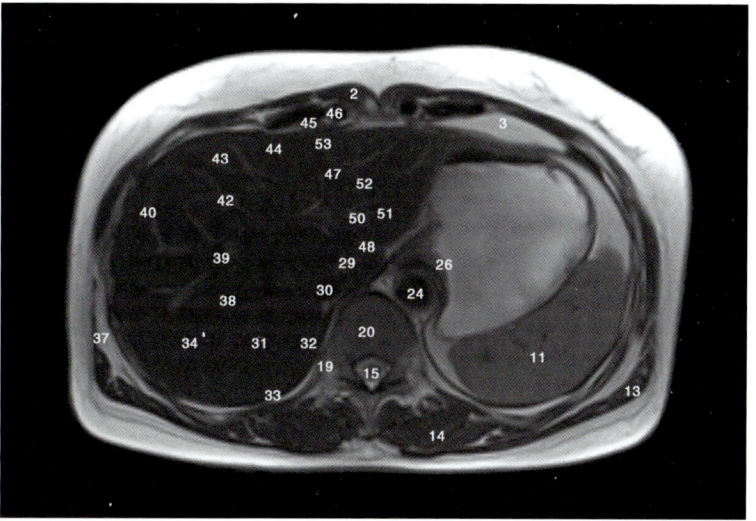

E. MR T2WI

关键结构：肝门静脉右前支，肝门静脉左外上支。

此断面经第 11 胸椎椎体上份。

肝脏断面逐渐变大，肝右前上段和左外上段内分别可见较粗大的肝门静脉右前上支和左外上支，并有相应的肝动脉和肝管伴行。肝门静脉右前支分布于肝的右前叶。研究发现几乎所有肝门静脉右前支发出的 3 级分支都分为腹侧和背侧方向，据此将门静脉右前支分成腹侧段和背侧段。在腹侧段门静脉 3 级分支和背侧段门静脉 3 级分支之间，存在一缺少血管的垂直裂，并且在这一垂直裂中有一肝静脉走行，此静脉一般为肝中静脉或肝右静脉 1 级属支[16]。肝门静脉左外上支起自角部，分布于左外叶上段。大网膜内横结肠首次出现，正常情况下，结肠的悬韧带和固有韧带能阻止结肠进入肝和横膈之间。然而，解剖位的异常改变会导致结肠病理性的插入肝脏与膈之间，患者可无症状，也可出现右季肋部隐痛、腹胀甚至消化道梗阻，由此引发的症状称为间位结肠综合征，也称为 Chilaiditi 综合征。另外，肝硬化患者肝脏体积缩小，右侧膈下空间增大，发生间位结肠综合征的概率高于正常人[17]。

腹部连续横断层 25（FH.11430）

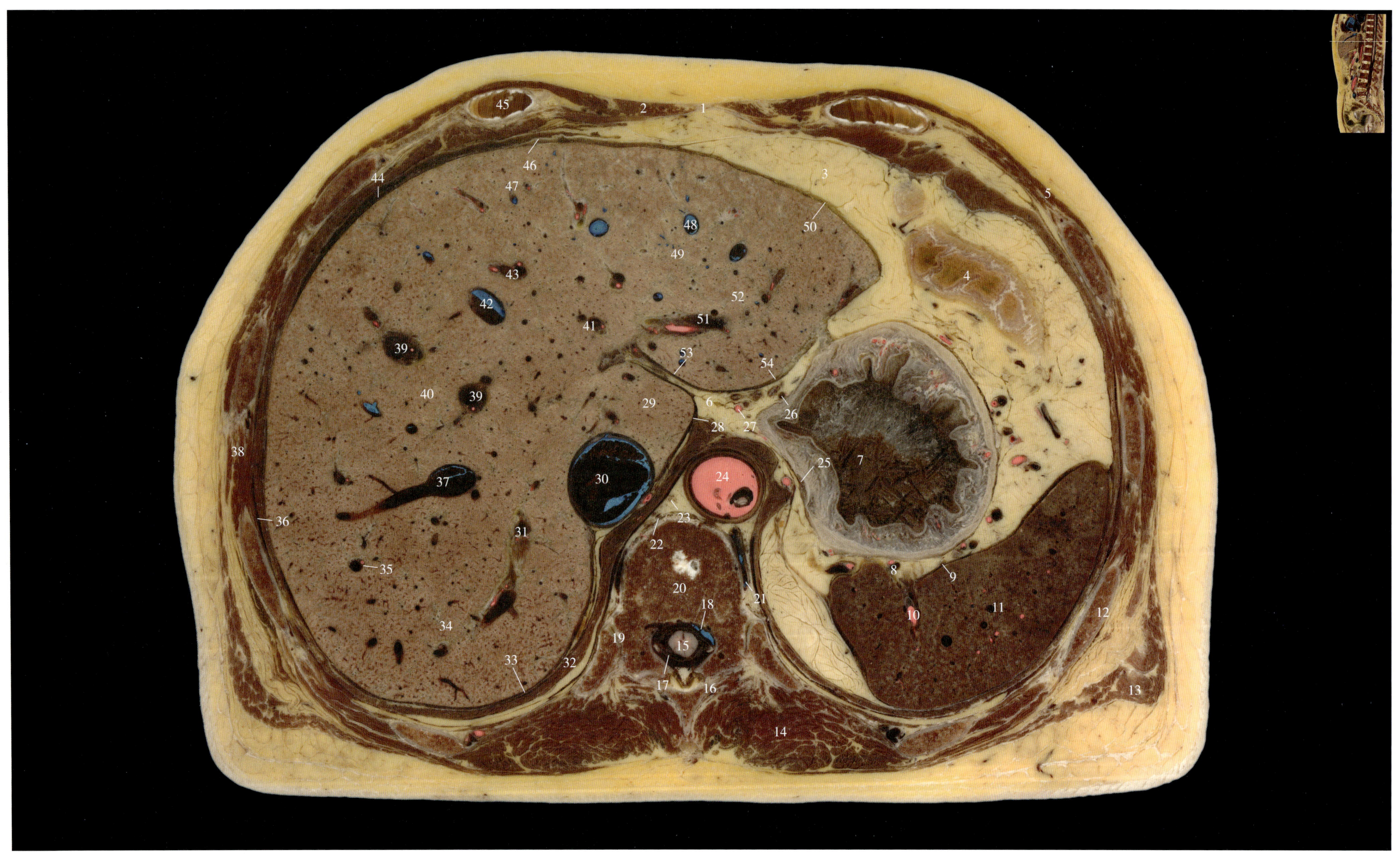

A. 断层标本图像

1. 腹白线 linea alba
2. 腹直肌 rectus abdominis
3. 大网膜 greater omentum
4. 横结肠 transverse colon
5. 腹外斜肌 obliquus externus abdominis
6. 小网膜 lesser omentum
7. 胃 stomach
8. 脾静脉 splenic vein
9. 网膜囊脾隐窝 splenic recess omental bursa
10. 脾动脉 splenic artery
11. 脾 spleen
12. 第9肋骨 9th costal bone
13. 背阔肌 latissimus dorsi
14. 竖脊肌 erector spinae
15. 脊髓 spinal cord
16. 第11胸椎横突 transverse process of 11th thoracic vertebra
17. 硬脊膜 spinal dura matter
18. 椎内静脉丛 internal vertebral venous plexus
19. 肋头关节 joint of costal head
20. 第11胸椎椎体 body of 11th thoracic vertebra
21. 肋间后静脉 posterior intercostal vein
22. 奇静脉 azygos vein
23. 胸导管 thoracic duct
24. 胸主动脉 thoracic aorta
25. 胃裸区 bara area of stomach
26. 胃左静脉 left gastric vein
27. 胃左动脉 left gastric artery
28. 网膜囊上隐窝 superior omental recess
29. 肝尾状叶 caudate lobe of liver
30. 下腔静脉 inferior vena cava
31. 肝门静脉右后支 right posterior branch of hepatic portal vein
32. 膈 diaphragm
33. 肝裸区 bare area of liver
34. 肝右后叶上段 superior segment of right posterior lobe of liver
35. 肝门静脉右后上支及肝动脉 right posterosuperior branch of hepatic portal vein and corresponding hepatic artery
36. 肋膈隐窝 costodiaphragmatic recess
37. 肝右静脉 right hepatic vein
38. 肋间内肌 intercostale interni
39. 肝门静脉右前上支 right anterosuperior branch of hepatic portal vein
40. 肝右前叶上段 superior segment of right anterior lobe of liver
41. 肝门静脉左外下支 left lateroinferior branch of hepatic portal vein
42. 肝中静脉 middle hepatic vein
43. 肝门静脉左内支 left medial branch of hepatic portal vein
44. 右肝上间隙 right suprahepatic space
45. 第6肋软骨 6th costal cartilage
46. 肝镰状韧带 falciform ligament of liver
47. 肝左内叶 left medial lobe of liver
48. 肝左静脉 left hepatic vein
49. 肝左外叶下段 inferior segment of left lateral lobe of liver
50. 左肝上前间隙 anterior left suprahepatic space
51. 肝门静脉左外上支 left laterosuperior branch of hepatic portal vein
52. 肝左外叶上段 superior segment of left lateral lobe of liver
53. 静脉韧带裂 fissure for ligamentum venosum
54. 左肝下前间隙 anterior left subrahepatic space

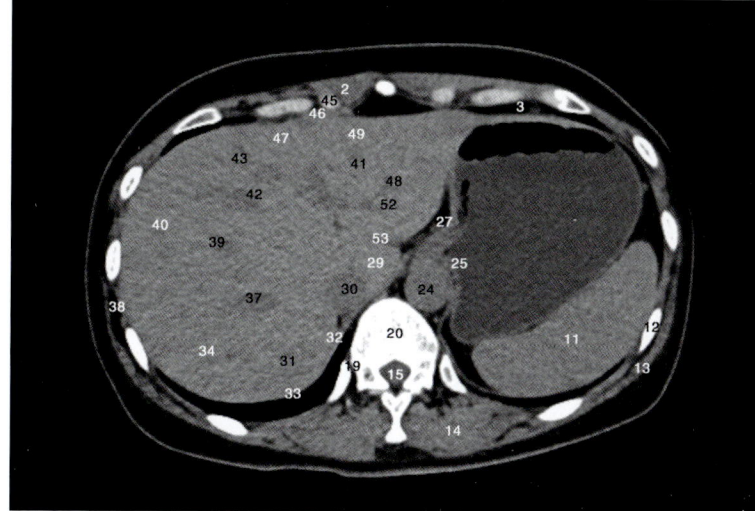

B. CT 平扫图像

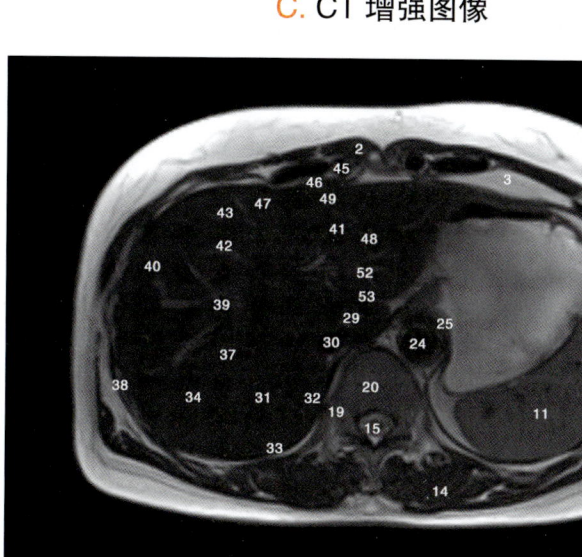

C. CT 增强图像

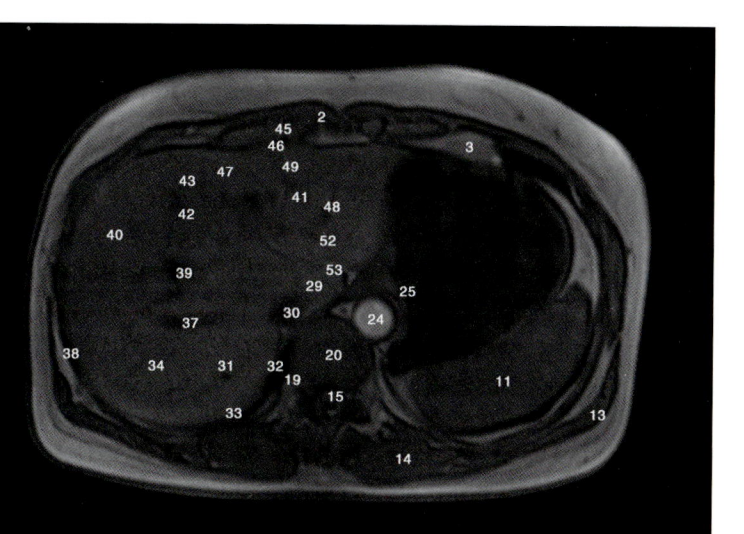

D. MR T1WI

E. MR T2WI

关键结构：脾，脾动、静脉。

此断面经第11胸椎椎体上份。

腹腔内的主要结构由右往左分别为肝、胃和脾。脾位于左季肋区的肋弓深处，后端平左侧第9肋的上缘，距后正中线4~5 cm；前端平左侧第11肋达腋中线；长轴与左侧第10肋平行。脾与膈紧邻，故脾的位置可随呼吸和体位的不同而变化。脾的膈面与膈、膈结肠韧带接触；脏面前上份与胃底相贴，后下部与左肾、左肾上腺为邻；脾门邻近胰尾。脾动脉起自腹腔干，沿胰背侧面的上缘左行，其远侧段入脾肾韧带内，并在韧带内发出各级分支，终末支经脾门入脾内。脾动脉起源变异较为常见，但对其变异率的报道差异较大，为4.10%~14.00% 不等[18]。脾静脉由脾门处的2~6条属支组成，其管径比脾动脉大一倍，走行较直，与弯曲的脾动脉形成鲜明对照。脾静脉的行程较恒定，位于脾动脉的后下方，走行在胰后面的横沟中。脾静脉沿途收纳胃短静脉、胃网膜左静脉、胃后静脉、肠系膜下静脉及来自胰的一些小静脉，向右达胰颈处与肠系膜上静脉汇合成肝门静脉。在正常情况下腹部一般摸不到脾，如在仰卧位或侧卧位时能摸到脾边缘即认为脾大。脾大是重要的病理体征，原因可为两类：一类是感染性脾大，如病毒、细菌、寄生虫等；另一类是非感染性脾大，即继发于一些疾病，如肝硬化门脉高压所致淤血性脾大、血液系统疾病、结缔组织病等。在CT或MR图像上一般可通过测量脾的厚度等径线、肋单元计数等方法来诊断脾大。

腹部连续横断层 26 (FH.11410)

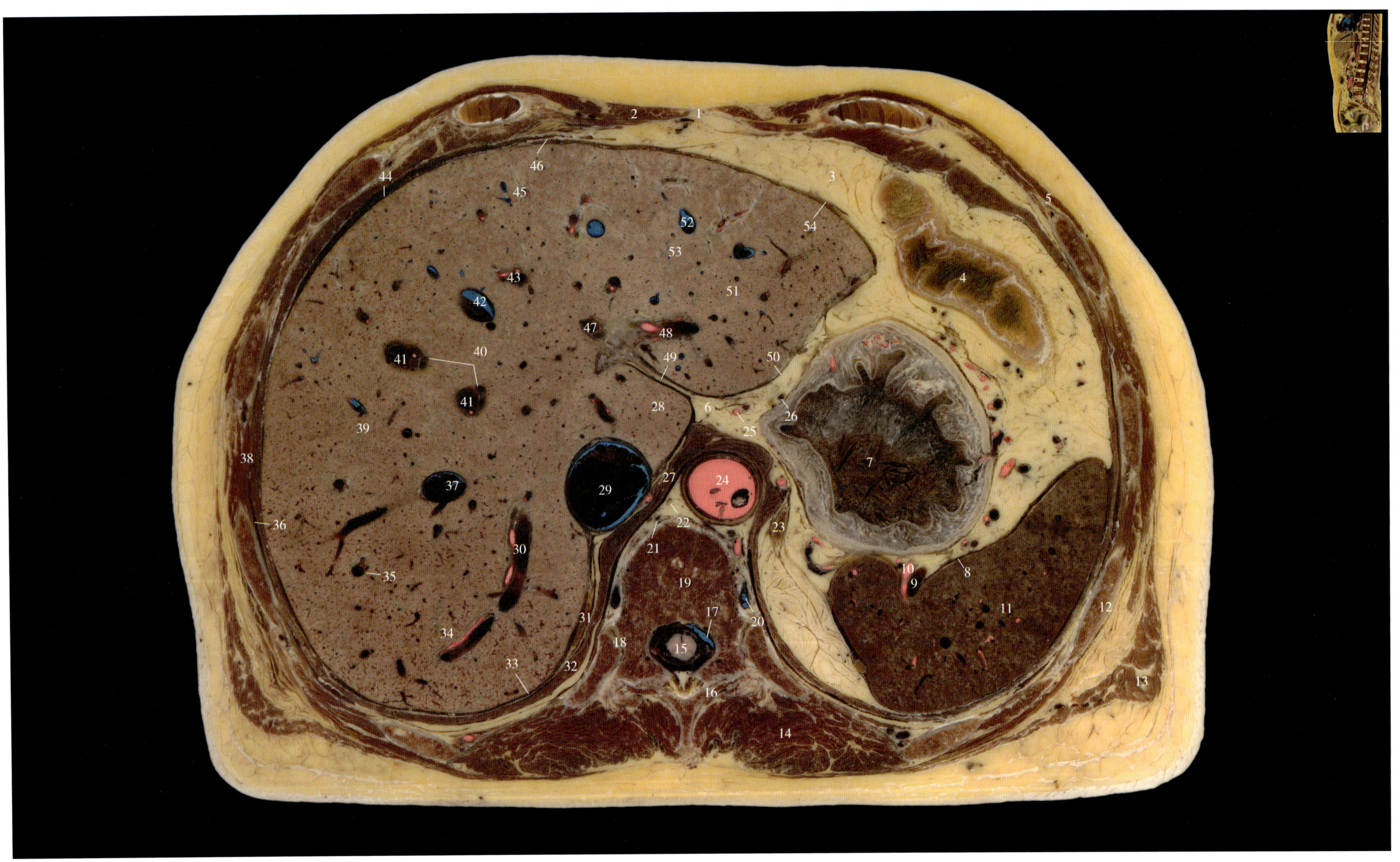

A. 断层标本图像

1. 腹白线 linea alba
2. 腹直肌 rectus abdominis
3. 大网膜 greater omentum
4. 横结肠 transverse colon
5. 腹外斜肌 obliquus externus abdominis
6. 小网膜 lesser omentum
7. 胃 stomach
8. 网膜囊脾隐窝 splenic recess omental bursa
9. 脾静脉 splenic vein
10. 脾动脉 splenic artery
11. 脾 spleen
12. 第 9 肋骨 9th costal bone
13. 背阔肌 latissimus dorsi
14. 竖脊肌 erector spinae
15. 脊髓 spinal cord
16. 第 11 胸椎横突 transverse process of 11th thoracic vertebra
17. 椎内静脉丛 internal vertebral venous plexus
18. 肋头关节 joint of costal head
19. 第 11 胸椎椎体 body of 11th thoracic vertebra
20. 肋间后静脉 posterior intercostal vein
21. 奇静脉 azygos vein
22. 胸导管 thoracic duct
23. 左肾上腺 left suprarenal gland
24. 胸主动脉 thoracic aorta
25. 胃左动脉 left gastric artery
26. 胃左静脉 left gastric vein
27. 右膈脚 right crus of diaphragm
28. 肝尾状叶 caudate lobe of liver
29. 下腔静脉 inferior vena cava
30. 肝门静脉右后支 right posterior branch of hepatic portal vein
31. 右肾上腺 right suprarenal gland
32. 膈 diaphragm
33. 肝裸区 bare area of liver
34. 肝右后叶上段 superior segment of right posterior lobe of liver
35. 肝门静脉右后上支及肝动脉 right posterosuperior branch of hepatic portal vein and corresponding hepatic artery
36. 肋膈隐窝 costodiaphragmatic recess
37. 肝右静脉 right hepatic vein
38. 肋间内肌 intercostale interni
39. 肝右前叶上段 superior segment of right anterior lobe of liver
40. 肝右管 right hepatic duct
41. 肝门静脉右前上支 right anterosuperior branch of hepatic portal vein
42. 肝中静脉 middle hepatic vein
43. 肝门静脉左内支 left medial branch of hepatic portal vein
44. 右肝上间隙 right suprahepatic space
45. 肝左内叶 left medial lobe of liver
46. 肝镰状韧带 falciform ligament of liver
47. 肝门静脉左外下支 left lateroinferior branch of hepatic portal vein
48. 肝门静脉左外上支 left laterosuperior branch of hepaticportal vein
49. 静脉韧带裂 fissure for ligamentum venosum
50. 左肝下前间隙 anterior left subrahepatic space
51. 肝左外叶上段 superior segment of left lateral lobe of liver
52. 肝左静脉 left hepatic vein
53. 肝左外叶下段 inferior segment of left lateral lobe of liver
54. 左肝上前间隙 anterior left suprahepatic space

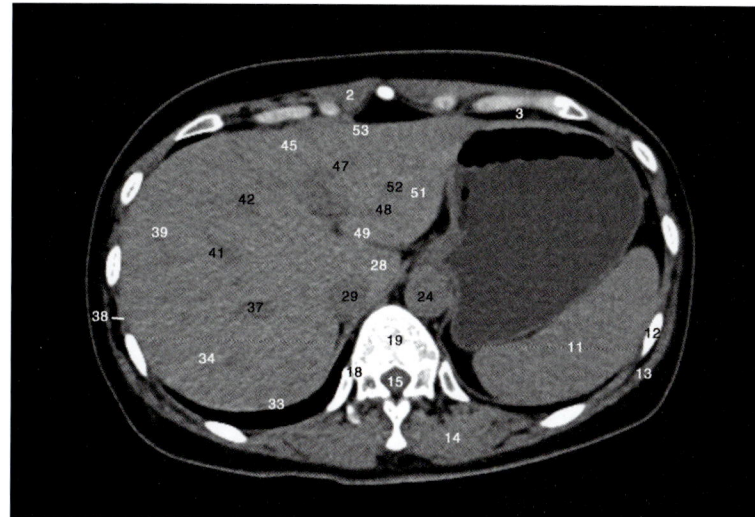

B. CT 平扫图像

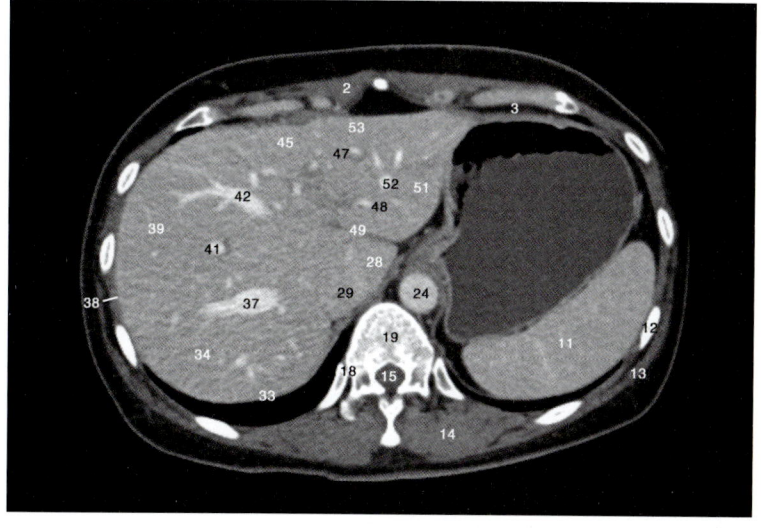

C. CT 增强图像

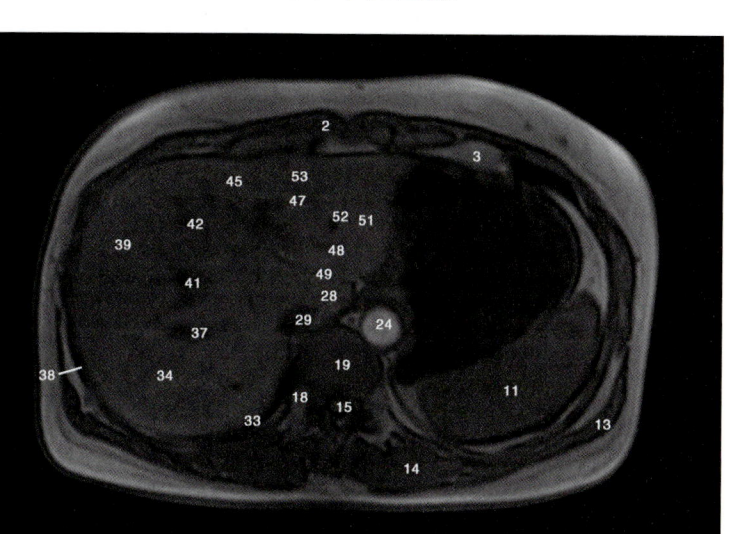

D. MR T1WI

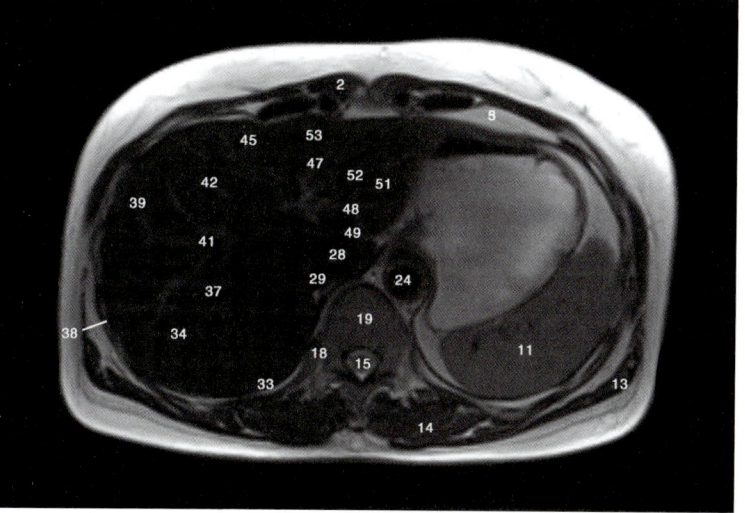

E. MR T2WI

关键结构：肝胃韧带，胃脾韧带。

此断面经第 11 胸椎椎体中份。

左肾上腺首次出现，位于左膈脚、胃和脾围成的左肾上腺三角内。肝胃韧带从膈和静脉韧带裂连于胃小弯，是小网膜的一部分，其前方为肝胃隐窝，后方为网膜囊上隐窝。肝胃隐窝绕过肝左外叶外侧缘和后缘分别与左肝上前间隙和左肝上后间隙相通，与网膜囊上隐窝之间则因隔以肝胃韧带而不相通。肝胃韧带后层在胃小弯附近向右后反折至右侧膈脚形成内侧胃膈韧带。而其在膈肌附着部位正对食管前方或右前方部分则称之为肝膈韧带。肝胃韧带前层沿膈肌前面向左侧延续，后层在此处反折至膈肌前面向右延伸走行，在下腔静脉的左缘反折至肝尾状叶，与覆盖肝尾状叶后面的腹膜相续。肝胃韧带与覆盖肝尾状叶和膈的腹膜围成网膜囊上隐窝。胃脾韧带由胃大弯左侧部连于脾门，为双层腹膜结构，其上部内有胃短血管，下份有胃网膜左动、静脉。

53

腹部连续横断层 27 (FH.11390)

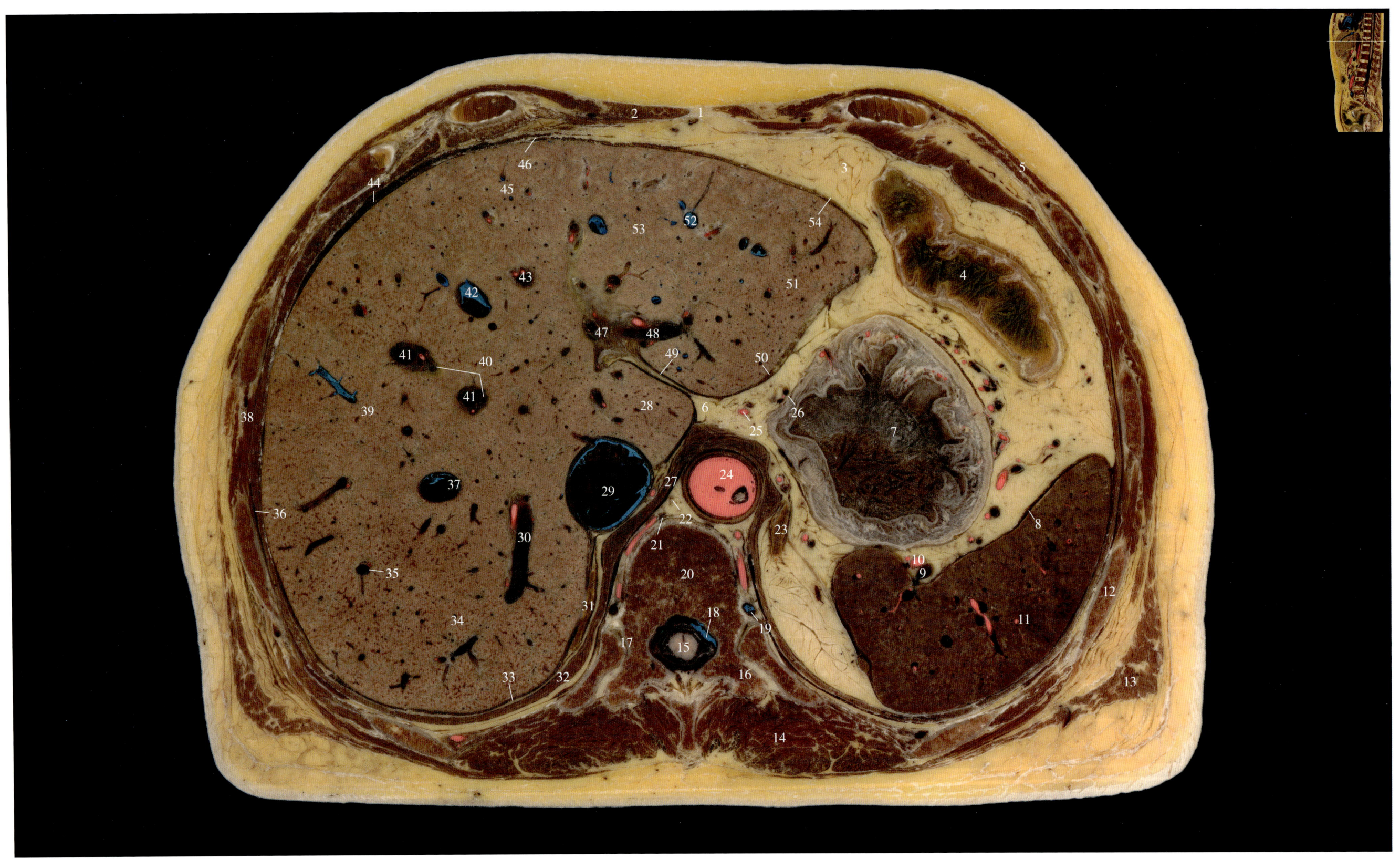

A. 断层标本图像

1. 腹白线 linea alba
2. 腹直肌 rectus abdominis
3. 大网膜 greater omentum
4. 横结肠 transverse colon
5. 腹外斜肌 obliquus externus abdominis
6. 小网膜 lesser omentum
7. 胃 stomach
8. 网膜囊脾隐窝 splenic recess omental bursa
9. 脾静脉 splenic vein
10. 脾动脉 splenic artery
11. 脾 spleen
12. 第9肋骨 9th costal bone
13. 背阔肌 latissimus dorsi
14. 竖脊肌 erector spinae
15. 脊髓 spinal cord
16. 第11胸椎横突 transverse process of 11th thoracic vertebra
17. 肋头关节 joint of costal head
18. 椎内静脉丛 internal vertebral venous plexus
19. 肋间后静脉 posterior intercostal vein
20. 第11胸椎椎体 body of 11th thoracic vertebra
21. 奇静脉 azygos vein
22. 胸导管 thoracic duct
23. 左肾上腺 left suprarenal gland
24. 胸主动脉 thoracic aorta
25. 胃左动脉 left gastric artery
26. 胃左静脉 left gastric vein
27. 右膈脚 right crus of diaphragm
28. 肝尾状叶 caudate lobe of liver
29. 下腔静脉 inferior vena cava
30. 肝门静脉右后支 right posterior branch of hepatic portal vein
31. 右肾上腺 right suprarenal gland
32. 膈 diaphragm
33. 肝裸区 bare area of liver
34. 肝右后叶上段 superior segment of right posterior lobe of liver
35. 肝门静脉右后上支及肝动脉 right posterosuperior branch of hepatic portal vein and corresponding hepatic artery
36. 肋膈隐窝 costodiaphragmatic recess
37. 肝右静脉 right hepatic vein
38. 肋间内肌 intercostale interni
39. 肝右前叶上段 superior segment of right anterior lobe of liver
40. 肝右管 right hepatic duct
41. 肝门静脉右前上支 right anterosuperior branch of hepatic portal vein
42. 肝中静脉 middle hepatic vein
43. 肝门静脉左内支 left medial branch of hepatic portal vein
44. 右肝上间隙 right suprahepatic space
45. 肝左内叶 left medial lobe of liver
46. 肝镰状韧带 falciform ligament of liver
47. 肝门静脉左支角部 angular part of left hepatic portal vein
48. 肝门静脉左外上支 left laterosuperior branch of hepatic portal vein
49. 静脉韧带裂和肝胃韧带 fissure for ligamentum venosum and hepatogastric ligament
50. 左肝下前间隙 anterior left subhepatic space
51. 肝左外叶上段 superior segment of left lateral lobe of liver
52. 肝左静脉 left hepatic vein
53. 肝左外叶下段 inferior segment of left lateral lobe of liver
54. 左肝上前间隙 anterior left suprahepatic space

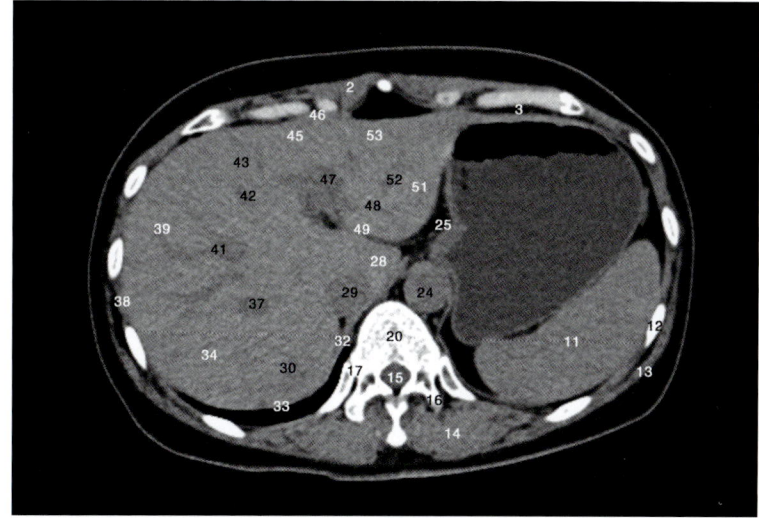

B. CT 平扫图像

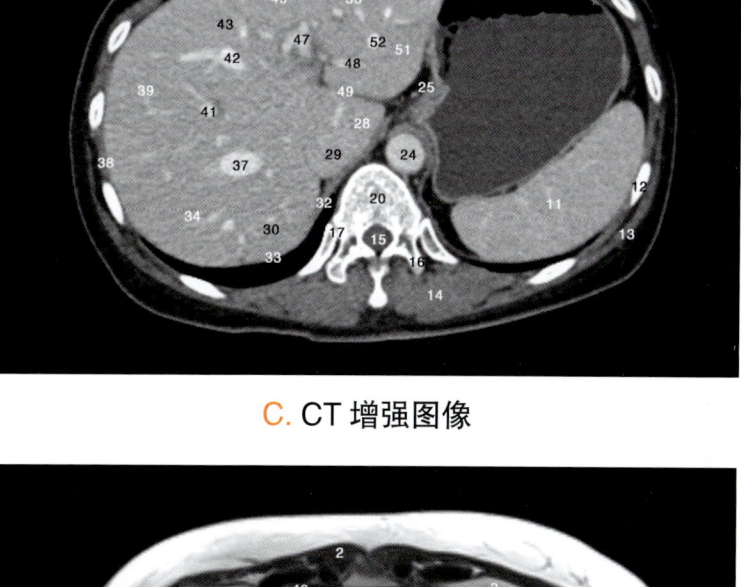

C. CT 增强图像

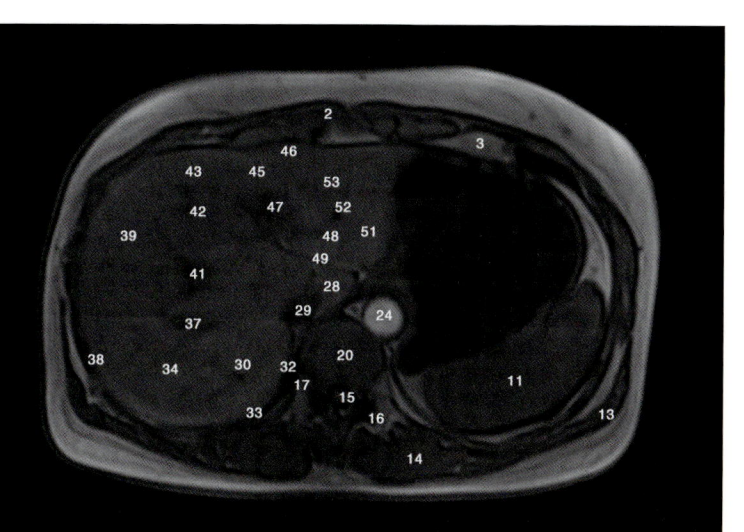

D. MR T1WI

E. MR T2WI

关键结构：横结肠，左、右膈脚。

此断面经第11胸椎椎体中份。

肝门静脉左支角部首次出现，位于静脉韧带裂的右前方，并向左侧发出肝门静脉左外上支，胃前方的大网膜内可见横结肠的断面。横结肠自结肠右曲开始，向左呈下垂的弓形，横过腹腔中部，至脾前端折转下行续为降结肠，折转处称结肠左曲又称脾曲。横结肠长40~50cm，几乎完全被腹膜包裹形成横结肠系膜，该系膜根附着于十二指肠降部、胰与左肾的前面。横结肠左、右两端的系膜较短，位置较固定，中间部因系膜长而活动度较大。横结肠上方与肝、胃相邻，下方与空、回肠相邻，故横结肠常随肝、胃的充盈变化而升降。胃充盈或直立时，横结肠中部大多降至脐下，甚至垂入盆腔。结肠左曲较右曲高，相当于第10~11肋水平，借膈结肠韧带附于膈下，后方贴靠胰尾与左肾，前方通过胃结肠韧带附着于胃大弯并为肋弓所掩盖。因此，结肠左曲处的肿瘤不易被扪及。膈脚，即膈肌的终点，分左、右2个膈脚，位于约第12胸椎体前方，左右两个膈脚在此区域与脊柱共同围成主动脉裂孔，在CT上位于主动脉两侧且贴近脊柱，表现为类圆形的软组织密度影。膈脚后间隙位于脊柱前方的左膈脚与右膈脚之间，其两侧为纵隔胸膜，内有胸主动脉、胸导管、奇静脉和半奇静脉等，是后纵隔的最低部分。膈脚移位征也是鉴别胸腹水的一种征象：胸腔积液聚集在膈脚与脊柱间，可使膈脚向前外侧移位，而腹水集聚在膈脚的前外侧，可将膈脚推向后内侧。

55

腹部连续横断层 28（FH.11370）

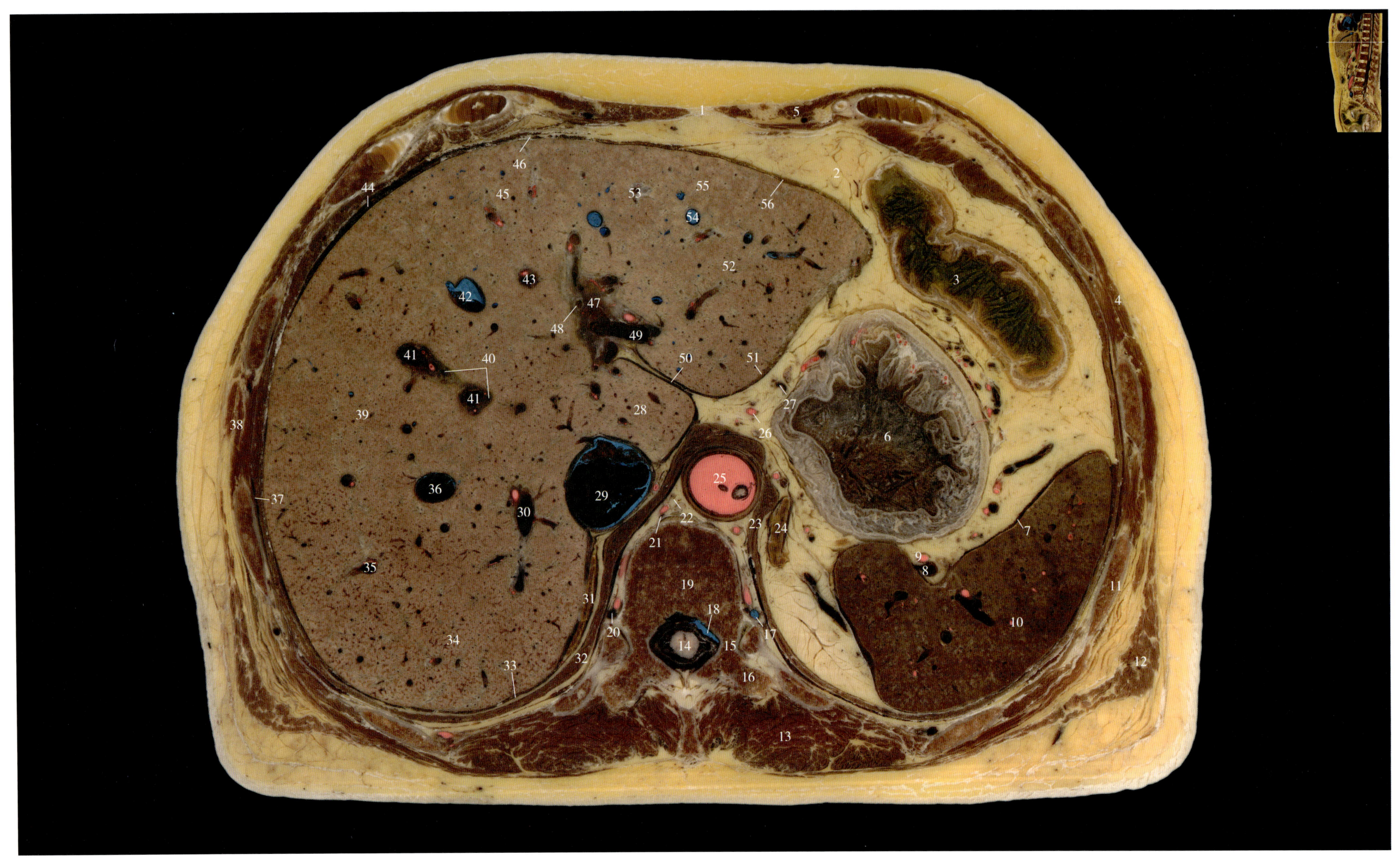

A. 断层标本图像

1. 腹白线 linea alba
2. 大网膜 greater omentum
3. 横结肠 transverse colon
4. 腹外斜肌 obliquus externus abdominis
5. 腹直肌 rectus abdominis
6. 胃 stomach
7. 网膜囊脾隐窝 splenic recess omental bursa
8. 脾静脉 splenic vein
9. 脾动脉 splenic artery
10. 脾 spleen
11. 第 9 肋骨 9th costal bone
12. 背阔肌 latissimus dorsi
13. 竖脊肌 erector spinae
14. 脊髓 spinal cord
15. 椎弓峡部 isthmus of vertebral arch
16. 第 11 胸椎横突 transverse process of 11th thoracic vertebra
17. 肋间后静脉 posterior intercostal vein
18. 椎内静脉丛 internal vertebral venous plexus
19. 第 11 胸椎椎体 body of 11th thoracic vertebra
20. 肋间后动脉 posterior intercostal artery
21. 奇静脉 azygos vein
22. 胸导管 thoracic duct
23. 左膈脚 left crus of diaphragm
24. 左肾上腺 left suprarenal gland
25. 胸主动脉 thoracic aorta
26. 胃左动脉 left gastric artery
27. 胃左静脉 left gastric vein
28. 肝尾状叶 caudate lobe of liver
29. 下腔静脉 inferior vena cava
30. 肝门静脉右后支 right posterior branch of hepatic portal vein
31. 右肾上腺 right suprarenal gland
32. 膈 diaphragm
33. 肝裸区 bare area of liver
34. 肝右后叶上段 superior segment of right posterior lobe of liver
35. 肝门静脉右后上支及肝动脉 right posterosuperior branch of hepatic portal vein and corresponding hepatic artery
36. 肝右静脉 right hepatic vein
37. 肋膈隐窝 costodiaphragmatic recess
38. 肋间外肌 intercostale externi
39. 肝右前叶上段 superior segment of right anterior lobe of liver
40. 肝右管 right hepatic duct
41. 肝门静脉右前上支 right anterosuperior branch of hepatic portal vein
42. 肝中静脉 middle hepatic vein
43. 肝门静脉左内支 left medial branch of hepatic portal vein
44. 右肝上间隙 right suprahepatic space
45. 肝左内叶 left medial lobe of liver
46. 肝镰状韧带 falciform ligament of liver
47. 肝门静脉左支角部 angular part of left hepatic portal vein
48. 肝左管 left hepatic duct
49. 肝门静脉左外上支 left laterosuperior branch of hepatic portal vein
50. 静脉韧带裂 fissure for ligamentum venosum
51. 左肝下前间隙 anterior left subrahepatic space
52. 肝左外叶上段 superior segment of left lateral lobe of liver
53. 肝门静脉左外下支 left lateroinferior branch of hepatic portal vein
54. 肝左静脉 left hepatic vein
55. 肝左外叶下段 inferior segment of left lateral lobe of liver
56. 左肝上前间隙 anterior left suprahepatic space

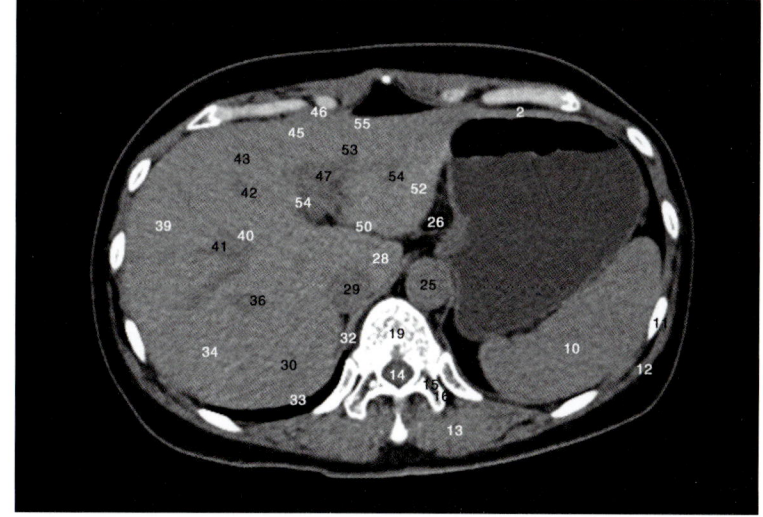

B. CT 平扫图像

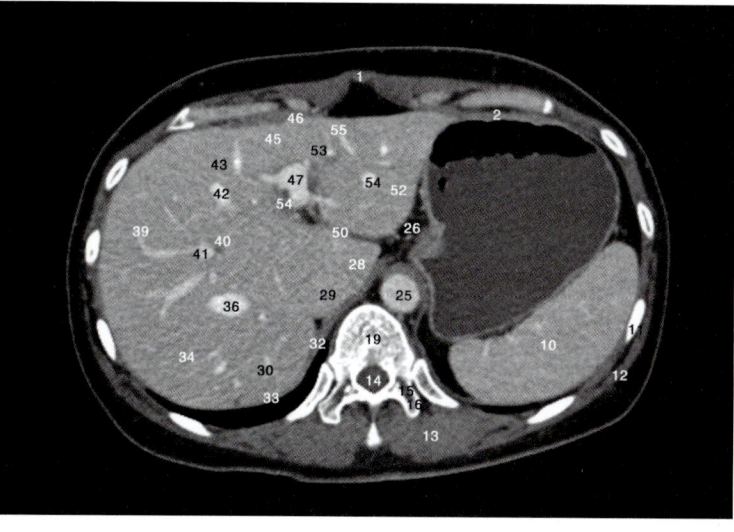

C. CT 增强图像

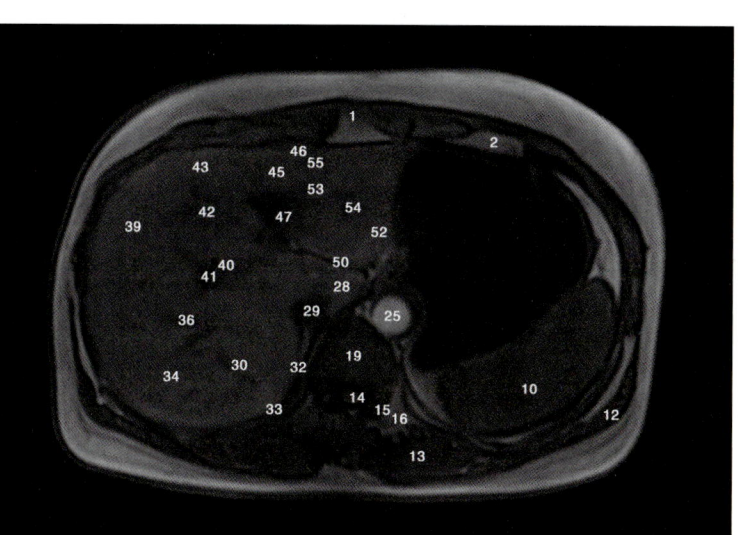

D. MR T1WI

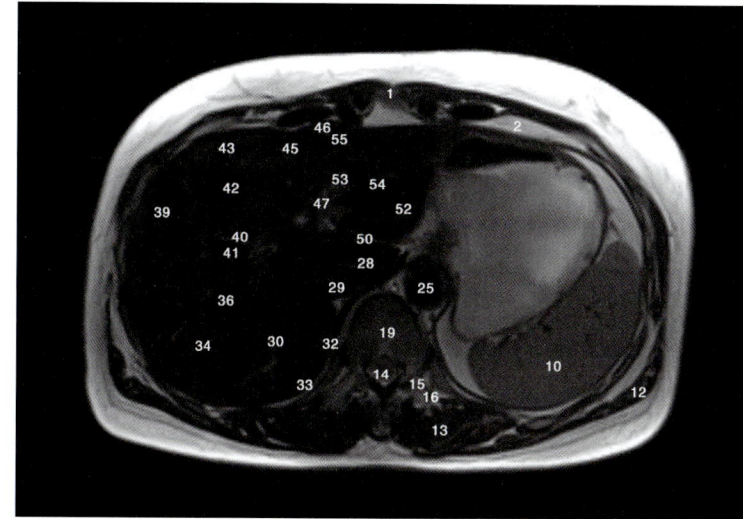

E. MR T2WI

关键结构：肝门静脉左支角部，大网膜。

此断面经第 11 胸椎椎体中份。

肝门静脉左支角部是本断面的重要特征，其右侧可见细小的肝左管。在横断面上，自上而下，肝门静脉左支先出现角部，稍低水平可切及横部的起始部和矢状部，囊部可与矢状部同层或稍低一个层面出现。大网膜连接于胃大弯与横结肠之间，呈围裙状下垂，覆盖于横结肠和小肠的前面，其长度因人而异。成人大网膜前两层和后两层通常愈着，使前两层上部直接由胃大弯连至横结肠，形成胃结肠韧带。大网膜具有很大的活动性，当腹腔器官发生炎症（如阑尾炎）时，大网膜能迅速将其包绕以限制炎症的蔓延。晚期腹盆腔恶性肿瘤易种植性转移至大网膜，CT 图像上可见大网膜脂肪间隙模糊，见结节状、索条状高密度灶，后期甚至呈饼状改变，实性成分可见强化。MR 扩散加权成像（DWI）显示大网膜呈高信号，ADC 低信号，结合肿瘤病史，常提示转移。但是，需要与大网膜感染性病变如结核等进行鉴别。

腹部连续横断层 29（FH.11350）

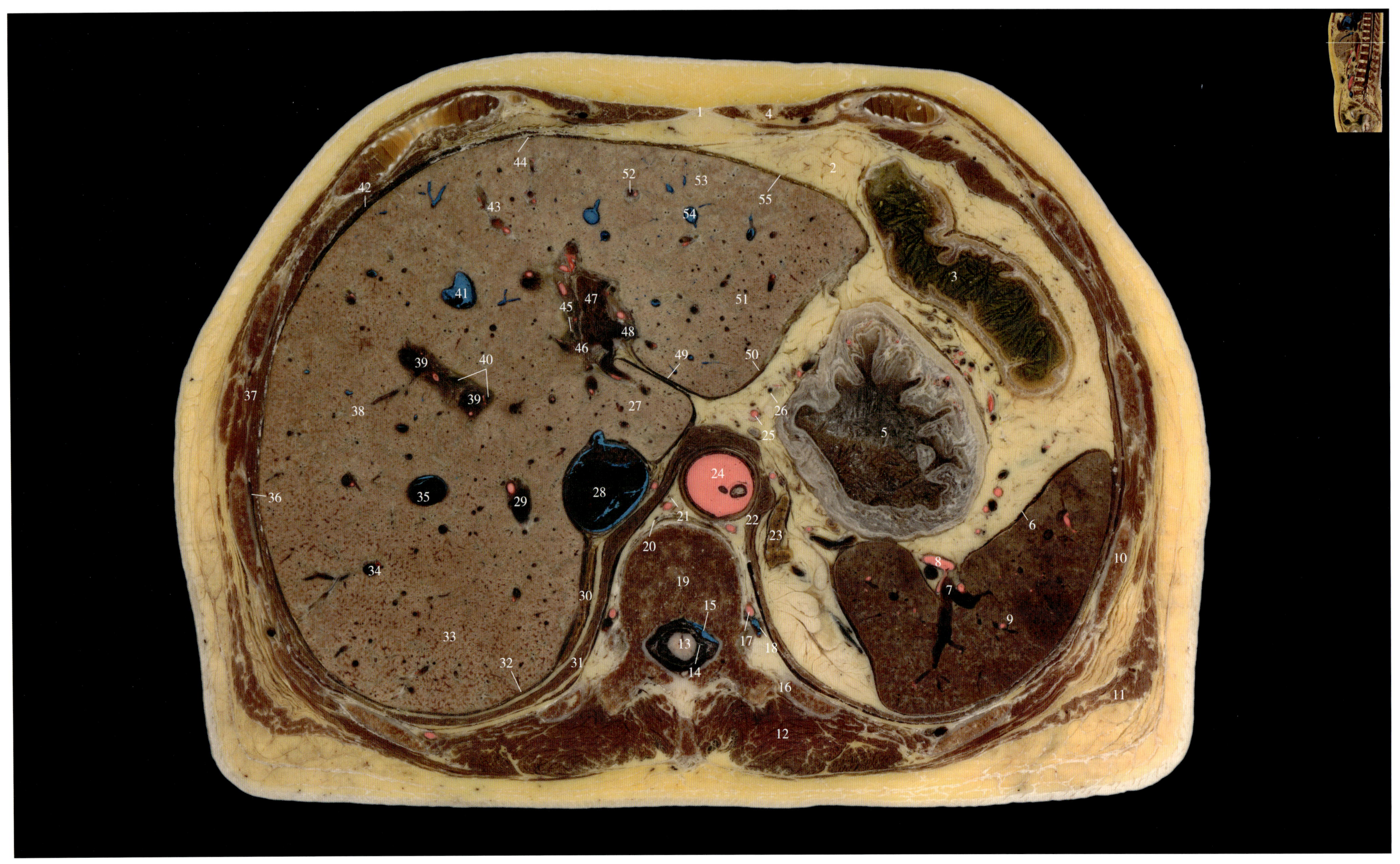

A. 断层标本图像

1. 腹白线 linea alba
2. 大网膜 greater omentum
3. 横结肠 transverse colon
4. 腹直肌 rectus abdominis
5. 胃 stomach
6. 网膜囊脾隐窝 splenic recess omental bursa
7. 脾静脉 splenic vein
8. 脾动脉 splenic artery
9. 脾 spleen
10. 第9肋骨 9th costal bone
11. 背阔肌 latissimus dorsi
12. 竖脊肌 erector spinae
13. 脊髓 spinal cord
14. 脊神经前根 anterior root of spinal nerve
15. 椎内静脉丛 internal vertebral venous plexus
16. 肋横突关节 costal transverse process joint
17. 肋间后动脉 posterior intercostal artery
18. 肋间后静脉 posterior intercostal vein
19. 第11胸椎椎体 body of 11th thoracic vertebra
20. 奇静脉 azygos vein
21. 胸导管 thoracic duct
22. 左膈脚 left crus of diaphragm
23. 左肾上腺 left suprarenal gland
24. 胸主动脉 thoracic aorta
25. 胃左动脉 left gastric artery
26. 胃左静脉 left gastric vein
27. 肝尾状叶 caudate lobe of liver
28. 下腔静脉 inferior vena cava
29. 肝门静脉右后支 right posterior branch of hepatic portal vein
30. 右肾上腺 right suprarenal gland
31. 膈 diaphragm
32. 肝裸区 bare area of liver
33. 肝右后叶上段 superior segment of right posterior lobe of liver
34. 肝门静脉右后上支及肝右动脉 right posterosuperior branch of hepatic portal vein and corresponding hepatic artery
35. 肝右静脉 right hepatic vein
36. 肋膈隐窝 costodiaphragmatic recess
37. 肋间内肌 intercostale interni
38. 肝右前叶上段 superior segment of right anterior lobe of liver
39. 肝门静脉右前上支 right anterosuperior branch of hepatic portal vein
40. 肝右管 right hepatic duct
41. 肝中静脉 middle hepatic vein
42. 右肝上间隙 right suprahepatic space
43. 肝左内叶 left medial lobe of liver
44. 肝镰状韧带 falciform ligament of liver
45. 肝左管 left hepatic duct
46. 肝门静脉左支横部 transverse part of left hepatic portal vein
47. 肝门静脉左支矢状部 sagittal part of left hepatic portal vein
48. 肝门静脉左外上支 left laterosuperior branch of hepatic portal vein
49. 静脉韧带裂 fissure for ligamentum venosum
50. 左肝下间隙 anterior left subrahepatic space
51. 肝左外叶上段 superior segment of left lateral lobe of liver
52. 肝门静脉左外下支 left lateroinferior branch of hepatic portal vein
53. 肝左外叶下段 inferior segment of left lateral lobe of liver
54. 肝左静脉 left hepatic vein
55. 左肝上前间隙 anterior left suprahepatic space

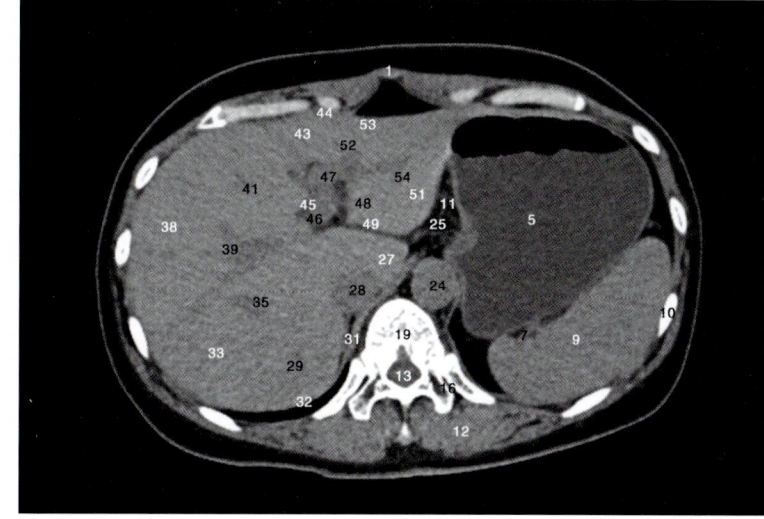

B. CT 平扫图像　　　　C. CT 增强图像

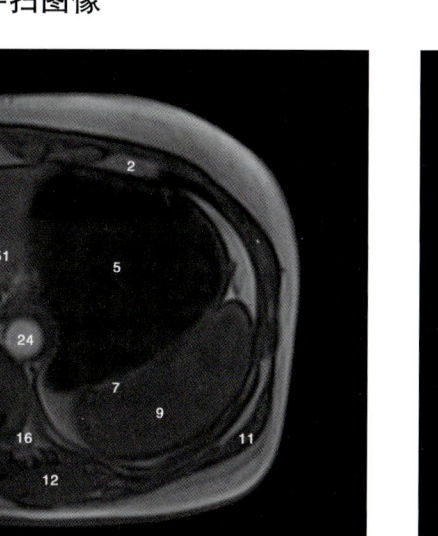
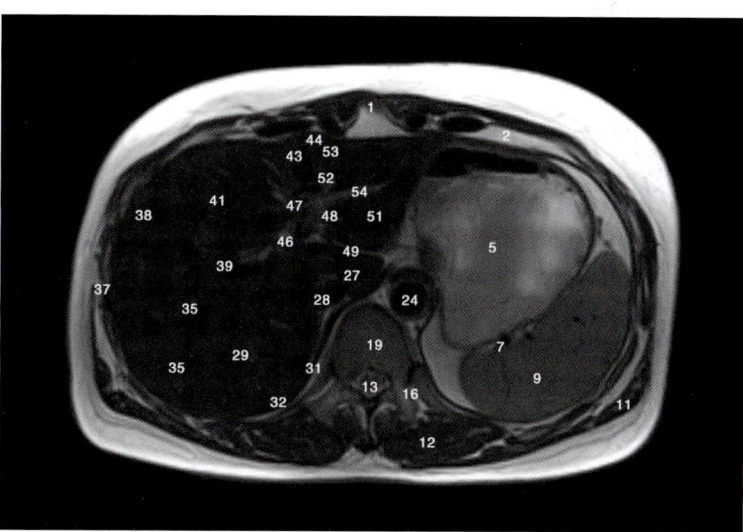

D. MR T1WI　　　　E. MR T2WI

关键结构：左肾上腺，肋间后动、静脉。

此断面经第11胸椎椎体中份。

左肾上腺位于由左膈脚、胃和脾围成的充满脂肪的左肾上腺三角内，其后方左肾即将出现，脊柱两侧可见肋间动、静脉。左肾上腺为半月形，高约5 cm，宽约3 cm，厚为0.5~1 cm，重5~7 g。左肾上腺前面的上部借网膜囊与胃相邻，下部与胰尾和脾血管相邻，内侧缘接近腹主动脉，后面为膈。左肾上腺门位于其前面的下部，有肾上腺中央静脉自门穿出注入左肾静脉。肋间后动脉除第1、2肋间后动脉来自锁骨下动脉的分支肋颈干外，其余9对肋间后动脉和1对肋下动脉均发自胸主动脉。各肋间后动脉走行于相应的肋间隙内，在肋间隙后部，行于胸内筋膜与肋间内膜之间。至肋角附近，穿行于肋间最内肌与肋间内肌之间，并紧贴肋沟前行。至腋前线前则在相应肋骨下缘下方的肋间内肌与胸内筋膜之间走行。肋间后动脉行至脊柱两旁在肋骨小头下缘附近发出后支，向后穿到背部至脊髓、背部肌和皮肤。肋间后动脉在近肋角处还分出一肋间侧副支，向前下走行，继而沿下位肋骨的上缘前行。上9对肋间后动脉及其侧副支的末端在肋间隙内与胸廓内动脉和膈动脉的肋间前支（又叫肋间前动脉）相吻合。如在肋间隙前部穿刺时，进针部位应在上、下肋之间刺入，而在肋角的内侧部位穿刺时，应在下肋骨的上缘刺入。各肋间后静脉与同序数的肋间后动脉伴行，位于动脉上方。肋间后静脉向后汇入奇静脉、半奇静脉或副半奇静脉。

腹部连续横断层 30（FH.11330）

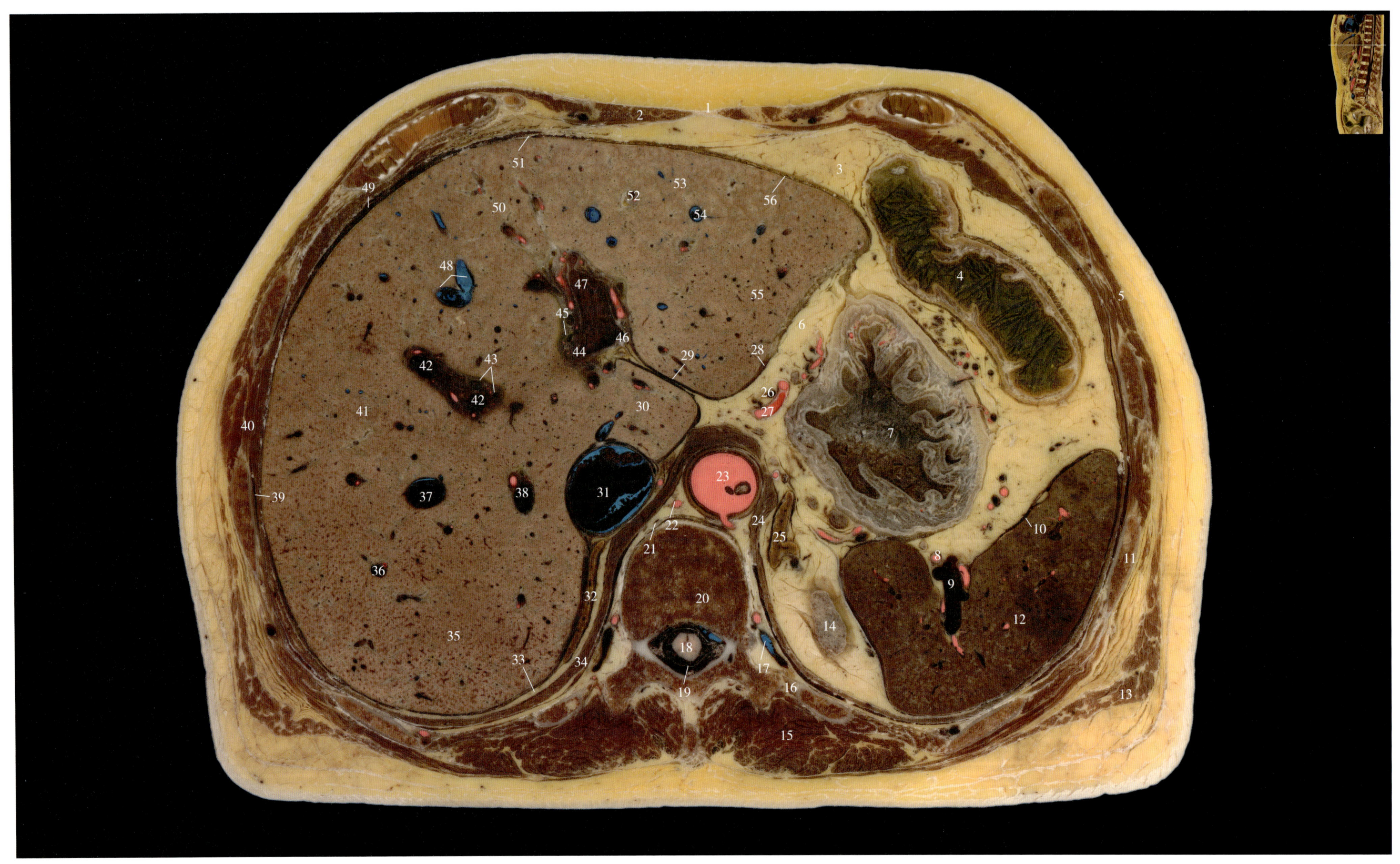

A. 断层标本图像

1. 腹白线 linea alba
2. 腹直肌 rectus abdominis
3. 大网膜 greater omentum
4. 横结肠 transverse colon
5. 腹外斜肌 obliquus externus abdominis
6. 小网膜 lesser omentum
7. 胃 stomach
8. 脾动脉 splenic artery
9. 脾静脉 splenic vein
10. 网膜囊脾隐窝 splenic recess omental bursa
11. 第9肋骨 9th costal bone
12. 脾 spleen
13. 背阔肌 latissimus dorsi
14. 左肾 left kidney
15. 竖脊肌 erector spinae
16. 肋横突关节 costal transverse process joint
17. 肋间后静脉 posterior intercostal vein
18. 脊髓 spinal cord
19. 硬脊膜 spinal dura matter
20. 第11胸椎椎体 body of 11th thoracic vertebra
21. 奇静脉 azygos vein
22. 胸导管 thoracic duct
23. 胸主动脉 thoracic aorta
24. 左膈脚 left crus of diaphragm
25. 左肾上腺 left suprarenal gland
26. 胃左静脉 left gastric vein
27. 胃左动脉 left gastric artery
28. 左肝下前间隙 anterior left subrahepatic space
29. 静脉韧带裂 fissure for ligamentum venosum
30. 肝尾状叶 caudate lobe of liver
31. 下腔静脉 inferior vena cava
32. 右肾上腺 right suprarenal gland
33. 肝裸区 bare area of liver
34. 膈 diaphragm
35. 肝右后叶上段 superior segment of right posterior lobe of liver
36. 肝门静脉右后上支及肝动脉 right posterosuperior branch of hepatic portal vein and corresponding hepatic artery
37. 肝右静脉 right hepatic vein
38. 肝门静脉右后支 right posterior branch of hepatic portal vein
39. 肋膈隐窝 costodiaphragmatic recess
40. 肋间内肌 intercostale interni
41. 肝右前叶上段 superior segment of right anterior lobe of liver
42. 肝门静脉右前上支 right anterosuperior branch of hepatic portal vein
43. 肝右管 right hepatic duct
44. 肝门静脉左支横部 transverse part of left hepatic portal vein
45. 肝左管 left hepatic duct
46. 肝门静脉左外上支 left laterosuperior branch of hepatic portal vein
47. 肝门静脉左支矢状部 sagittal part of left hepatic portal vein
48. 肝中静脉属支 tributary of middle hepatic vein
49. 右肝上间隙 right suprahepatic space
50. 肝左内叶 left medial lobe of liver
51. 肝镰状韧带 falciform ligament of liver
52. 肝门静脉左外下支 left lateroinferior branch of hepatic portal vein
53. 肝左外叶下段 inferior segment of left lateral lobe of liver
54. 肝左静脉 left hepatic vein
55. 肝左外叶上段 superior segment of left lateral lobe of liver
56. 左肝上前间隙 anterior left suprahepatic space

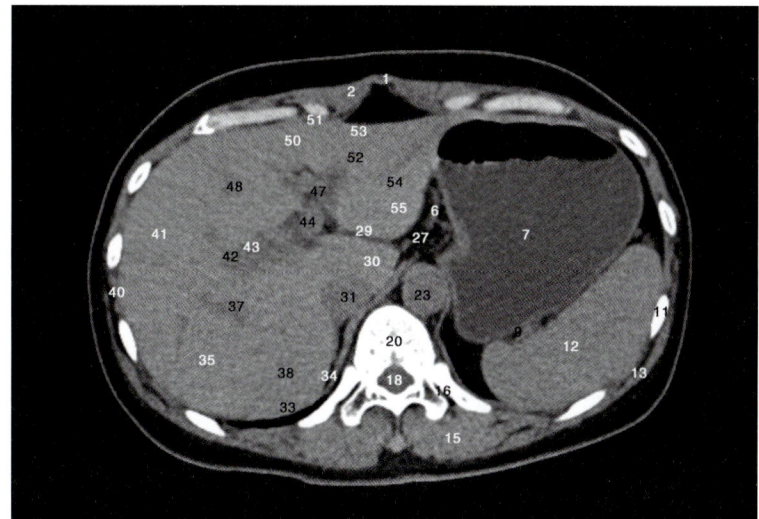

B. CT 平扫图像

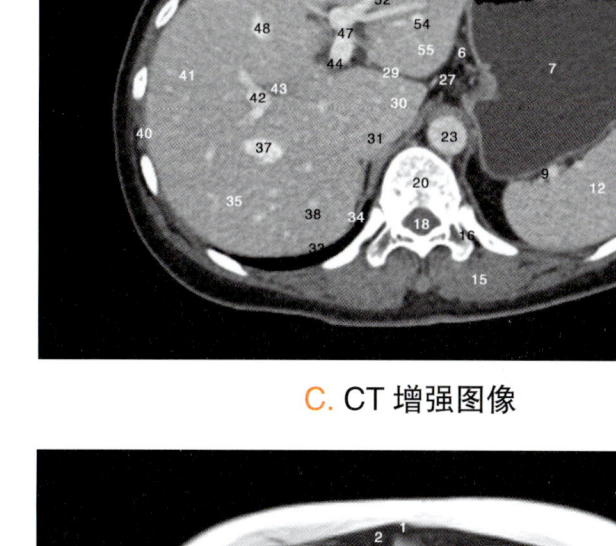

C. CT 增强图像

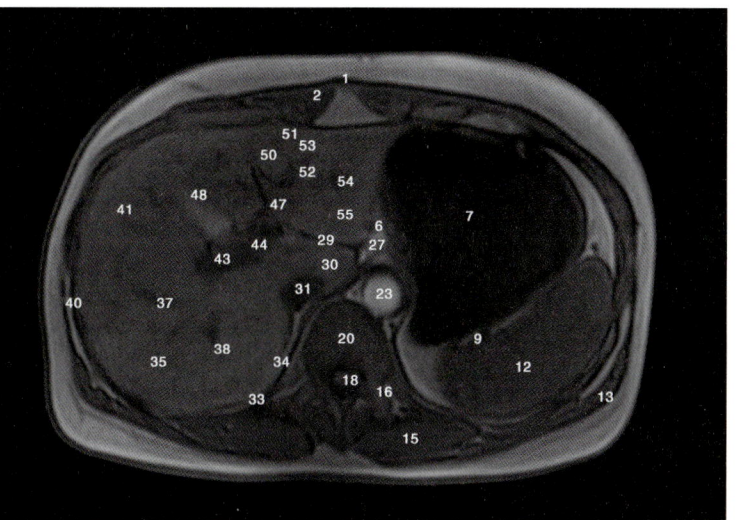

D. MR T1WI

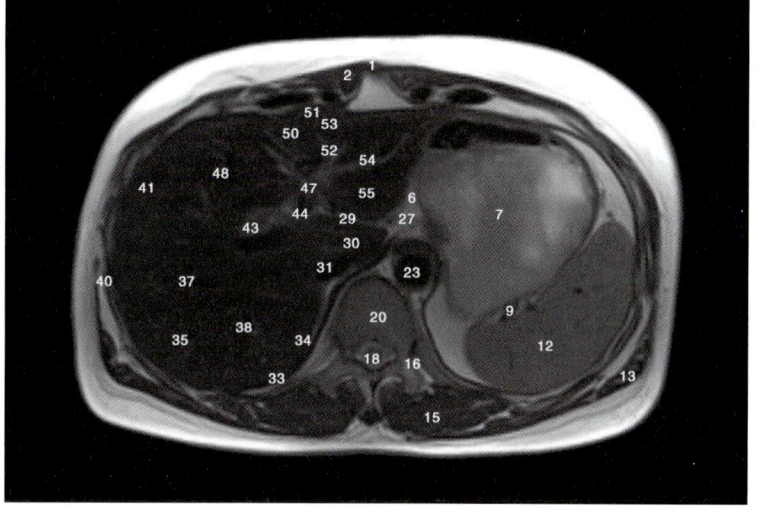

E. MR T2WI

关键结构：肝门静脉左支矢状部，左肾上极。

此断面经第11胸椎椎体下份。

左肾上极出现，位于脊柱左侧、左肾上腺后方。肝门静脉左支矢状部出现是本断面的重要特征。它标志着：①肝门已经出现或在下一个断层内出现；②肝圆韧带裂即将出现；③左叶间裂出现，其左侧为肝左外叶，右侧为肝左内叶；④肝左管内支的出现及肝管的合成，81%的肝左管内支经左支矢状部右侧上升，而肝左管在左支角部合成后一般沿横部往右。CT 平扫对肝脏的很多疾病鉴别能力较差，甚至可能造成误诊。如囊肿与血管瘤、血管瘤与肝癌、肝岛（弥漫性脂肪肝中残留的较正常肝组织）与肿瘤等，有时难以鉴别。而CT增强扫描可鉴别出大多数病变。例如在动态增强图像上，肝癌为"快进快出"，而肝血管瘤为"早出晚归"，囊肿则无强化。MRI 的多序列多参数扫描能提供更多的鉴别诊断信息，逐渐成为肝脏影像诊断的主力，尤其是 MR 肝特异性对比剂（钆塞酸二钠）的应用，显著提高了肝癌等疾病的诊断和鉴别诊断能力。

腹部连续横断层 31（FH.11310）

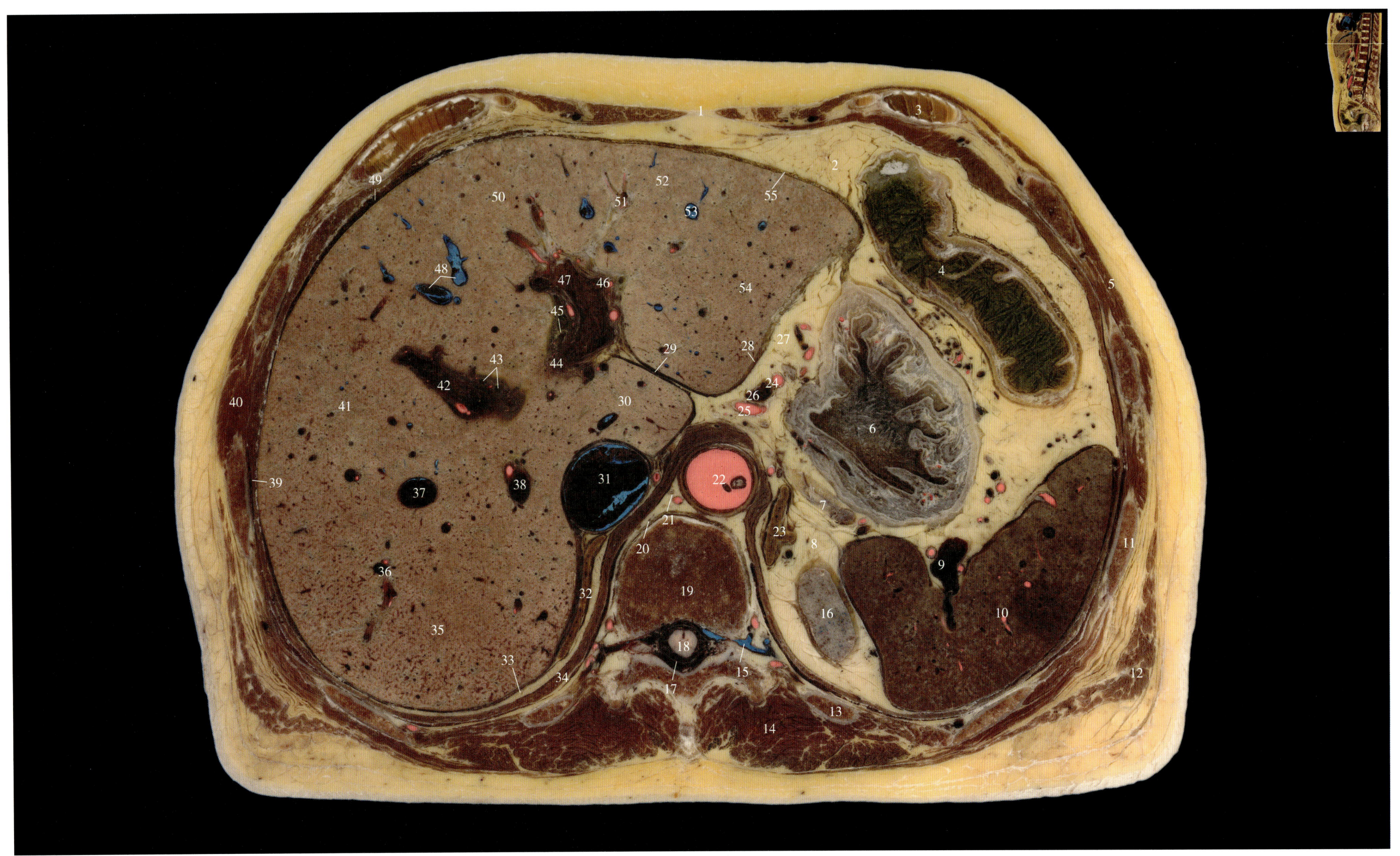

A. 断层标本图像

1. 腹白线 linea alba
2. 大网膜 greater omentum
3. 肋弓 costal arch
4. 横结肠 transverse colon
5. 腹外斜肌 obliquus externus abdominis
6. 胃 stomach
7. 脾动脉 splenic artery
8. 膈脾韧带 phrenicosplenic ligament
9. 脾静脉 splenic vein
10. 脾 spleen
11. 第9肋骨 9th costal bone
12. 背阔肌 latissimus dorsi
13. 第11肋骨 11th costal bone
14. 竖脊肌 erector spinae
15. 肋间后静脉 posterior intercostal vein
16. 左肾 left kidney
17. 硬脊膜 spinal dura matter
18. 脊髓 spinal cord
19. 第11胸椎椎体 body of 11th thoracic vertebra
20. 奇静脉 azygos vein
21. 胸导管 thoracic duct
22. 胸主动脉 thoracic aorta
23. 左肾上腺 left suprarenal gland
24. 胃动、静脉 gastric artery and vein
25. 胃左动脉 left gastric artery
26. 胃左静脉 left gastric vein
27. 小网膜 lesser omentum
28. 左肝下前间隙 anterior left subrahepatic space
29. 静脉韧带裂 fissure for ligamentum venosum
30. 肝尾状叶 caudate lobe of liver
31. 下腔静脉 inferior vena cava
32. 右肾上腺 right suprarenal gland
33. 肝裸区 bare area of liver
34. 膈 diaphragm
35. 肝右后叶上段 superior segment of right posterior lobe of liver
36. 肝门静脉右后上支及肝动脉 right posterosuperior branch of hepatic portal vein and corresponding hepatic artery
37. 肝右静脉 right hepatic vein
38. 肝门静脉右后支 right posterior branch of hepatic portal vein
39. 肋膈隐窝 costodiaphragmatic recess
40. 肋间外肌 intercostale externi
41. 肝右前叶上段 superior segment of right anterior lobe of liver
42. 肝门静脉右前支 right anterior branch of hepatic portal vein
43. 肝右管 right hepatic duct
44. 肝门静脉左支横部 transverse part of left hepatic portal vein
45. 肝左管 left hepatic duct
46. 肝门静脉左外下支及动脉、肝管 left lateroinferior branch of hepatic portal vein and corresponding artery and hepatic duct
47. 肝门静脉左支矢状部 sagittal part of left hepatic portal vein
48. 肝中静脉属支 tributary of middle hepatic vein
49. 右肝上间隙 right suprahepatic space
50. 肝左内叶 left medial lobe of liver
51. 肝门静脉左外下支 left lateroinferior branch of hepatic portal vein
52. 肝左外叶下段 inferior segment of left lateral lobe of liver
53. 肝左静脉 left hepatic vein
54. 肝左外叶上段 superior segment of left lateral lobe of liver
55. 左肝上前间隙 anterior left suprahepatic space

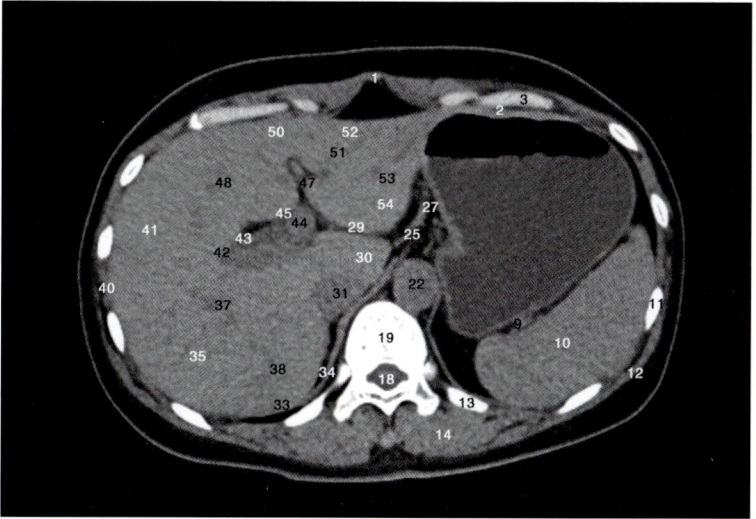

B. CT 平扫图像

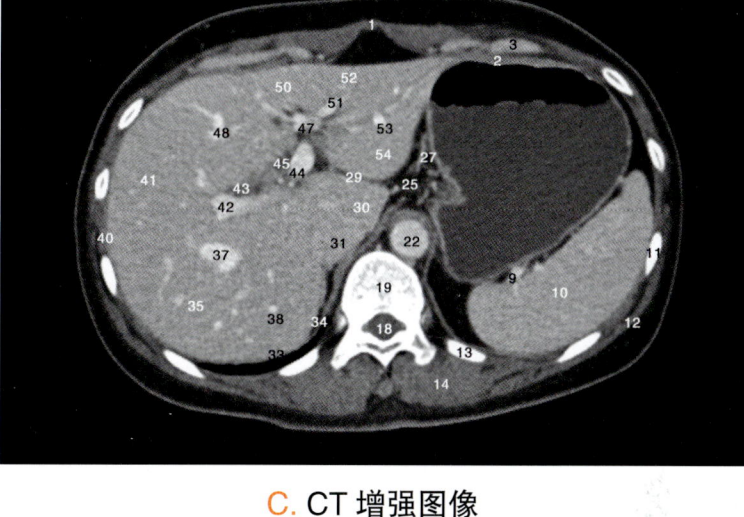

C. CT 增强图像

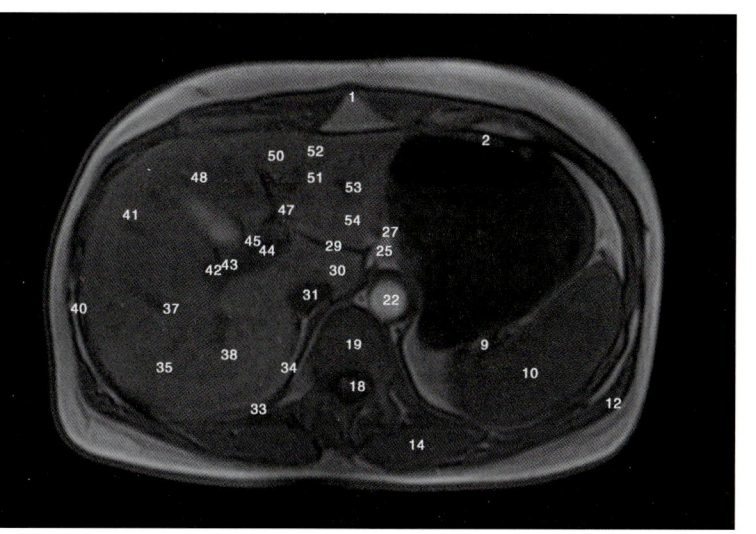

D. MR T1WI

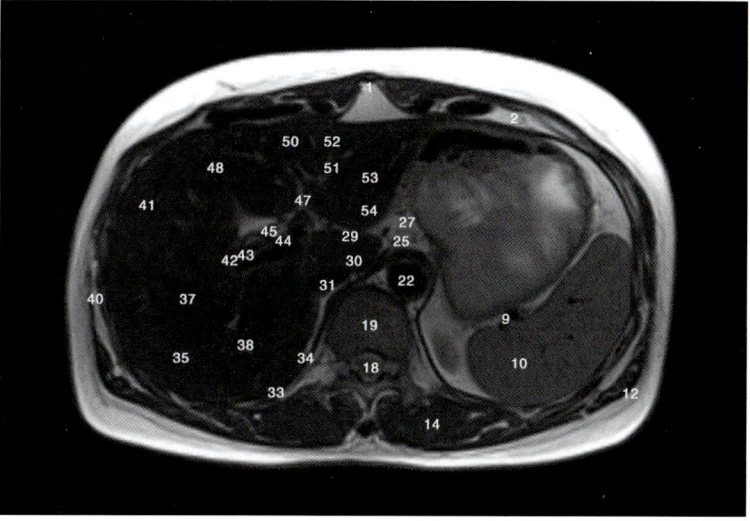

E. MR T2WI

关键结构：肋弓，左肾，脾动、静脉。

此断面经第11胸椎椎体下份。

脾门附近可见脾动、静脉，左肾位于左侧膈肌和脾之间。第8～10对肋骨不直接与胸骨相连，其前端借肋软骨和上位肋软骨连结，形成肋弓。肋弓常作为腹部触诊确定肝、脾大小的标志。肾脏为成对的扁豆状器官，呈红褐色，位于腹膜后脊柱两旁浅窝中，长10～12 cm、宽5～6 cm、厚3～4 cm、重120～150 g。左肾较右肾稍大，上端平第11胸椎下缘，下端平第2腰椎下缘。肾纵轴上端向内、下端向外，因此两肾上极相距较近，下极较远，肾纵轴与脊柱所成角度为30°左右[7]。肾和脾都是富血器官，其动静脉较为粗大，尤其是脾，有一定"血库"作用：当人体休息、安静时储存一定量血液，当运动、失血、缺氧等应激状态时，又将所储存血液排送到血循环中以增加血容量。脾质软而脆，当局部受暴力打击时易破裂出血。

腹部连续横断层 32（FH.11290）

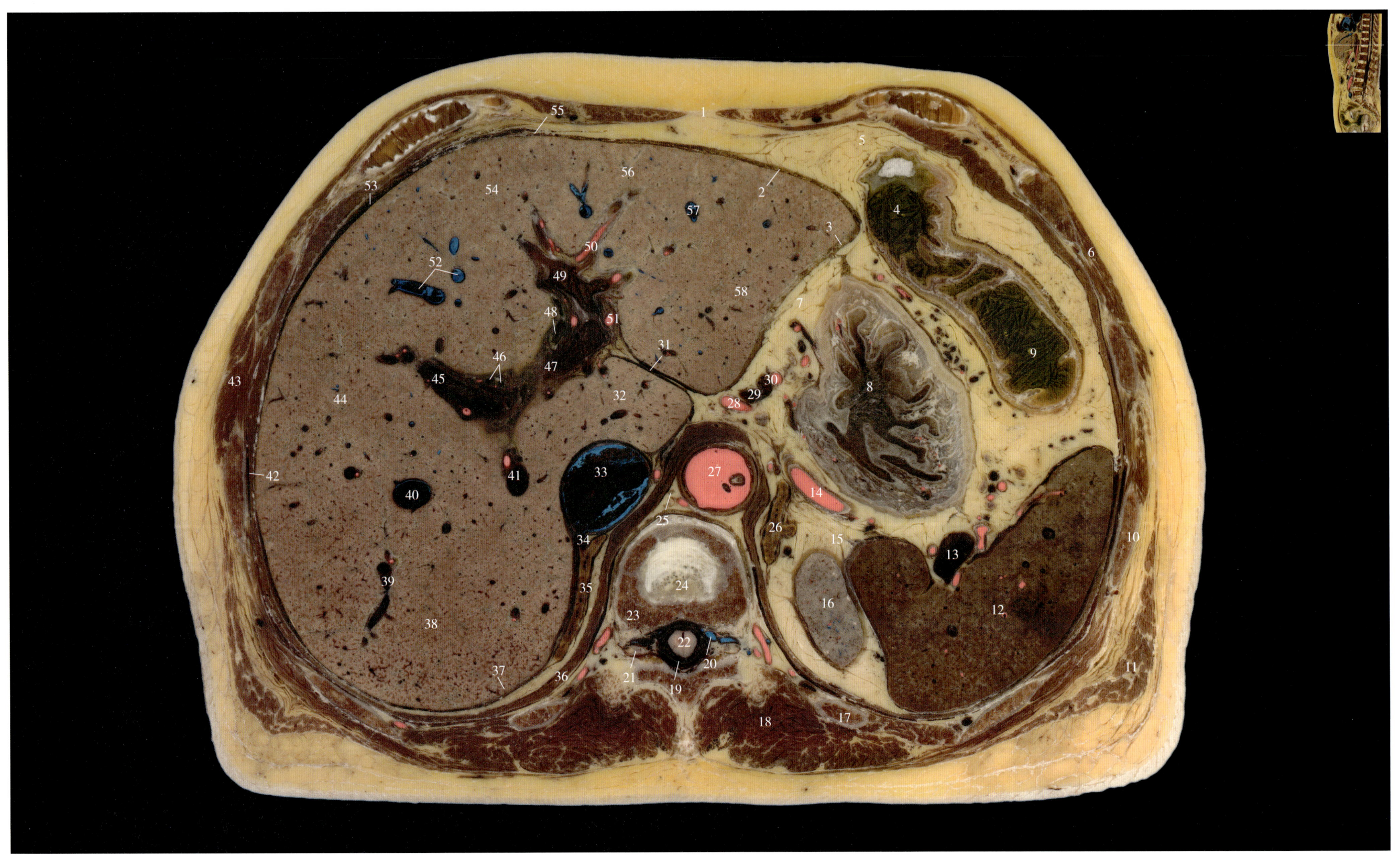

A. 断层标本图像

1. 腹白线 linea alba
2. 左肝上前间隙 anterior left suprahepatic space
3. 左肝下前间隙 anterior left subrahepatic space
4. 横结肠 transverse colon
5. 大网膜 greater omentum
6. 腹外斜肌 obliquus externus abdominis
7. 小网膜 lesser omentum
8. 胃 stomach
9. 降结肠 descending colon
10. 第 9 肋骨 9th costal bone
11. 背阔肌 latissimus dorsi
12. 脾 spleen
13. 脾静脉 splenic vein
14. 脾动脉 splenic artery
15. 膈韧带脾 phrenicosplenic ligament
16. 左肾 left kidney
17. 第 11 肋骨 11th costal bone
18. 竖脊肌 erector spinae
19. 硬脊膜 spinal dura matter
20. 椎内静脉丛 internal vertebral venous plexus
21. 脊神经根 spinal nerve root
22. 脊髓 spinal cord
23. 第 11 胸椎椎体 body of 11th thoracic vertebra
24. T11-12 椎间盘 T11-12 intervertebral disc
25. 胸导管 thoracic duct
26. 左肾上腺 left suprarenal gland
27. 胸主动脉 thoracic aorta
28. 胃左动脉 left gastric artery
29. 胃左静脉 left gastric vein
30. 胃动、静脉 gastric artery and vein
31. 静脉韧带裂 fissure for ligamentum venosum
32. 肝尾状叶 caudate lobe of liver
33. 下腔静脉 inferior vena cava
34. 副肝静脉 accessory hepatic veins
35. 右肾上腺 right suprarenal gland
36. 膈 diaphragm
37. 肝裸区 bare area of liver
38. 肝右后叶上段 superior segment of right posterior lobe of liver
39. 肝门静脉右后上支及肝动脉 right posterosuperior branch of hepatic portal vein and corresponding hepatic artery
40. 肝右静脉 right hepatic vein
41. 肝门静脉右后支 right posterior branch of hepatic portal vein
42. 肋膈隐窝 costodiaphragmatic recess
43. 肋间外肌 intercostale externi
44. 肝右前叶上段 superior segment of right anterior lobe of liver
45. 肝门静脉右前支 right anterior branch of hepatic portal vein
46. 肝右管 right hepatic duct
47. 肝门静脉左支横部 transverse part of left hepatic portal vein
48. 肝左管 left hepatic duct
49. 肝门静脉左支矢状部 sagittal part of left hepatic portal vein
50. 肝门静脉左外下支 left lateroinferior branch of hepatic portal vein
51. 肝门静脉左外上支及动脉、肝管 left laterosuperior branch of hepatic portal vein and corresponding artery and hepatic duct
52. 肝中静脉属支 tributary of middle hepatic vein
53. 右肝上间隙 right suprahepatic space
54. 肝左内叶 left medial lobe of liver
55. 肝镰状韧带 falciform ligament of liver
56. 肝左外叶下段 inferior segment of left lateral lobe of liver
57. 肝左静脉 left hepatic vein
58. 肝左外叶上段 superior segment of left lateral lobe of liver

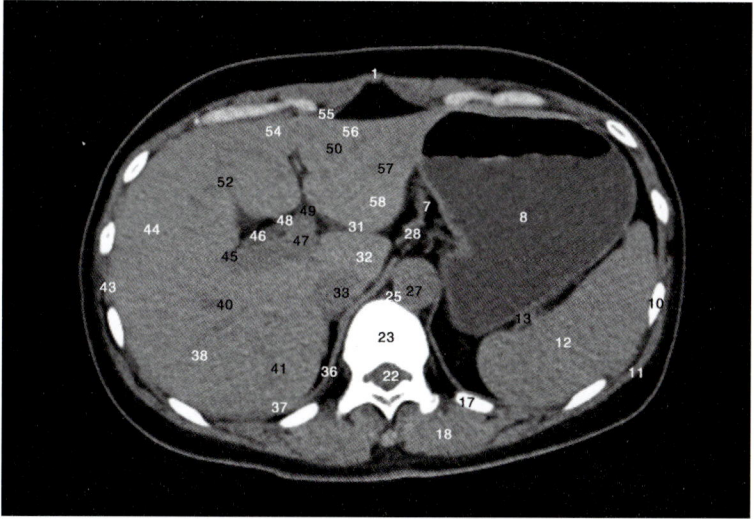

B. CT 平扫图像

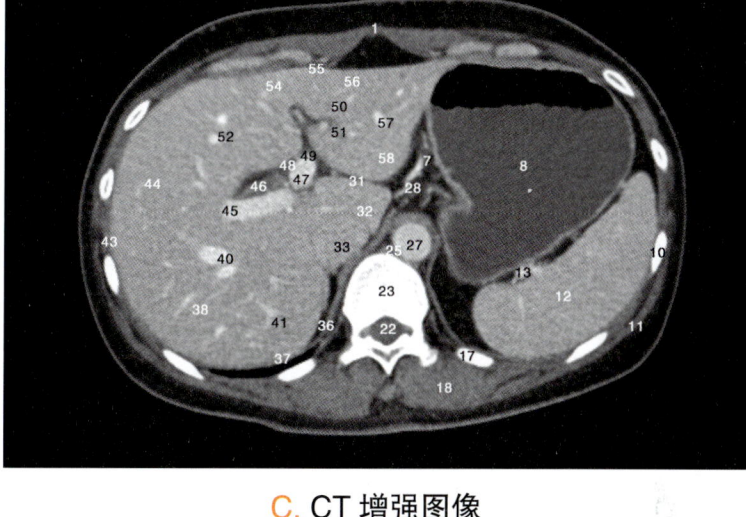

C. CT 增强图像

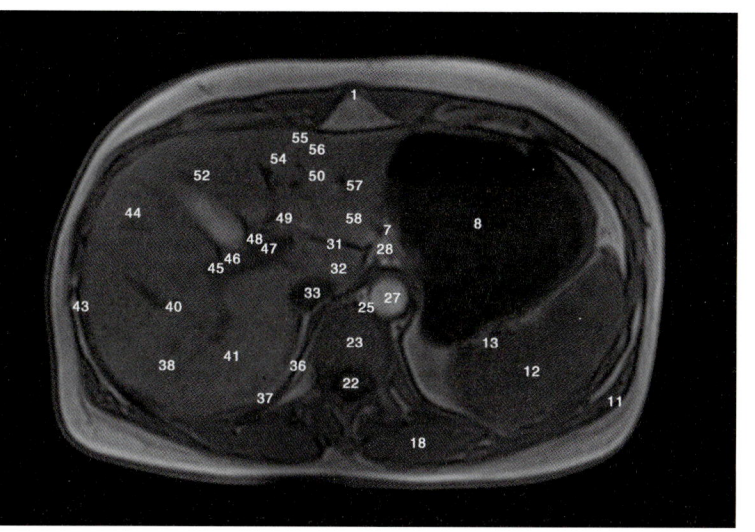

D. MR T1WI

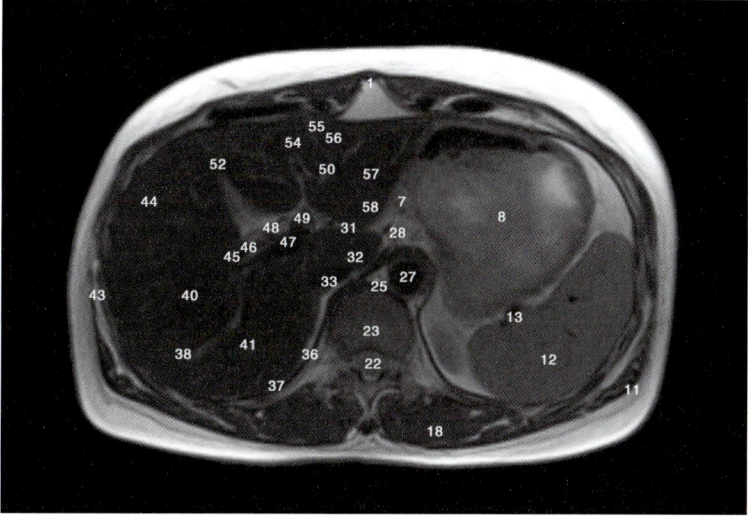

E. MR T2WI

关键结构：肝门静脉左支横部、矢状部，肝门静脉右支。

此断面经第 11 胸椎椎体下份。

切及肝门静脉左支横部和右支是本断面的特征，这也是肝门出现的标志。肝门静脉于下腔静脉前方的横沟内分出左支横部和右支主干，此分叉点多位于第 11、12 胸椎椎体水平。肝门静脉分叉点是识别肝门区结构和肝分叶分段的重要标志，通常行于下腔静脉的前方或稍偏右，二者隔以肝尾状突。原发性肝癌可并发肝门静脉癌栓，这是影响预后的一个极为重要的因素。超声、CT、MRI 等对肝门静脉癌栓的检出率都较高。并发肝门静脉癌栓的肝癌，因门脉压力升高、侧支循环所致食管胃底静脉曲张破裂出血的发生率增高。在治疗方面可行扩大肝叶切除、肝门静脉切开取栓、介入化疗等，但预后不良。

腹部连续横断层 33（FH.11270）

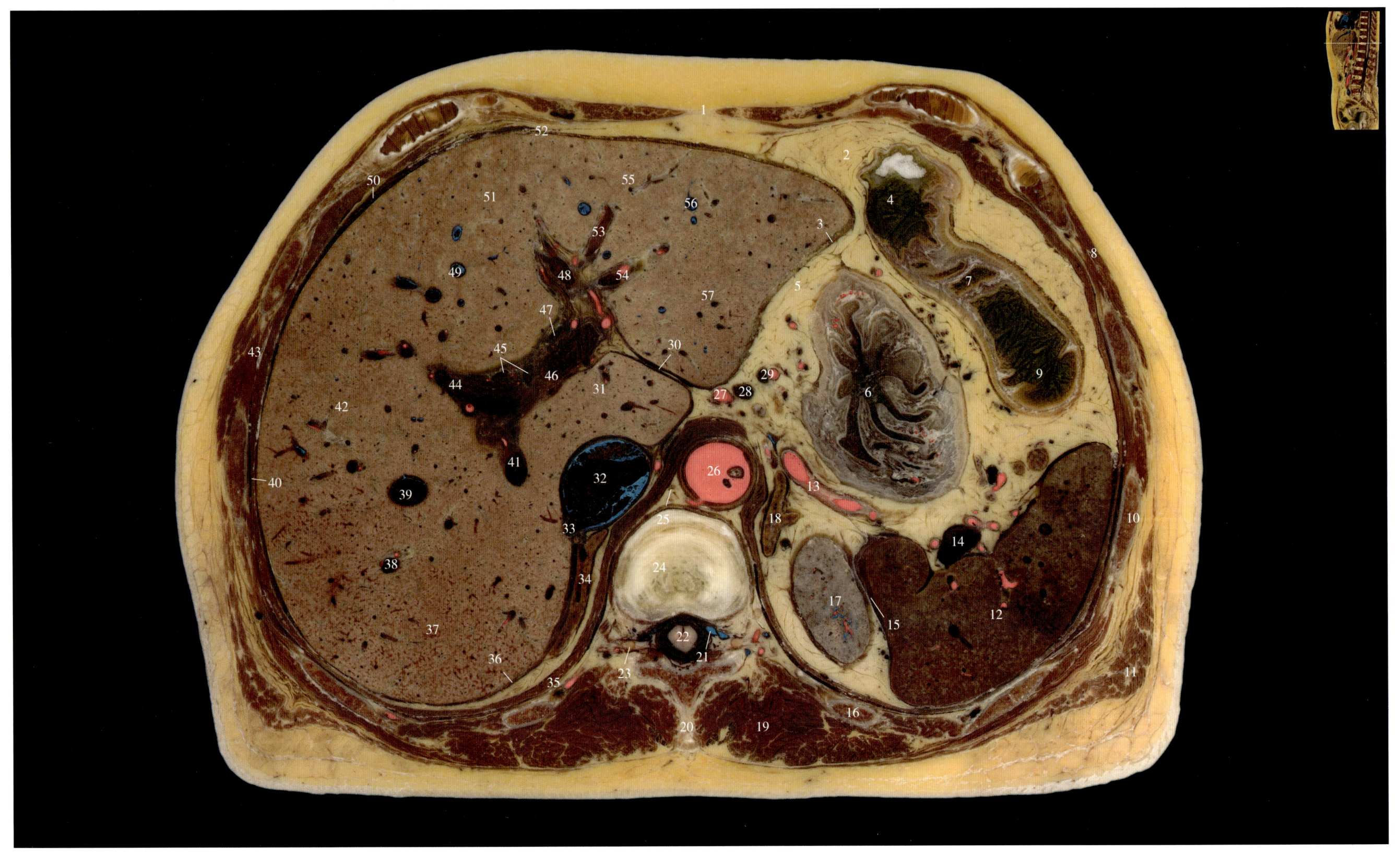

A. 断层标本图像

1. 腹白线 linea alba
2. 大网膜 greater omentum
3. 左肝下前间隙 anterior left subrahepatic space
4. 横结肠 transverse colon
5. 小网膜 lesser omentum
6. 胃 stomach
7. 结肠左曲 left colic flexure
8. 腹外斜肌 obliquus externus abdominis
9. 降结肠 descending colon
10. 第9肋骨 9th costal bone
11. 背阔肌 latissimus dorsi
12. 脾 spleen
13. 脾动脉 splenic artery
14. 脾静脉 splenic vein
15. 脾肾隐窝 splenorenal recess
16. 第11肋骨 11th costal bone
17. 左肾 left kidney
18. 左肾上腺 left suprarenal gland
19. 竖脊肌 erector spinae
20. 棘间韧带 interspinous ligament
21. 椎内静脉丛 internal vertebral venous plexus
22. 脊髓 spinal cord
23. 脊神经根 spinal nerve root
24. T11-12椎间盘 T11-12 intervertebral disc
25. 胸导管 thoracic duct
26. 胸主动脉 thoracic aorta
27. 胃左动脉 left gastric artery
28. 胃左静脉 left gastric vein
29. 胃动、静脉 gastric artery and vein
30. 静脉韧带裂 fissure for ligamentum venosum
31. 肝尾状叶 caudate lobe of liver
32. 下腔静脉 inferior vena cava
33. 副肝静脉 accessory hepatic veins
34. 右肾上腺 right suprarenal gland
35. 膈 diaphragm
36. 肝裸区 bare area of liver
37. 肝右后叶上段 superior segment of right posterior lobe of liver
38. 肝门静脉右后上支及肝动脉 right posterosuperior branch of hepatic portal vein and corresponding hepatic artery
39. 肝右静脉 right hepatic vein
40. 肋膈隐窝 costodiaphragmatic recess
41. 肝门静脉右后支 right posterior branch of hepatic portal vein
42. 肝右前叶上段 superior segment of right anterior lobe of liver
43. 肋间外肌 intercostale externi
44. 肝门静脉右前支 right anterior branch of hepatic portal vein
45. 肝右管 right hepatic duct
46. 肝门静脉左支横部 transverse part of left hepatic portal vein
47. 肝左管 left hepatic duct
48. 肝门静脉左支矢状部 sagittal part of left hepatic portal vein
49. 肝中静脉属支 tributary of middle hepatic vein
50. 右肝上间隙 right suprahepatic space
51. 肝左内叶 left medial lobe of liver
52. 肝镰状韧带 falciform ligament of liver
53. 肝门静脉左外下支 left lateroinferior branch of hepatic portal vein
54. 肝门静脉左外下支及动脉、肝管 left lateroinferior branch of hepatic portal vein and corresponding artery and hepatic duct
55. 肝左外叶下段 inferior segment of left lateral lobe of liver
56. 肝左静脉 left hepatic vein
57. 肝左外叶上段 superior segment of left lateral lobe of liver

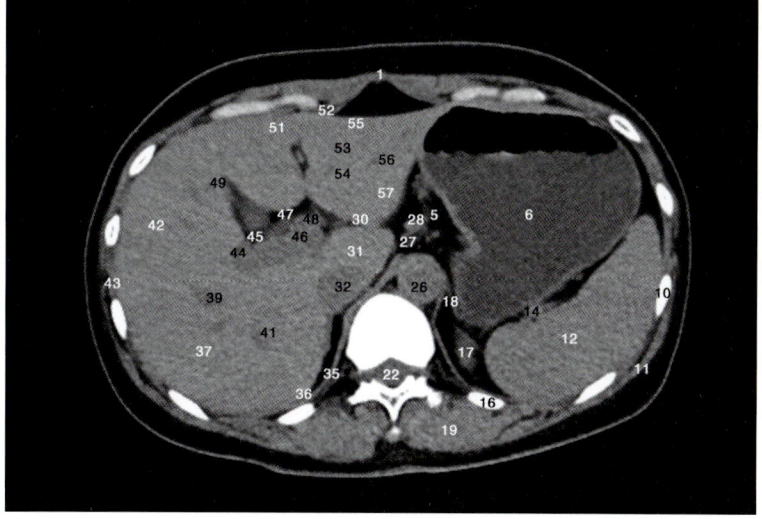

B. CT 平扫图像

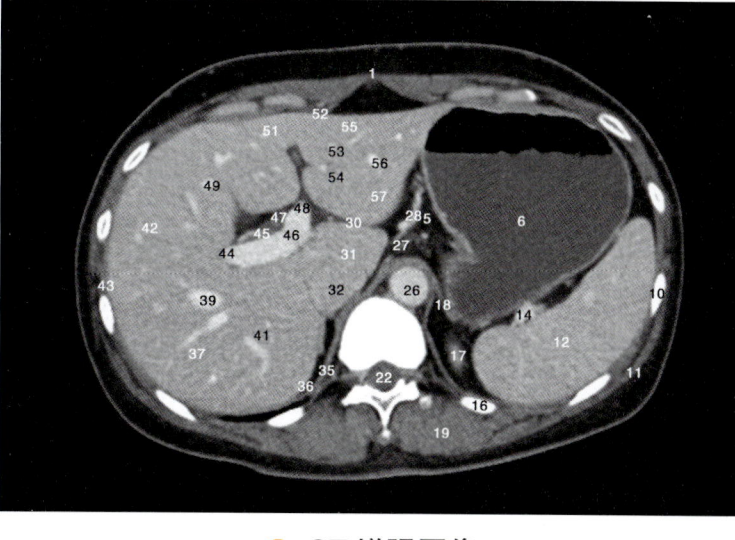

C. CT 增强图像

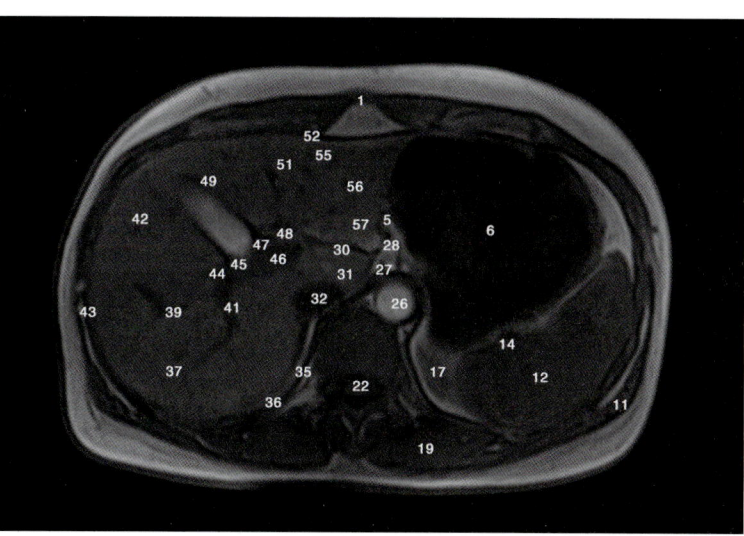

D. MR T1WI

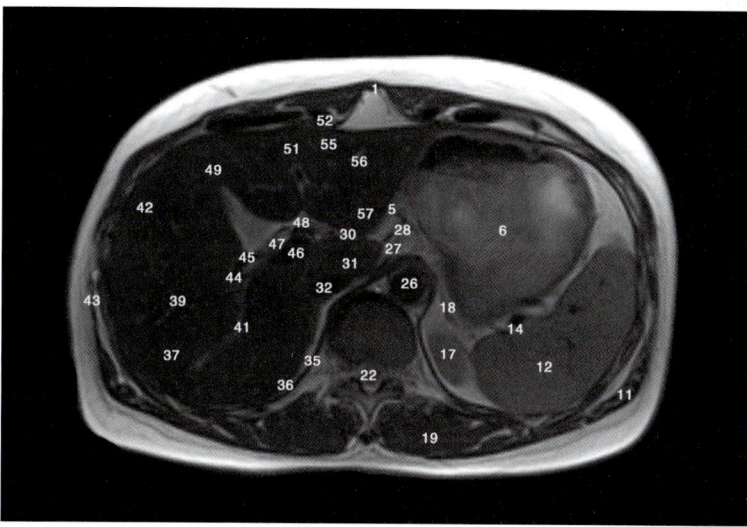

E. MR T2WI

关键结构：肝门平面，肝门静脉右前支，肝门静脉右后支。

此断面经 T11-12 椎间盘。

肝门区结构清晰可见，包括肝门静脉左支横部、矢状部，肝门静脉右支及其发出的右前支和右后支。肝门平面具有重要的标志性意义：①是腹腔结构配布发生较大变化的转折平面，平面以上的腹腔结构配布相对简单，自右向左主要为肝、胃和脾，平面以下的腹腔结构渐多且配布复杂；②该平面下方的第一个断面往往是胆囊、左肾、胰体和网膜孔等结构首次出现的层面；③往下肝的断面逐渐变小，肝内管道明显变细；④为右段间裂的标志平面；⑤是第三肝门的标志平面，肝右后下静脉多位于此层面或其上、下层面，出肝注入下腔静脉；⑥是识别肝左、右管的关键平面，肝门静脉分叉处的前方可见肝左、右管，常用来判断肝内胆管是否扩张。肝门是肝脏最重要的门户性结构，肝门区有肝固有动脉、门静脉、胆管系统共同构成的 Glisson 管道系统，还有淋巴管和神经等。肝门静脉由左下向右上进入肝脏，分支为左支和右支。肝左管、肝右管汇合成肝总管，肝总管和胆囊管汇合成胆总管。

67

腹部连续横断层 34 (FH.11250)

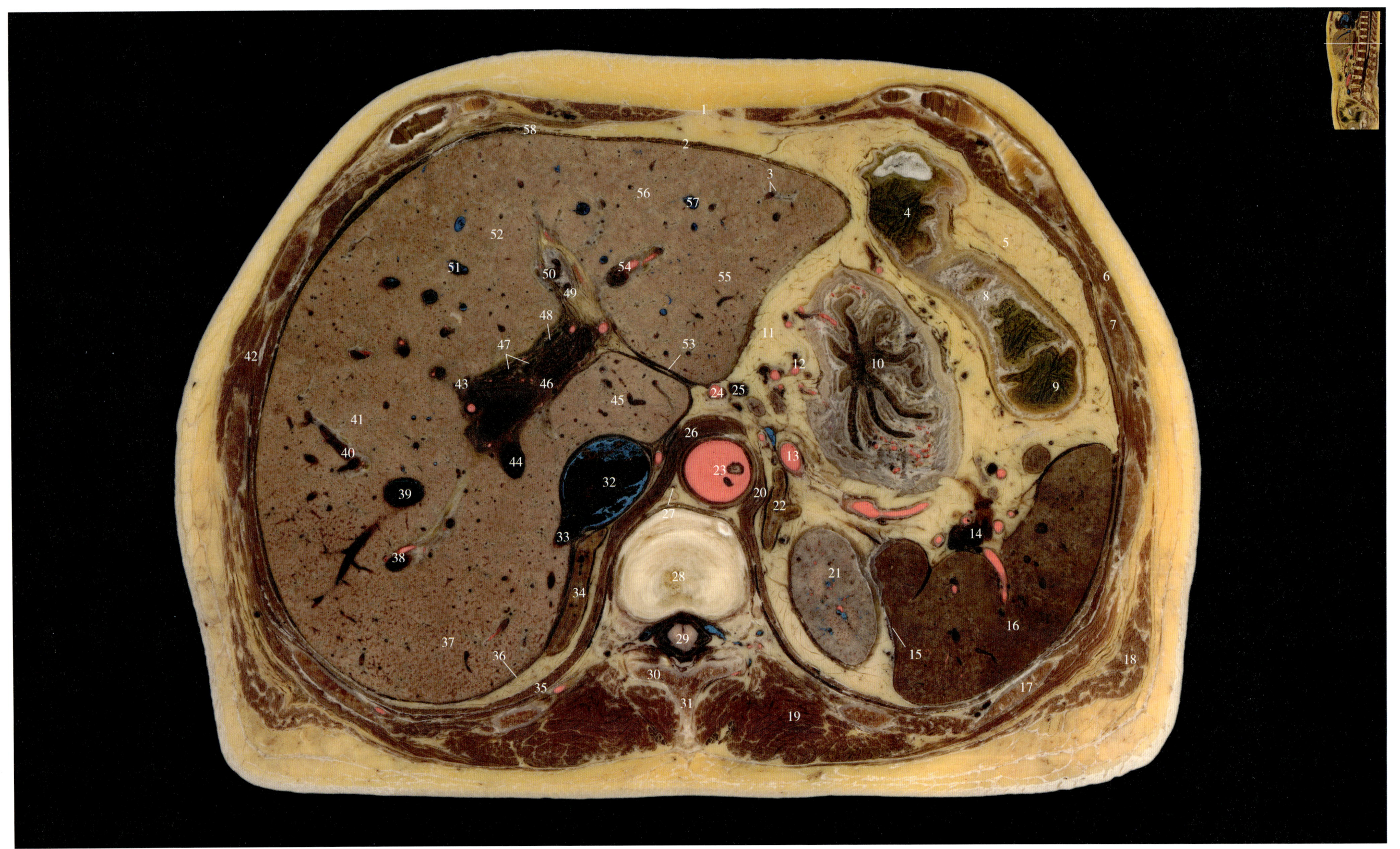

A. 断层标本图像

1. 腹白线 linea alba
2. 左肝上前间隙 anterior left suprahepatic space
3. 肝门静脉左外上支及肝动脉 left laterosuperior branch of hepatic portal vein and corresponding hepatic artery
4. 横结肠 transverse colon
5. 大网膜 greater omentum
6. 腹外斜肌 obliquus externus abdominis
7. 第 8 肋骨 8th costal bone
8. 结肠左曲 left colic flexure
9. 降结肠 descending colon
10. 胃 stomach
11. 小网膜 lesser omentum
12. 胃动、静脉 gastric artery and vein
13. 脾动脉 splenic artery
14. 脾静脉 splenic vein
15. 脾肾隐窝 splenorenal recess
16. 脾 spleen
17. 第 10 肋骨 10th costal bone
18. 背阔肌 latissimus dorsi
19. 竖脊肌 erector spinae
20. 左膈脚 left crus of diaphragm
21. 左肾 left kidney
22. 左肾上腺 left suprarenal gland
23. 胸主动脉 thoracic aorta
24. 胃左动脉 left gastric artery
25. 胃左静脉 left gastric vein
26. 右膈脚 right crus of diaphragm
27. 胸导管 thoracic duct
28. T11-12 椎间盘 T11-12 intervertebral disc
29. 脊髓 spinal cord
30. 第 12 胸椎横突 transverse process of 12th thoracic vertebra
31. 第 12 胸椎棘突 spinous process of 12th thoracic vertebra
32. 下腔静脉 inferior vena cava
33. 副肝静脉 accessory hepatic veins
34. 右肾上腺 right suprarenal gland
35. 膈 diaphragm
36. 肝裸区 bare area of liver
37. 肝右后叶上段 superior segment of right posterior lobe of liver
38. 肝门静脉右后上支及肝动脉 right posterosuperior branch of hepatic portal vein and corresponding hepatic artery
39. 肝右静脉 right hepatic vein
40. 肝门静脉右前支及动脉 right anterior branch of hepatic portal vein and corresponding artery
41. 肝右前叶上段 superior segment of right anterior lobe of liver
42. 肋间外肌 intercostale externi
43. 肝门静脉右前支 right anterior branch of hepatic portal vein
44. 肝门静脉右后支 right posterior branch of hepatic portal vein
45. 肝尾状叶 caudate lobe of liver
46. 肝门静脉左支横部 transverse part of left hepatic portal vein
47. 肝右管 right hepatic duct
48. 肝左管 left hepatic duct
49. 肝门静脉左支矢状部 sagittal part of left hepatic portal vein
50. 肝门静脉左内叶支 left medial branch of hepatic portal vein
51. 肝中静脉属支 tributary of middle hepatic vein
52. 肝左内叶 left medial lobe of liver
53. 静脉韧带裂 fissure for ligamentum venosum
54. 肝门静脉左外下支及动脉、肝管 left lateroinferior branch of hepatic portal vein and corresponding artery and hepatic duct
55. 肝左外叶上段 superior segment of left lateral lobe of liver
56. 肝左外叶下段 inferior segment of left lateral lobe of liver
57. 肝左静脉 left hepatic vein
58. 肝镰状韧带 falciform ligament of liver

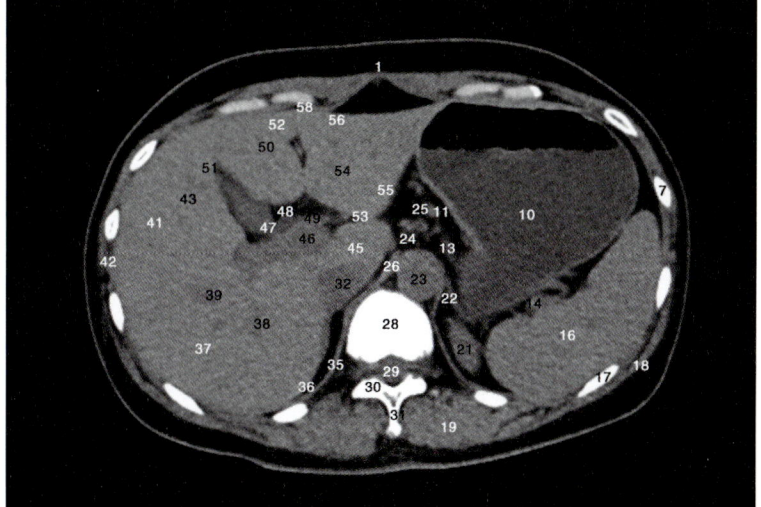

B. CT 平扫图像　　　　C. CT 增强图像

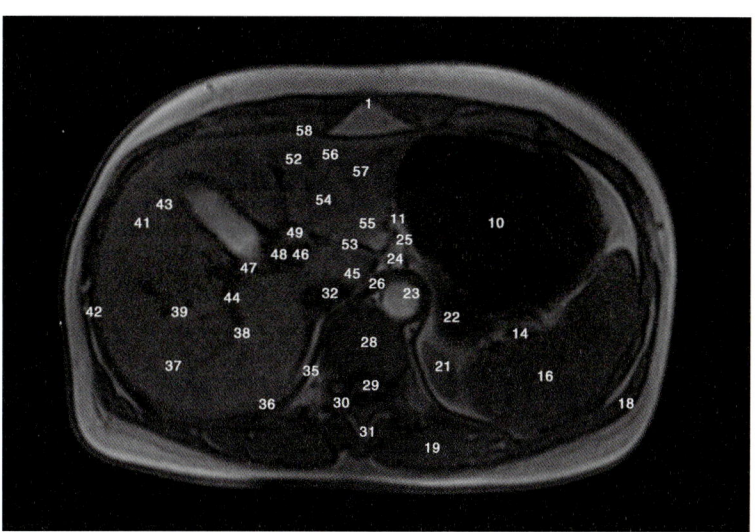

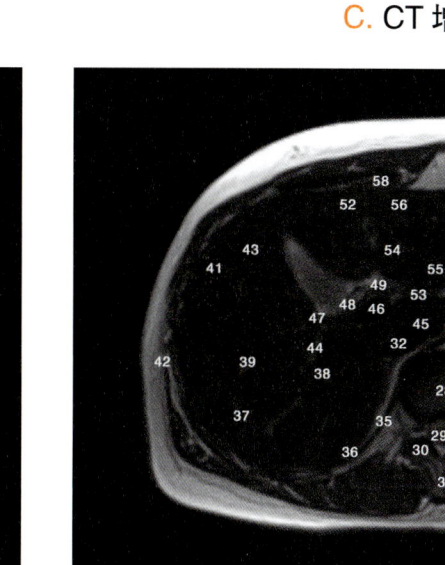

D. MR T1WI　　　　E. MR T2WI

关键结构：肝门静脉左内叶支，肝左、右管。

此断面经 T11-12 椎间盘。

肝门静脉左内叶支从囊部发出，肝左、右管位于肝门静脉前方。左外叶所产生的胆汁由左外上、下段肝管引流，49% 的左外下段肝管经肝门静脉左支矢状部左份深面上行至角部深面，与左外上段肝管汇合成左外叶肝管。左外叶肝管经肝门静脉左支角部凹侧或深面同左内叶肝管合成肝左管。81% 的左内叶肝管沿肝门静脉左支矢状部右侧上升，而肝左管一般沿肝门静脉左支横部方叶侧缘或前上方往右行。肝左管主要引流左半肝的胆汁。右前叶肝管由右前上、下段肝管汇合而成，大部分行经肝门静脉右前支根部左侧（62%）或深面（25%）。右后叶肝管由右后上、下段肝管汇合而成，大部分位于肝门静脉右后支上方，越过肝门静脉右支分叉处或肝门静脉右前支起始部深面，至肝门静脉右支的前上方，再与右前叶肝管合成肝右管。肝右管主要引流右半肝的胆汁。肝内胆管细胞癌是发病率仅次于肝细胞肝癌的原发恶性肿瘤，近年来发病率呈上升趋势，早期一般无症状，进展期可出现持续的梗阻性黄疸或胆管炎性症状。该病恶性程度高，预后与其大体分型相关，管周浸润型预后最差，肿块型次之，管内生长型预后较好。总体而言，胆管细胞癌的预后远不及肝细胞肝癌。尾状叶肝管可汇入肝左、右管及肝左、右管汇合处，但以汇入肝左管为主（47%）。尾状叶胆汁的这种混合性引流特点，致使肝门区胆管细胞癌常侵及尾状叶，故该区胆管细胞癌的根治应常规切除尾状叶。

69

腹部连续横断层 35（FH.11230）

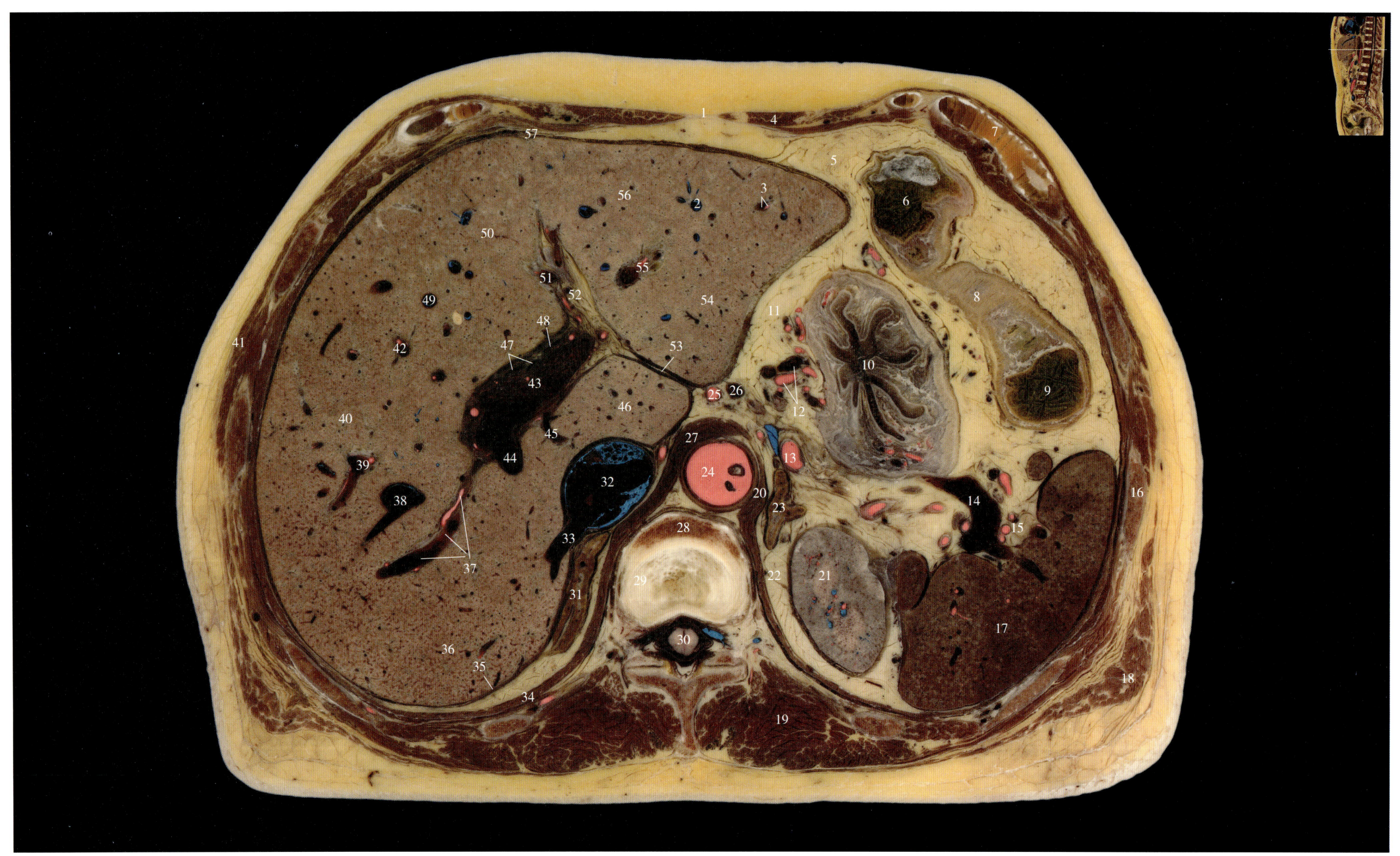

A. 断层标本图像

1. 腹白线 linea alba
2. 肝左静脉 left hepatic vein
3. 肝门静脉左外上支及肝动脉 left laterosuperior branch of hepatic portal vein and corresponding hepatic artery
4. 腹直肌 rectus abdominis
5. 大网膜 greater omentum
6. 横结肠 transverse colon
7. 第7肋软骨 7th costal cartilage
8. 结肠左曲 left colic flexure
9. 降结肠 descending colon
10. 胃 stomach
11. 小网膜 lesser omentum
12. 胃动、静脉 gastric artery and vein
13. 脾动脉 splenic artery
14. 脾静脉 splenic vein
15. 脾门 hilum of spleen
16. 第9肋骨 9th costal bone
17. 脾 spleen
18. 背阔肌 latissimus dorsi
19. 竖脊肌 erector spinae
20. 左膈脚 left crus of diaphragm
21. 左肾 left kidney
22. 左肾上腺三角 left adrenal triangle
23. 左肾上腺 left suprarenal gland
24. 胸主动脉 thoracic aorta
25. 胃左动脉 left gastric artery
26. 胃左静脉 left gastric vein
27. 右膈脚 right crus of diaphragm
28. 第12胸椎椎体 body of 12th thoracic vertebra
29. T11-12椎间盘 T11-12 intervertebral disc
30. 脊髓 spinal cord
31. 右肾上腺 right suprarenal gland
32. 下腔静脉 inferior vena cava
33. 副肝静脉 accessory hepatic veins
34. 膈 diaphragm
35. 肝裸区 bare area of liver
36. 肝右后叶上段 superior segment of right posterior lobe of liver
37. 肝门静脉右后上支及肝动脉 right posterosuperior branch of hepatic portal vein and corresponding hepatic artery
38. 肝右静脉 right hepatic vein
39. 肝门静脉右前支及动脉 right anterior branch of hepatic portal vein and corresponding artery
40. 肝右前叶上段 superior segment of right anterior lobe of liver
41. 肋间外肌 intercostale externi
42. 肝门静脉右前支 right anterior branch of hepatic portal vein
43. 肝门静脉左支横部 transverse part of left hepatic portal vein
44. 肝门静脉右后支 right posterior branch of hepatic portal vein
45. 肝门静脉尾状叶支 caudate branch of hepatic portal vein
46. 肝尾状叶 caudate lobe of liver
47. 肝右管 right hepatic duct
48. 肝左管 left hepatic duct
49. 肝中静脉属支 tributary of middle hepatic vein
50. 肝内叶 left medial lobe of liver
51. 肝门静脉内叶支 left medial branch of hepatic portal vein
52. 肝门静脉左支矢状部 sagittal part of left hepatic portal vein
53. 静脉韧带裂 fissure for ligamentum venosum
54. 肝左外叶上段 superior segment of left lateral lobe of liver
55. 肝门静脉左外下支及动脉、肝管 left lateroinferior branch of hepatic portal vein and corresponding artery and hepatic duct
56. 肝左外叶下段 inferior segment of left lateral lobe of liver
57. 肝镰状韧带 falciform ligament of liver

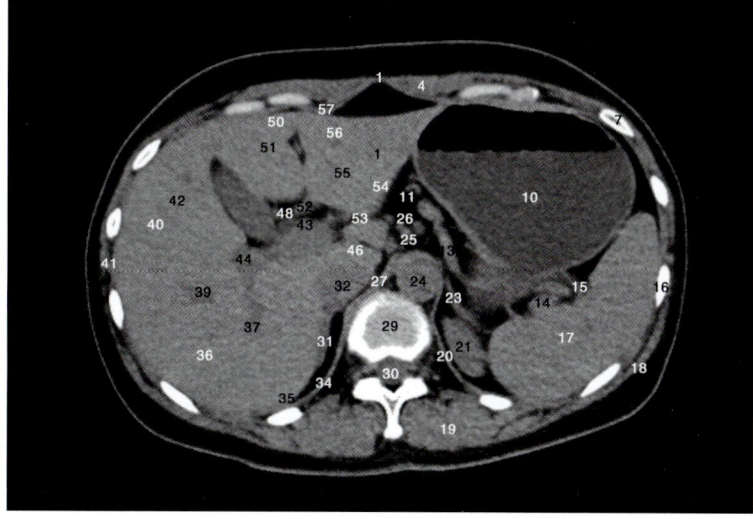

B. CT 平扫图像

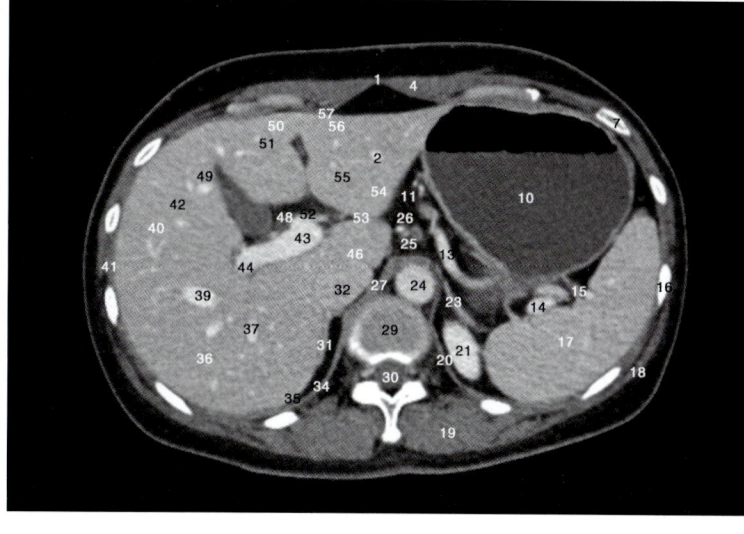

C. CT 增强图像

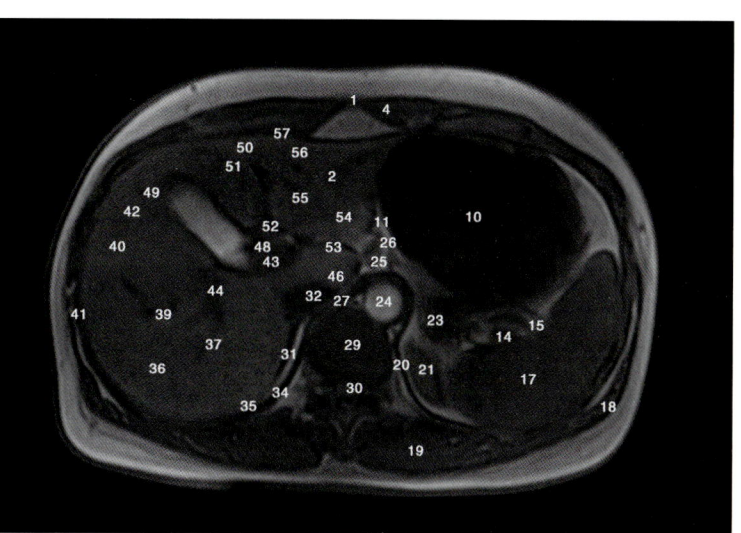

D. MR T1WI

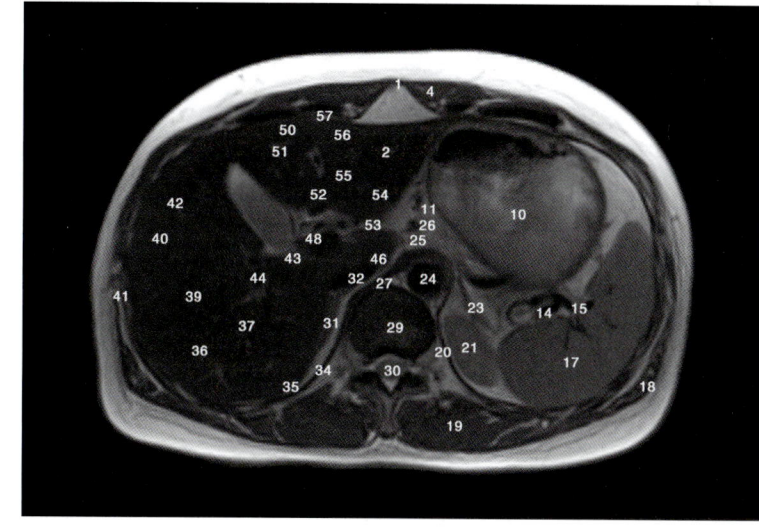

E. MR T2WI

关键结构：降结肠，结肠左曲。

此断面经 T11-12 椎间盘。

肝内结构与上一断面相似，胃左前方的大网膜内可见横结肠、结肠左曲和降结肠。结肠左曲又称脾曲，横结肠起始于结肠右曲后先行向左前下方，后略转向左后上方，至脾脏面下转折成的弯曲称结肠左曲，其位置较结肠右曲高。结肠左曲综合征指结肠左曲处的弯曲部积聚过多的气体或粪便引起腹胀、腹痛及顽固性不全结肠梗阻的一种临床综合征。本征与痉挛性结肠功能紊乱性疾病类似，是一种精神躯体性疾病，多见于神经官能症和自主神经功能失调者。降结肠始于结肠左曲，沿腹腔左外侧贴腹后壁下行，至左髂嵴处续于乙状结肠。降结肠长25~30 cm，内侧为左结肠系膜窦及空肠袢，外侧为左结肠旁沟。由于左膈结肠韧带的阻隔，左结肠旁沟内的积液只能向下流入盆腔。在儿童，有一种较常见的结肠相关的先天性疾病—先天性巨结肠，又称希尔施普龙病（Hirschsprung disease），是由于结肠缺乏神经节细胞导致肠管持续痉挛，粪便淤滞于近端结肠，近端结肠肥厚、扩张，病因尚未完全清楚，多认为与遗传有密切关系。

腹部连续横断层 36（FH.11210）

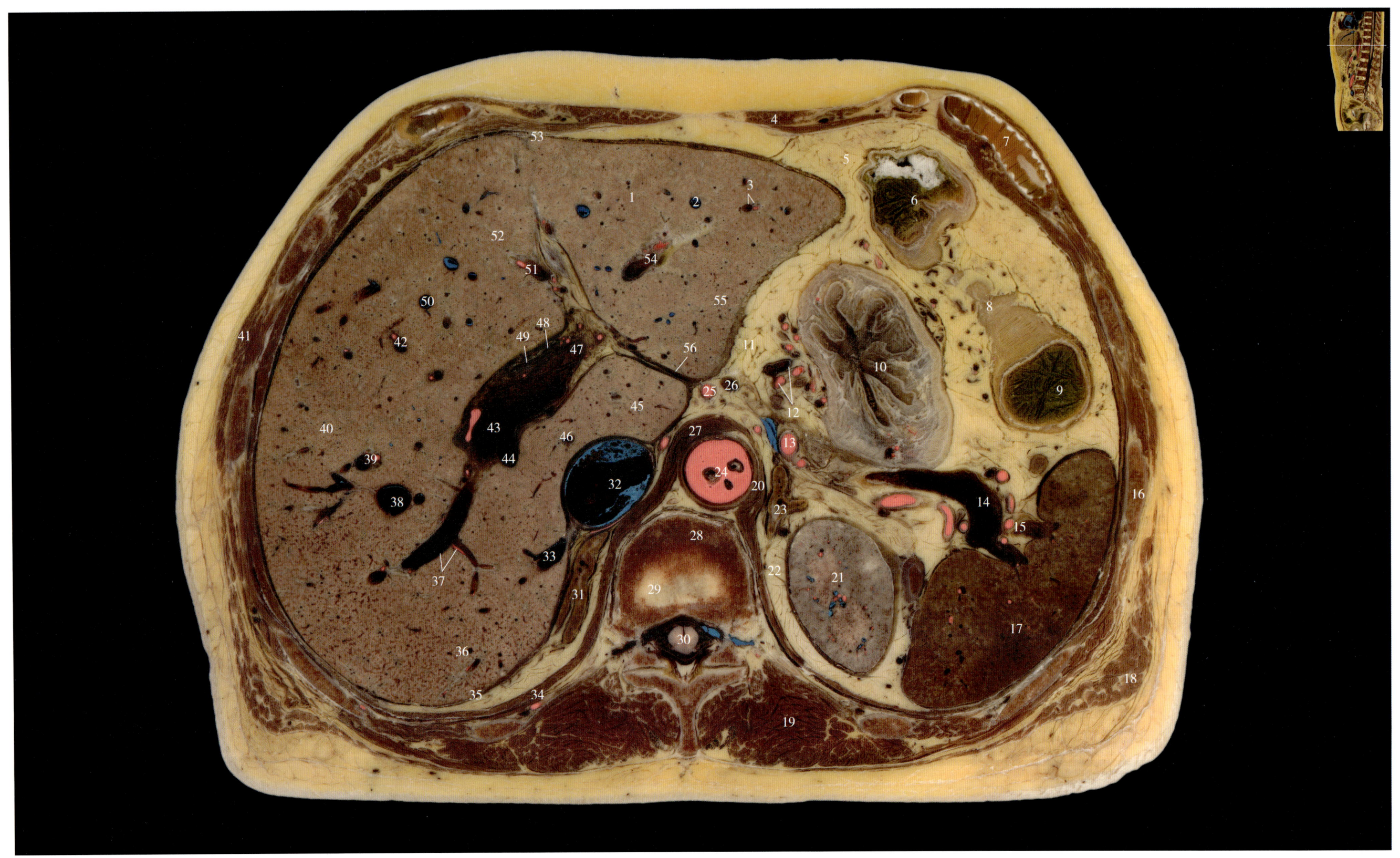

A. 断层标本图像

1. 肝左外叶下段 inferior segment of left lateral lobe of liver
2. 肝左静脉 left hepatic vein
3. 肝门静脉左外上支及肝动脉 left laterosuperior branch of hepatic portal vein and corresponding hepatic artery
4. 腹直肌 rectus abdominis
5. 大网膜 greater omentum
6. 横结肠 transverse colon
7. 第 7 肋软骨 7th costal cartilage
8. 结肠左曲 left colic flexure
9. 降结肠 descending colon
10. 胃 stomach
11. 肝胃韧带 hepatogastric ligament
12. 胃动、静脉 gastric artery and vein
13. 脾动脉 splenic artery
14. 脾静脉 splenic vein
15. 脾门 hilum of spleen
16. 第 9 肋骨 9th costal bone
17. 脾 spleen
18. 背阔肌 latissimus dorsi
19. 竖脊肌 erector spinae
20. 左膈脚 left crus of diaphragm
21. 左肾 left kidney
22. 左肾上腺三角 left adrenal triangle
23. 左肾上腺 left suprarenal gland
24. 胸主动脉 thoracic aorta
25. 胃左动脉 left gastric artery
26. 胃左静脉 left gastric vein
27. 右膈脚 right crus of diaphragm
28. 第 12 胸椎椎体 body of 12th thoracic vertebra
29. T11-12 椎间盘 T11-12 intervertebral disc
30. 脊髓 spinal cord
31. 右肾上腺 right suprarenal gland
32. 下腔静脉 inferior vena cava
33. 副肝静脉 accessory hepatic veins
34. 膈 diaphragm
35. 肝裸区 bare area of liver
36. 肝右后叶上段 superior segment of right posterior lobe of liver
37. 肝门静脉右后上支及肝动脉 right posterosuperior branch of hepatic portal vein and corresponding hepatic artery
38. 肝右静脉 right hepatic vein
39. 肝门静脉右前支及动脉 right anterior branch of hepatic portal vein and corresponding artery
40. 肝右前叶上段 superior segment of right anterior lobe of liver
41. 肋间外肌 intercostale externi
42. 肝门静脉右前支 right anterior branch of hepatic portal vein
43. 肝门静脉右支 right hepatic portal vein
44. 肝门静脉右后支 right posterior branch of hepatic portal vein
45. 肝尾状叶 caudate lobe of liver
46. 肝门静脉尾状叶支 caudate branch of hepatic portal vein
47. 肝门静脉左支横部 transverse part of left hepatic portal vein
48. 肝左管 left hepatic duct
49. 肝右管 right hepatic duct
50. 肝中静脉属支 tributary of middle hepatic vein
51. 肝门静脉左内叶支 left medial branch of hepatic portal vein
52. 肝左内叶 left medial lobe of liver
53. 肝镰状韧带 falciform ligament of liver
54. 肝门静脉左外下支及动脉、肝管 left lateroinferior branch of hepatic portal vein and corresponding artery and hepatic duct
55. 肝左外叶上段 superior segment of left lateral lobe of liver
56. 静脉韧带裂 fissure for ligamentum venosum

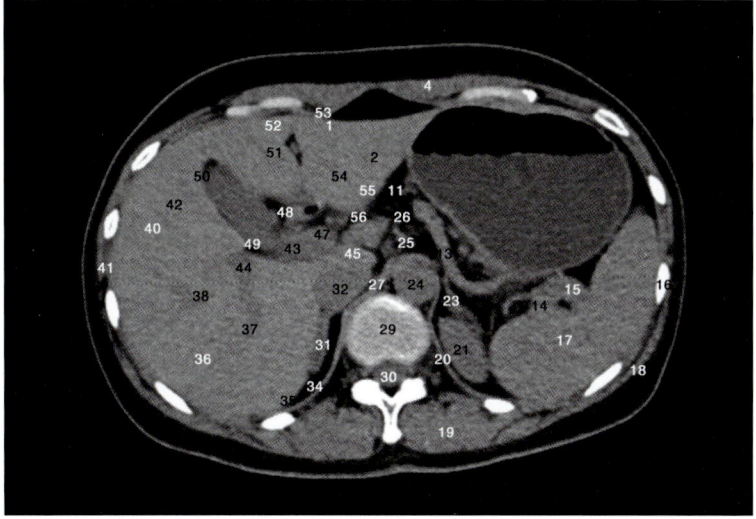

B. CT 平扫图像　　　　C. CT 增强图像

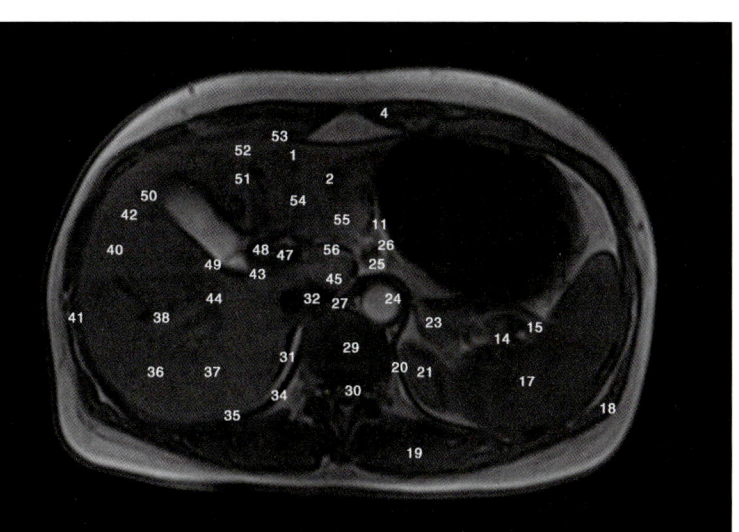

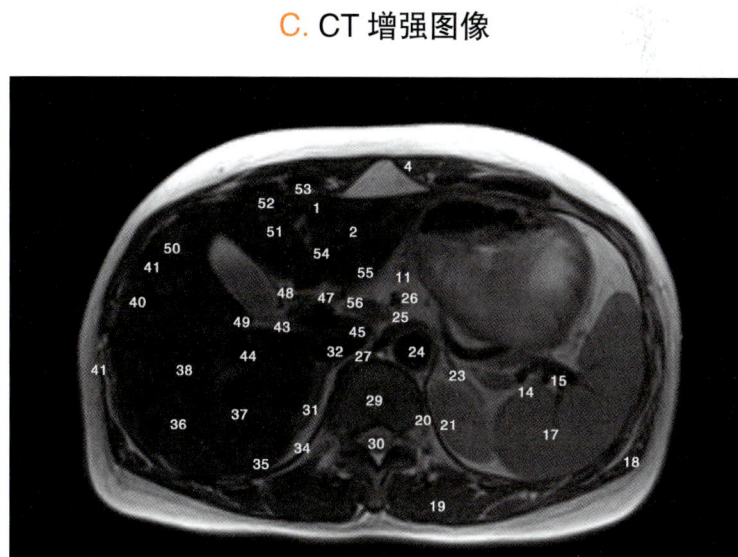

D. MR T1WI　　　　E. MR T2WI

关键结构：右肾上腺，肝门静脉尾状叶支。

此断面经第 12 胸椎椎体上份。

脊柱右侧可见由右膈肌、下腔静脉和肝右后叶围成的右肾上腺三角，内有脂肪和右肾上腺，其右侧副肝静脉正汇入下腔静脉，尾状叶内可见肝门静脉尾状叶支。尾状叶接受肝门静脉左、右支的双重供血，以发自左支横部的为主，而尾状突主要接受肝门静脉右后支的供血。该断面在标本及 CT、MR 图像上，双侧肾上腺均清晰地显示。肾上腺由肾上腺上、中、下动脉供给，它们分别发自下动脉、腹主动脉和肾动脉。3 组动脉分成小支至肾上腺的纤维囊，互相吻合成丛，由丛发出皮质支和髓质支。一些恶性肿瘤，如肺癌，瘤细胞可经血液发生肾上腺转移，表现为肾上腺的不规则增粗或形成肿块，强化不均匀。肾上腺常见的原发肿瘤有腺瘤、嗜铬细胞瘤等，良性居多，恶性如皮质腺癌等较少见。肾上腺为重要的内分泌器官，当肾上腺增生或发生肿瘤时，可能会导致相应内分泌异常。如肾上腺皮质束状带增生或发生腺瘤等病变时，可分泌过量糖皮质激素，从而发生 Cushing（库欣）综合征；如发生于皮质球状带，可分泌过多的盐皮质激素导致 Conn 综合征；发生于皮质网状带时，可分泌过多的雄激素等，导致男性化等。肾上腺髓质则可看作是一种神经–内分泌转换器，在应激状态下受交感神经支配能迅速分泌肾上腺素、去甲肾上腺素等。嗜铬细胞瘤、神经源性肿瘤亦可发生于肾上腺髓质。

腹部连续横断层 37（FH.11190）

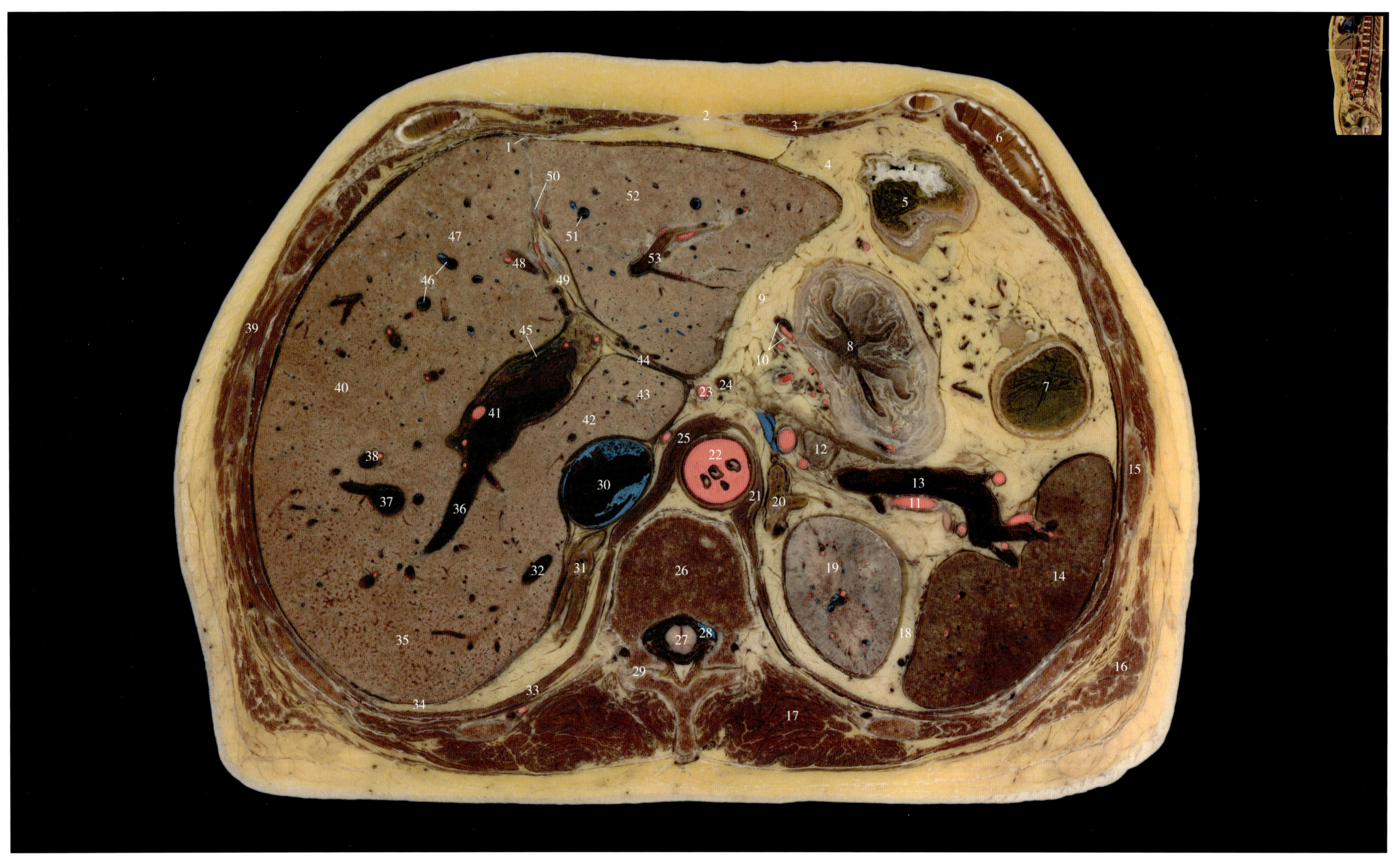

A. 断层标本图像

1. 肝镰状韧带 falciform ligament of liver
2. 腹白线 linea alba
3. 腹直肌 rectus abdominis
4. 大网膜 greater omentum
5. 横结肠 transverse colon
6. 第7肋软骨 7th costal cartilage
7. 降结肠 descending colon
8. 胃 stomach
9. 肝胃韧带 hepatogastric ligament
10. 胃动、静脉 gastric artery and vein
11. 脾动脉 splenic artery
12. 胰体 body of pancreas
13. 脾静脉 splenic vein
14. 脾 spleen
15. 第9肋骨 9th costal bone
16. 背阔肌 latissimus dorsi
17. 竖脊肌 erector spinae
18. 脾肾韧带 lienorenal ligament
19. 左肾 left kidney
20. 左肾上腺 left suprarenal gland
21. 左膈脚 left crus of diaphragm
22. 胸主动脉 thoracic aorta
23. 胃左动脉 left gastric artery
24. 胃左静脉 left gastric vein
25. 右膈脚 right crus of diaphragm
26. 第12胸椎椎体 body of 12th thoracic vertebra
27. 脊髓 spinal cord
28. 椎内静脉丛 internal vertebral venous plexus
29. 关节突关节 zygapophysial joint
30. 下腔静脉 inferior vena cava
31. 右肾上腺 right suprarenal gland
32. 副肝静脉 accessory hepatic veins
33. 膈 diaphragm
34. 肝裸区 bare area of liver
35. 肝右后叶上段 superior segment of right posterior lobe of liver
36. 肝门静脉右后上支 right posterosuperior branch of hepatic portal vein
37. 肝右静脉 right hepatic vein
38. 肝门静脉右前支及动脉 right anterior branch of hepatic portal vein and corresponding artery
39. 肋间外肌 intercostale externi
40. 肝右前叶上段 superior segment of right anterior lobe of liver
41. 肝门静脉右支 right hepatic portal vein
42. 尾状突 caudate process
43. 乳头突 papillary process
44. 静脉韧带裂 fissure for ligamentum venosum
45. 肝总管 common hepatic duct
46. 肝中静脉属支 tributary of middle hepatic vein
47. 肝左内叶 left medial lobe of liver
48. 肝门静脉左内叶支 left medial branch of hepatic portal vein
49. 肝圆韧带 ligamentum teres hepatis
50. 肝圆韧带裂 fissure for ligamentum teres hepatis
51. 肝左静脉属支 tributary of left hepatic vein
52. 肝左外叶下段 inferior segment of left lateral lobe of liver
53. 肝门静脉左外下支及肝动脉 left lateroinferior branch of hepatic portal vein and corresponding hepatic artery

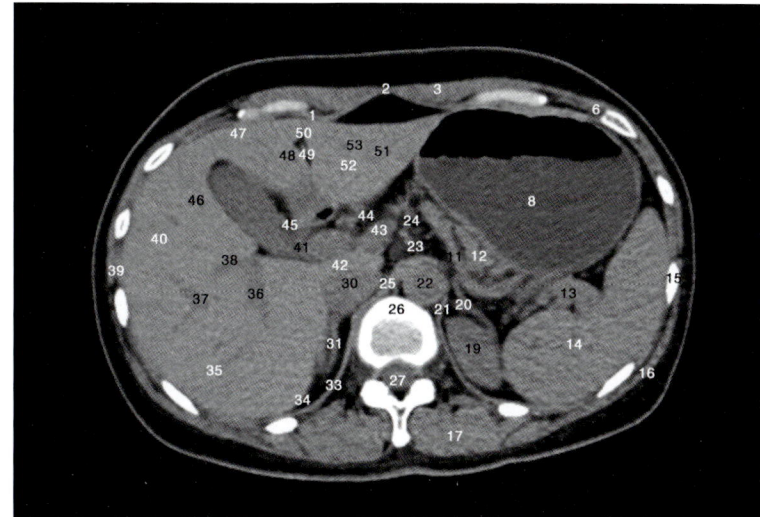

B. CT 平扫图像

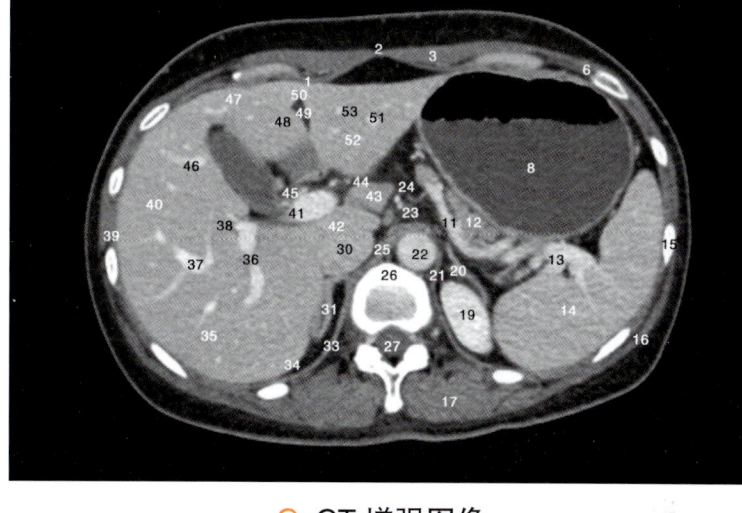

C. CT 增强图像

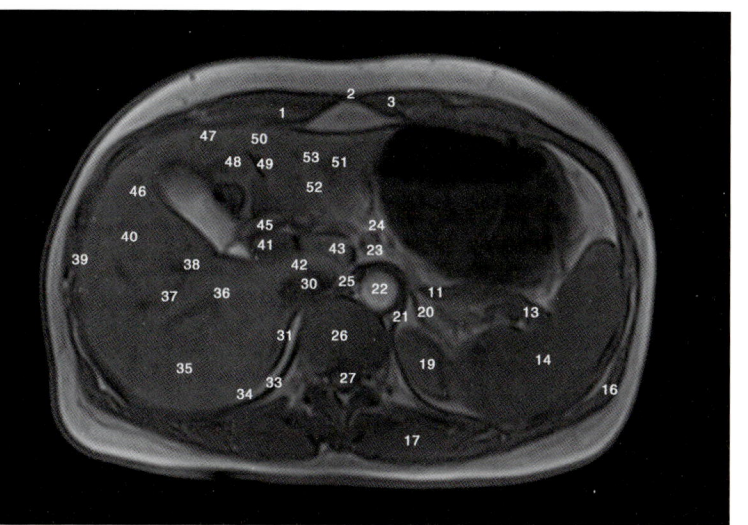

D. MR T1WI

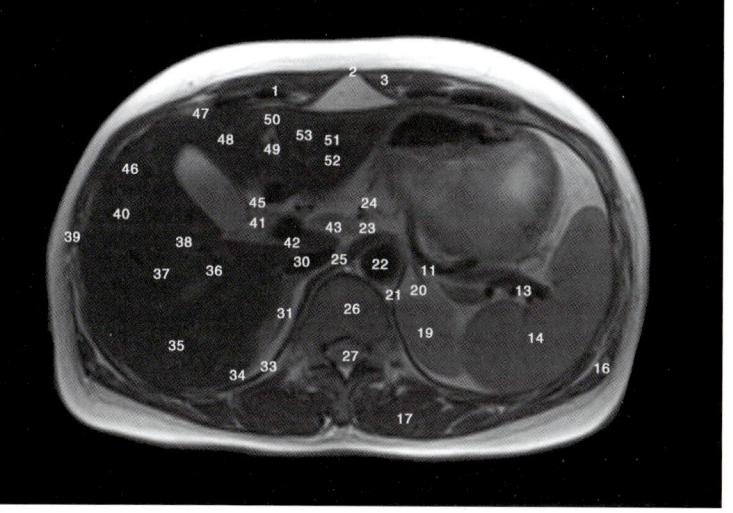

E. MR T2WI

关键结构：副肝静脉，第三肝门。

此断面经第12胸椎椎体上份。

肝右后上段内可见副肝静脉，与右侧的肝门静脉右后上支和肝右静脉连成一线。副肝静脉主要来源于左侧的尾状叶或者右侧的肝Ⅵ、Ⅶ段，直接汇入下腔静脉。人均 6.12 ± 1.13（2~10）支，内径范围为 0.1~1.0 cm，平均为 0.36 cm ± 0.11 cm[19]。副肝静脉管径粗者则血管数量少，否则血管数量多，呈此消彼长的关系。

在肝尾状叶肿瘤切除术中，最大风险在于术中损伤紧贴下腔静脉的副肝静脉，出血凶险，止血困难。临床上提及肝脏的3个肝门：第一肝门即解剖学上的肝门，为肝门静脉、肝固有动脉、肝管组成的Glisson管道系统出入肝脏处；第二肝门是肝左、中、右静脉汇入下腔静脉处，是划分肝叶和肝段的关键平面；第三肝门即副肝静脉汇入下腔静脉处，主要是在腔静脉旁，右侧为主。

75

腹部连续横断层 38（FH.11170）

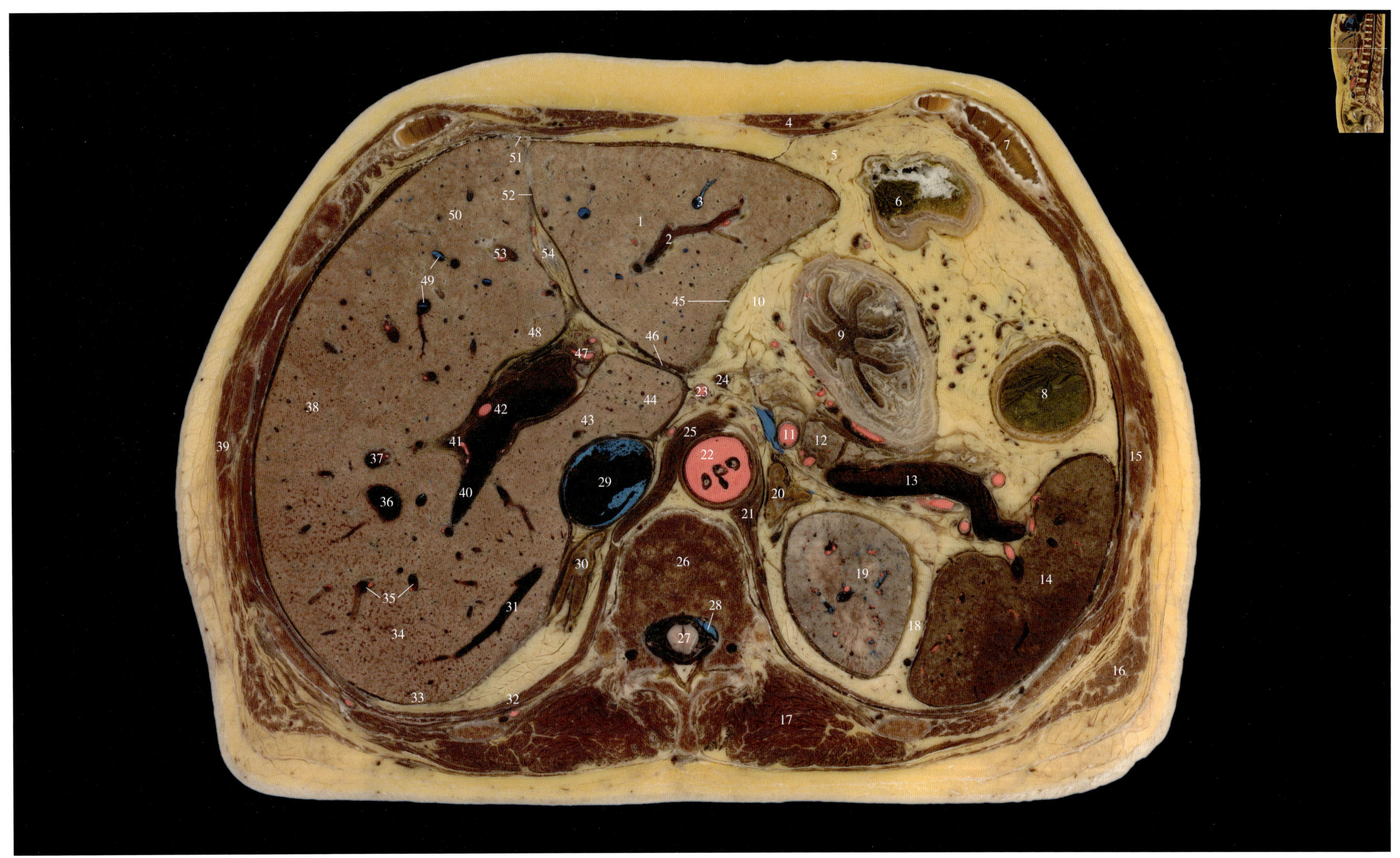

A. 断层标本图像

1. 肝左外叶下段 inferior segment of left lateral lobe of liver
2. 肝门静脉左外下支及肝动脉 left lateroinferior branch of hepatic portal vein and corresponding hepatic artery
3. 肝左静脉下根 inferior root of left hepatic vein
4. 腹直肌 rectus abdominis
5. 大网膜 greater omentum
6. 横结肠 transverse colon
7. 第 7 肋软骨 7th costal cartilage
8. 降结肠 descending colon
9. 胃 stomach
10. 肝胃韧带 hepatogastric ligament
11. 脾动脉 splenic artery
12. 胰体 body of pancreas
13. 脾静脉 splenic vein
14. 脾 spleen
15. 第 9 肋骨 9th costal bone
16. 背阔肌 latissimus dorsi
17. 竖脊肌 erector spinae
18. 脾肾韧带 lienorenal ligament
19. 左肾 left kidney
20. 左肾上腺 left suprarenal gland
21. 左膈脚 left crus of diaphragm
22. 腹主动脉 abdominal aorta
23. 胃左动脉 left gastric artery
24. 胃左静脉 left gastric vein
25. 右膈脚 right crus of diaphragm
26. 第 12 胸椎椎体 body of 12th thoracic vertebra
27. 脊髓 spinal cord
28. 椎内静脉丛 internal vertebral venous plexus
29. 下腔静脉 inferior vena cava
30. 右肾上腺 right suprarenal gland
31. 副肝静脉 accessory hepatic veins
32. 膈 diaphragm
33. 肝裸区 bare area of liver
34. 肝右后叶上段 superior segment of right posterior lobe of liver
35. 肝门静脉右后下支及肝动脉、肝管 right posteroinferior branch of hepatic portal vein and corresponding hepatic artery and hepatic duct
36. 肝右静脉 right hepatic vein
37. 肝门静脉右前支及动脉 right anterior branch of hepatic portal vein and corresponding artery
38. 肝右前叶上段 superior segment of right anterior lobe of liver
39. 肋间外肌 intercostale externi
40. 肝门静脉右后上支 right posterosuperior branch of hepatic portal vein
41. 肝门静脉右前支 right anterior branch of hepatic portal vein
42. 肝门静脉右支 right hepatic portal vein
43. 尾状突 caudate process
44. 乳头突 papillary process
45. 左肝下前间隙 anterior left subrahepatic space
46. 静脉韧带裂 fissure for ligamentum venosum
47. 肝左动脉 left hepatic artery
48. 肝总管 common hepatic duct
49. 肝中静脉属支 tributary of middle hepatic vein
50. 肝左内叶 left medial lobe of liver
51. 肝镰状韧带 falciform ligament of liver
52. 肝圆韧带裂 fissure for ligamentum teres hepatis
53. 肝门静脉左内叶支 left medial branch of hepatic portal vein
54. 肝圆韧带 ligamentum teres hepatis

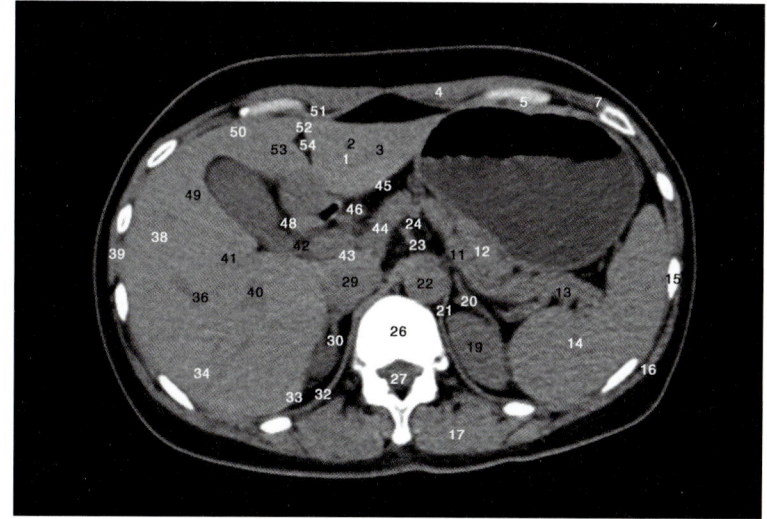

B. CT 平扫图像　　C. CT 增强图像

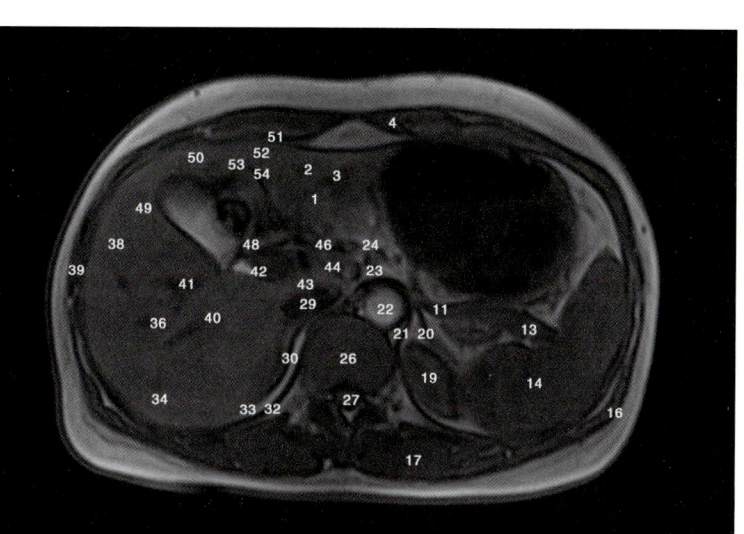

D. MR T1WI

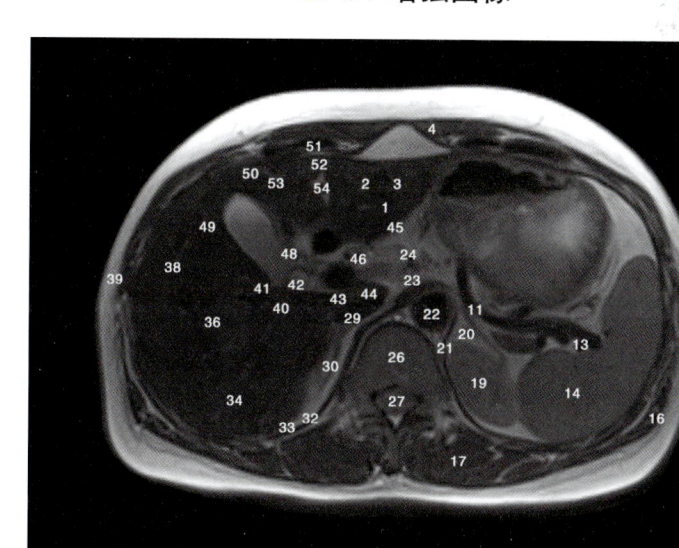

E. MR T2WI

关键结构：肝镰状韧带，肝圆韧带，脾肾韧带。

此断面经第 12 胸椎椎体上份。

腹腔右侧前方可见镰状韧带及其后方的肝圆韧带裂、肝圆韧带。镰状韧带是一个由前腹壁连于肝的比较薄的腹膜反折，向下延至脐平面，止于肝圆韧带索。从解剖结构上看，它与静脉韧带裂和肝胃韧带是相连续的。肝圆韧带是脐静脉闭锁后形成的，经过镰状韧带游离缘的两层腹膜间达到脐静脉窝，止于肝门静脉左支的囊部，与静脉韧带相连。正常情况下，肝圆韧带内的血管是闭锁的，而当肝硬化门静脉高压时，肝圆韧带有可能出现病理性再通。对于再通的肝圆韧带，还可以通过肝圆韧带 - 下腔静脉转流术来实现门腔分流，从而达到减轻门静脉高压的作用。脾肾韧带脾与肾之间形成的双层腹膜皱襞，脾动、静脉及胰尾位于其内。在胃背侧系膜的后部，网膜囊的后方，介于脾与腹膜后壁之间。CT 平扫图像显示镰状韧带旁的肝左内叶和 / 或肝左外叶前缘有时见局限性略低密度灶，增强扫描呈相对低强化，以门静脉期更明显，考虑为没有临床意义的"肝镰状韧带旁假病灶"，易被误认为肝内占位性病变。目前多认为其形成是由于镰旁肝局部特殊血供因素[20]，或镰旁肝局部脂肪浸润所致[21]。但也应注意镰状韧带旁是否存在真性病灶而漏诊，MRI 可予以鉴别。如真性病灶的 DWI 多呈高信号。应用肝胆特异性对比剂时，真性病灶肝胆期信号多有明显下降，而假病灶不下降或仅轻微下降[22]。

77

腹部连续横断层 39（FH.11150）

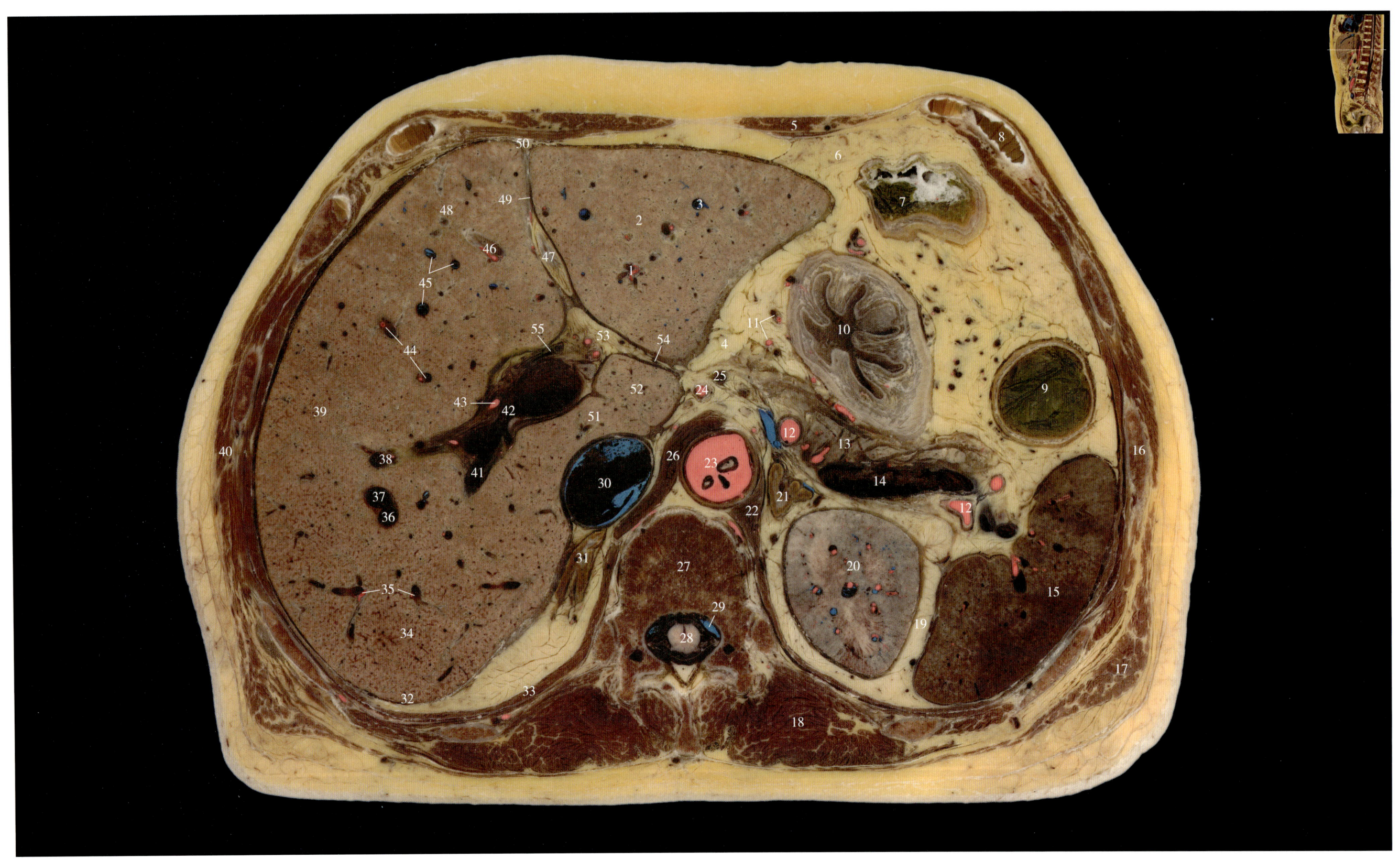

A. 断层标本图像

1. 肝门静脉左外下支及肝动脉 left lateroinferior branch of hepatic portal vein and corresponding hepatic artery
2. 肝左外叶下段 inferior segment of left lateral lobe of liver
3. 肝左静脉下根 inferior root of left hepatic vein
4. 肝胃韧带 hepatogastric ligament
5. 腹直肌 rectus abdominis
6. 大网膜 greater omentum
7. 横结肠 transverse colon
8. 第 7 肋软骨 7th costal cartilage
9. 降结肠 descending colon
10. 胃体 body of stomach
11. 胃动、静脉 gastric artery and vein
12. 脾动脉 splenic artery
13. 胰体 body of pancreas
14. 脾静脉 splenic vein
15. 脾 spleen
16. 第 9 肋骨 9th costal bone
17. 背阔肌 latissimus dorsi
18. 竖脊肌 erector spinae
19. 脾肾韧带 lienorenal ligament
20. 左肾 left kidney
21. 左肾上腺 left suprarenal gland
22. 左膈脚 left crus of diaphragm
23. 腹主动脉 abdominal aorta
24. 胃左动脉 left gastric artery
25. 胃左静脉 left gastric vein
26. 右膈脚 right crus of diaphragm
27. 第 12 胸椎椎体 body of 12th thoracic vertebra
28. 脊髓 spinal cord
29. 椎内静脉丛 internal vertebral venous plexus
30. 下腔静脉 inferior vena cava
31. 右肾上腺 right suprarenal gland
32. 肝裸区 bare area of liver
33. 膈 diaphragm
34. 肝右后叶上段 superior segment of right posterior lobe of liver
35. 肝门静脉右后下支及肝动脉、肝管 right posteroinferior branch of hepatic portal vein and corresponding hepatic artery and hepatic duct
36. 肝右静脉后根 posterior root of right hepatic vein
37. 肝右静脉前根 anterior root of right hepatic vein
38. 肝门静脉右前支及动脉 right anterior branch of hepatic portal vein and corresponding artery
39. 肝右前叶上段 superior segment of right anterior lobe of liver
40. 肋间外肌 intercostale externi
41. 肝门静脉右后上支 right posterosuperior branch of hepatic portal vein
42. 肝门静脉右支 right hepatic portal vein
43. 肝右动脉 right hepatic artery
44. 肝门静脉右前下支及肝动脉、肝管 right anteroinferior branch of hepatic portal vein and corresponding hepatic artery and hepatic duct
45. 肝中静脉属支 tributary of middle hepatic vein
46. 肝门静脉左内叶支 left medial branch of hepatic portal vein
47. 肝圆韧带 ligamentum teres hepatis
48. 肝左内叶 left medial lobe of liver
49. 肝圆韧带裂 fissure for ligamentum teres hepatis
50. 肝镰状韧带 falciform ligament of liver
51. 尾状突 caudate process
52. 乳头突 papillary process
53. 肝胃韧带 hepatogastric ligament
54. 静脉韧带裂 fissure for ligamentum venosum
55. 肝总管 common hepatic duct

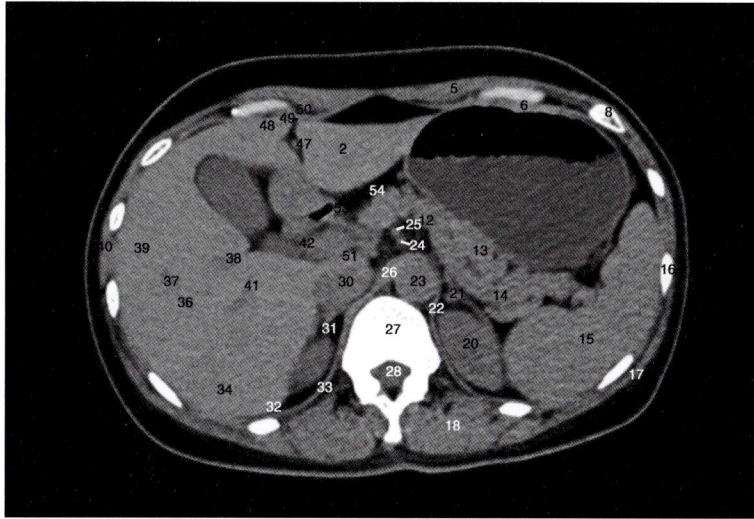

B. CT 平扫图像

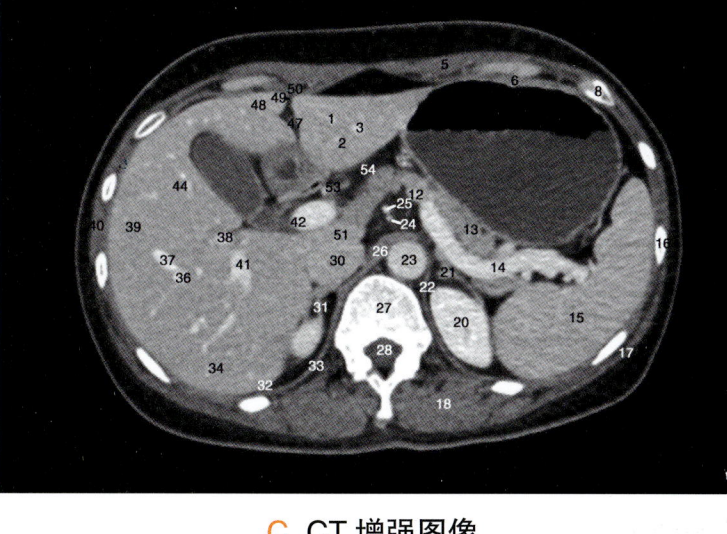

C. CT 增强图像

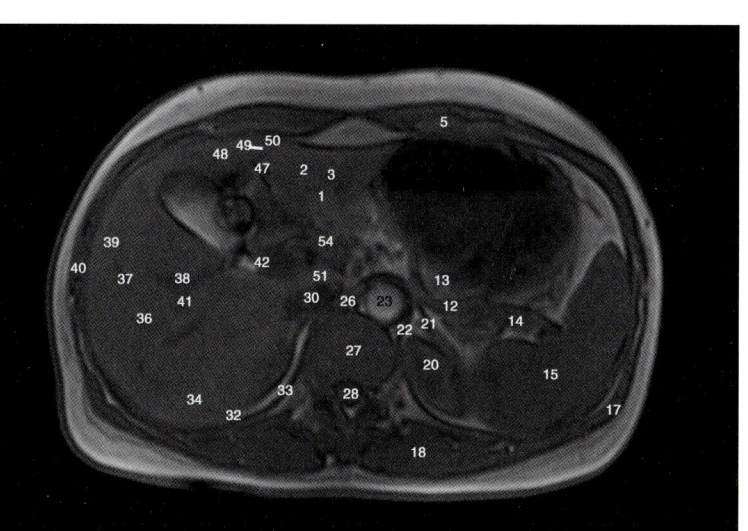

D. MR T1WI

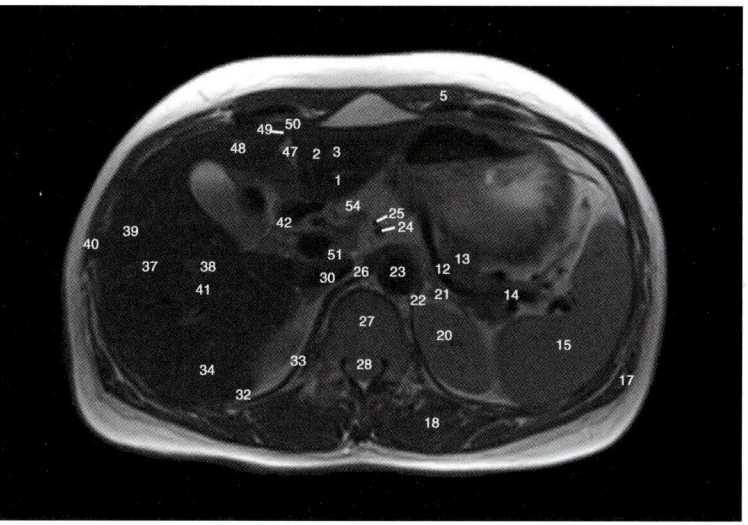

E. MR T2WI

关键结构：胰体，右肾上腺。

此断面经第 12 胸椎椎体中份。

胃后方，脾动、静脉前方可见胰体，右肾上腺位于下腔静脉后方的右肾上腺三角内。胰体位于胰颈与胰尾之间，占胰的大部分，略呈三棱柱形。胰体的前面隔网膜囊与胃后壁相邻，故胃后壁肿瘤或溃疡穿孔常与胰体粘连。胰体癌症状以疼痛为主，因为胰体与腹腔神经丛相邻，病变容易侵及神经，疼痛为间歇性或持续性，夜间加重。胰体为腹膜后位器官，受其前面腹腔脏器及后方脊柱周围肌肉的相对保护，外伤较少见，占腹腔脏器损伤的 2%~5%[23]。但近年来由于交通事故增多，胰腺外伤有增多的趋势，损伤的原因往往由于汽车方向盘等撞击上腹部所致，故又称"方向盘伤"。如暴力直接作用于上腹中线，损伤常在胰颈、体部；如暴力作用于脊柱左侧，则多伤及胰尾。胰腺外伤易被其他脏器外伤掩盖而不易发现，但胰腺破裂后具有消化作用的胰液外渗，亦造成周围脏器和组织的严重伤害，死亡率 5%~30%[24]，应予以重视。肾上腺位于脊柱两侧的腹膜后间隙内，属于腹膜外位器官。右肾上腺呈三角形，较左肾上腺稍短。其前面的内侧直接与下腔静脉接触，外侧与肝相邻接，后面稍凸与膈相贴，底凹陷叫作肾面，紧卧于右肾的上端，内侧缘邻腹腔神经节。右肾上腺门位于腺的前面内上方，肾上腺中央静脉经门穿出汇入下腔静脉或右肾静脉。

腹部连续横断层 40（FH.11130）

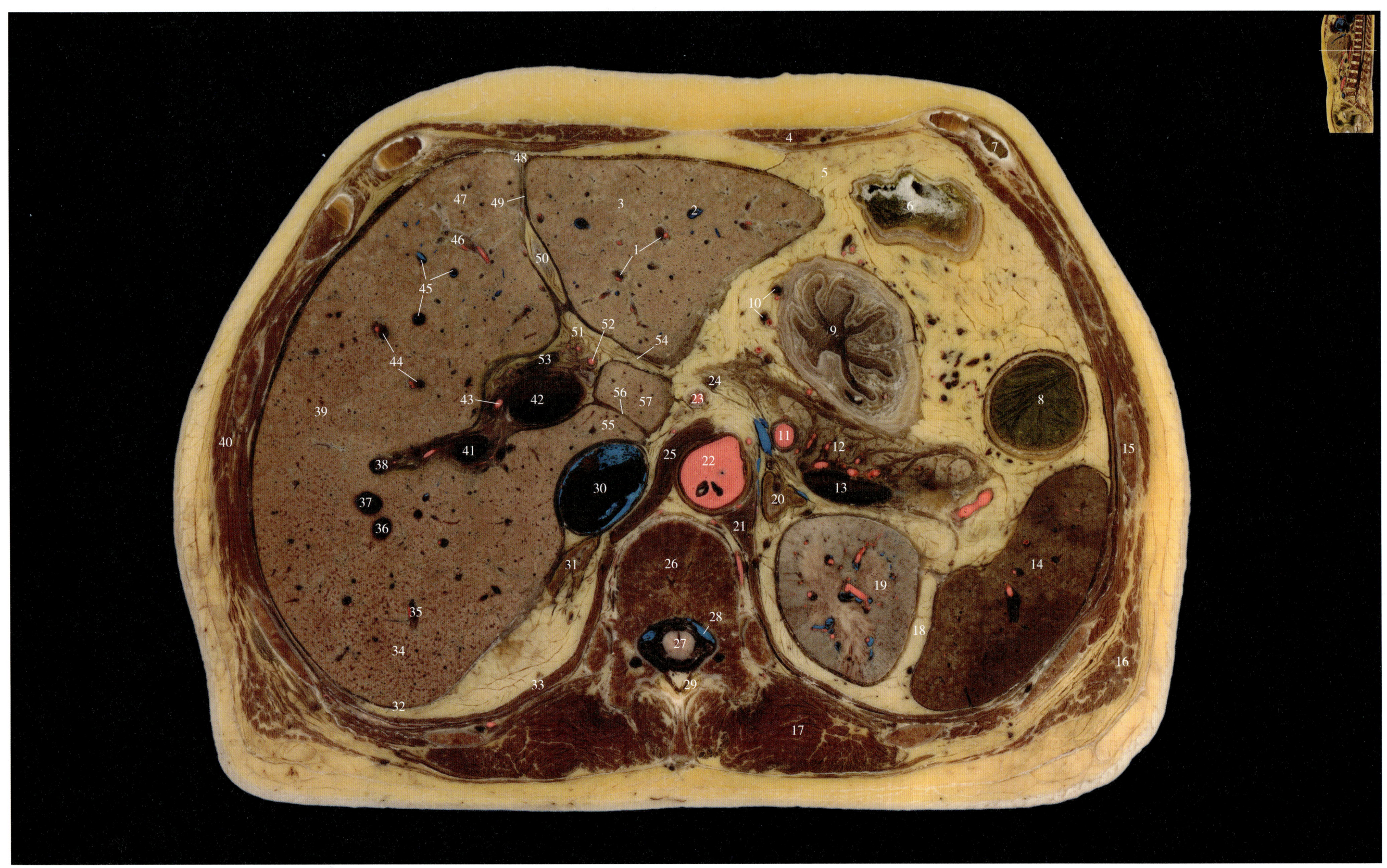

A. 断层标本图像

1. 肝门静脉左外下支及肝动脉 left lateroinferior branch of hepatic portal vein and corresponding hepatic artery
2. 肝左静脉下根 inferior root of left hepatic vein
3. 肝左外叶下段 inferior segment of left lateral lobe of liver
4. 腹直肌 rectus abdominis
5. 大网膜 greater omentum
6. 横结肠 transverse colon
7. 第 7 肋软骨 7th costal cartilage
8. 降结肠 descending colon
9. 胃体 body of stomach
10. 胃动、静脉 gastric artery and vein
11. 脾动脉 splenic artery
12. 胰体 body of pancreas
13. 脾静脉 splenic vein
14. 脾 spleen
15. 第 9 肋骨 9th costal bone
16. 背阔肌 latissimus dorsi
17. 竖脊肌 erector spinae
18. 脾肾韧带 lienorenal ligament
19. 左肾 left kidney
20. 左肾上腺 left suprarenal gland
21. 左膈脚 left crus of diaphragm
22. 腹主动脉 abdominal aorta
23. 胃左动脉 left gastric artery
24. 胃左静脉 left gastric vein
25. 右膈脚 right crus of diaphragm
26. 第 12 胸椎椎体 body of 12th thoracic vertebra
27. 脊髓 spinal cord
28. 椎内静脉丛 internal vertebral venous plexus
29. 黄韧带 ligamenta flava
30. 下腔静脉 inferior vena cava
31. 右肾上腺 right suprarenal gland
32. 肝裸区 bare area of liver
33. 膈 diaphragm
34. 肝右后叶上段 superior segment of right posterior lobe of liver
35. 肝门静脉右后下支及肝动脉、肝管 right posteroinferior branch of hepatic portal vein and corresponding hepatic artery and hepatic duct
36. 肝右静脉后根 posterior root of right hepatic vein
37. 肝右静脉前根 anterior root of right hepatic vein
38. 肝门静脉右前支及动脉 right anterior branch of hepatic portal vein and corresponding artery
39. 肝右前叶上段 superior segment of right anterior lobe of liver
40. 肋间外肌 intercostale externi
41. 肝门静脉右支 right hepatic portal vein
42. 肝门静脉 hepatic portal vein
43. 肝右动脉 right hepatic artery
44. 肝门静脉右前下支及肝动脉、肝管 right anteroinferior branch of hepatic portal vein and corresponding hepatic artery and hepatic duct
45. 肝中静脉属支 tributary of middle hepatic vein
46. 肝门静脉左内叶支 left medial branch of hepatic portal vein
47. 肝左内叶 left medial lobe of liver
48. 肝镰状韧带 falciform ligament of liver
49. 肝圆韧带裂 fissure for ligamentum teres hepatis
50. 肝圆韧带 ligamentum teres hepatis
51. 肝胃韧带 hepatogastric ligament
52. 肝左动脉 left hepatic artery
53. 肝总管 common hepatic duct
54. 静脉韧带裂 fissure for ligamentum venosum
55. 尾状突 caudate process
56. 弓状切迹 arcuate notch
57. 乳头突 papillary process

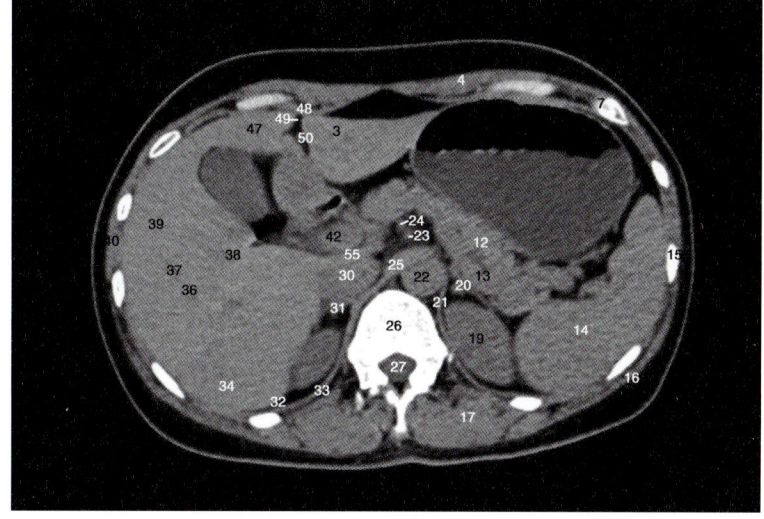

B. CT 平扫图像

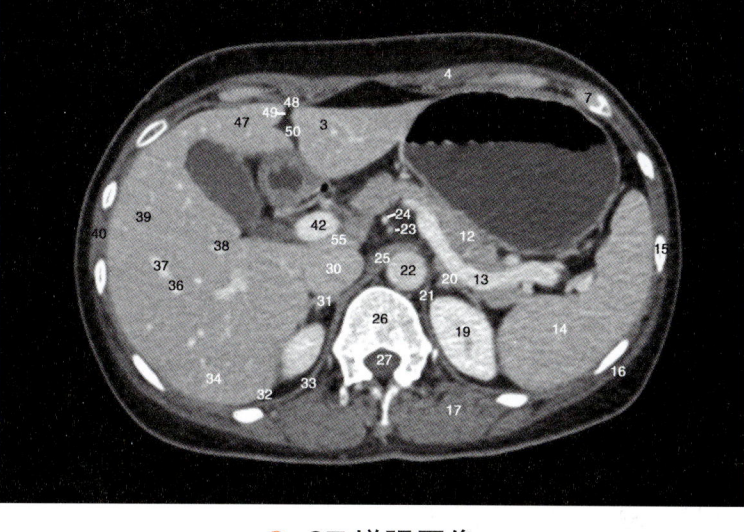

C. CT 增强图像

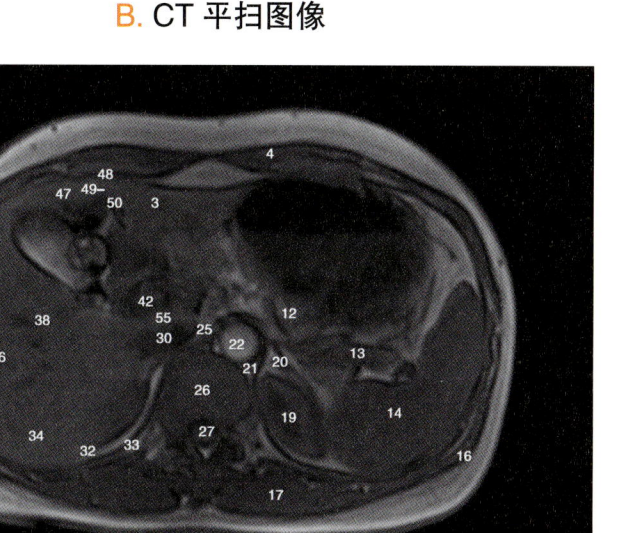

D. MR T1WI

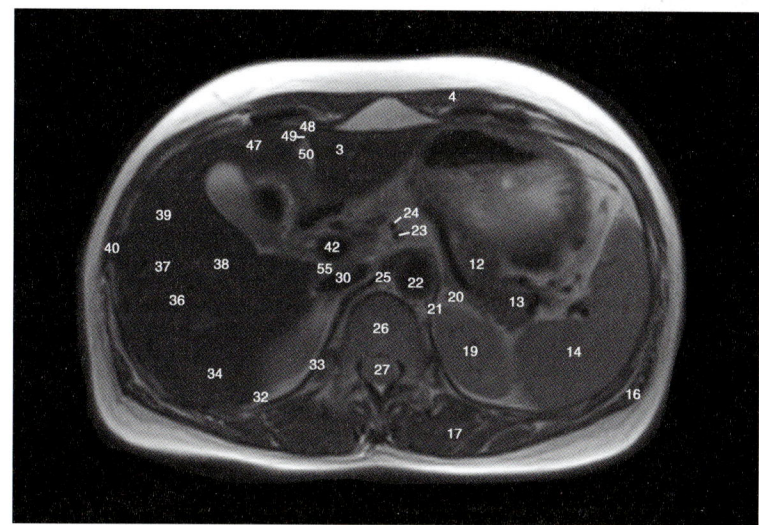

E. MR T2WI

关键结构：第 12 胸椎椎体，黄韧带，脊髓。

此断面经第 12 胸椎椎体中份。

椎体呈心形，位于断面中间靠后部，其后方脊髓和黄韧带清晰可见，前方腹主动脉即将发出腹腔干。黄韧带参与构成椎管后壁，连接相邻的上下位椎弓板，起于第 2 颈椎，止于第 1 骶椎，分节存在。黄韧带向上附着于上位椎板前面的下半部，向下附着于下位椎板后面及上缘，外侧附着部可延伸到椎间关节囊，向内可延伸到中线椎板形成棘突处。两侧黄韧带在中线汇合处留下一窄长纵行间隙，内有静脉经此间隙回流到脊柱后外侧的椎静脉丛。脊髓位于椎管内，呈前后稍扁的圆柱体，全长粗细不等，上端在枕骨大孔处与延髓相连，下端尖削呈圆锥状，称脊髓圆锥，成人脊髓全长 42~45 cm。脊髓有两个膨大，上方者称颈膨大，位于颈髓第三段到胸髓第二段，在颈髓第六段处最粗；下方为腰膨大，始自胸髓第九段到脊髓圆锥，在第 12 胸椎水平处最粗。这两个膨大的形成与四肢的出现有关，因此处脊髓内部神经元的增多所致。黄韧带是脊柱椎管内维持脊柱稳定的结构，属于脊柱后柱的支持结构之一。长期坐位或弯腰工作可导致肥厚，常引起椎管狭窄，严重出现腰痛和下肢疼痛和麻木。MRI 可清晰地显示黄韧带，由于纤维成分较多，在 T1WI 及 T2WI 上均呈低信号。

腹部连续横断层 41（FH.11110）

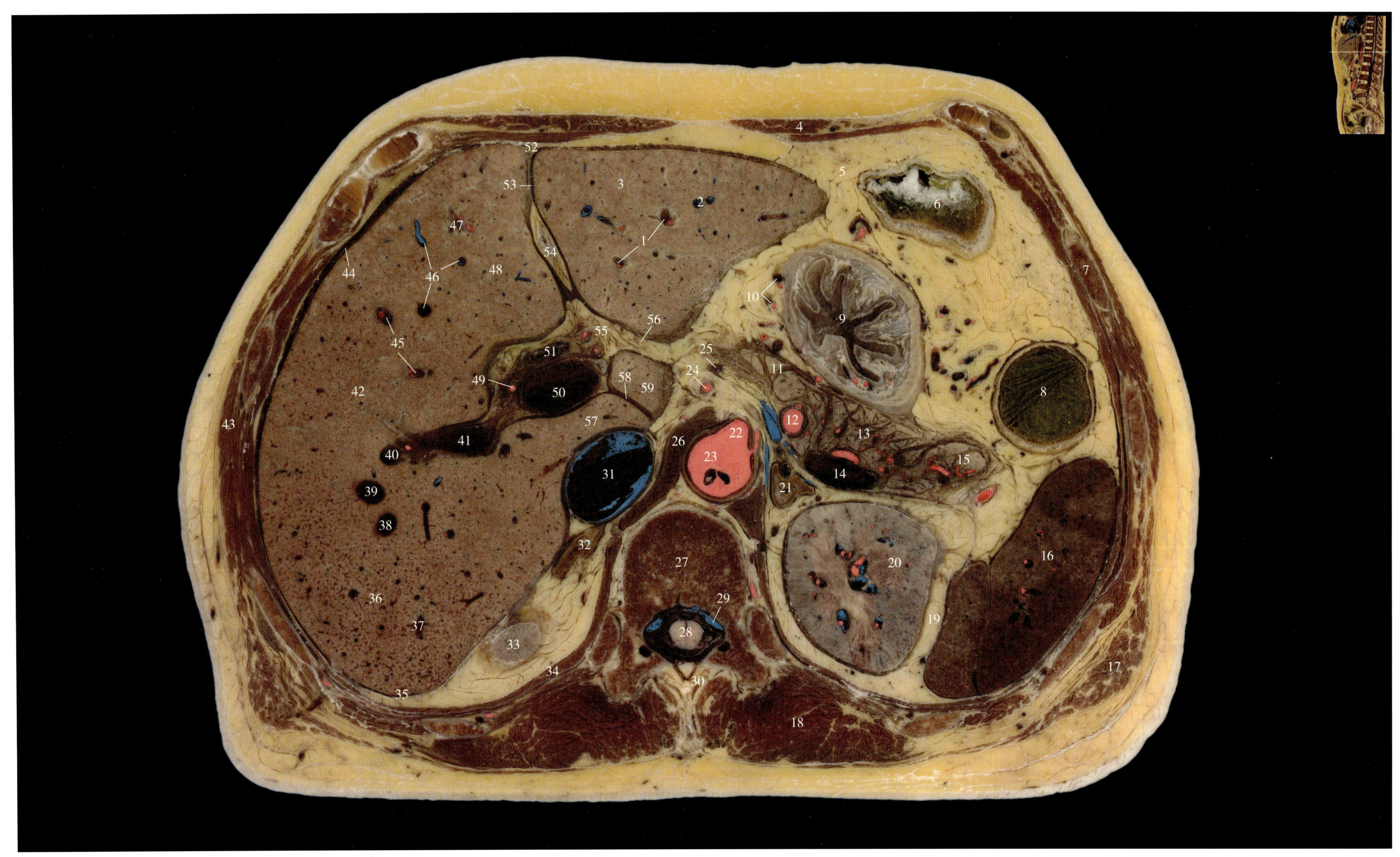

A. 断层标本图像

1. 肝门静脉左外下支及肝动脉 left lateroinferior branch of hepatic portal vein and corresponding hepatic artery
2. 肝左静脉下根 inferior root of left hepatic vein
3. 肝左外叶下段 inferior segment of left lateral lobe of liver
4. 腹直肌 rectus abdominis
5. 大网膜 greater omentum
6. 横结肠 transverse colon
7. 第8肋骨 8th costal bone
8. 降结肠 descending colon
9. 胃体 body of stomach
10. 胃动、静脉 gastric artery and vein
11. 胰颈 neck of pancreas
12. 脾动脉 splenic artery
13. 胰体 body of pancreas
14. 脾静脉 splenic vein
15. 胰尾 tail of pancreas
16. 脾 spleen
17. 背阔肌 latissimus dorsi
18. 竖脊肌 erector spinae
19. 脾肾韧带 lienorenal ligament
20. 左肾 left kidney
21. 左肾上腺 left suprarenal gland
22. 腹腔干 celiac trunk
23. 腹主动脉 abdominal aorta
24. 胃左动脉 left gastric artery
25. 胃左静脉 left gastric vein
26. 右膈脚 right crus of diaphragm
27. 第12胸椎椎体 body of 12th thoracic vertebra
28. 脊髓 spinal cord
29. 椎内静脉丛 internal vertebral venous plexus
30. 黄韧带 ligamenta flava
31. 下腔静脉 inferior vena cava
32. 右肾上腺 right suprarenal gland
33. 右肾上极 the upper pole of right kidney
34. 膈 diaphragm
35. 肝裸区 bare area of liver
36. 肝右后叶下段 inferior segment of right posterior lobe of liver
37. 肝门静脉右后下支及肝动脉、肝管 right posteroinferior branch of hepatic portal vein and corresponding hepatic artery and hepatic duct
38. 肝右静脉后根 posterior root of right hepatic vein
39. 肝右静脉前根 anterior root of right hepatic vein
40. 肝门静脉右前支及动脉 right anterior branch of hepatic portal vein and corresponding artery
41. 肝门静脉右支 right hepatic portal vein
42. 肝右前叶下段 inferior segment of right anterior lobe of liver
43. 肋间外肌 intercostale externi
44. 右肝上间隙 right suprahepatic space
45. 肝门静脉右前下支及肝动脉、肝管 right anteroinferior branch of hepatic portal vein and corresponding hepatic artery and hepatic duct
46. 肝中静脉属支 tributary of middle hepatic vein
47. 肝门静脉左内叶支 left medial branch of hepatic portal vein
48. 肝左内叶 left medial lobe of liver
49. 肝右动脉 right hepatic artery
50. 肝门静脉 hepatic portal vein
51. 肝总管 common hepatic duct
52. 肝镰状韧带 falciform ligament of liver
53. 肝圆韧带裂 fissure for ligamentum teres hepatis
54. 肝圆韧带 ligamentum teres hepatis
55. 肝胃韧带 hepatogastric ligament
56. 静脉韧带裂 fissure for ligamentum venosum
57. 尾状突 caudate process
58. 弓状切迹 arcuate notch
59. 乳头突 papillary process

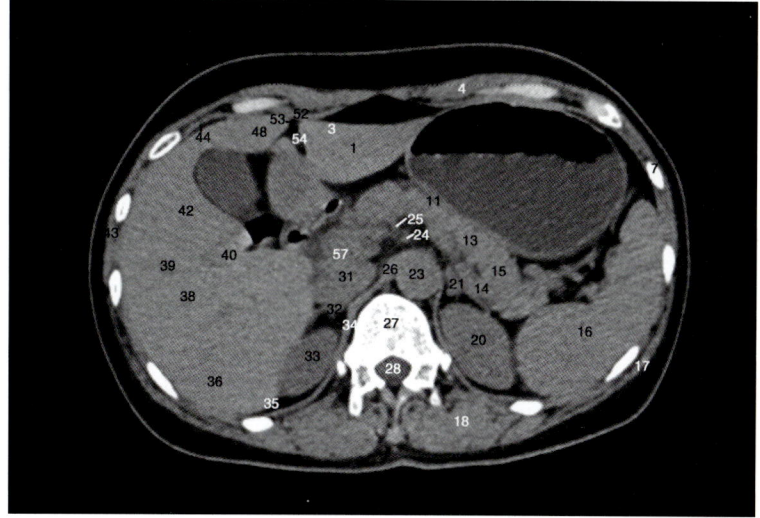

B. CT 平扫图像　　　　C. CT 增强图像

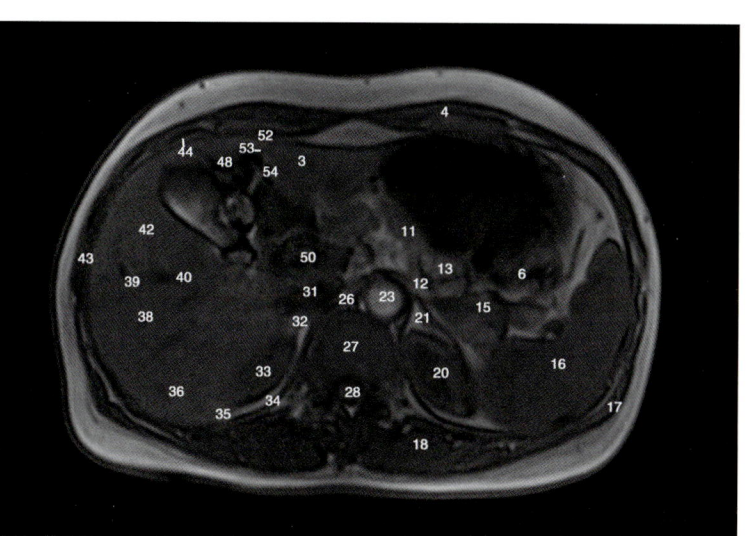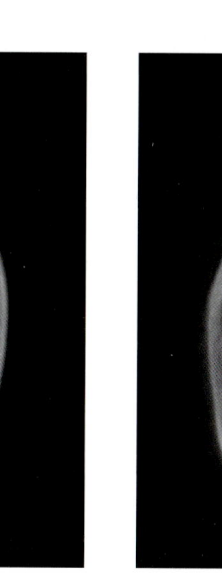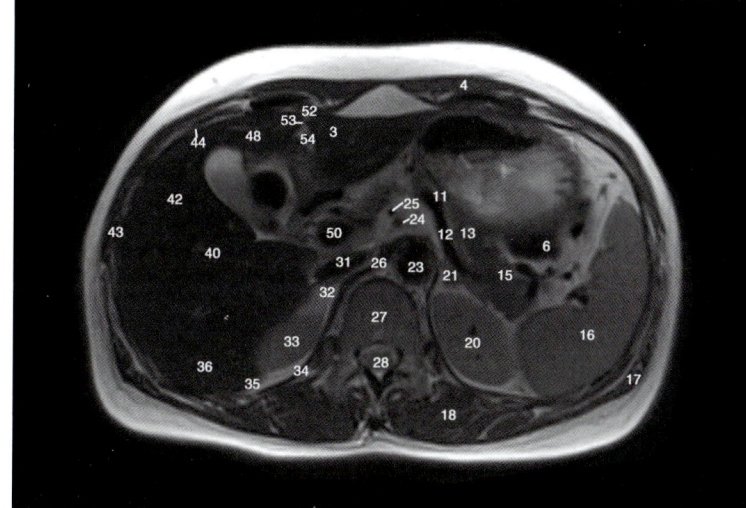

D. MR T1WI　　　　E. MR T2WI

关键结构：肝门静脉，肝尾状突。

此断面经第12胸椎椎体中份。

粗大的肝门静脉位于断面中央偏右处，其前方可见肝右动脉和肝总管，向后与下腔静脉之间形成门腔间隙，内有肝尾状叶的尾状突。肝门静脉分为左、右两支主干，分别进入肝左、右叶。其中，左支主干较长，按行程分为4部：横部，行于肝后下面的横沟内，其长度平均为 29.50 mm ± 6.51 mm，内径平均为 7.70 mm ± 1.55 mm；角部，自横沟左侧端呈弧形转折，转折角度平均为 118.16° ± 13.73°；矢状部，转折后继续向前下方走行在肝圆韧带裂的直部内，长度平均为 18.74 mm ± 4.22 mm，内径平均为 6.98 mm ± 1.41 mm；左外叶下段支长为 28.46 mm ± 13.56 mm，内径为 3.21 mm ± 0.87 mm。左内叶支形态变化较大[25]。肝门静脉高压症是一组由门静脉压力持久增高引起的症候群，大多数由肝硬化引起。当门静脉血不能顺利通过肝脏回流入下腔静脉就会引起门静脉压力增高，表现为门-体静脉间交通支开放，一般会出现3组重要的侧支循环：①食管静脉丛曲张，增强CT图像可清晰地显示食管下段-胃底迂曲增粗的静脉，肝硬化患者在进食较锐利食物时可能划破上述静脉，出现急性上消化道出血，严重者可危及生命；②直肠静脉丛曲张，主要是指门静脉系的直肠上静脉与下腔静脉系的直肠下静脉和肛静脉等沟通；③脐周静脉网曲张，门静脉高压时脐静脉重新开放，在脐周腹壁可以见到迂曲的静脉，外观似"水母头"。

腹部连续横断层 42（FH.11090）

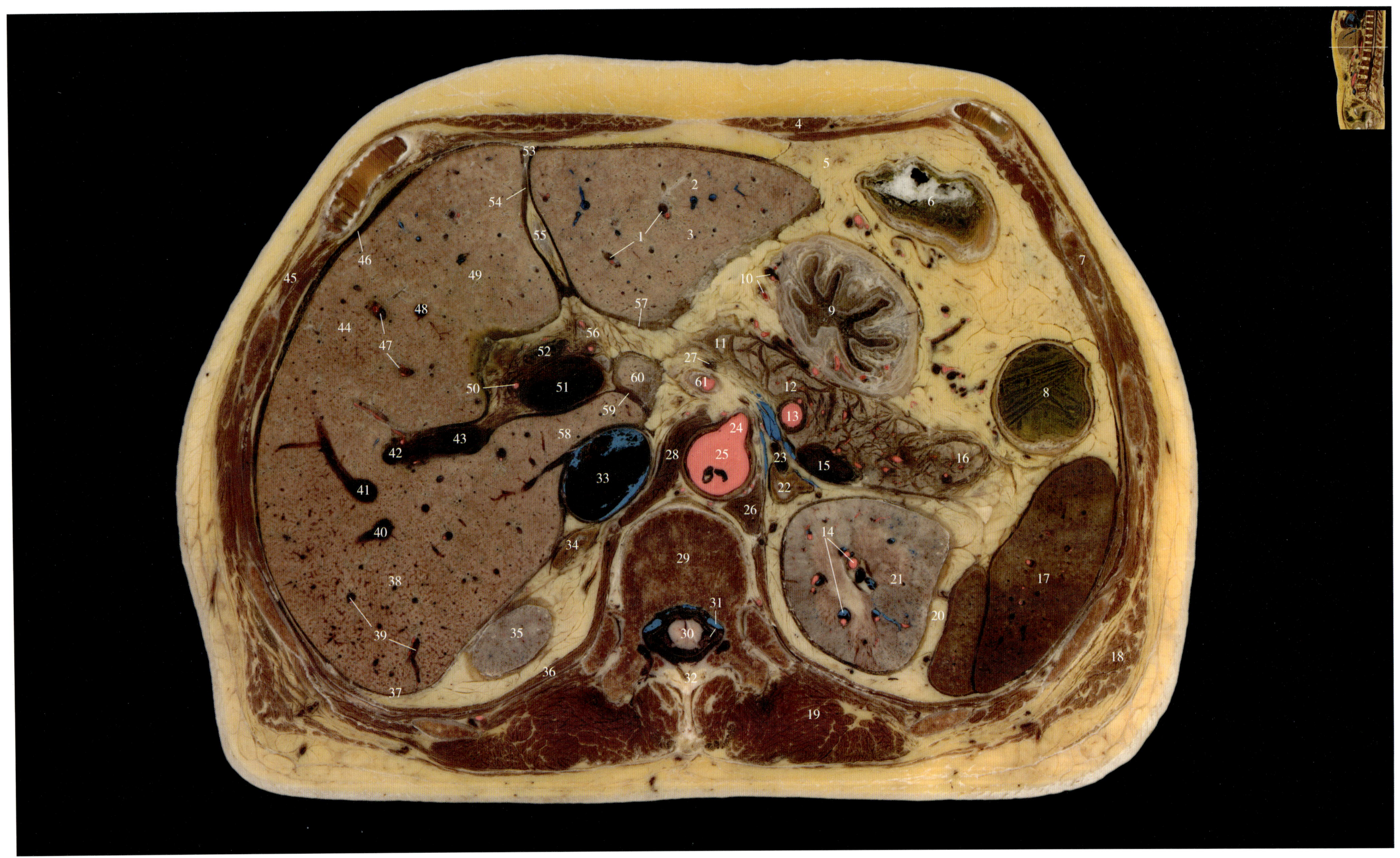

A. 断层标本图像

1. 肝门静脉左外下支及肝动脉 left lateroinferior branch of hepatic portal vein and corresponding hepatic artery
2. 肝左静脉下根 inferior root of left hepatic vein
3. 肝左外叶下段 inferior segment of left lateral lobe of liver
4. 腹直肌 rectus abdominis
5. 大网膜 greater omentum
6. 横结肠 transverse colon
7. 第8肋骨 8th costal bone
8. 降结肠 descending colon
9. 胃体 body of stomach
10. 胃动、静脉 gastric artery and vein
11. 胰颈 neck of pancreas
12. 胰体 body of pancreas
13. 脾动脉 splenic artery
14. 肾动、静脉 renal artery and vein
15. 脾静脉 splenic vein
16. 胰尾 tail of pancreas
17. 脾 spleen
18. 背阔肌 latissimus dorsi
19. 竖脊肌 erector spinae
20. 脾肾韧带 lienorenal ligament
21. 左肾 left kidney
22. 左肾上腺 left suprarenal gland
23. 肾上腺静脉 adrenal vein
24. 腹腔干 celiac trunk
25. 腹主动脉 abdominal aorta
26. 左膈脚 left crus of diaphragm
27. 胃左静脉 left gastric vein
28. 右膈脚 right crus of diaphragm
29. 第12胸椎椎体 body of 12th thoracic vertebra
30. 脊髓 spinal cord
31. 椎内静脉丛 internal vertebral venous plexus
32. 黄韧带 ligamenta flava
33. 下腔静脉 inferior vena cava
34. 右肾上腺 right suprarenal gland
35. 右肾上极 the upper pole of right kidney
36. 膈 diaphragm
37. 肝裸区 bare area of liver
38. 肝右后叶下段 inferior segment of right posterior lobe of liver
39. 肝门静脉右后下支及肝动脉、肝管 right posteroinferior branch of hepatic portal vein and corresponding hepatic artery and hepatic duct
40. 肝右静脉后根 posterior root of right hepatic vein
41. 肝右静脉前根 anterior root of right hepatic vein
42. 肝门静脉右前支及动脉 right anterior branch of hepatic portal vein and corresponding artery
43. 肝门静脉右支 right hepatic portal vein
44. 肝右前叶下段 inferior segment of right anterior lobe of liver
45. 肋间外肌 intercostale externi
46. 右肝上间隙 right suprahepatic space
47. 肝门静脉右前下支及肝动脉、肝管 right anteroinferior branch of hepatic portal vein and corresponding hepatic artery and hepatic duct
48. 肝中静脉属支 tributary of middle hepatic vein
49. 肝左内叶 left medial lobe of liver
50. 肝右动脉 right hepatic artery
51. 肝门静脉 hepatic portal vein
52. 肝总管 common hepatic duct
53. 肝镰状韧带 falciform ligament of liver
54. 肝圆韧带裂 fissure for ligamentum teres hepatis
55. 肝圆韧带 ligamentum teres hepatis
56. 肝胃韧带 hepatogastric ligament
57. 静脉韧带裂 fissure for ligamentum venosum
58. 尾状突 caudate process
59. 弓状切迹 arcuate notch
60. 乳头突 papillary process
61. 胃左动脉 left gastric artery

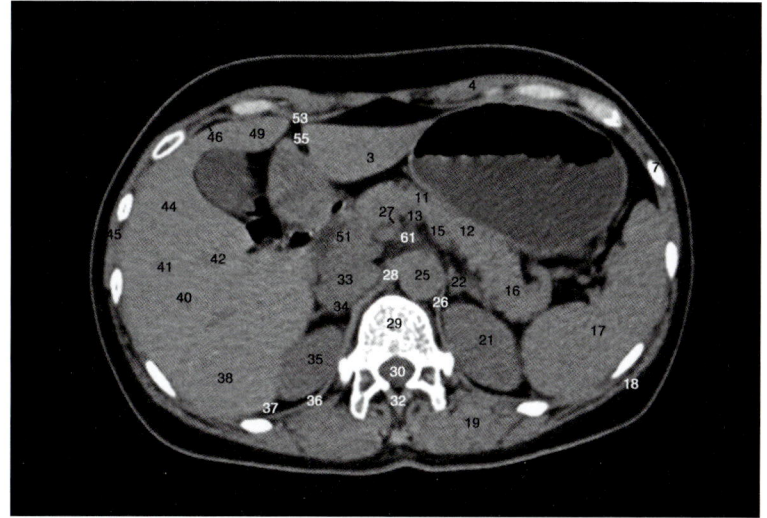

B. CT 平扫图像　　　　C. CT 增强图像

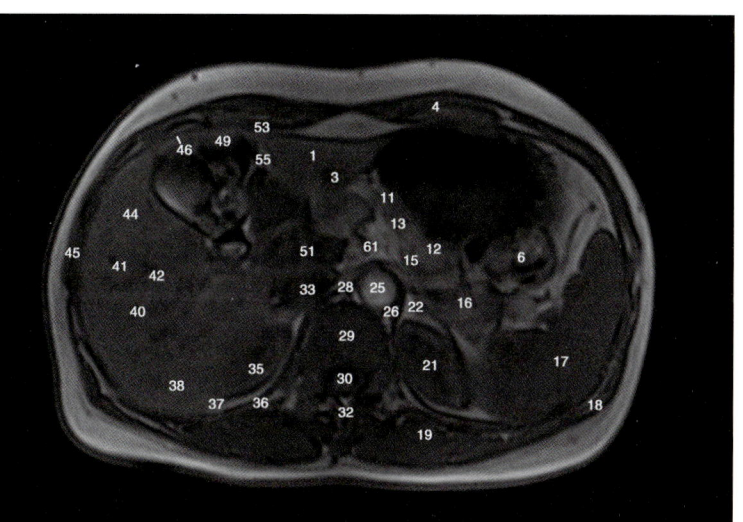

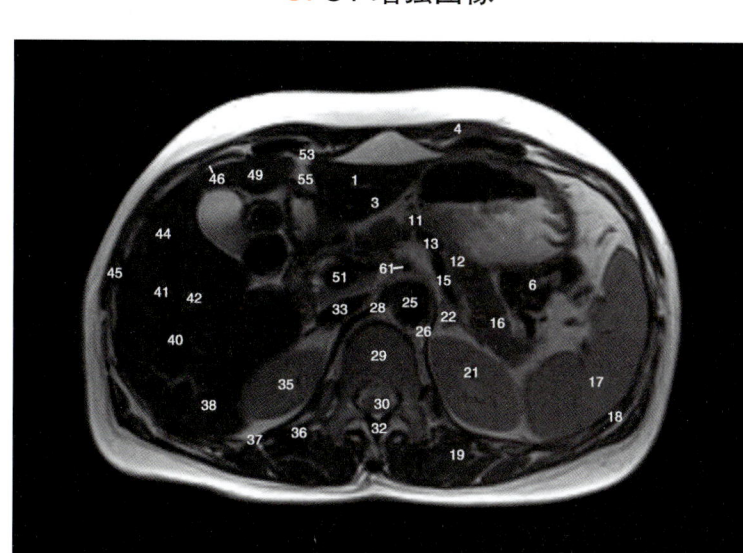

D. MR T1WI　　　　E. MR T2WI

关键结构：肝尾状叶，肝总管。

此断面经第12胸椎椎体中份。

下腔静脉前方可见肝尾状叶，被弓状切迹分隔为乳头突和尾状突。胰的断面逐渐增大，其后方为脾动、静脉及从腹主动脉发出的腹腔干。肝尾状叶位于肝左、右叶背部中央，右侧连于肝右后段，向左伸入第一肝门、第二肝门、第三肝门及下腔静脉之间，左缘游离并突入小网膜囊内。肝尾状叶整体呈左大右小的不规则靴形。尾状叶从外形上有4面、3个突起和3个缘。4面：即横沟面、腔静脉面、静脉韧带裂面和脏面，从脏面上可观测到3个突起：即尾状突、乳头突和腔静脉后突。乳头突和尾状突位于肝尾状叶的最下方，二者向前邻近第一肝门，乳头突位于左侧，变异较大，向左下突出。

尾状突位于右侧，位置较恒定，向右前方伸至第一肝门与下腔静脉之间，将尾状叶连至肝右叶。腔静脉后突自左向右经下腔静脉后壁包绕下腔静脉，有韧带连至下腔静脉和肝右叶，该韧带与肝右叶向左的突起汇合，部分人体的腔静脉后突完全包绕下腔静脉与肝右叶相遇。肝门静脉前方可见肝总管，由左、右肝管出肝后在肝门附近汇合而成，其汇合点多位于肝门平面以下，偶有高位者。肝总管下行2.5~4 cm后，与其右侧的胆囊管汇合，形成胆总管。肝总管管壁由内膜、肌层和外膜3层构成，其功能为输送胆汁。肝总管如因结石或邻近肿瘤压迫影响胆汁输送，可发生梗阻性黄疸。

腹部连续横断层 43（FH.11070）

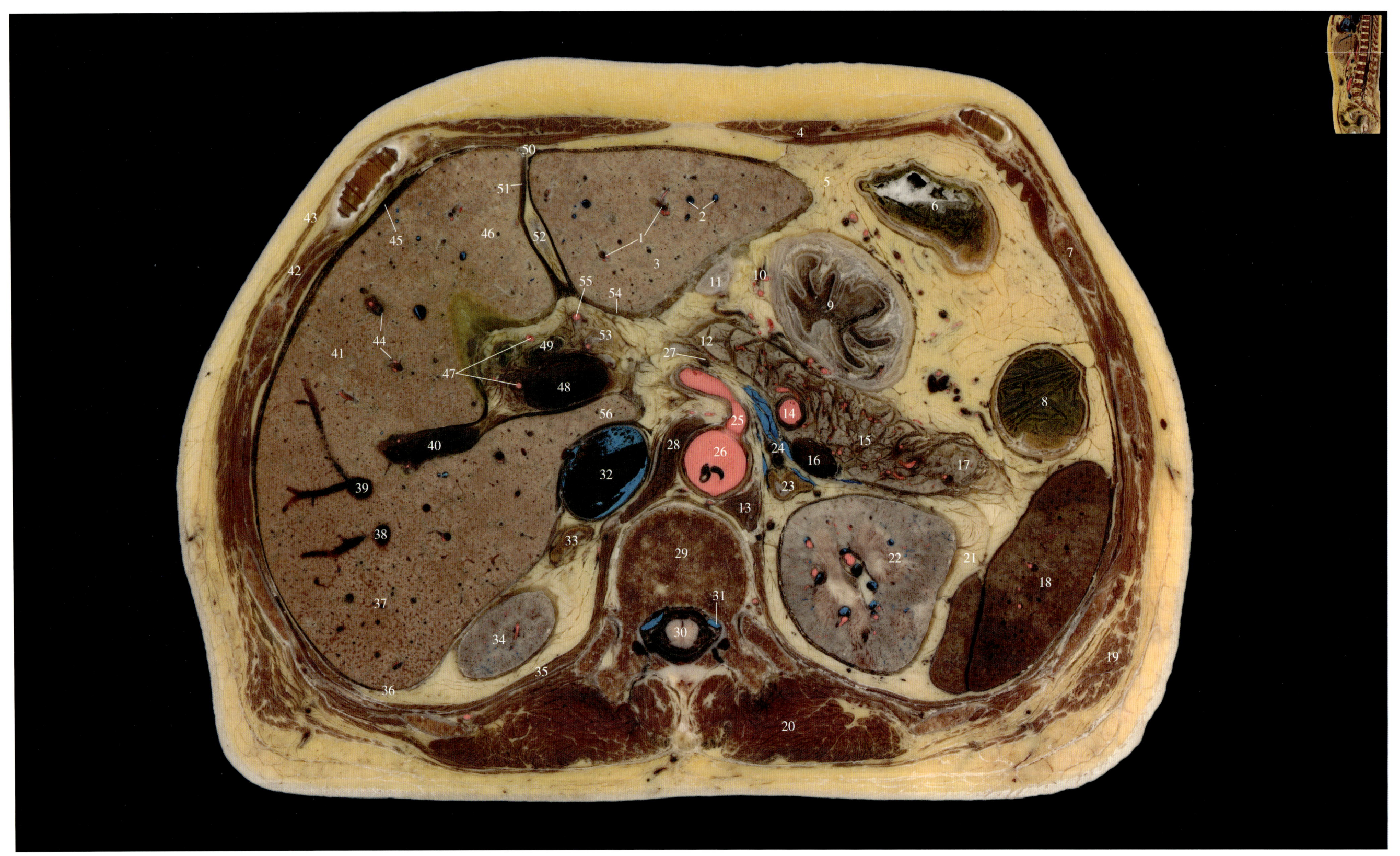

A. 断层标本图像

1. 肝门静脉左外下支及肝动脉 left lateroinferior branch of hepatic portal vein and corresponding hepatic artery
2. 肝左静脉下根 inferior root of left hepatic vein
3. 肝左外叶下段 inferior segment of left lateral lobe of liver
4. 腹直肌 rectus abdominis
5. 大网膜 greater omentum
6. 横结肠 transverse colon
7. 第 8 肋骨 8th costal bone
8. 降结肠 descending colon
9. 胃体 body of stomach
10. 胃动、静脉 gastric artery and vein
11. 胃幽门部 pyloric part of stomach
12. 胰颈 neck of pancreas
13. 左膈脚 left crus of diaphragm
14. 脾动脉 splenic artery
15. 胰体 body of pancreas
16. 脾静脉 splenic vein
17. 胰尾 tail of pancreas
18. 脾 spleen
19. 背阔肌 latissimus dorsi
20. 竖脊肌 erector spinae
21. 脾肾韧带 lienorenal ligament
22. 左肾 left kidney
23. 左肾上腺 left suprarenal gland
24. 肾上腺静脉 adrenal vein
25. 腹腔干 celiac trunk
26. 腹主动脉 abdominal aorta
27. 胃左静脉 left gastric vein
28. 右膈脚 right crus of diaphragm
29. 第 12 胸椎椎体 body of 12th thoracic vertebra
30. 脊髓 spinal cord
31. 椎内静脉丛 internal vertebral venous plexus
32. 下腔静脉 inferior vena cava
33. 右肾上腺 right suprarenal gland
34. 右肾上极 the upper pole of right kidney
35. 膈 diaphragm
36. 肝裸区 bare area of liver
37. 肝右后叶下段 inferior segment of right posterior lobe of liver
38. 肝静脉后根 posterior root of right hepatic vein
39. 肝静脉前根 anterior root of right hepatic vein
40. 肝门静脉右支 right hepatic portal vein
41. 肝右前叶下段 inferior segment of right anterior lobe of liver
42. 肋间外肌 intercostale externi
43. 腹外斜肌 obliquus externus abdominis
44. 肝门静脉右前下支及肝动脉、肝管 right anteroinferior branch of hepatic portal vein and corresponding hepatic artery and hepatic duct
45. 右肝上间隙 right suprahepatic space
46. 肝左内叶 left medial lobe of liver
47. 肝右动脉 right hepatic artery
48. 肝门静脉 hepatic portal vein
49. 肝总管 common hepatic duct
50. 肝镰状韧带 falciform ligament of liver
51. 肝圆韧带裂 fissure for ligamentum teres hepatis
52. 肝圆韧带 ligamentum teres hepatis
53. 肝胃韧带 hepatogastric ligament
54. 静脉韧带裂 fissure for ligamentum venosum
55. 肝左动脉 left hepatic artery
56. 肝尾状叶 caudate lobe of liver

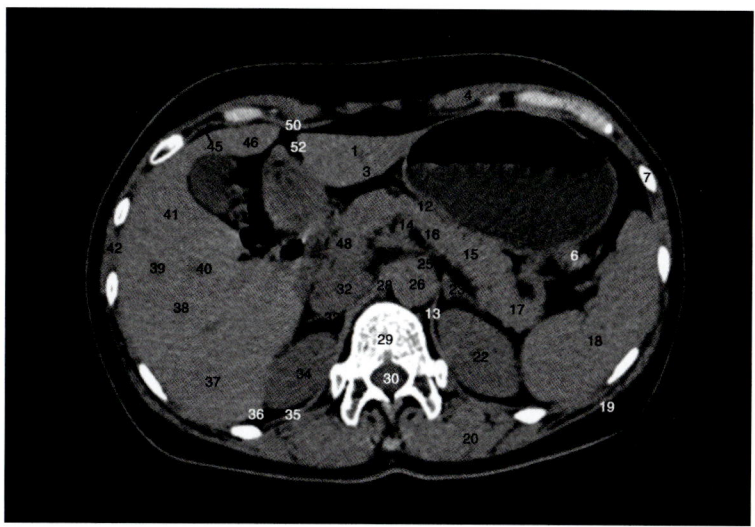

B. CT 平扫图像

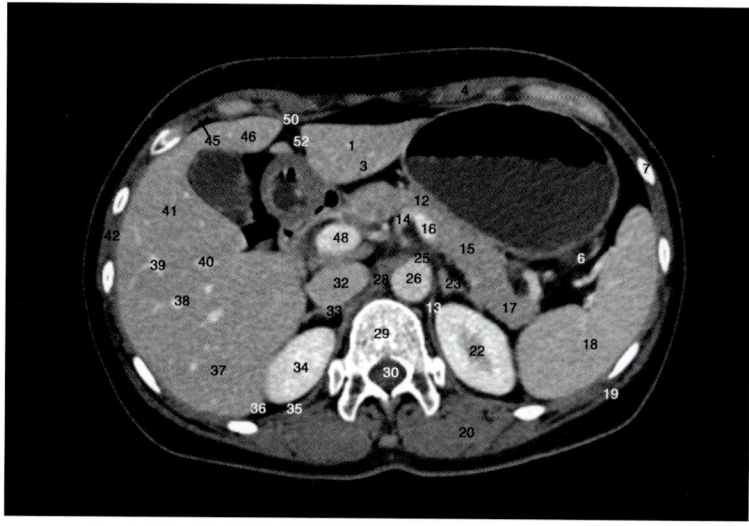

C. CT 增强图像

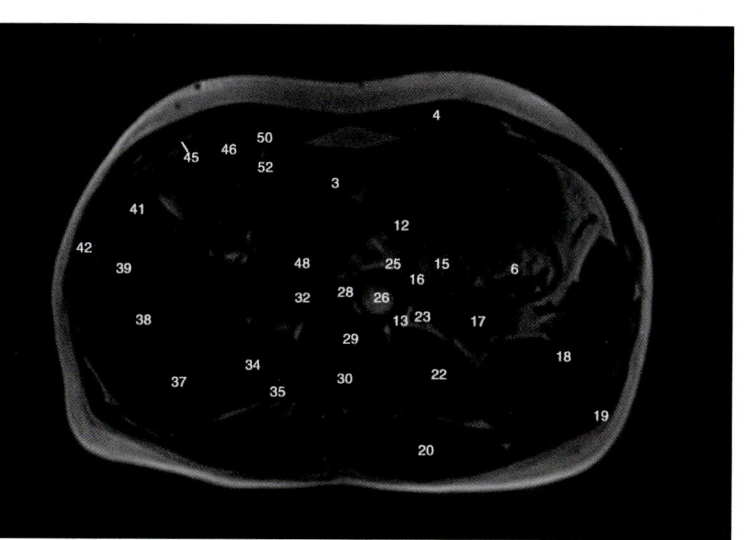

D. MR T1WI

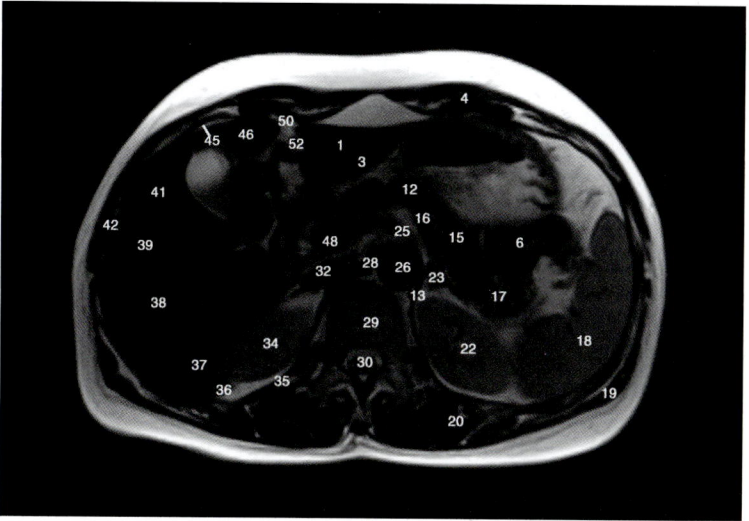

E. MR T2WI

关键结构：腹主动脉，腹腔干，肝右动脉，肝左动脉。

此断面经第 12 胸椎椎体下份。

腹腔干从腹主动脉发出为本断面的主要特征，肝门静脉周围可见肝左、右动脉。腹主动脉又称主动脉腹部，在第 12 胸椎下缘前方略偏左侧，经膈的主动脉裂孔进入腹膜后隙，沿脊柱的左前方下行，至第 4 腰椎下缘水平分为左、右髂总动脉。腹主动脉全长 14~15 cm，周径 2.9~3.0 cm。腹主动脉的前面为胰、十二指肠水平部及肠系膜根等；后面为第 1~4 腰椎及椎间盘；右侧为下腔静脉；左侧为左交感干。腹主动脉周围还有腰淋巴结、腹腔淋巴结和神经丛等。腹腔干为一短干，平均长约 24.5 mm，在膈的主动脉裂孔稍下方自腹主动脉前壁，起点多在第 1 腰椎水平，少数在第 1 腰椎以上。其分支可有变异，但以分出肝总动脉、脾动脉和胃左动脉为多。肝右动脉 43% 起源于肝固有动脉，31% 来于肝总动脉，余为异位起源，称为迷走肝右动脉。肝右动脉多数经胆道后方入胆囊三角，在此分出胆囊动脉支。此后它行走在肝总管后面（80%），少数在肝总管之前（20%），绕肝门静脉右支和肝管的浅面，在肝门右切迹内发出右尾状叶动脉、右前叶动脉和右后叶动脉，后者再分成上、下两段支，分布于相应的肝叶和肝段。肝右动脉平均长度为 3.5~4.5 cm，直径 0.3~0.42 cm。肝左动脉 40% 起源于肝固有动脉，32% 起于肝总动脉，其他起源于异位者为迷走肝左动脉。肝左动脉一般沿肝门静脉左支横部及肝左管的浅面向左走行，其叶、段分支大部在肝外发出。通常先发出尾状叶动脉，再发出左内叶动脉和左外叶动脉，而左外叶动脉又分成上、下段支，分布于相应的肝叶和肝段。肝左动脉直径为 0.25~0.35 cm，少数可达 0.4~0.45 cm[26]。

87

腹部连续横断层 44（FH.11050）

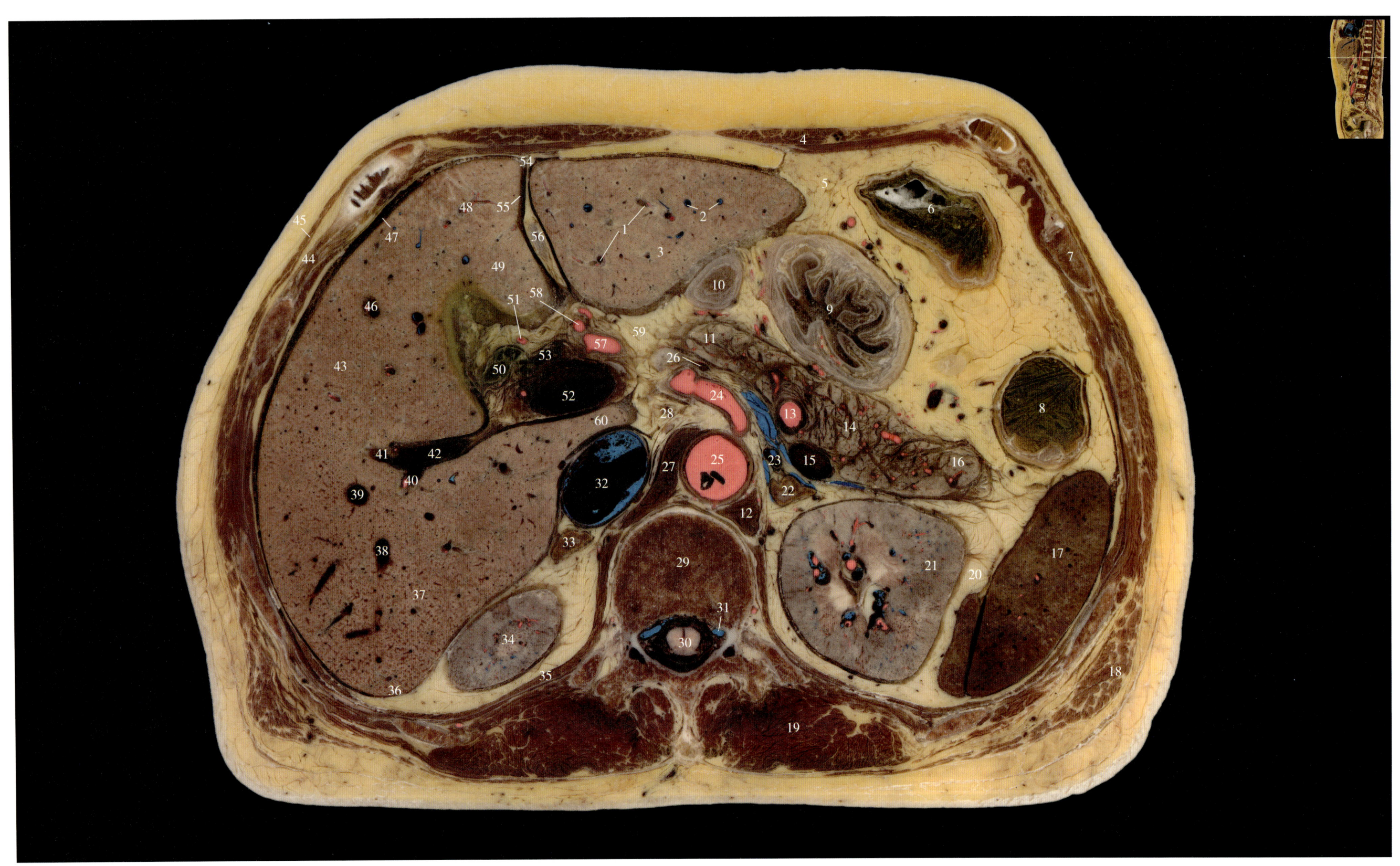

A. 断层标本图像

1. 肝门静脉左外下支及肝动脉 left lateroinferior branch of hepatic portal vein and corresponding hepatic artery
2. 肝左静脉下根属支 tributary of inferior root of left hepatic vein
3. 肝左外叶下段 inferior segment of left lateral lobe of liver
4. 腹直肌 rectus abdominis
5. 大网膜 greater omentum
6. 横结肠 transverse colon
7. 第 8 肋骨 8th costal bone
8. 降结肠 descending colon
9. 胃体 body of stomach
10. 胃幽门部 pyloric part of stomach
11. 胰颈 neck of pancreas
12. 左膈脚 left crus of diaphragm
13. 脾动脉 splenic artery
14. 胰体 body of pancreas
15. 脾静脉 splenic vein
16. 胰尾 tail of pancreas
17. 脾 spleen
18. 背阔肌 latissimus dorsi
19. 竖脊肌 erector spinae
20. 脾肾韧带 lienorenal ligament
21. 左肾 left kidney
22. 左肾上腺 left suprarenal gland
23. 肾上腺静脉 adrenal vein
24. 腹腔干 celiac trunk
25. 腹主动脉 abdominal aorta
26. 胃左静脉 left gastric vein
27. 右膈脚 right crus of diaphragm
28. 淋巴结 lymph node
29. 第 12 胸椎椎体 body of 12th thoracic vertebra
30. 脊髓 spinal cord
31. 椎内静脉丛 internal vertebral venous plexus
32. 下腔静脉 inferior vena cava
33. 右肾上腺 right suprarenal gland
34. 右肾 right kidney
35. 膈 diaphragm
36. 肝裸区 bare area of liver
37. 肝右后叶下段 inferior segment of right posterior lobe of liver
38. 肝右静脉后根 posterior root of right hepatic vein
39. 肝右静脉前根 anterior root of right hepatic vein
40. 肝门静脉右后支 right posterior branch of hepatic portal vein
41. 肝门静脉右前支 right anterior branch of hepatic portal vein
42. 肝门静脉右支 right hepatic portal vein
43. 肝右前叶下段 inferior segment of right anterior lobe of liver
44. 肋间外肌 intercostale externi
45. 腹外斜肌 obliquus externus abdominis
46. 肝门静脉右前下支及肝动脉、肝管 right anteroinferior branch of hepatic portal vein and corresponding hepatic artery and hepatic duct
47. 右肝上间隙 right suprahepatic space
48. 肝门静脉左内叶支 left medial branch of hepatic portal vein
49. 肝左内叶 left medial lobe of liver
50. 胆囊底 fundus of gallbladder
51. 肝右动脉 right hepatic artery
52. 肝门静脉 hepatic portal vein
53. 肝总管 common hepatic duct
54. 肝镰状韧带 falciform ligament of liver
55. 肝圆韧带裂 fissure for ligamentum teres hepatis
56. 肝圆韧带 ligamentum teres hepatis
57. 肝总动脉 common hepatic artery
58. 肝左动脉 left hepatic artery
59. 肝胃韧带 hepatogastric ligament
60. 肝尾状叶 caudate lobe of liver

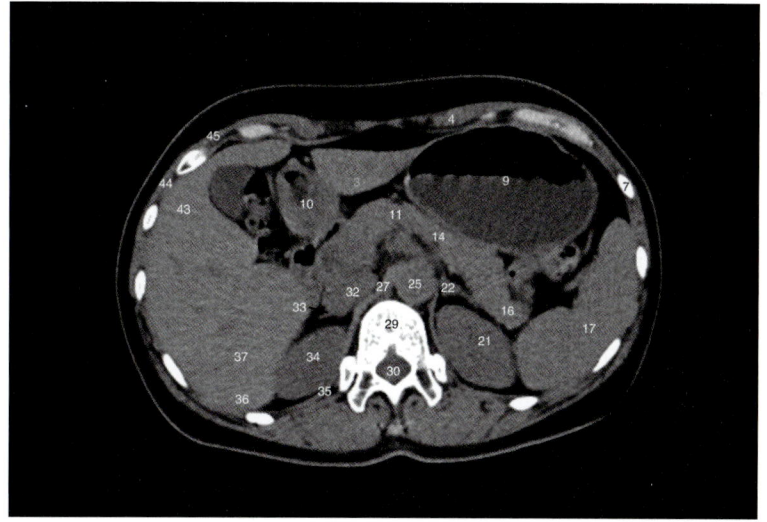

B. CT 平扫图像

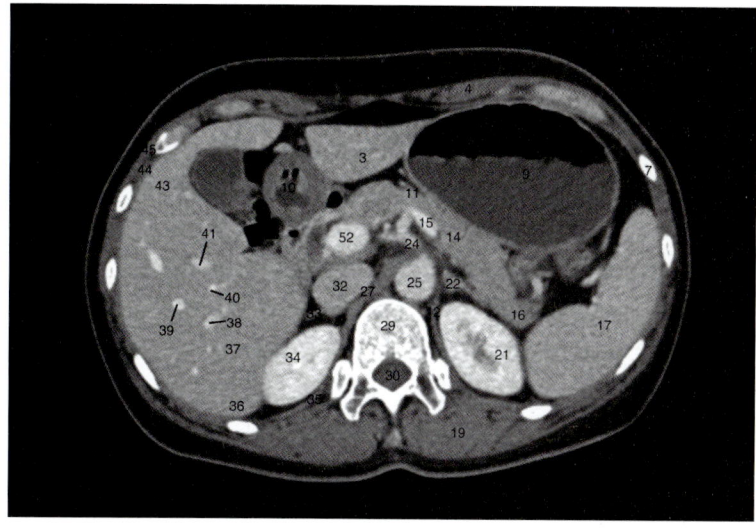

C. CT 增强图像

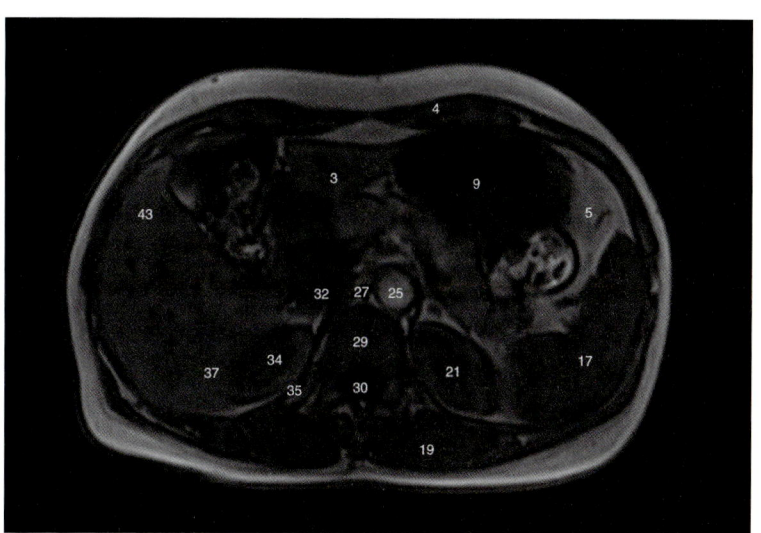

D. MR T1WI

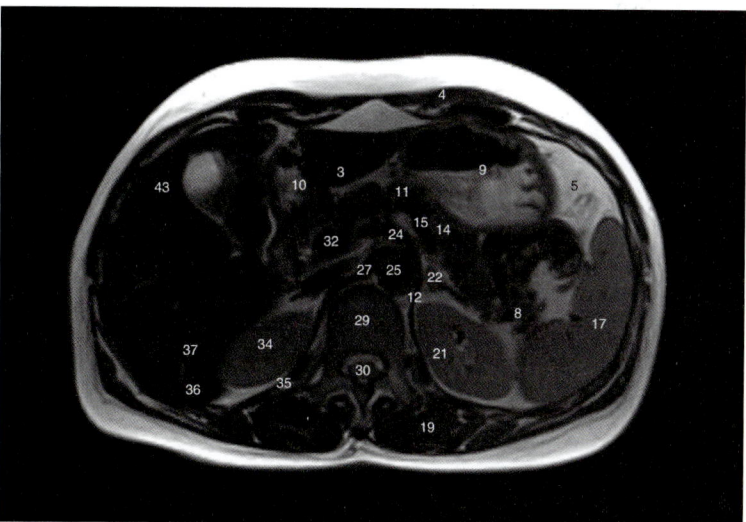

E. MR T2WI

关键结构：右肾，腹腔淋巴结，肝总动脉。

此断面经过第 12 胸椎椎体。

腹主动脉行于脊柱左前方，右侧为下腔静脉，胰居左肾与胃体之间，脊柱两侧可见左肾及右肾上极。右肾从前面观位于第 12 胸椎椎体上缘至第 3 腰椎椎体上缘之间，从背面观位于第 11~12 胸椎棘突之间，或第 12 胸椎棘突至第 2~3 腰椎棘突之间，或第 3 腰椎棘突平面[2]。右肾前方上部为肝右叶，下部为结肠右曲，内侧为十二指肠降部。肾与周边器官关系密切，当发生肿瘤或炎性疾病时可累及邻近结构，甚至出现远处淋巴结的转移。腹腔淋巴结位于腹腔干周围[27,28]，数目较恒定，一般为 1~3 个，平均 1.3 个[27~29]。腹腔淋巴结与腹腔神经节相似，蔡昌平等[30]发现在尸体标本的 CT 图像上二者很难区分，而 MRI 却比较容易进行鉴别，这是因为尸体标本由于甲醛灌注导致周围液体密度增加，但正常人 CT 图像中腹腔淋巴结与周围脂肪存在较大的密度差而容易识别[31~33]。在 MR 图像中，腹腔神经节较腹腔淋巴结更薄，位置贴近膈脚、位于腹腔后内方而易于识别。肝总动脉一般起自腹腔干，然后又分为胃十二指肠动脉和肝固有动脉，肝固有动脉再分出左、右肝动脉，这种分支类型通常被称为正常型。但肝动脉解剖有很多变异，Michels[34] 和 Hitta 分型[35] 是目前国际学术界常用的肝动脉解剖变异分型，其中 Michels 分型常用，仅该分型目前就有 10 种肝动脉变异类型。肝动脉变异率高且表现形式复杂多样。在肝疾病影像诊断、手术和介入治疗之前，需充分了解肝动脉的解剖变异，避免手术或穿刺误伤，从而精准栓塞肿瘤血管，减少并发症，缩短治疗时间，最终提高诊治效果[36]。

腹部连续横断层 45（FH.11030）

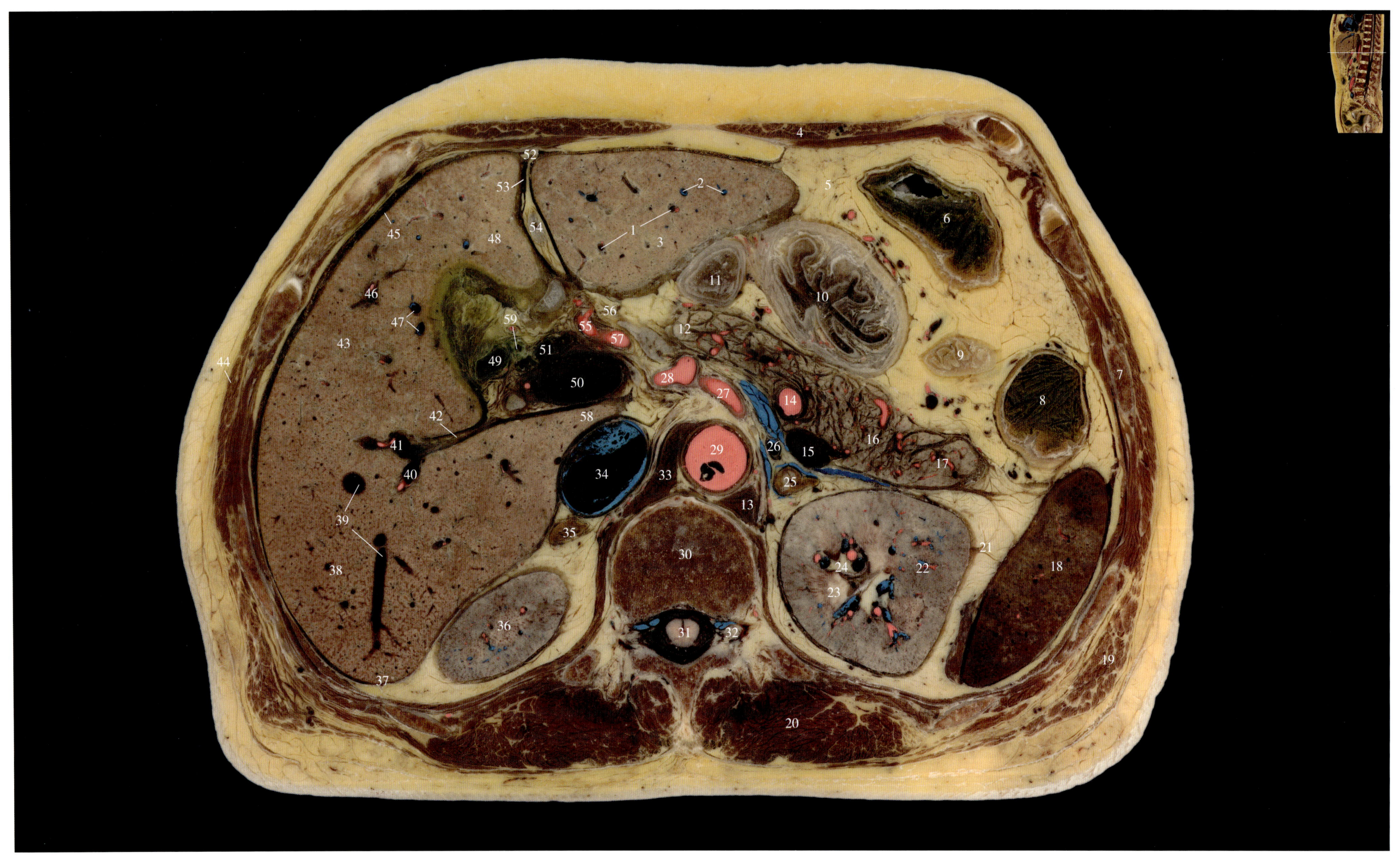

A. 断层标本图像

1. 肝门静脉左外下支及肝动脉 left lateroinferior branch of hepatic portal vein and corresponding hepatic artery
2. 肝左静脉下根属支 tributary of inferior root of left hepatic vein
3. 肝左外叶下段 inferior segment of left lateral lobe of liver
4. 腹直肌 rectus abdominis
5. 大网膜 greater omentum
6. 横结肠 transverse colon
7. 第9肋骨 9th costal bone
8. 降结肠 descending colon
9. 空肠 jejunum
10. 胃体 body of stomach
11. 胃幽门部 pyloric part of stomach
12. 胰颈 neck of pancreas
13. 左膈脚 left crus of diaphragm
14. 脾动脉 splenic artery
15. 脾静脉 splenic vein
16. 胰体 body of pancreas
17. 胰尾 tail of pancreas
18. 脾 spleen
19. 背阔肌 latissimus dorsi
20. 竖脊肌 erector spinae
21. 脾肾韧带 lienorenal ligament
22. 左肾 left kidney
23. 肾锥体 renal pyramid
24. 肾小盏 minor renal calices
25. 左肾上腺 left suprarenal gland
26. 肾上腺静脉 adrenal vein
27. 腹腔干 celiac trunk
28. 肝总动脉 common hepatic artery
29. 腹主动脉 abdominal aorta
30. 第12胸椎椎体 body of 12th thoracic vertebra
31. 脊髓 spinal cord
32. 脊神经根 root of spinal nerve
33. 右膈脚 right crus of diaphragm
34. 下腔静脉 inferior vena cava
35. 右肾上腺 right suprarenal gland
36. 右肾 right kidney
37. 肝裸区 bare area of liver
38. 肝右后叶下段 inferior segment of right posterior lobe of liver
39. 肝右静脉属支 tributary of right hepatic vein
40. 肝门静脉右后支 right posterior branch of hepatic portal vein
41. 肝门静脉右前支 right anterior branch of hepatic portal vein
42. 肝门右切迹 right notch of porta hepatis
43. 肝右前叶下段 inferior segment of right anterior lobe of liver
44. 腹外斜肌 obliquus externus abdominis
45. 右肝上间隙 right suprahepatic space
46. 肝门静脉右前下支及肝动脉、肝管 right anteroinferior branch of hepatic portal vein and corresponding hepatic artery and hepatic duct
47. 肝中静脉属支 tributary of middle hepatic vein
48. 肝左内叶 left medial lobe of liver
49. 胆囊底 fundus of gallbladder
50. 肝门静脉 hepatic portal vein
51. 肝总管 common hepatic duct
52. 肝镰状韧带 falciform ligament of liver
53. 肝圆韧带裂 fissure for ligamentum teres hepatis
54. 肝圆韧带 ligamentum teres hepatis
55. 肝左动脉 left hepatic artery
56. 肝胃韧带 hepatogastric ligament
57. 肝固有动脉 proper hepatic artery
58. 肝尾状叶 caudate lobe of liver
59. 胆囊管 cystic duct

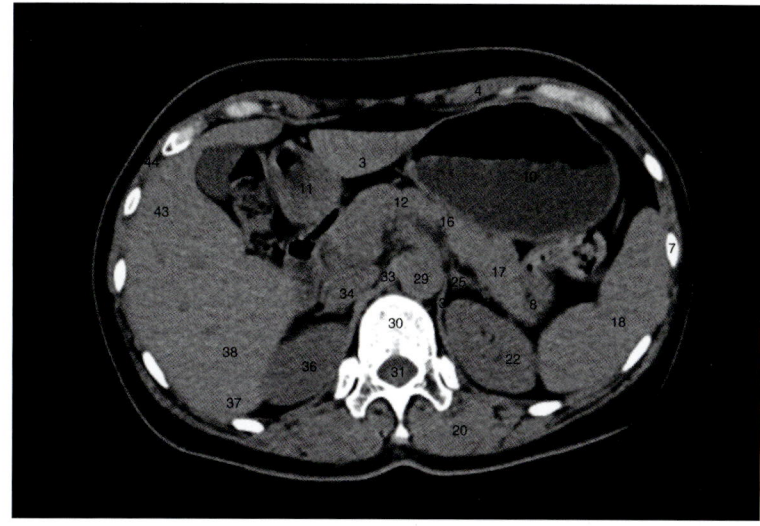

B. CT 平扫图像

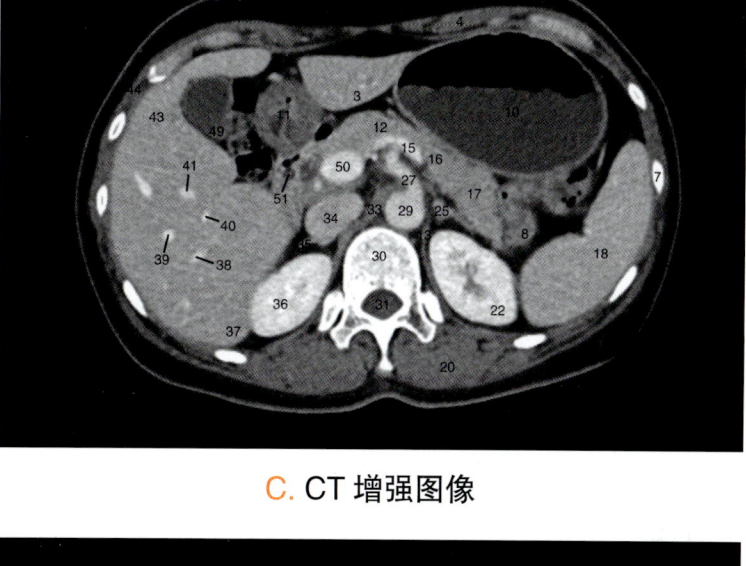

C. CT 增强图像

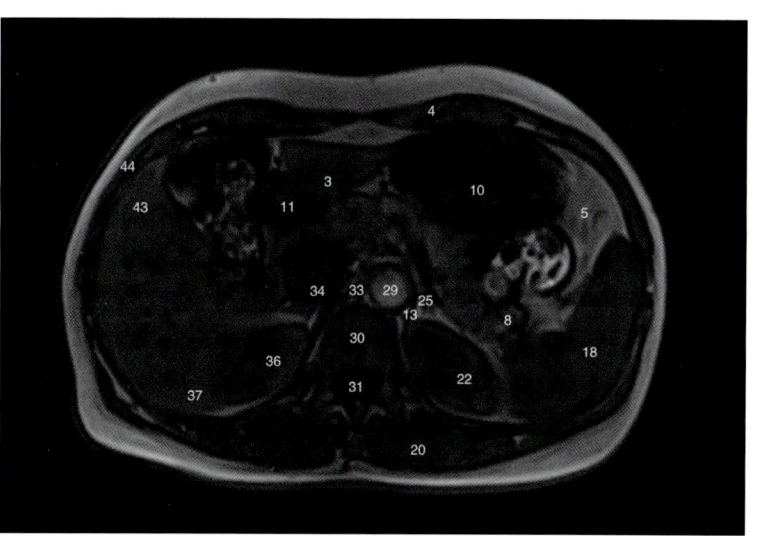

D. MR T1WI

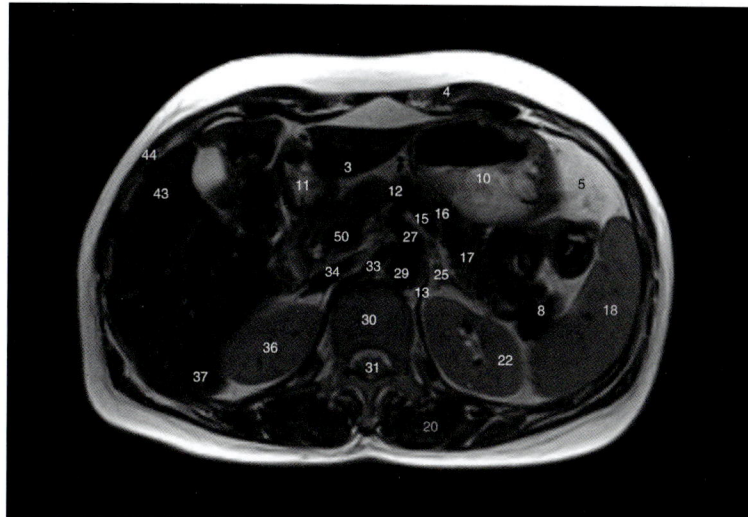

E. MR T2WI

关键结构：胆囊底，胆囊管，肝固有动脉。

此断面经过第12胸椎椎体。

肝门静脉右前方可见胆囊底、胆囊管和肝总管。胆囊底前缘与腹前壁相接触，位于右侧第9肋软骨与锁骨中线交点的稍下方，后缘与横结肠的起始部相邻。临床上常以右侧腹直肌的外侧缘与右肋弓的交点作为胆囊触诊区[2]。胆囊管由胆囊颈向左后下方延续而成，长为1.6~3.5 cm，直径为0.2~0.3 cm。胆囊管多汇入肝总管右侧壁再延续成胆总管，二者汇合的形式可分为3种，即角型、平行型、螺旋型。黄瀛等[37]研究发现：角型约占47%；平行型约占43%；螺旋型较少见，约占10%。解剖学上将胆囊管、肝总管及肝脏脏面三者构成的三角形区域称为胆囊三角（又叫Calot三角、卡洛氏三角或胆囊动脉三角）。该三角内常有发自肝右动脉的胆囊动脉经过，并常见胆囊颈部的淋巴结。胆囊三角是临床解剖上的主要标志，在行胆囊切除时要在该三角内寻找到胆囊动脉并加以结扎切断，要仔细甄别出较粗的肝右动脉，以免发生误伤导致出血或因结扎导致右半肝缺血。肝固有动脉在肝十二指肠韧带内与肝门静脉、胆总管同行，有文献报道肝固有动脉及其分支变异率为19.7%~46.5%[38-40]。魏桢杰等[41]在标本解剖中发现肝左动脉变异合并肝固有动脉、胃右动脉阙如的情况。此种变异在临床上极为少见，提示临床医生在进行肝脏以及胃部手术时要充分考虑血管变异的可能性，选择合理的治疗手段。

腹部连续横断层 46（FH.11010）

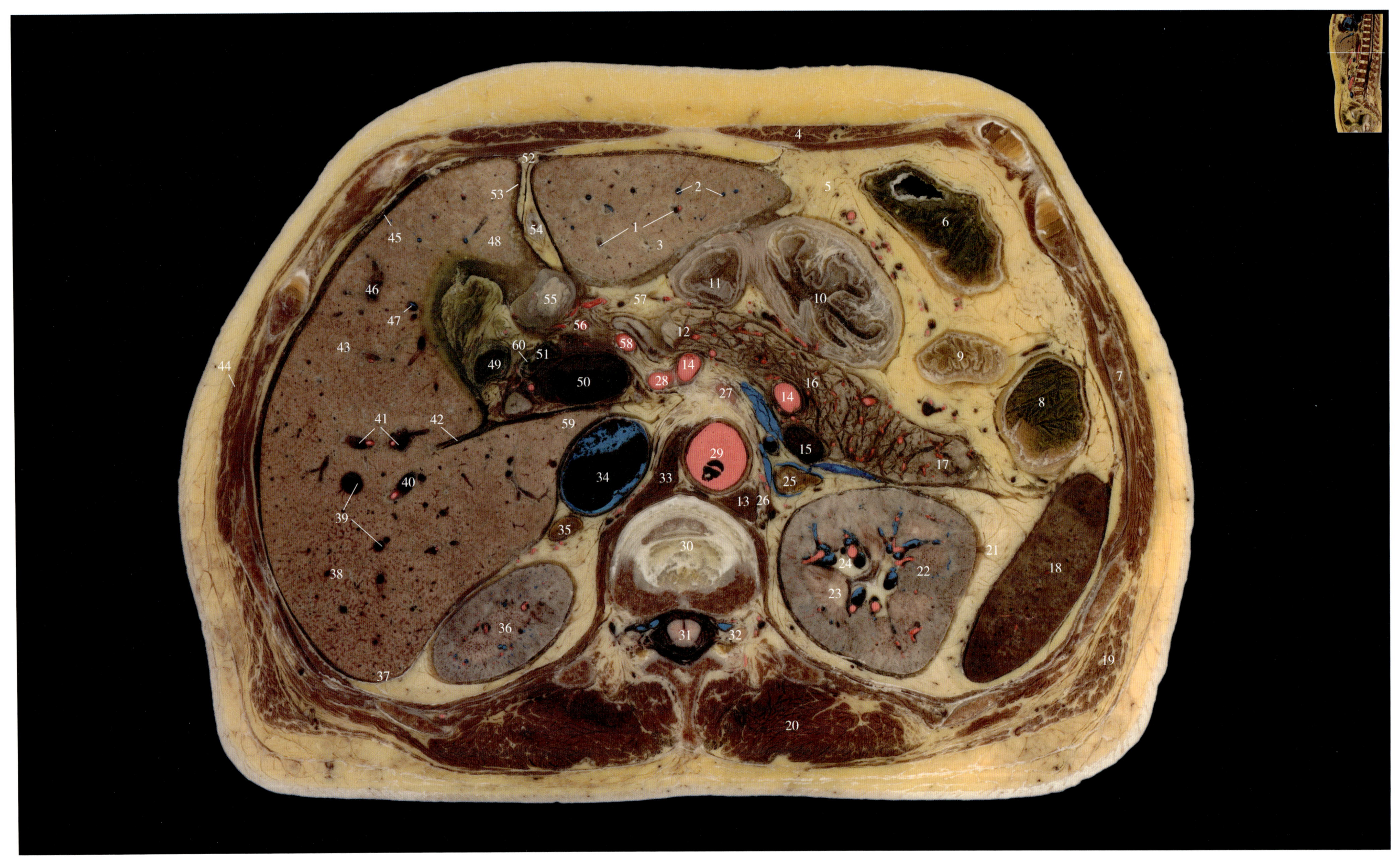

A. 断层标本图像

1. 肝门静脉左外下支及肝动脉 left lateroinferior branch of hepatic portal vein and corresponding hepatic artery
2. 肝左静脉下根属支 tributary of inferior root of left hepatic vein
3. 肝左外叶下段 inferior segment of left lateral lobe of liver
4. 腹直肌 rectus abdominis
5. 大网膜 greater omentum
6. 横结肠 transverse colon
7. 第9肋骨 9th costal bone
8. 降结肠 descending colon
9. 空肠 jejunum
10. 胃体 body of stomach
11. 胃幽门部 pyloric part of stomach
12. 胰颈 neck of pancreas
13. 左膈脚 left crus of diaphragm
14. 脾动脉 splenic artery
15. 脾静脉 splenic vein
16. 胰体 body of pancreas
17. 胰尾 tail of pancreas
18. 脾 spleen
19. 背阔肌 latissimus dorsi
20. 竖脊肌 erector spinae
21. 脾肾韧带 lienorenal ligament
22. 左肾 left kidney
23. 肾锥体 renal pyramid
24. 肾小盏 minor renal calices
25. 左肾上腺 left suprarenal gland
26. 交感干 sympathetic trunk
27. 腹腔干 celiac trunk
28. 肝总动脉 common hepatic artery
29. 腹主动脉 abdominal aorta
30. T12-L1 椎间盘 T12-L1 intervertebral disc
31. 脊髓 spinal cord
32. 脊神经根 root of spinal nerve
33. 右膈脚 right crus of diaphragm
34. 下腔静脉 inferior vena cava
35. 右肾上腺 right suprarenal gland
36. 右肾 right kidney
37. 肝裸区 bare area of liver
38. 肝右后叶下段 inferior segment of right posterior lobe of liver
39. 肝右静脉属支 tributary of right hepatic vein
40. 肝门静脉右后支 right posterior branch of hepatic portal vein
41. 肝门静脉右前支 right anterior branch of hepatic portal vein
42. 肝门右切迹 right notch of porta hepatis
43. 肝右前叶下段 inferior segment of right anterior lobe of liver
44. 腹外斜肌 obliquus externus abdominis
45. 右肝上间隙 right suprahepatic space
46. 肝门静脉右前下支及肝动脉、肝管 right anteroinferior branch of hepatic portal vein and corresponding hepatic artery and hepatic duct
47. 肝中静脉属支 tributary of middle hepatic vein
48. 肝左内叶 left medial lobe of liver
49. 胆囊 gallbladder
50. 肝门静脉 hepatic portal vein
51. 肝总管 common hepatic duct
52. 肝镰状韧带 falciform ligament of liver
53. 肝圆韧带裂 fissure for ligamentum teres hepatis
54. 肝圆韧带 ligamentum teres hepatis
55. 十二指肠上部 superior part of duodenum
56. 肝左动脉 left hepatic artery
57. 肝胃韧带 hepatogastric ligament
58. 肝固有动脉 proper hepatic artery
59. 肝尾状叶 caudate lobe of liver
60. 胆囊管 cystic duct

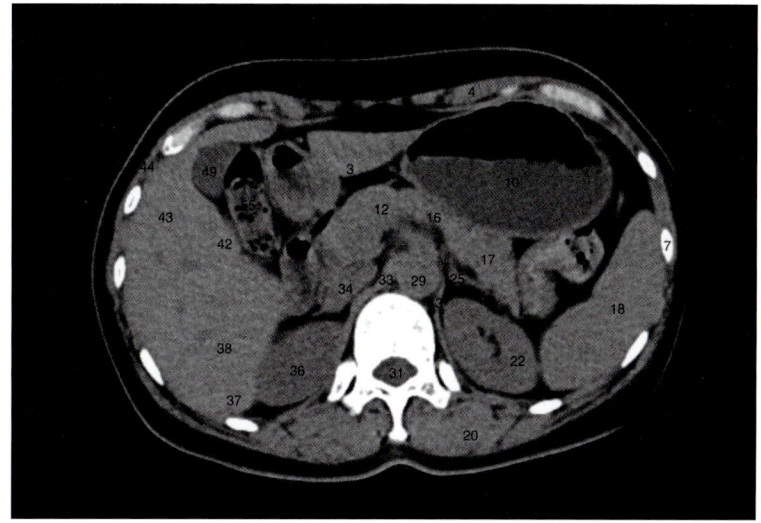

B. CT 平扫图像

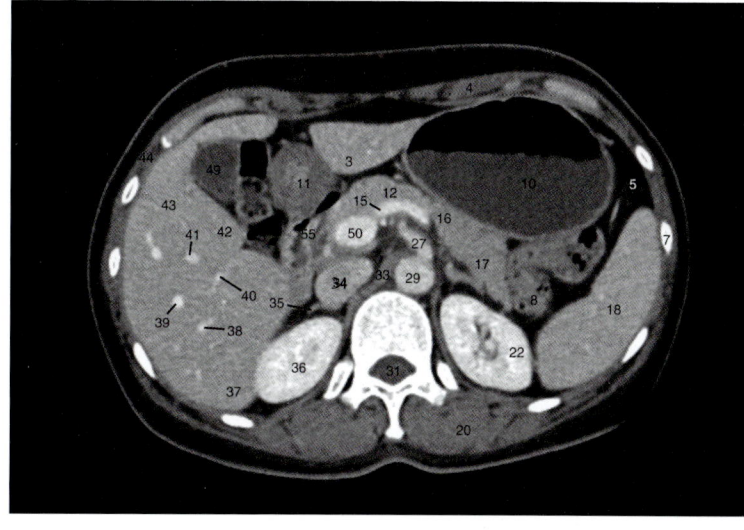

C. CT 增强图像

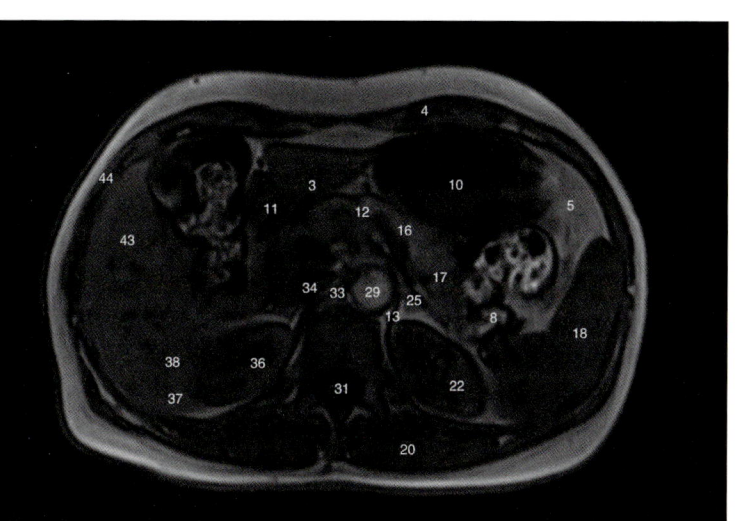

D. MR T1WI

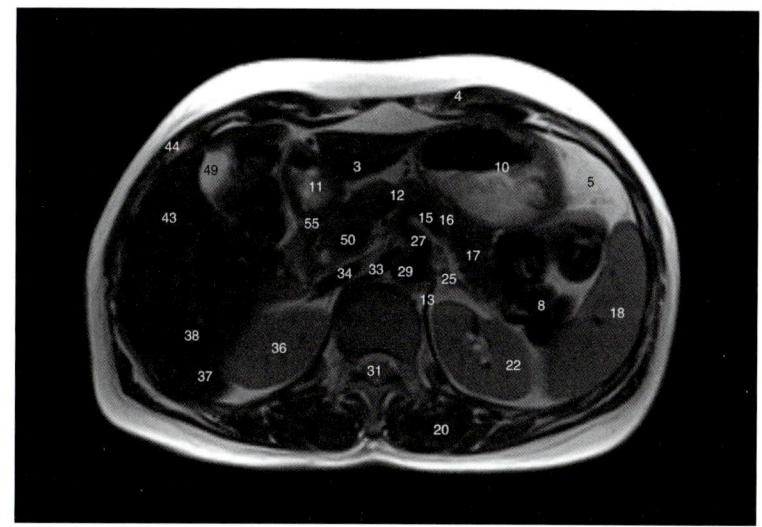

E. MR T2WI

关键结构：胃幽门部，横结肠，降结肠。

此断面经过 T12-L1 椎间盘。

腹腔内由右向左依次为肝、胆囊、胰、胃、横结肠、降结肠、脾等结构，肝左叶与胃之间可见胃幽门部。胃幽门部是溃疡好发部位，且易发生梗阻。幽门前面有 1 条幽门前静脉，手术时是识别幽门的重要标志。发生胃潴留时钡餐检查可见胃影扩大、张力减低，钡剂入胃后下沉出现气、液、钡 3 层现象，钡餐后 6 小时钡剂存留超过 25% 或 24 小时后仍有钡剂残留者提示有瘢痕性的幽门梗阻存在。横结肠起自结肠右曲，先向左下横过腹中部再向左后上至脾下方，形成开口向上的弓形，在脾的内下方急转向下形成结肠左曲，与降结肠相续。横结肠长 40~50 cm，为腹膜内位器官，前方被大网膜覆盖，后方与胰腺及十二指肠水平部相邻，上方与肝右叶、胆囊、胃和脾相邻，下方与空、回肠相邻，是结肠最长、活动度最大的部分。其中部有不同程度下垂，老年或瘦长体型者可达脐下，甚至盆腔，横结肠常随胃肠的充盈变化而升降。降结肠沿肾外侧缘向下达左侧髂嵴水平，下端移行为乙状结肠。降结肠长 20~25 cm，属腹膜间位器官，其内侧为左侧肠系膜窦和空肠肠袢，后方借疏松结缔组织与腹后壁相连，外侧为左侧结肠旁沟，此沟上端被膈结肠韧带阻隔，向下与盆腔相通，因此沟内积液只能向下流入盆腔。

腹部连续横断层 47（FH.10990）

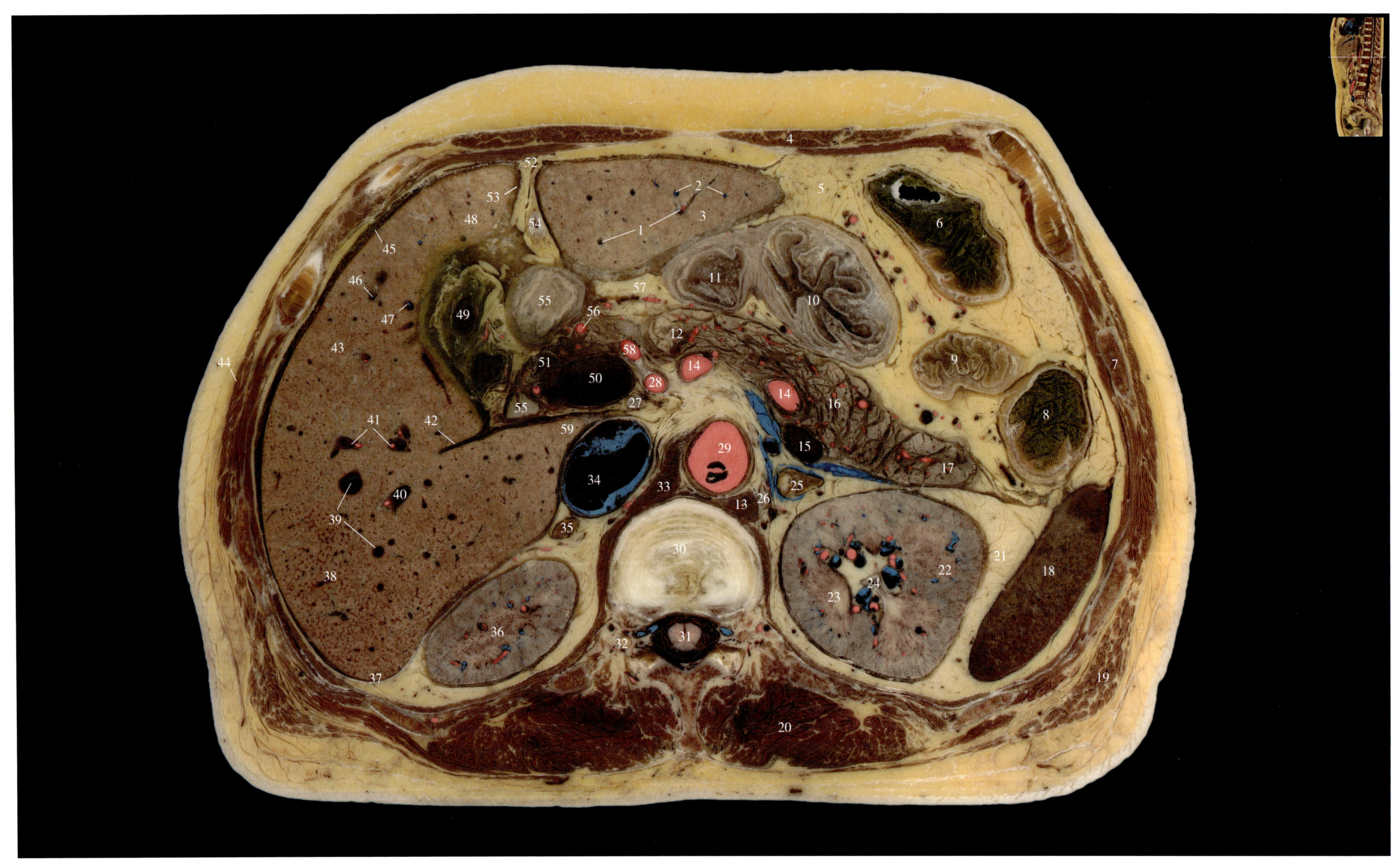

A. 断层标本图像

1. 肝门静脉左外下支及肝动脉 left lateroinferior branch of hepatic portal vein and corresponding hepatic artery
2. 肝左静脉下根属支 tributary of inferior root of left hepatic vein
3. 肝左外叶下段 inferior segment of left lateral lobe of liver
4. 腹直肌 rectus abdominis
5. 大网膜 greater omentum
6. 横结肠 transverse colon
7. 第9肋骨 9th costal bone
8. 降结肠 descending colon
9. 空肠 jejunum
10. 胃体 body of stomach
11. 胃幽门部 pyloric part of stomach
12. 胰颈 neck of pancreas
13. 左膈脚 left crus of diaphragm
14. 脾动脉 splenic artery
15. 脾静脉 splenic vein
16. 胰体 body of pancreas
17. 胰尾 tail of pancreas
18. 脾 spleen
19. 背阔肌 latissimus dorsi
20. 竖脊肌 erector spinae
21. 脾肾韧带 lienorenal ligament
22. 左肾 left kidney
23. 肾锥体 renal pyramid
24. 肾小盏 minor renal calices
25. 左肾上腺 left suprarenal gland
26. 交感干 sympathetic trunk
27. 门腔淋巴结 portocaval lymph node
28. 肝总动脉 common hepatic artery
29. 腹主动脉 abdominal aorta
30. T12-L1椎间盘 T12-L1 intervertebral disc
31. 脊髓 spinal cord
32. 第12胸神经 12th thoracic nerve
33. 右膈脚 right crus of diaphragm
34. 下腔静脉 inferior vena cava
35. 右肾上腺 right suprarenal gland
36. 右肾 right kidney
37. 肝裸区 bare area of liver
38. 肝右后叶下段 inferior segment of right posterior lobe of liver
39. 肝右静脉属支 tributary of right hepatic vein
40. 肝门静脉右后支 right posterior branch of hepatic portal vein
41. 肝门静脉右前支 right anterior branch of hepatic portal vein
42. 肝门右切迹 right notch of porta hepatis
43. 肝右前叶下段 inferior segment of right anterior lobe of liver
44. 腹外斜肌 obliquus externus abdominis
45. 右肝上间隙 right suprahepatic space
46. 肝门静脉右前下支及肝动脉、肝管 right anteroinferior branch of hepatic portal vein and corresponding hepatic artery and hepatic duct
47. 肝中静脉属支 tributary of middle hepatic vein
48. 肝左内叶 left medial lobe of liver
49. 胆囊 gallbladder
50. 肝门静脉 hepatic portal vein
51. 胆总管 common bile duct
52. 肝镰状韧带 falciform ligament of liver
53. 肝圆韧带裂 fissure for ligamentum teres hepatis
54. 肝圆韧带 ligamentum teres hepatis
55. 十二指肠上部 superior part of duodenum
56. 肝左动脉 left hepatic artery
57. 肝胃韧带 hepatogastric ligament
58. 肝固有动脉 proper hepatic artery
59. 肝尾状叶 caudate lobe of liver

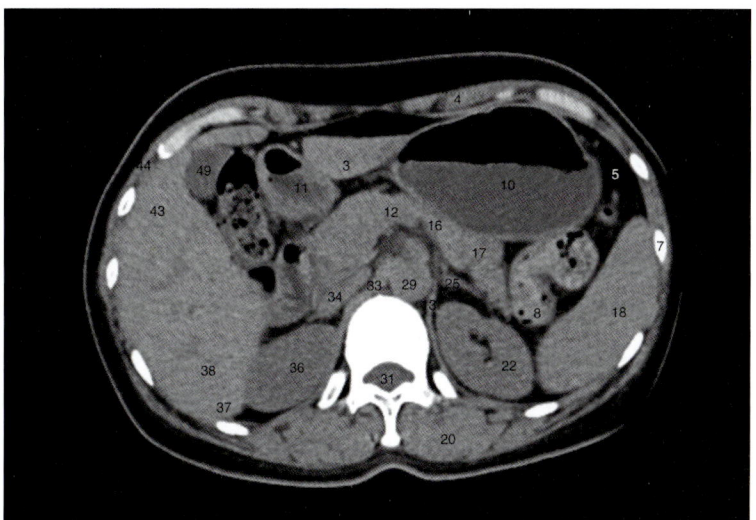

B. CT 平扫图像

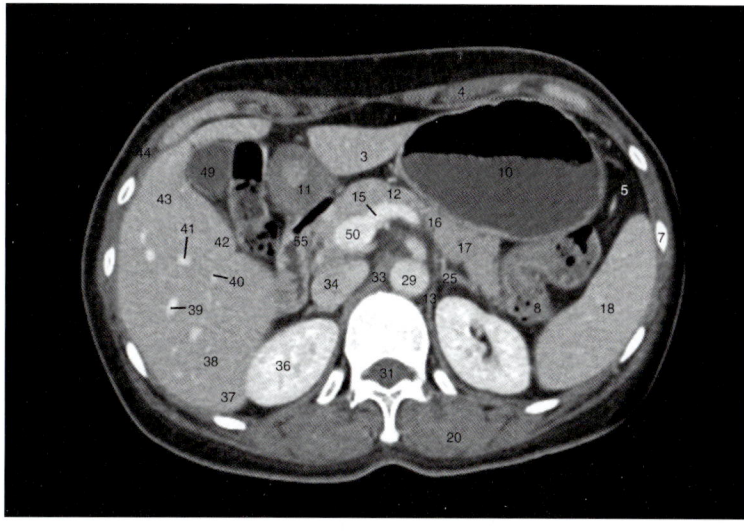

C. CT 增强图像

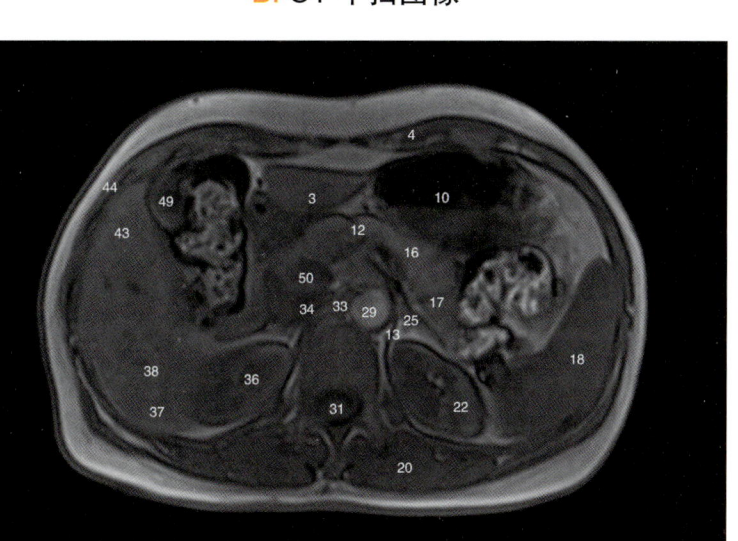

D. MR T1WI

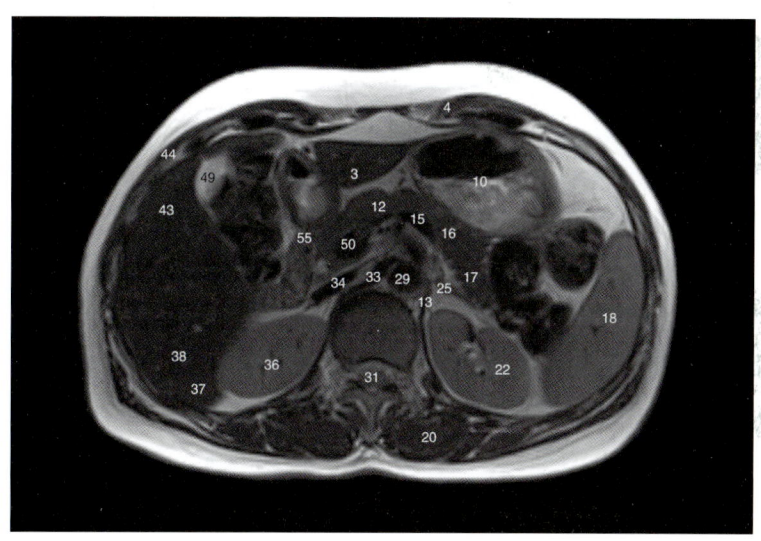

E. MR T2WI

关键结构：左、右膈脚，肝门右切迹，空肠。

此断面经过T12-L1椎间盘。

脊柱两侧为左、右膈脚，后方为竖脊肌，前方为下腔静脉和腹主动脉。肝门静脉稍右后方可见肝门右切迹。空肠行于横结肠和降结肠之间。膈脚是膈肌的终点，位于椎体前方，居腹主动脉两侧。左、右膈脚在此区域与脊柱共同围成主动脉裂孔。在CT图像上表现为位于主动脉两侧且贴近脊柱的类圆形的软组织密度影，此时须结合上下层连续断面图像与肿大淋巴结相鉴别。膈脚的后方可见交感干上的腰交感神经节，注意与淋巴结进行鉴别。肝门右切迹位于胆囊右后方，伸向肝右叶呈右后下走行，其内含肝右后叶下段鞘系，故此切迹可作为区分肝右前叶和右后叶的标志。该切迹见于70%~80%的解剖标本中，但在CT图像中仅能显示50%，所以在影像诊断中，应当注意此切迹与疾病的鉴别。

腹部连续横断层 48（FH.10970）

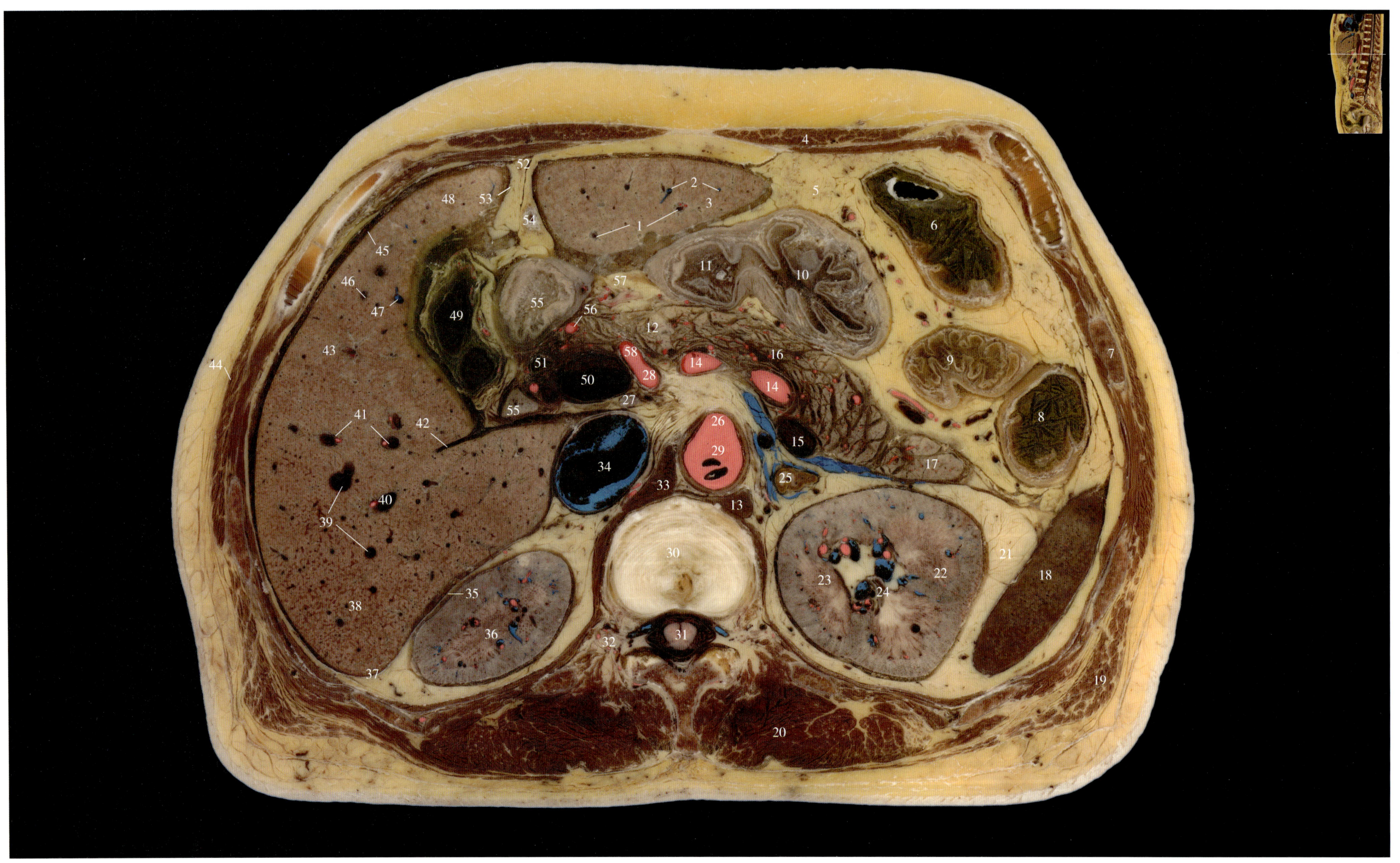

A. 断层标本图像

1. 肝门静脉左外下支及肝动脉 left lateroinferior branch of hepatic portal vein and corresponding hepatic artery
2. 肝左静脉下根属支 tributary of inferior root of left hepatic vein
3. 肝左外叶下段 inferior segment of left lateral lobe of liver
4. 腹直肌 rectus abdominis
5. 大网膜 greater omentum
6. 横结肠 transverse colon
7. 第 9 肋骨 9th costal bone
8. 降结肠 descending colon
9. 空肠 jejunum
10. 胃体 body of stomach
11. 胃幽门部 pyloric part of stomach
12. 胰颈 neck of pancreas
13. 左膈脚 left crus of diaphragm
14. 脾动脉 splenic artery
15. 脾静脉 splenic vein
16. 胰体 body of pancreas
17. 胰尾 tail of pancreas
18. 脾 spleen
19. 背阔肌 latissimus dorsi
20. 竖脊肌 erector spinae
21. 脾肾韧带 lienorenal ligament
22. 左肾 left kidney
23. 肾锥体 renal pyramid
24. 肾小盏 minor renal calices
25. 左肾上腺 left suprarenal gland
26. 肠系膜上动脉 superior mesenteric artery
27. 门腔淋巴结 portocaval lymph node
28. 肝总动脉 common hepatic artery
29. 腹主动脉 abdominal aorta
30. T12-L1 椎间盘 T12-L1 intervertebral disc
31. 脊髓 spinal cord
32. 第 12 胸神经 12th thoracic nerve
33. 右膈脚 right crus of diaphragm
34. 下腔静脉 inferior vena cava
35. 肝肾隐窝 hepatorenal recess
36. 右肾 right kidney
37. 肝裸区 bare area of liver
38. 肝右后叶下段 inferior segment of right posterior lobe of liver
39. 肝右静脉属支 tributary of right hepatic vein
40. 肝门静脉右后支 right posterior branch of hepatic portal vein
41. 肝门静脉右前支 right anterior branch of hepatic portal vein
42. 肝门右切迹 right notch of porta hepatis
43. 肝右前叶下段 inferior segment of right anterior lobe of liver
44. 腹外斜肌 obliquus externus abdominis
45. 右肝上间隙 right suprahepatic space
46. 肝门静脉右前下支及肝动脉、肝管 right anteroinferior branch of hepatic portal vein and corresponding hepatic artery and hepatic duct
47. 肝中静脉属支 tributary of middle hepatic vein
48. 肝左内叶 left medial lobe of liver
49. 胆囊 gallbladder
50. 肝门静脉 hepatic portal vein
51. 胆总管 common bile duct
52. 肝镰状韧带 falciform ligament of liver
53. 肝圆韧带裂 fissure for ligamentum teres hepatis
54. 肝圆韧带 ligamentum teres hepatis
55. 十二指肠上部 superior part of duodenum
56. 肝左动脉 left hepatic artery
57. 肝胃韧带 hepatogastric ligament
58. 肝固有动脉 proper hepatic artery

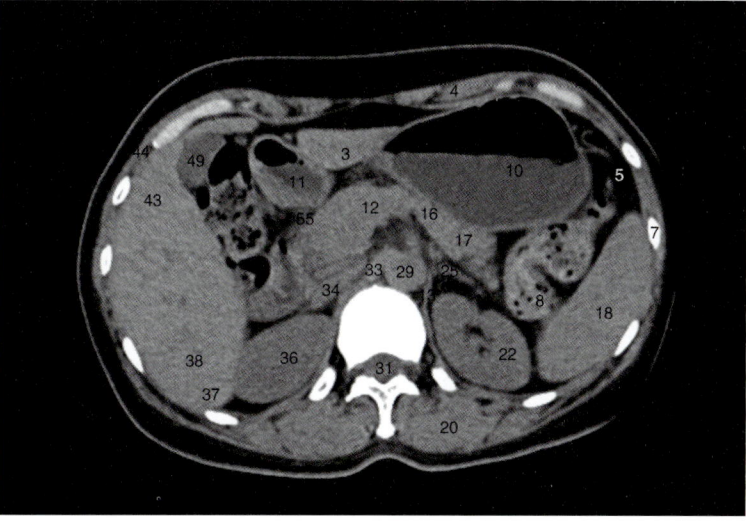

B. CT 平扫图像

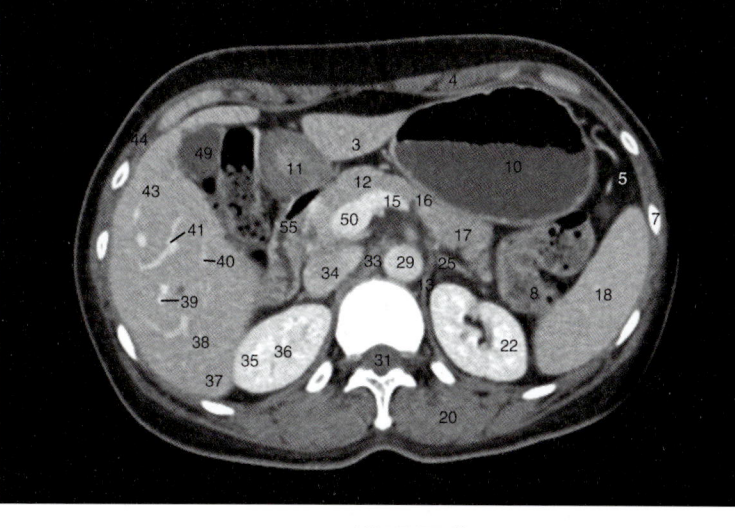

C. CT 增强图像

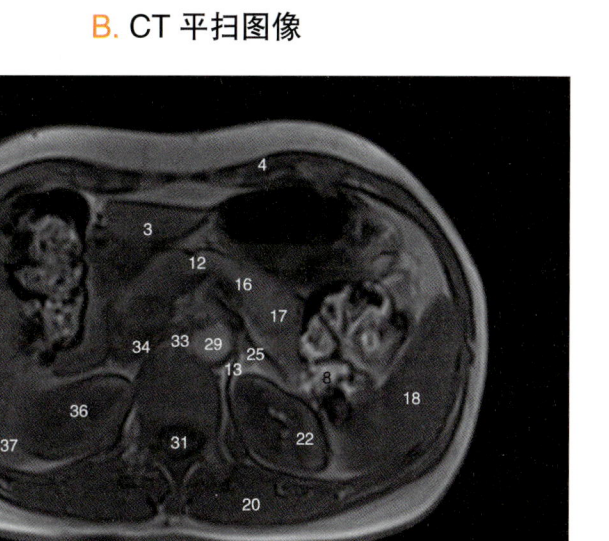

D. MR T1WI

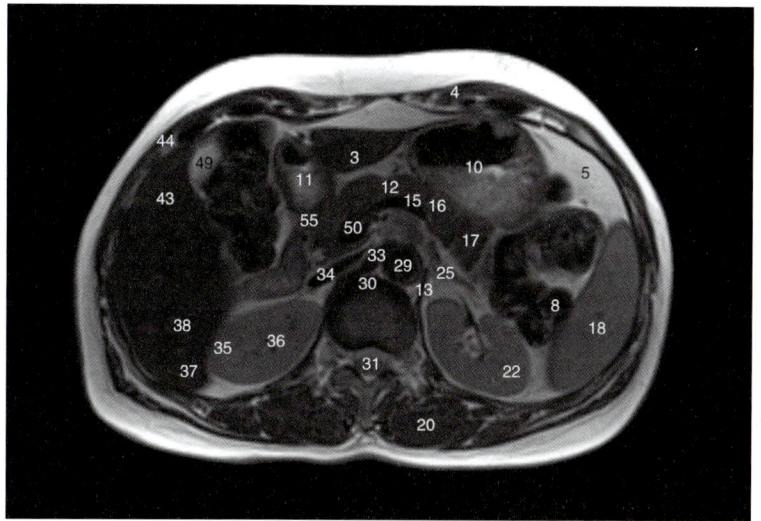

E. MR T2WI

关键结构：十二指肠上部，T12-L1 椎间盘。

此断面经过 T12-L1 椎间盘。

腹主动脉向前发出肠系膜上动脉，其后方为 T12-L1 椎间盘，右前方肝总动脉正移行为肝固有动脉。肝门静脉右前方为十二指肠上部，胰腺横于胃与腹主动脉之间。十二指肠上部为小肠最上端与胃幽门相连接的部分，被肝脏和胆囊覆盖，长约 4.3 cm。十二指肠起自幽门，其末端至十二指肠空肠曲移行为空肠，全段肠管呈蹄铁状弯曲，其突凸侧向右，凹侧向左上方，环抱于胰头周围。当发生十二指肠溃疡时，临近脂肪组织密度增高、边界模糊，合并穿孔时，可见腹腔游离气体。胆囊结石时，结石可能从慢性发炎的胆囊底部挤压到十二指肠内，结石到回肠时可造成肠梗阻（胆结石肠梗阻）[42]。椎间盘由髓核、纤维环、Sharpey 纤维和透明软骨终板组成。髓核位于椎间盘的中央偏后方，纤维环则围绕于髓核的周围，透明软骨终板紧贴于椎体的上、下面，构成髓核的上、下界，最外层则由 Sharpey 纤维包绕。CT 图像上髓核和纤维环显示不清，但 MR T1WI 图像上可清晰地显示：髓核和内纤维环呈较高信号，外纤维环和 Sharpey 纤维呈低信号。临床上以颈、腰椎间盘突出较为常见，而胸椎间盘突出少见。感染性病变如结核等可累及胸椎间盘。

腹部连续横断层 49（FH.10950）

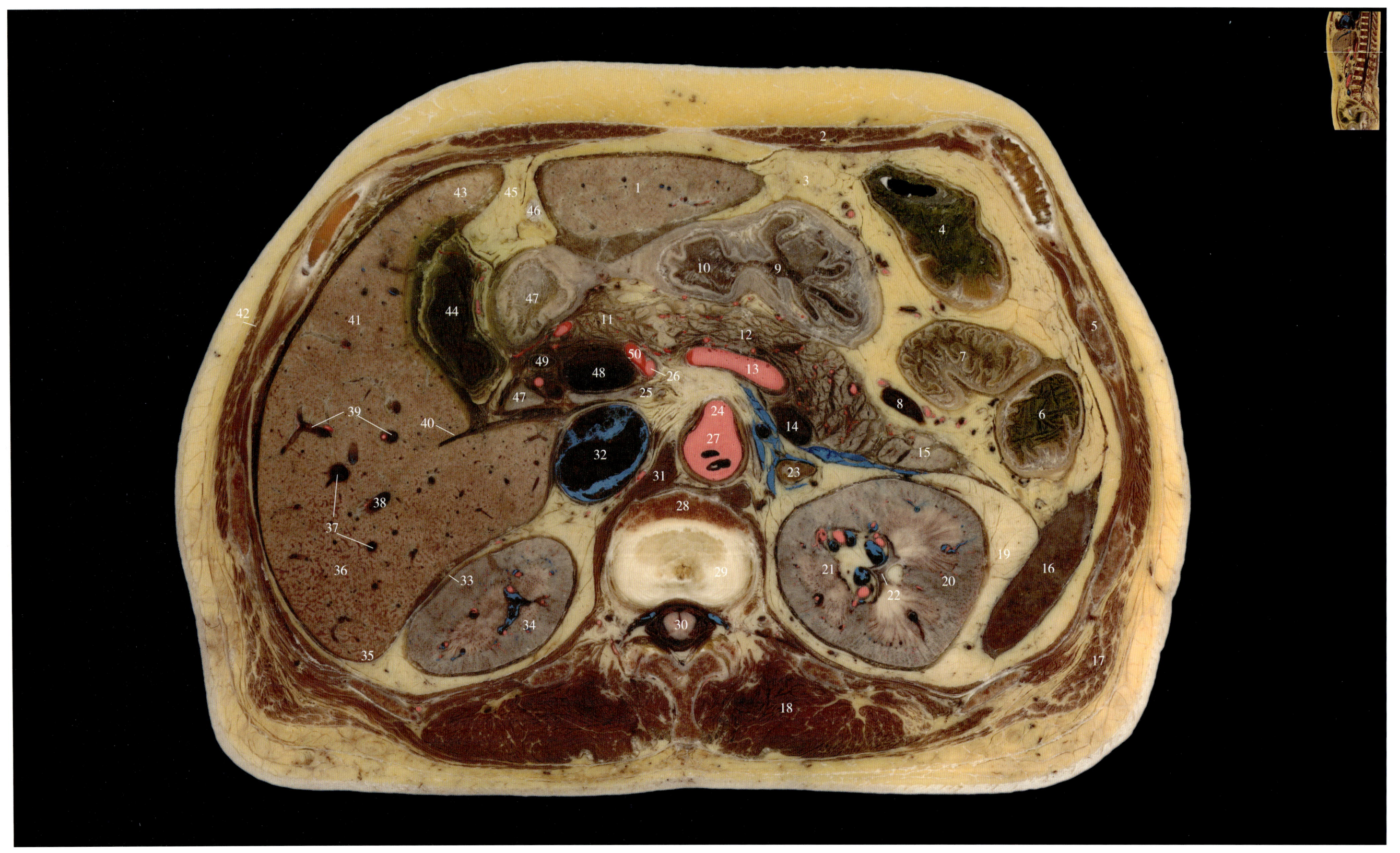

A. 断层标本图像

1. 肝左外叶下段 inferior segment of left lateral lobe of liver
2. 腹直肌 rectus abdominis
3. 大网膜 greater omentum
4. 横结肠 transverse colon
5. 第9肋骨 9th costal bone
6. 降结肠 descending colon
7. 空肠 jejunum
8. 空肠静脉 jejunal vein
9. 胃体 body of stomach
10. 胃幽门部 pyloric part of stomach
11. 胰颈 neck of pancreas
12. 胰体 body of pancreas
13. 脾动脉 splenic artery
14. 脾静脉 splenic vein
15. 胰尾 tail of pancreas
16. 脾 spleen
17. 背阔肌 latissimus dorsi
18. 竖脊肌 erector spinae
19. 脾肾韧带 lienorenal ligament
20. 左肾 left kidney
21. 肾锥体 renal pyramid
22. 肾大盏 major renal calices
23. 左肾上腺 left suprarenal gland
24. 肠系膜上动脉 superior mesenteric artery
25. 门腔淋巴结 portocaval lymph node
26. 肝总动脉 common hepatic artery
27. 腹主动脉 abdominal aorta
28. 第1腰椎椎体 body of 1nd lumbar vertebra
29. T12-L1 椎间盘 T12-L1 intervertebral disc
30. 脊髓 spinal cord
31. 右膈脚 right crus of diaphragm
32. 下腔静脉 inferior vena cava
33. 肝肾隐窝 hepatorenal recess
34. 右肾 right kidney
35. 肝裸区 bare area of liver
36. 肝右后叶下段 inferior segment of right posterior lobe of liver
37. 肝右静脉属支 tributary of right hepatic vein
38. 肝门静脉右后下支 right posteroinferior branch of hepatic portal vein
39. 肝门静脉右前下支 right anteroinferior branch of hepatic portal vein
40. 肝门右切迹 right notch of porta hepatis
41. 肝右前叶下段 inferior segment of right anterior lobe of liver
42. 腹外斜肌 obliquus externus abdominis
43. 肝左内叶 left medial lobe of liver
44. 胆囊 gallbladder
45. 肝圆韧带裂 fissure for ligamentum teres hepatis
46. 肝圆韧带 ligamentum teres hepatis
47. 十二指肠上部 superior part of duodenum
48. 肝门静脉 hepatic portal vein
49. 胆总管 common bile duct
50. 肝固有动脉 proper hepatic artery

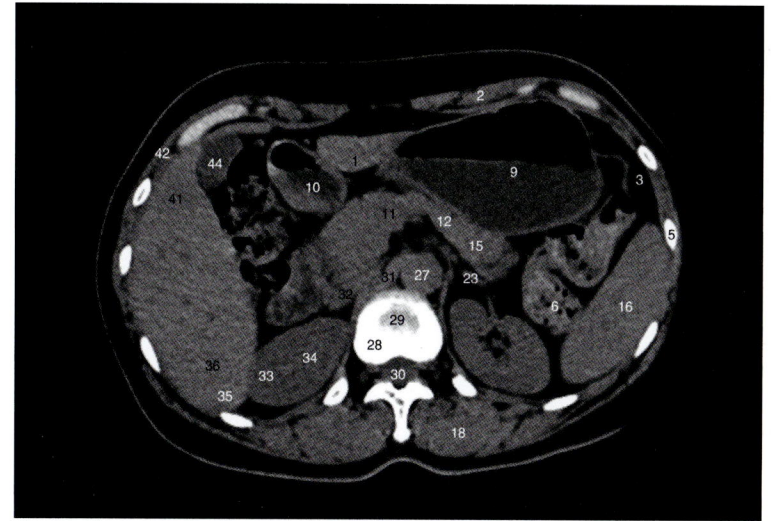

B. CT 平扫图像

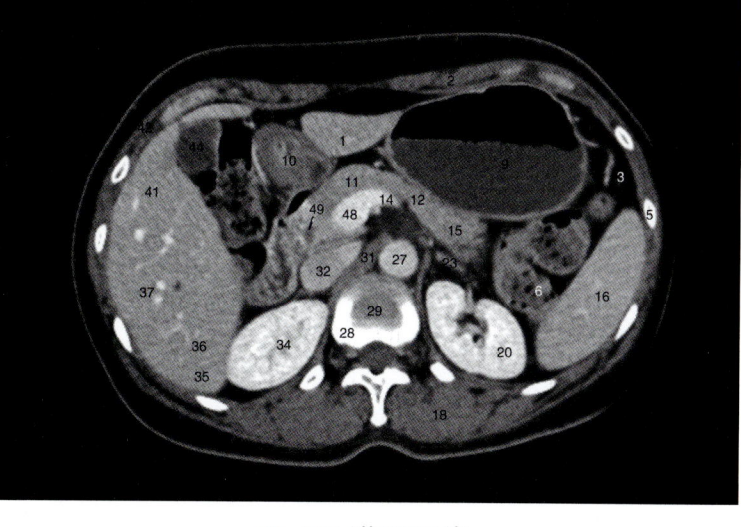

C. CT 增强图像

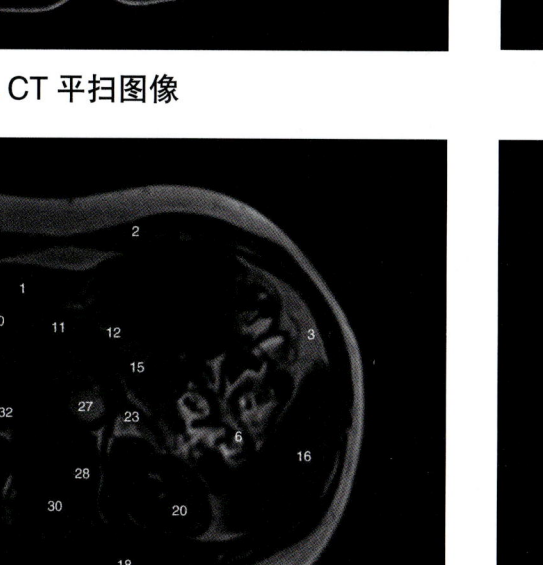

D. MR T1WI

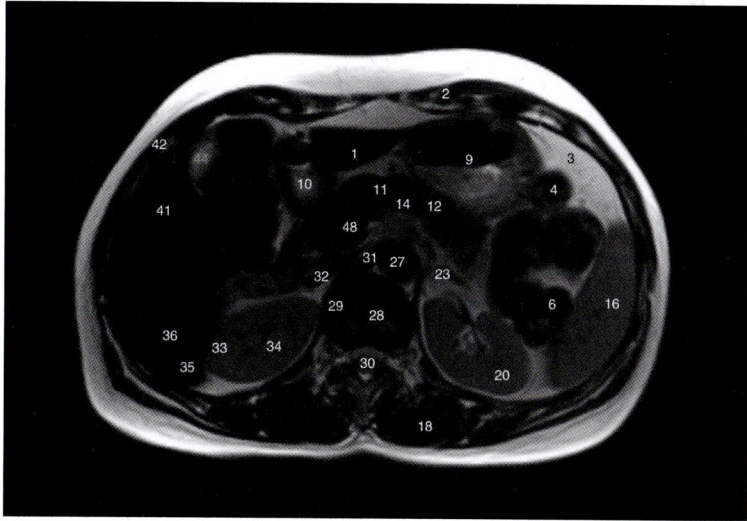

E. MR T2WI

关键结构：胰颈，门腔淋巴结。

此断面经过 T12-L1 椎间盘及第1腰椎椎体。

肝脏断面逐渐变小，胰腺位于断面中央，其前方胃幽门部与十二指肠上部相连，后方由右往左为肝门静脉、脾动脉、脾静脉、肠系膜上动脉等结构。胰颈是胰头与胰体之间的狭窄部分，长约2.5cm，宽约2.0cm，肠系膜上静脉和脾静脉在胰颈后方汇合成肝门静脉。肝门静脉或肠系膜上静脉右壁是区分胰头和胰颈的标志，肠系膜上动脉左壁是区分胰颈与胰体的标志。胰颈的下部在肠系膜下静脉汇入门静脉位置前方，这一解剖特点对胰腺癌切除非常关键，若肿瘤侵犯这些血管会导致肿瘤切除的难度增加或无法切除[43]。

门腔淋巴结位于门腔静脉间隙内，是该间隙的重要组成部分。门腔淋巴结由 Zirinsky 等于1985年提出[44]。Engel 等[45]认为网膜孔淋巴结即门腔淋巴结，测量门腔淋巴结时以前后径为主。Zirinsky 等[44]提出1.3cm是门腔淋巴结前后径的正常上限。Dorfman 等[46]则提出门腔淋巴结最短径的正常上限是1.0cm，Araki 等[47]认为门腔淋巴结的最短径大于1.5cm时才有临床意义，国外普遍接受以1.3cm作为前后径的正常上限值。正常门腔淋巴结在 CT 增强图像上表现为卵圆形或前后缘略呈凹面的结节影，密度低于门静脉和下腔静脉。邻近脏器的恶性肿瘤、感染或淋巴瘤时须观察此淋巴结的变化。

腹部连续横断层 50（FH.10930）

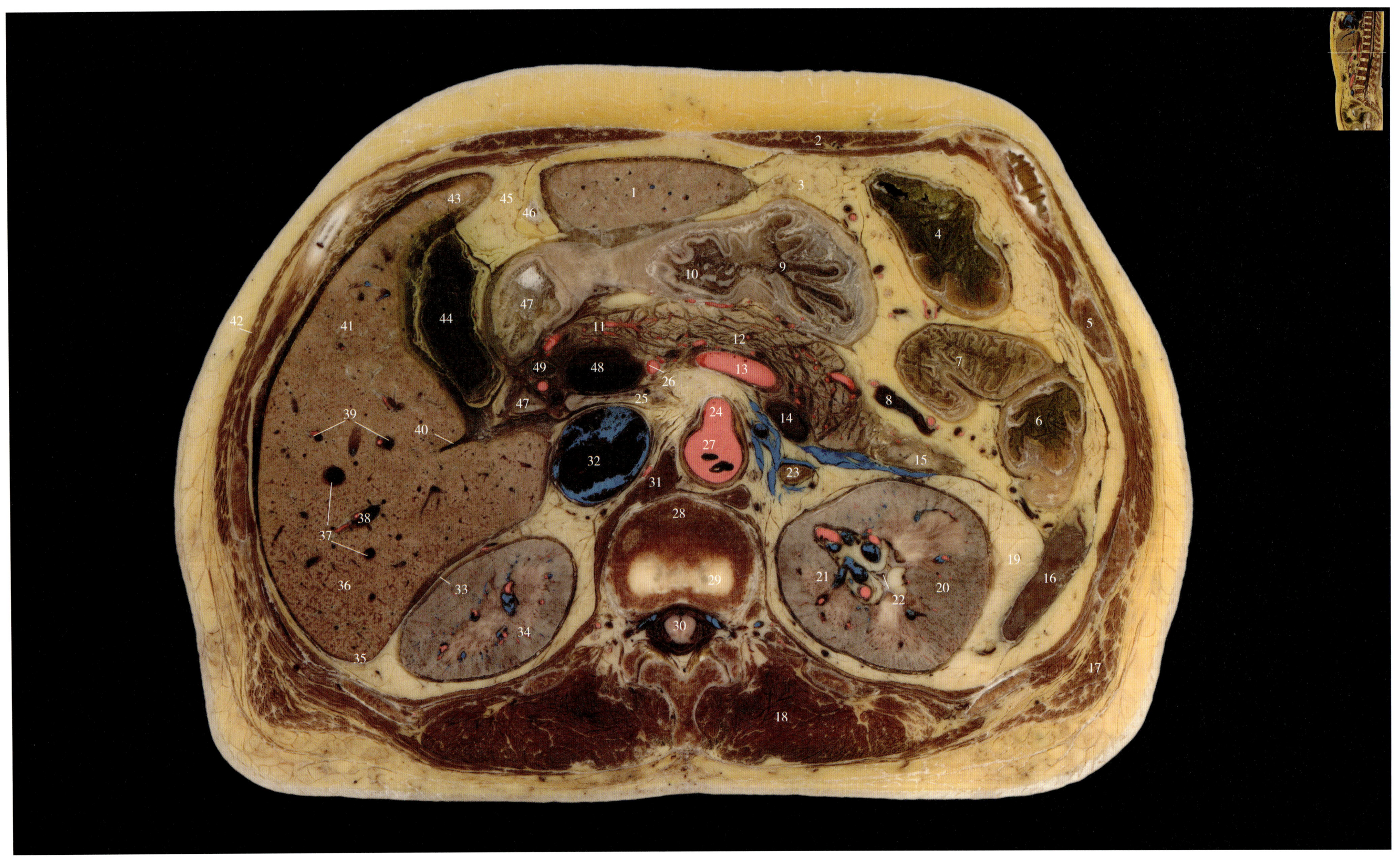

A. 断层标本图像

1. 肝左外叶下段 inferior segment of left lateral lobe of liver
2. 腹直肌 rectus abdominis
3. 大网膜 greater omentum
4. 横结肠 transverse colon
5. 第9肋骨 9th costal bone
6. 降结肠 descending colon
7. 空肠 jejunum
8. 空肠静脉 jejunal vein
9. 胃体 body of stomach
10. 胃幽门部 pyloric part of stomach
11. 胰颈 neck of pancreas
12. 胰体 body of pancreas
13. 脾动脉 splenic artery
14. 脾静脉 splenic vein
15. 胰尾 tail of pancreas
16. 脾 spleen
17. 背阔肌 latissimus dorsi
18. 竖脊肌 erector spinae
19. 脾肾韧带 lienorenal ligament
20. 左肾 left kidney
21. 肾锥体 renal pyramid
22. 肾大盏 major renal calices
23. 左肾上腺 left suprarenal gland
24. 肠系膜上动脉 superior mesenteric artery
25. 门腔淋巴结 portocaval lymph node
26. 肝总动脉 common hepatic artery
27. 腹主动脉 abdominal aorta
28. 第1腰椎椎体 body of 1st lumbar vertebra
29. T12-L1椎间盘 T12-L1 intervertebral disc
30. 脊髓 spinal cord
31. 右膈脚 right crus of diaphragm
32. 下腔静脉 inferior vena cava
33. 肝肾隐窝 hepatorenal recess
34. 右肾 right kidney
35. 肝裸区 bare area of liver
36. 肝右后叶下段 inferior segment of right posterior lobe of liver
37. 肝右静脉属支 tributary of right hepatic vein
38. 肝门静脉右后下支 right posteroinferior branch of hepatic portal vein
39. 肝门静脉右前下支 right anteroinferior branch of hepatic portal vein
40. 肝门右切迹 right notch of porta hepatis
41. 肝右前叶下段 inferior segment of right anterior lobe of liver
42. 腹外斜肌 obliquus externus abdominis
43. 肝左内叶 left medial lobe of liver
44. 胆囊 gallbladder
45. 肝圆韧带裂 fissure for ligamentum teres hepatis
46. 肝圆韧带 ligamentum teres hepatis
47. 十二指肠上部 superior part of duodenum
48. 肝门静脉 hepatic portal vein
49. 胆总管 common bile duct

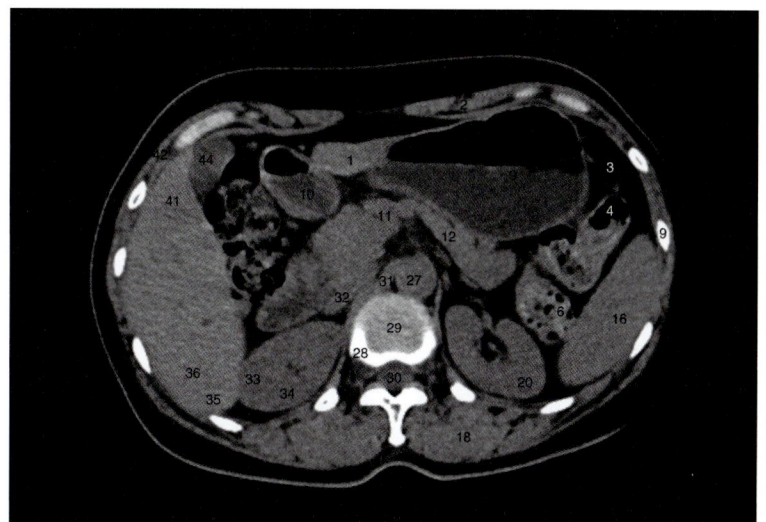

B. CT 平扫图像　　　　C. CT 增强图像

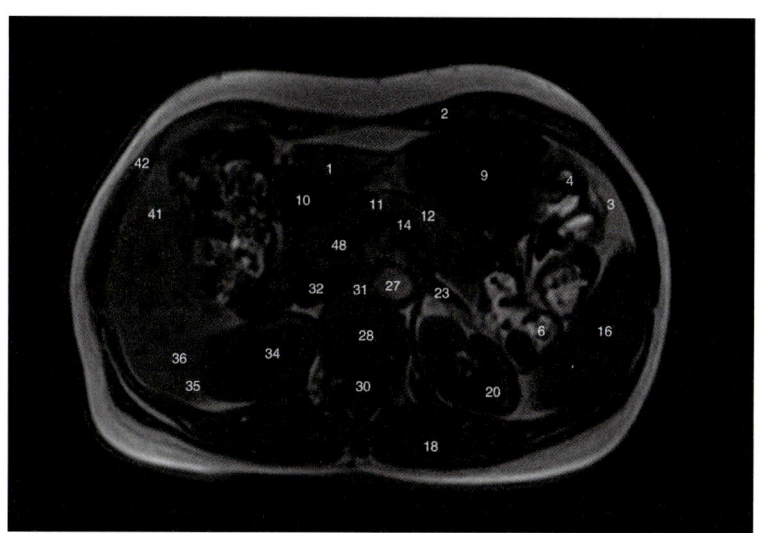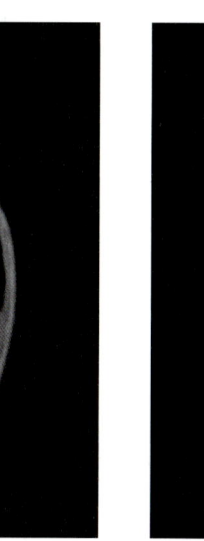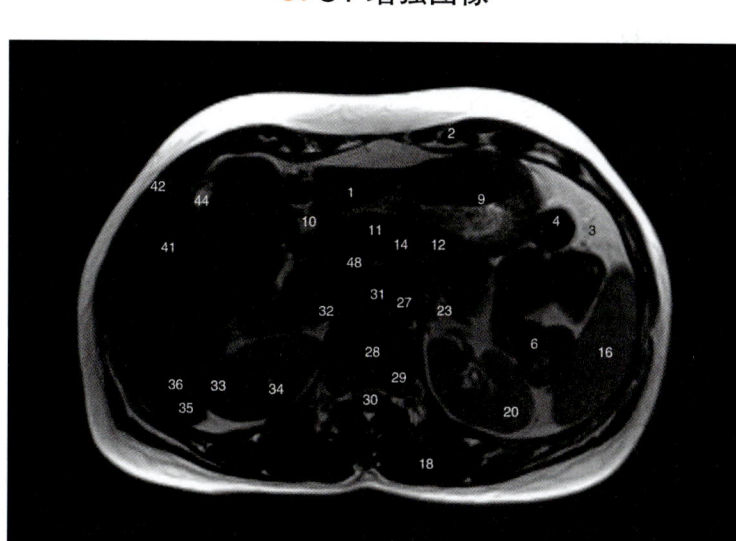

D. MR T1WI　　　　E. MR T2WI

关键结构：肠系膜上动脉，幽门，腹主动脉。

此断面经过T12-L1椎间盘及第1腰椎椎体。

肠系膜上动脉从腹主动脉发出，二者形成"水滴样"结构。胰腺居腹部中间，前方见幽门连接十二指肠和胃。肠系膜上动脉约在第1腰椎水平起自腹主动脉前壁，在脾静脉和胰头的后方下行，跨过胰腺钩突的前方，在胰腺下缘和十二指肠水平部之间进入小肠系膜根[48]，再斜行向右下，至右髂窝处其末端与回结肠动脉的回肠支吻合。肠系膜上动脉的主干呈向左侧稍凸的弓状，从弓的凸侧依次发出胰十二指肠动脉和十余支空、回肠动脉，从弓的凹侧依次发出中结肠动脉、右结肠动脉和回结肠动脉。腹主动脉从膈的主动脉裂孔起始，沿脊柱左前下行，至第4腰椎椎体下缘处分为左、右髂总动脉。腹主动脉前方自上而下为肝左叶、小网膜、腹腔丛、食管末端、横结肠系膜、脾静脉、胰、左肾静脉、十二指肠水平部、小肠系膜根及小肠袢、主动脉丛和主动脉前淋巴结；其后方与上位4个腰椎椎体及其椎间盘、前纵韧带及左侧第2~4腰静脉相邻；右侧为下腔静脉、右膈脚、右腹腔神经节、右内脏大神经、乳糜池和胸导管起始部等；左侧为左膈脚、左腹腔神经节及左内脏大神经等。在影像图像上，腹主动脉表现为椎体左前方的圆形断面，其分支根据走行表现为小圆形或细管状、分支状，老年人动脉硬化其管壁可见多发高密度钙化灶。如腹主动脉管径增粗呈囊状则为主动脉瘤，管壁广泛增厚可能为大动脉炎。腹主动脉的右侧扁管状影即下腔静脉，二者周围为腹膜后淋巴结所在区域，也是恶性肿瘤淋巴结转移的好发部位。

腹部连续横断层 51（FH.10910）

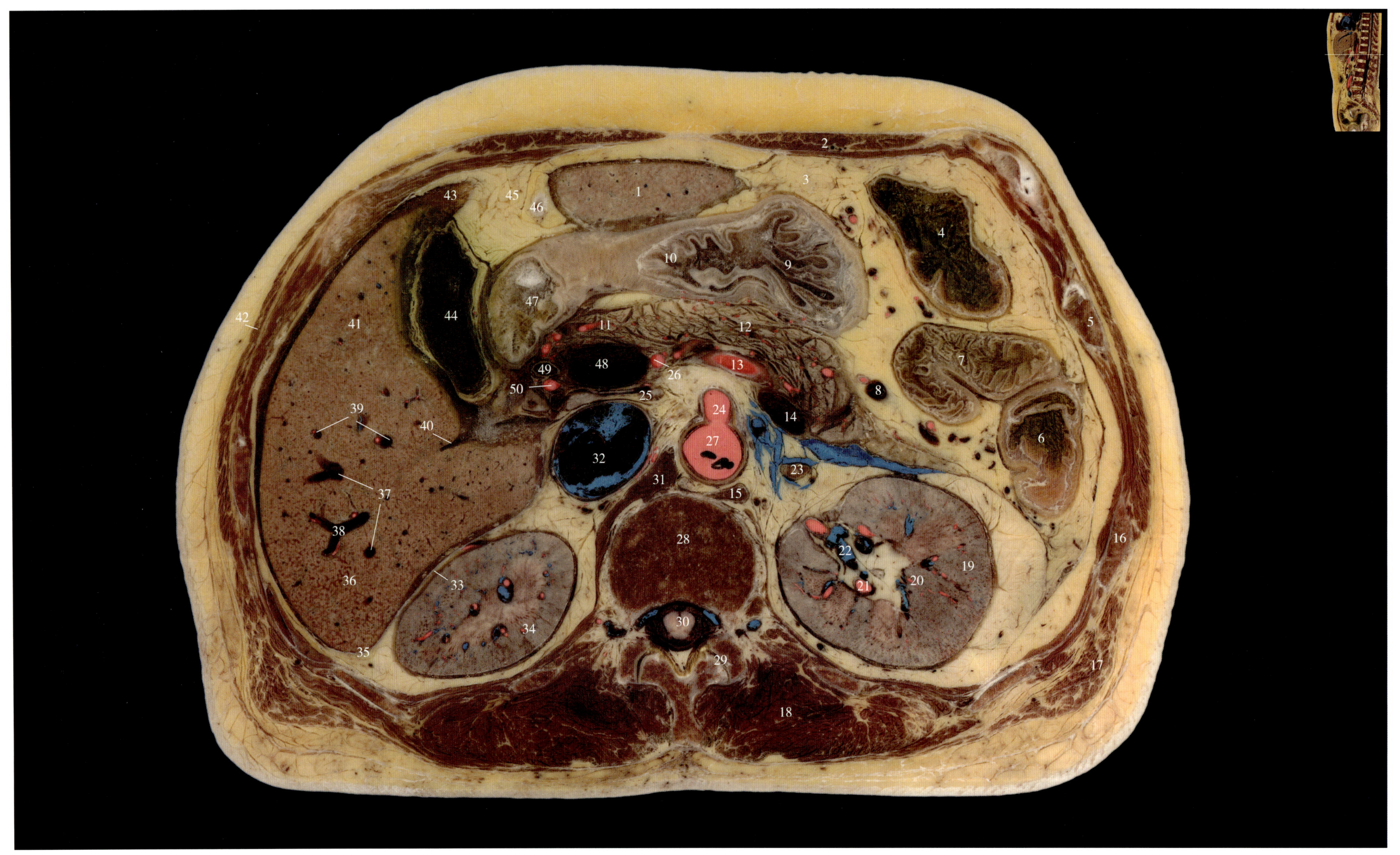

A. 断层标本图像

1. 肝左外叶下段 inferior segment of left lateral lobe of liver
2. 腹直肌 rectus abdominis
3. 大网膜 greater omentum
4. 横结肠 transverse colon
5. 第9肋骨 9th costal bone
6. 降结肠 descending colon
7. 空肠 jejunum
8. 空肠静脉 jejunal vein
9. 胃体 body of stomach
10. 胃幽门部 pyloric part of stomach
11. 胰颈 neck of pancreas
12. 胰体 body of pancreas
13. 脾动脉 splenic artery
14. 脾静脉 splenic vein
15. 左膈脚 left crus of diaphragm
16. 第10肋骨 10th costal bone
17. 背阔肌 latissimus dorsi
18. 竖脊肌 erector spinae
19. 左肾 left kidney
20. 肾锥体 renal pyramid
21. 肾动脉 renal artery
22. 肾静脉 renal vein
23. 左肾上腺 left suprarenal gland
24. 肠系膜上动脉 superior mesenteric artery
25. 门腔淋巴结 portocaval lymph node
26. 肝总动脉 common hepatic artery
27. 腹主动脉 abdominal aorta
28. 第1腰椎椎体 body of 1st lumbar vertebra
29. 关节突关节 zygapophysial joint
30. 脊髓 spinal cord
31. 右膈脚 right crus of diaphragm
32. 下腔静脉 inferior vena cava
33. 肝肾隐窝 hepatorenal recess
34. 右肾 right kidney
35. 肝裸区 bare area of liver
36. 肝右后叶下段 inferior segment of right posterior lobe of liver
37. 肝右静脉属支 tributary of right hepatic vein
38. 肝门静脉右后下支 right posteroinferior branch of hepatic portal vein
39. 肝门静脉右前下支 right anteroinferior branch of hepatic portal vein
40. 肝门右切迹 right notch of porta hepatis
41. 肝右前叶下段 inferior segment of right anterior lobe of liver
42. 腹外斜肌 obliquus externus abdominis
43. 肝左内叶 left medial lobe of liver
44. 胆囊 gallbladder
45. 肝圆韧带裂 fissure for ligamentum teres hepatis
46. 肝圆韧带 ligamentum teres hepatis
47. 十二指肠上部 superior part of duodenum
48. 肝门静脉 hepatic portal vein
49. 胆总管 common bile duct
50. 肝右动脉 right hepatic artery

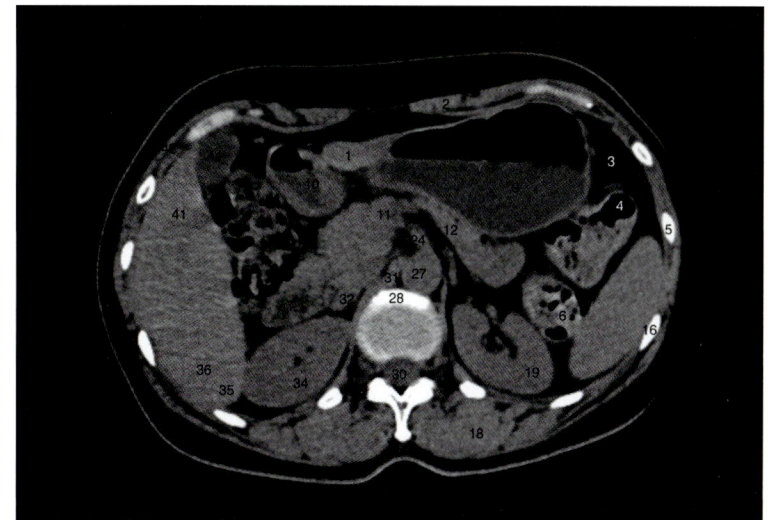

B. CT 平扫图像

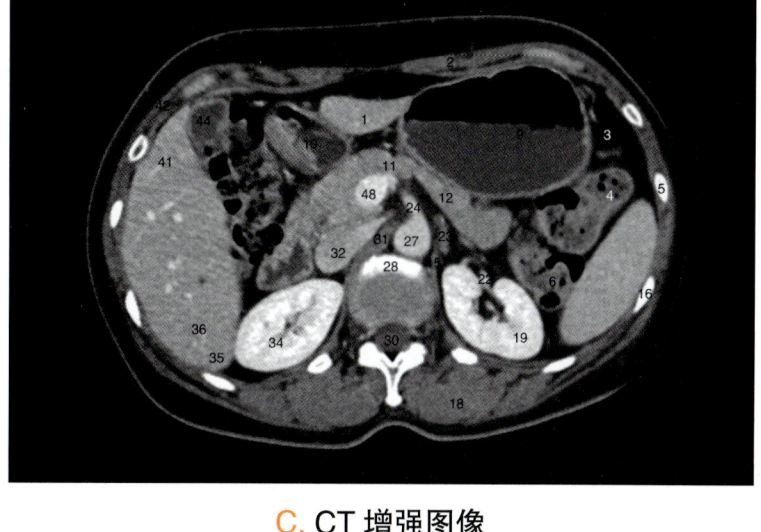

C. CT 增强图像

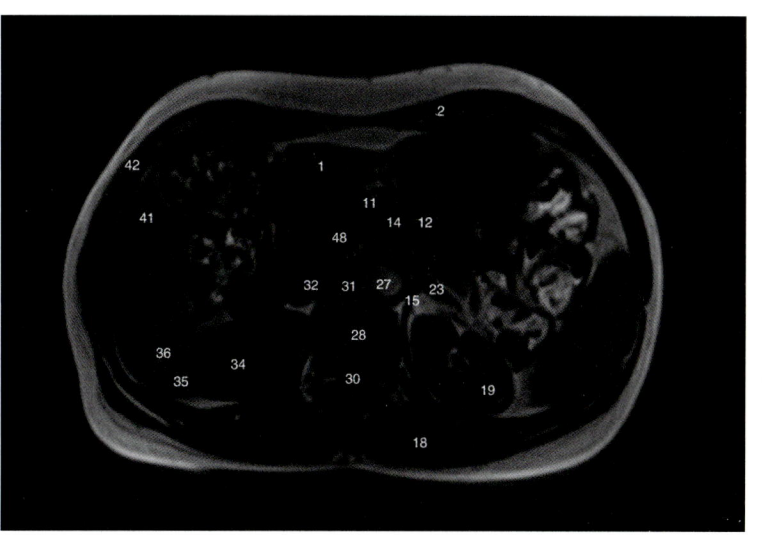

D. MR T1WI

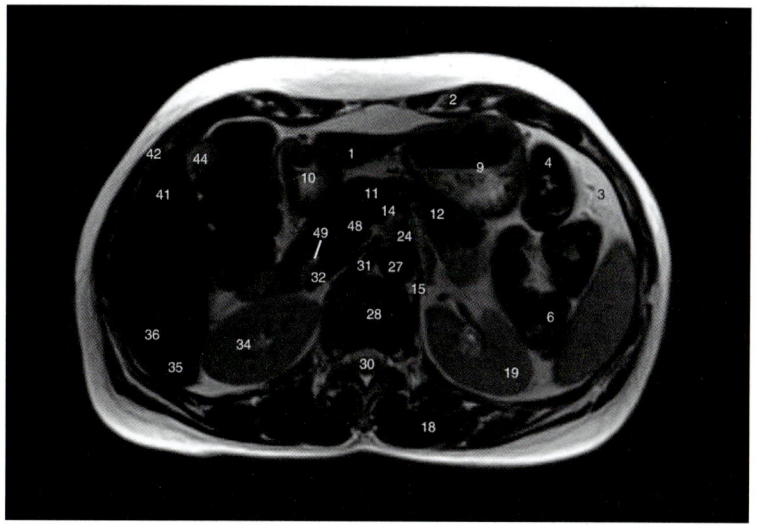

E. MR T2WI

关键结构：肝门静脉，下腔静脉，门腔间隙。

此断面经过第1腰椎椎体。

胰尾及脾消失，肝门静脉位于胰颈后方，其与下腔静脉之间为门腔间隙，内有门腔淋巴结。肝门静脉由脾静脉和肠系膜上静脉在胰颈后方汇合而成，其主干在肝十二指肠韧带内走行，并在肝门处分成左支和右支。在肝十二指肠韧带内走行的肝门静脉，其右前方为胆总管，左前方为肝固有动脉，后面隔网膜孔与下腔静脉相邻，多数门静脉与下腔静脉交叉成角，少数前后平行。门静脉与腔静脉之间有丰富的吻合支，门静脉高压时，吻合支静脉明显迂曲、扩张[48-51]，门静脉血流经过吻合支向周围引流，可形成脾－胃、脾－肾、门－体静脉等多种分流。下腔静脉沿腹主动脉的右侧上行，经腔静脉沟向上经膈穿腔静脉孔，到达胸腔后注入右心房。下腔静脉通过左、右髂总静脉及其他属支收集盆部、下肢和腹部的静脉血。布加综合征是由各种原因导致的肝静脉或上段下腔静脉阻塞，而伴有以下腔静脉高压为特点的一种肝后门静脉高压症病变。对比剂增强CT的特异性表现是下腔静脉肝后段及主肝静脉内出现充盈缺损，其下方静脉增粗或侧支血管开放。门腔间隙上至肝门静脉分叉处，下至肠系膜上静脉和脾静脉汇合处，内有很多重要的解剖结构，如门腔淋巴结、胆囊管、网膜孔、肝尾状突等。此结构比较深且隐匿，但腹部CT和MRI可以很好地显示其中的精细结构。

腹部连续横断层 52（FH.10890）

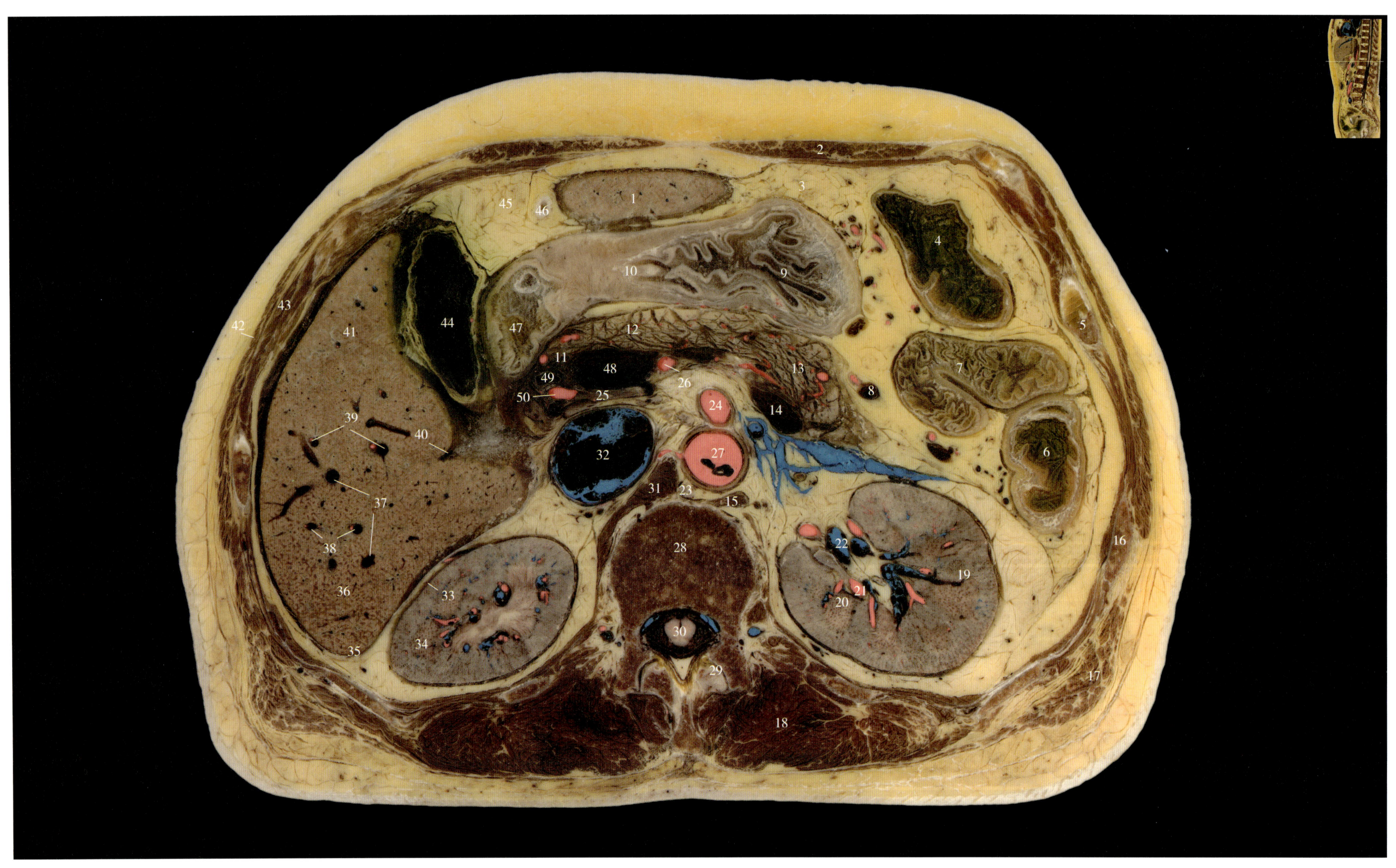

A. 断层标本图像

1. 肝左外叶下段 inferior segment of left lateral lobe of liver
2. 腹直肌 rectus abdominis
3. 大网膜 greater omentum
4. 横结肠 transverse colon
5. 第9肋骨 9th costal bone
6. 降结肠 descending colon
7. 空肠 jejunum
8. 空肠静脉 jejunal vein
9. 胃体 body of stomach
10. 胃幽门部 pyloric part of stomach
11. 胰头 head of pancreas
12. 胰颈 neck of pancreas
13. 胰体 body of pancreas
14. 脾静脉 splenic vein
15. 左膈脚 left crus of diaphragm
16. 第10肋骨 10th costal bone
17. 背阔肌 latissimus dorsi
18. 竖脊肌 erector spinae
19. 左肾 left kidney
20. 肾锥体 renal pyramid
21. 肾动脉 renal artery
22. 肾静脉 renal vein
23. 交感干 sympathetic trunk
24. 肠系膜上动脉 superior mesenteric artery
25. 门腔淋巴结 portocaval lymph node
26. 肝总动脉 common hepatic artery
27. 腹主动脉 abdominal aorta
28. 第1腰椎椎体 body of 1st lumbar vertebra
29. 关节突关节 zygapophysial joint
30. 脊髓 spinal cord
31. 右膈脚 right crus of diaphragm
32. 下腔静脉 inferior vena cava
33. 肝肾隐窝 hepatorenal recess
34. 右肾 right kidney
35. 肝裸区 bare area of liver
36. 肝右后叶下段 inferior segment of right posterior lobe of liver
37. 肝右静脉属支 tributary of right hepatic vein
38. 肝门静脉右后下支 right posteroinferior branch of hepatic portal vein
39. 肝门静脉右前下支 right anteroinferior branch of hepatic portal vein
40. 肝门右切迹 right notch of porta hepatis
41. 肝右前叶下段 inferior segment of right anterior lobe of liver
42. 腹外斜肌 obliquus externus abdominis
43. 腹内斜肌 obliquus internus abdominis
44. 胆囊 gallbladder
45. 肝圆韧带裂 fissure for ligamentum teres hepatis
46. 肝圆韧带 ligamentum teres hepatis
47. 十二指肠上部 superior part of duodenum
48. 肝门静脉 hepatic portal vein
49. 胆总管 common bile duct
50. 肝右动脉 right hepatic artery

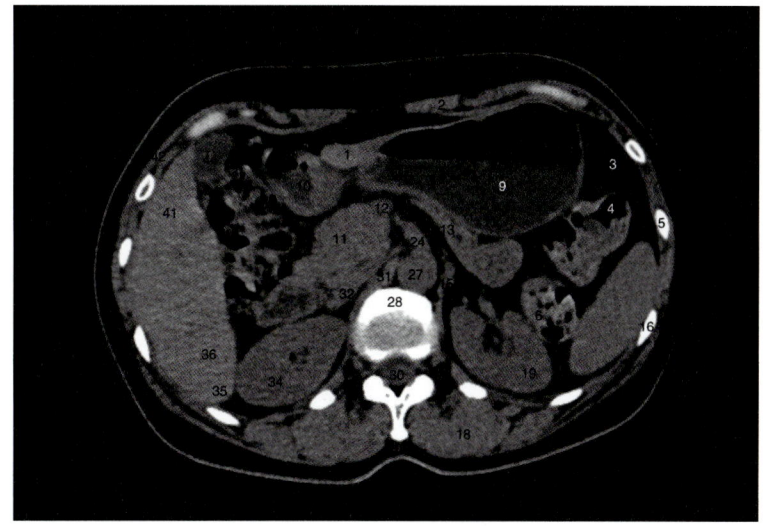

B. CT 平扫图像

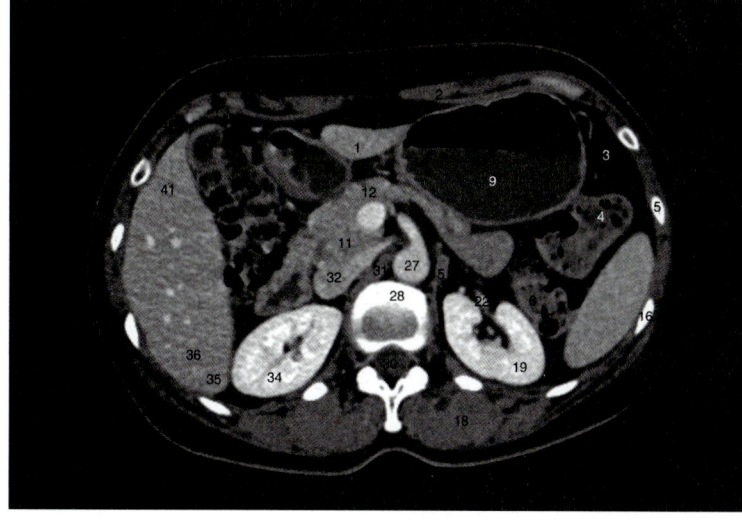

C. CT 增强图像

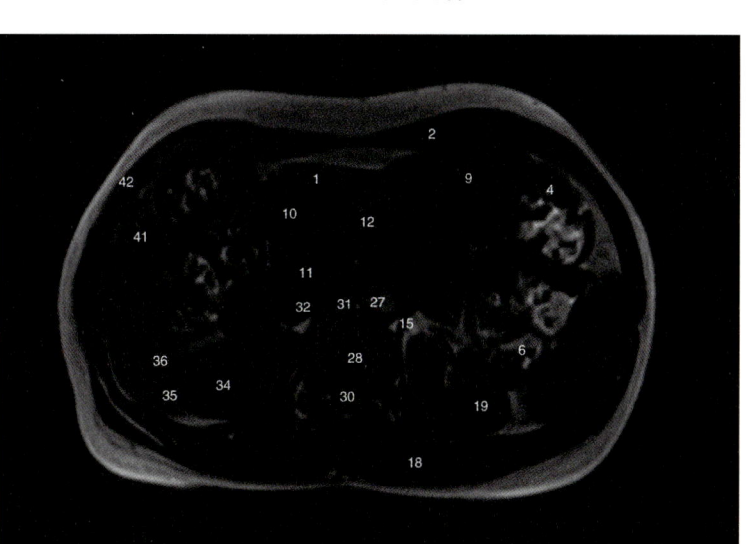

D. MR T1WI

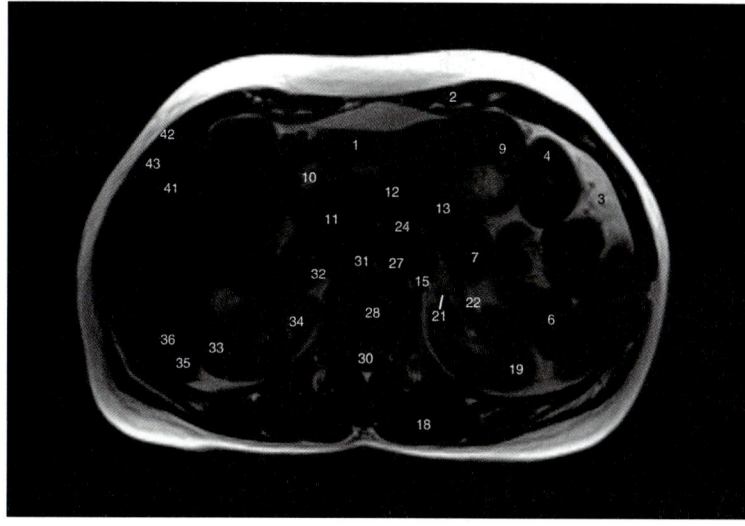

E. MR T2WI

关键结构：胆囊体，胆总管，胰头。

此断面经过第1腰椎椎体。

胆囊位于肝右叶与十二指肠上部之间，十二指肠上部的后方可见胆总管。胰头出现，居于十二指肠上部与肝门静脉之间。胆囊体为胆囊底向左右上方逐渐缩窄的部分，约至肝门的右端延续为胆囊颈。胆囊体与底和颈之间无明显的分界。胆囊体的上缘（肝面）借结缔组织连于肝的胆囊窝内，下缘（游离面）由前向后，依次与横结肠的右端、十二指肠上部及降部的上端相连接[2]。胆总管由胆囊管与肝总管汇合而成，长4~8 cm，直径6~8 mm，它位于肝固有动脉右侧、门静脉前方，下行于肝十二指肠韧带中，向下经十二指肠上部后方，穿过胰头与十二指肠降部间，进入十二指肠降部的左后壁，在此处与胰管汇合，形成略膨大的总管，叫肝胰壶腹，开口于十二指肠大乳头顶端，胆结石易在此处嵌顿。胆总管分为十二指肠上段、十二指肠后段、胰腺段和十二指肠壁内段四段。胆总管在CT断面图像上为低密度的小圆形断面，在MR T2WI图像呈高信号，MRCP可显示胆管胰管的全貌。正常胆总管直径在10 mm以内，超过12 mm时为胆总管扩张。胆总管结石及肿瘤、邻近的胰腺肿瘤等均可导致上游胆管的扩张，先天性胆总管囊肿也表现为胆总管的明显扩张，应注意鉴别。

105

腹部连续横断层 53（FH.10870）

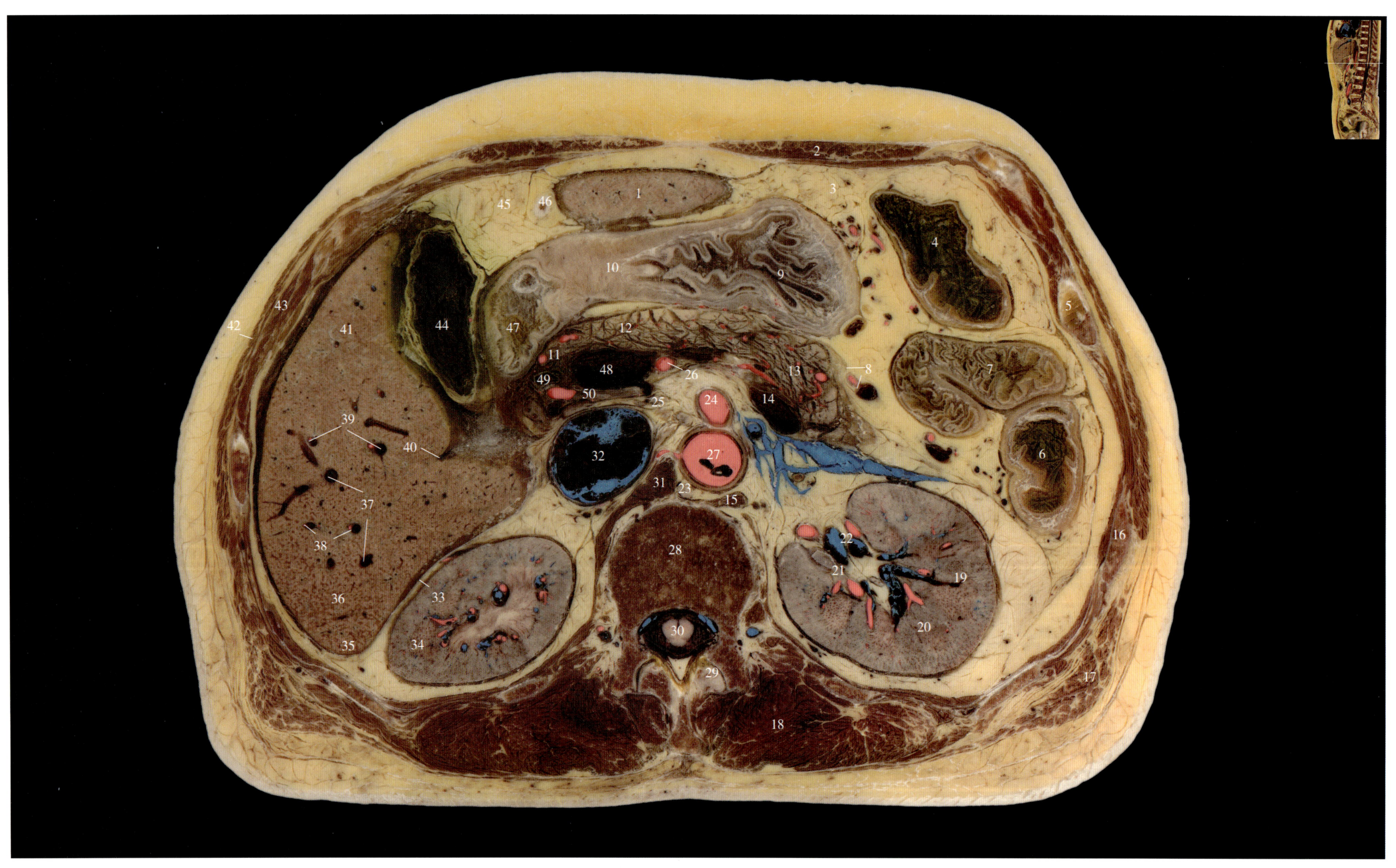

A. 断层标本图像

1. 肝左外叶下段 inferior segment of left lateral lobe of liver
2. 腹直肌 rectus abdominis
3. 大网膜 greater omentum
4. 横结肠 transverse colon
5. 第9肋软骨 9th costal cartilage
6. 降结肠 descending colon
7. 空肠 jejunum
8. 空肠动、静脉 jejunal artery and vein
9. 胃体 body of stomach
10. 胃幽门部 pyloric part of stomach
11. 胰头 head of pancreas
12. 胰颈 neck of pancreas
13. 胰体 body of pancreas
14. 脾静脉 splenic vein
15. 左膈脚 left crus of diaphragm
16. 第10肋骨 10th costal bone
17. 背阔肌 latissimus dorsi
18. 竖脊肌 erector spinae
19. 左肾 left kidney
20. 肾锥体 renal pyramid
21. 肾动脉 renal artery
22. 肾静脉 renal vein
23. 右交感干 right sympathetic trunk
24. 肠系膜上动脉 superior mesenteric artery
25. 门腔淋巴结 portocaval lymph node
26. 肝总动脉 common hepatic artery
27. 腹主动脉 abdominal aorta
28. 第1腰椎椎体 body of 1st lumbar vertebra
29. 关节突关节 zygapophysial joint
30. 脊髓 spinal cord
31. 右膈脚 right crus of diaphragm
32. 下腔静脉 inferior vena cava
33. 肝肾隐窝 hepatorenal recess
34. 右肾 right kidney
35. 肝裸区 bare area of liver
36. 肝右后叶下段 inferior segment of right posterior lobe of liver
37. 肝右静脉属支 tributary of right hepatic vein
38. 肝门静脉右后下支 right posteroinferior branch of hepatic portal vein
39. 肝门静脉右前下支 right anteroinferior branch of hepatic portal vein
40. 肝门右切迹 right notch of porta hepatis
41. 肝右前叶下段 inferior segment of right anterior lobe of liver
42. 腹外斜肌 obliquus externus abdominis
43. 腹内斜肌 obliquus internus abdominis
44. 胆囊 gallbladder
45. 肝圆韧带裂 fissure for ligamentum teres hepatis
46. 肝圆韧带 ligamentum teres hepatis
47. 十二指肠上部 superior part of duodenum
48. 肝门静脉 hepatic portal vein
49. 胆总管 common bile duct
50. 肝右动脉 right hepatic artery

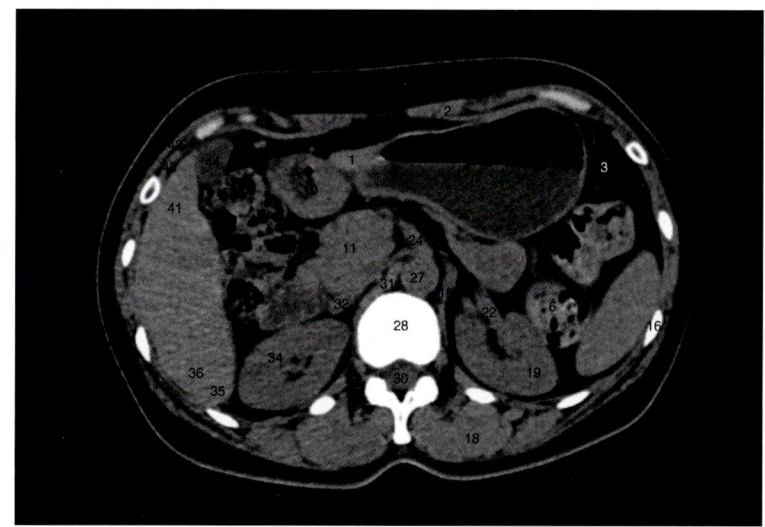

B. CT 平扫图像

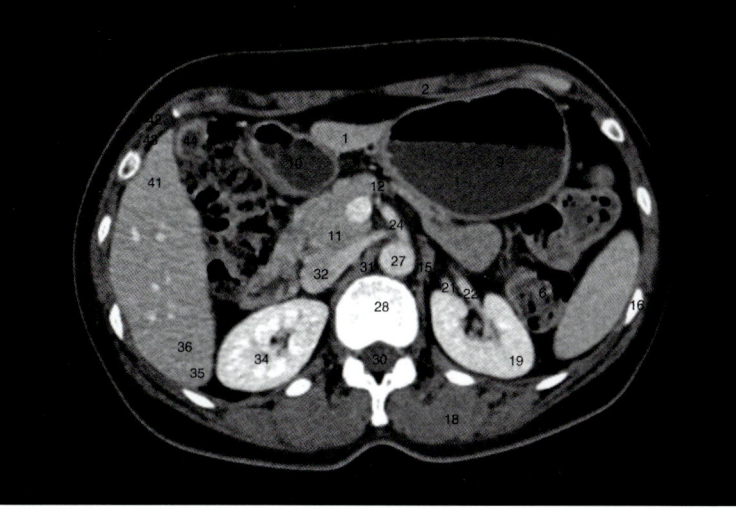

C. CT 增强图像

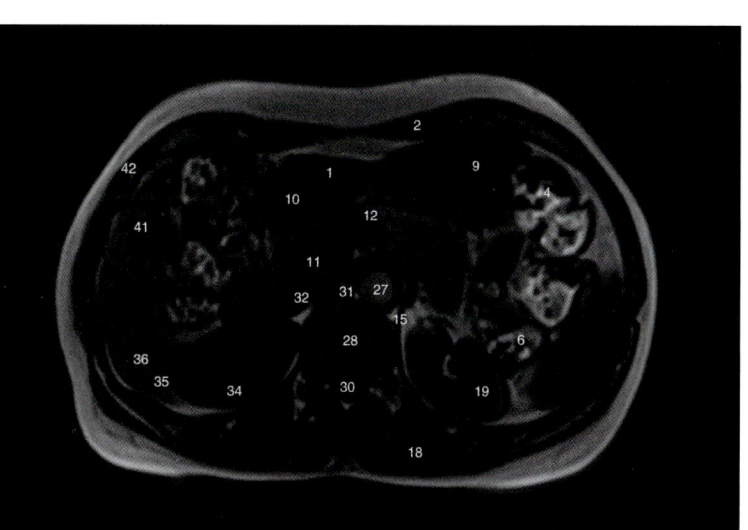

D. MR T1WI

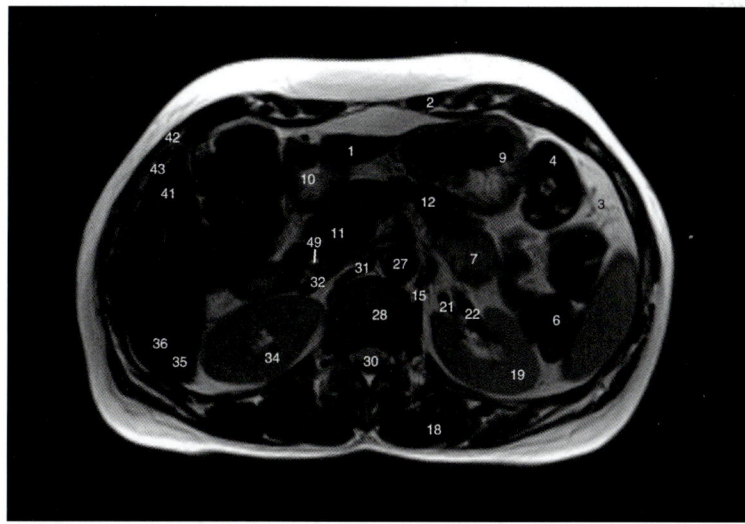

E. MR T2WI

关键结构：右交感干，肝肾隐窝，肾锥体。

此断面经过第1腰椎椎体。

脊柱与腹主动脉之间可见交感干走行，左、右膈脚纤维稀疏。胰腺体积变小，但仍能显示部分胰头、胰颈和胰体。十二指肠上部继续向下延伸，位于胆囊与胰之间，肝右后叶和右肾之间为肝肾隐窝。交感干由交感神经椎旁节借节间支相连而成，分布于椎体的前外侧，左右各一，上至第2颈椎，下至尾骨。腰交感干是胸交感干的延续，右腰交感干均位于下腔静脉外侧缘后方、腰大肌内侧与腰椎之间；生殖股神经穿出点与腰交感干很近，尤其是从腰大肌内侧缘处穿出的神经，在行腰交感神经切除时很容易损伤或误切该神经，导致手术失败或术后患者外阴部感觉迟钝[52]，因此手术中应格外小心。肝肾隐窝（又称Morison间隙）是肝右叶与右肾之间一潜在的间隙，在正常CT轴位图像上，该间隙表现为肝右叶后缘与右肾前外侧缘之间的带状形隐窝，其大小和形状依据肝肾的位置及肝大小和形态的变化而有所改变。腹腔积液时在此隐窝内易见。

肾锥体是位于肾髓质内的圆锥样结构，一般为15~20个。锥体的底朝向皮质，尖朝肾窦，有许多放射状条纹从锥体尖部向皮质方向扩展，这些条纹由肾直小管和血管平行排列而成。平扫CT和MR图像显示肾锥体困难，对比剂增强动脉期图像可清晰地显示肾锥体。

腹部连续横断层 54（FH.10850）

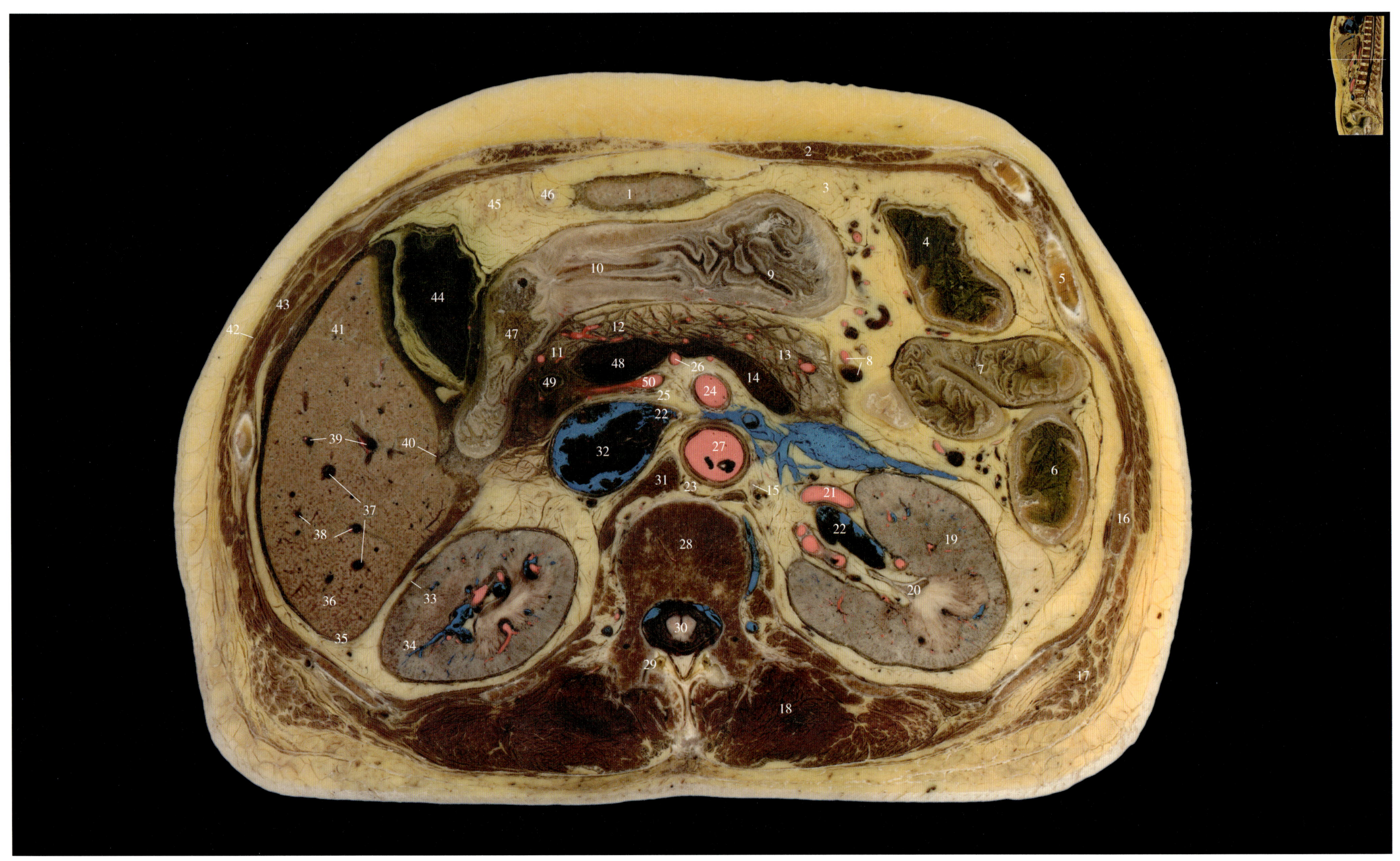

A. 断层标本图像

1. 肝左外叶下段 inferior segment of left lateral lobe of liver
2. 腹直肌 rectus abdominis
3. 大网膜 greater omentum
4. 横结肠 transverse colon
5. 第9肋软骨 9th costal cartilage
6. 降结肠 descending colon
7. 空肠 jejunum
8. 空肠动、静脉 jejunal artery and vein
9. 胃体 body of stomach
10. 胃幽门部 pyloric part of stomach
11. 胰头 head of pancreas
12. 胰颈 neck of pancreas
13. 胰体 body of pancreas
14. 脾静脉 splenic vein
15. 左交感干 left sympathetic trunk
16. 第10肋骨 10th costal bone
17. 背阔肌 latissimus dorsi
18. 竖脊肌 erector spinae
19. 左肾 left kidney
20. 左肾盂 left renal pelvis
21. 左肾动脉 left renal artery
22. 左肾静脉 left renal vein
23. 右交感干 right sympathetic trunk
24. 肠系膜上动脉 superior mesenteric artery
25. 门腔淋巴结 portocaval lymph node
26. 肝总动脉 common hepatic artery
27. 腹主动脉 abdominal aorta
28. 第1腰椎椎体 body of 1st lumbar vertebra
29. 关节突关节 zygapophysial joint
30. 脊髓 spinal cord
31. 右膈脚 right crus of diaphragm
32. 下腔静脉 inferior vena cava
33. 肝肾隐窝 hepatorenal recess
34. 右肾 right kidney
35. 肝裸区 bare area of liver
36. 肝右后叶下段 inferior segment of right posterior lobe of liver
37. 肝右静脉属支 tributary of right hepatic vein
38. 肝门静脉右后下支 right posteroinferior branch of hepatic portal vein
39. 肝门静脉右前下支 right anteroinferior branch of hepatic portal vein
40. 肝门右切迹 right notch of porta hepatis
41. 肝右前叶下段 inferior segment of right anterior lobe of liver
42. 腹外斜肌 obliquus externus abdominis
43. 腹内斜肌 obliquus internus abdominis
44. 胆囊 gallbladder
45. 肝圆韧带裂 fissure for ligamentum teres hepatis
46. 肝圆韧带 ligamentum teres hepatis
47. 十二指肠上部 superior part of duodenum
48. 肠系膜上静脉 superior mesenteric vein
49. 胆总管 common bile duct
50. 肝右动脉 right hepatic artery

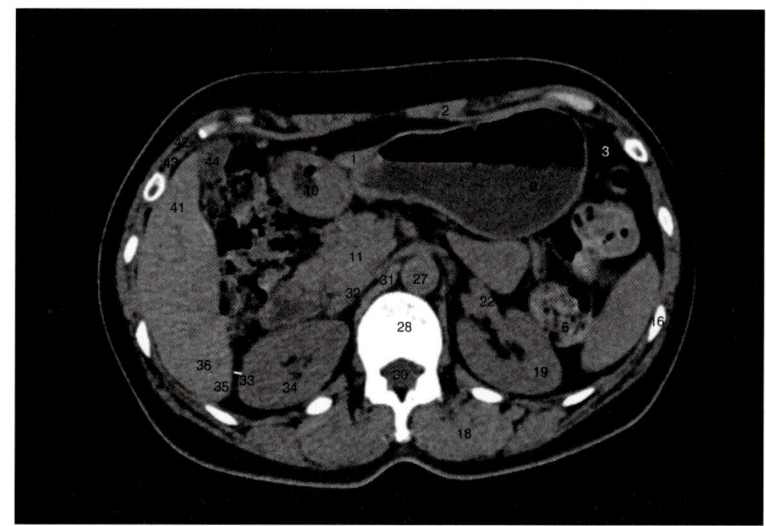

B. CT 平扫图像

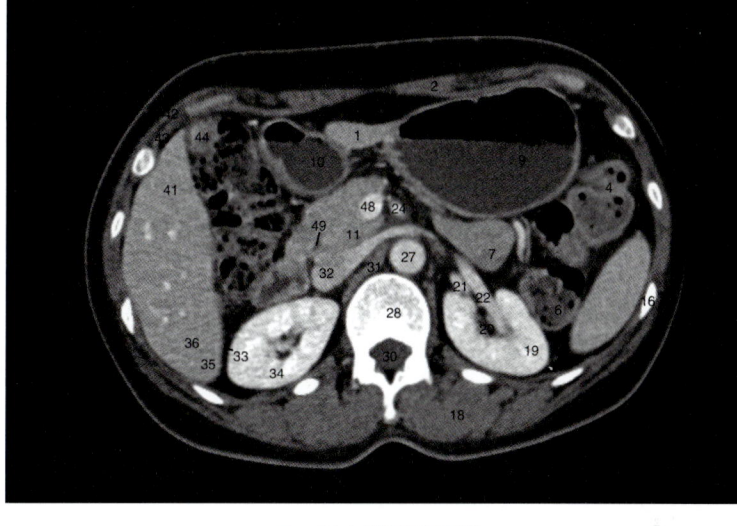

C. CT 增强图像

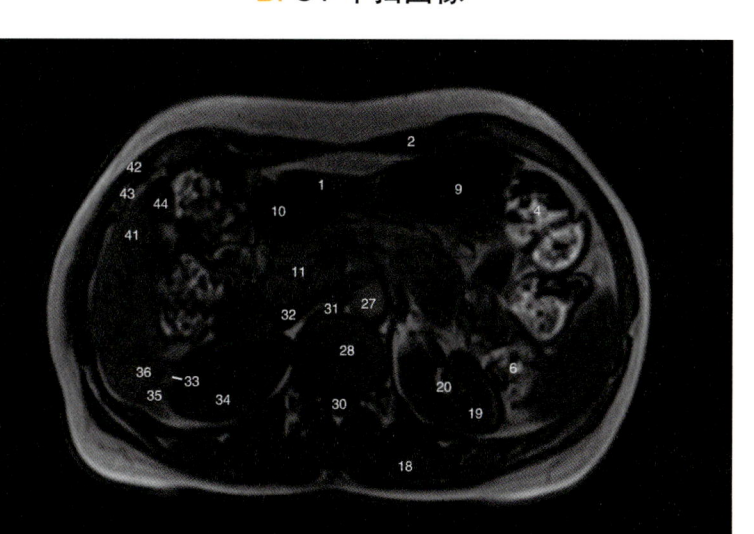

D. MR T1WI

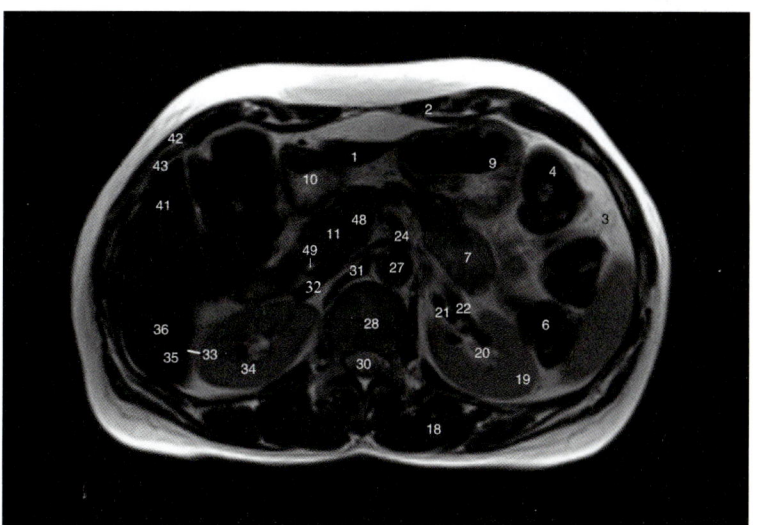

E. MR T2WI

关键结构：脾静脉，肠系膜上静脉，左肾盂。

此断面经过第1腰椎椎体。

肠系膜上静脉和脾静脉在胰腺后方汇成肝门静脉是本断面的主要特征。左肾静脉一端位于肾门附近，其左后方可见肾盂，另一端正在汇入下腔静脉。脾静脉由脾门处的2~6条（常见为3条）属支汇集而成，通过脾肾韧带，在脾动脉下方、胰腺后方右行，在胰颈后方与肠系膜上静脉汇合成肝门静脉。途中接受胃网膜左静脉、胃短静脉、胰腺的小静脉支及肠系膜下静脉汇入。脾静脉的管径常为脾动脉的2倍，在门静脉高压症时管径更大，且壁更加变薄。在巨脾切除术分离、结扎脾静脉时，应仔细操作，以免破裂出血。当脾静脉血运不畅或发生阻塞时，可导致充血性脾肿大及脾功能亢进。肾盂是由肾大盏合并成的漏斗状扁囊，位于肾窦内，出肾门后移行于输尿管。成人肾盂的容积3~10 mL。尿道逆行感染易引起该部的炎症、积脓乃至肾盂肾炎；肾结石多于该处集聚，其表面投影位于第12肋与骶棘肌（竖脊肌）外缘形成的夹角处，患者可于该部产生触压痛或叩击痛。依据肾盂与肾门的关系，国人肾盂可分3型，以门内型多见（54.76%），中间型次之（41.27%），门外型最少（3.97%）[37]。

腹部连续横断层 55（FH.10830）

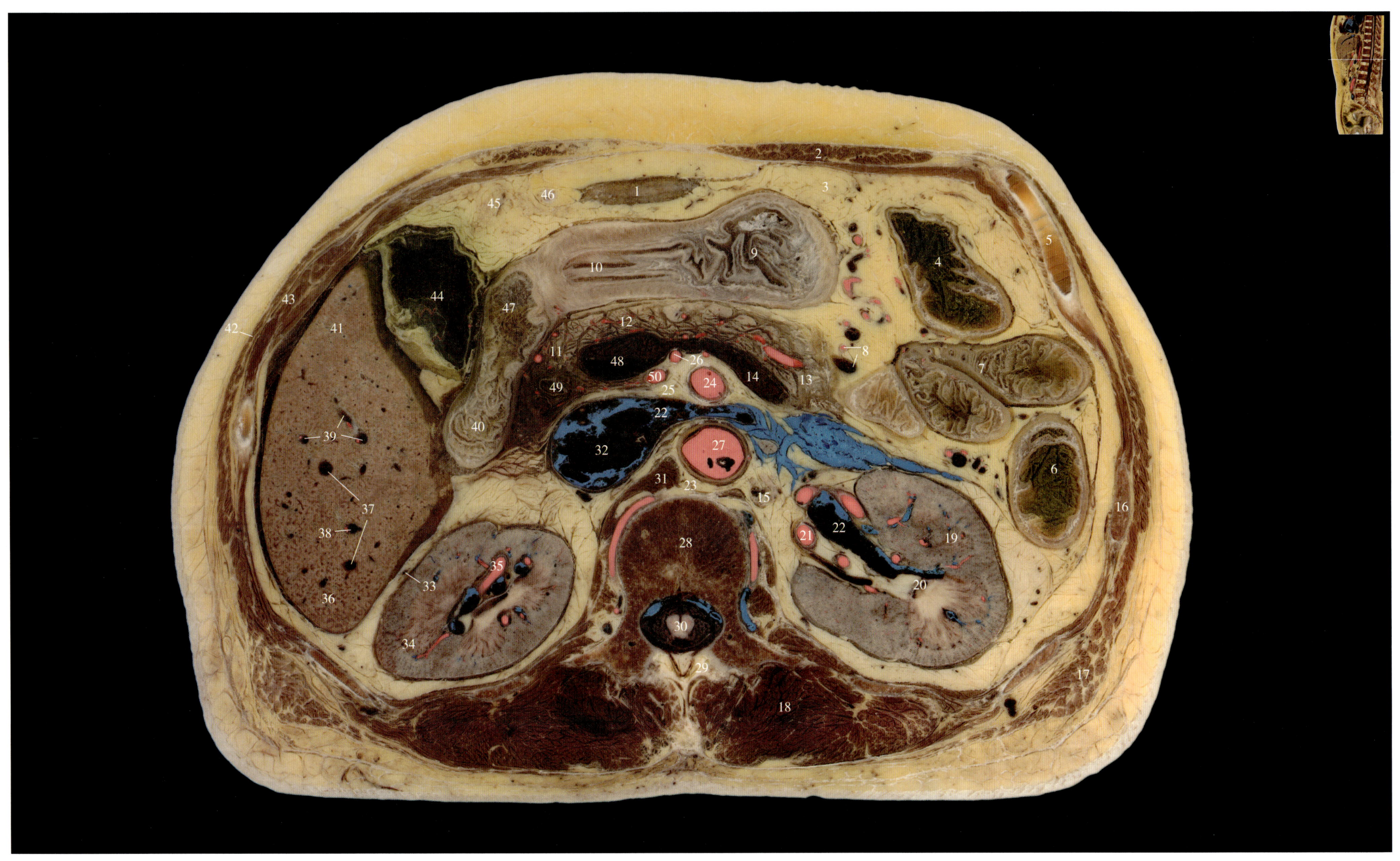

A. 断层标本图像

1. 肝左外叶下段 inferior segment of left lateral lobe of liver
2. 腹直肌 rectus abdominis
3. 大网膜 greater omentum
4. 横结肠 transverse colon
5. 第 9 肋软骨 9th costal cartilage
6. 降结肠 descending colon
7. 空肠 jejunum
8. 空肠动、静脉 jejunal artery and vein
9. 胃体 body of stomach
10. 胃幽门部 pyloric part of stomach
11. 胰头 head of pancreas
12. 胰颈 neck of pancreas
13. 胰体 body of pancreas
14. 脾静脉 splenic vein
15. 左交感干 left sympathetic trunk
16. 第 10 肋骨 10th costal bone
17. 背阔肌 latissimus dorsi
18. 竖脊肌 erector spinae
19. 左肾 left kidney
20. 左肾盂 left renal pelvis
21. 左肾动脉 left renal artery
22. 左肾静脉 left renal vein
23. 右交感干 right sympathetic trunk
24. 肠系膜上动脉 superior mesenteric artery
25. 门腔淋巴结 portocaval lymph node
26. 肝总动脉 common hepatic artery
27. 腹主动脉 abdominal aorta
28. 第 1 腰椎椎体 body of 1st lumbar vertebra
29. 关节突关节 zygapophysial joint
30. 脊髓 spinal cord
31. 右膈脚 right crus of diaphragm
32. 下腔静脉 inferior vena cava
33. 肝肾隐窝 hepatorenal recess
34. 右肾 right kidney
35. 右肾动脉 right renal artery
36. 肝右后叶下段 inferior segment of right posterior lobe of liver
37. 肝右静脉属支 tributary of right hepatic vein
38. 肝门静脉右后下支 right posteroinferior branch of hepatic portal vein
39. 肝门静脉右前下支 right anteroinferior branch of hepatic portal vein
40. 十二指肠降部 descending part of duodenum
41. 肝右前叶下段 inferior segment of right anterior lobe of liver
42. 腹外斜肌 obliquus externus abdominis
43. 腹内斜肌 obliquus internus abdominis
44. 胆囊 gallbladder
45. 肝圆韧带裂 fissure for ligamentum teres hepatis
46. 肝圆韧带 ligamentum teres hepatis
47. 十二指肠上部 superior part of duodenum
48. 肠系膜上静脉 superior mesenteric vein
49. 胆总管 common bile duct
50. 肝右动脉 right hepatic artery

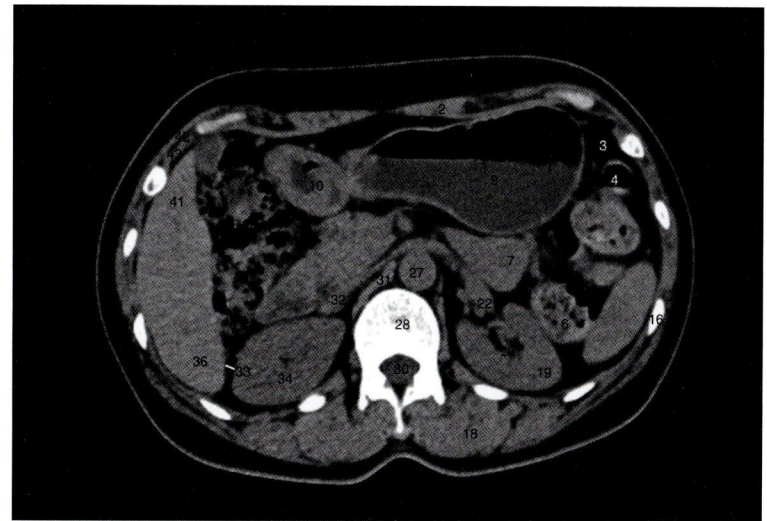

B. CT 平扫图像

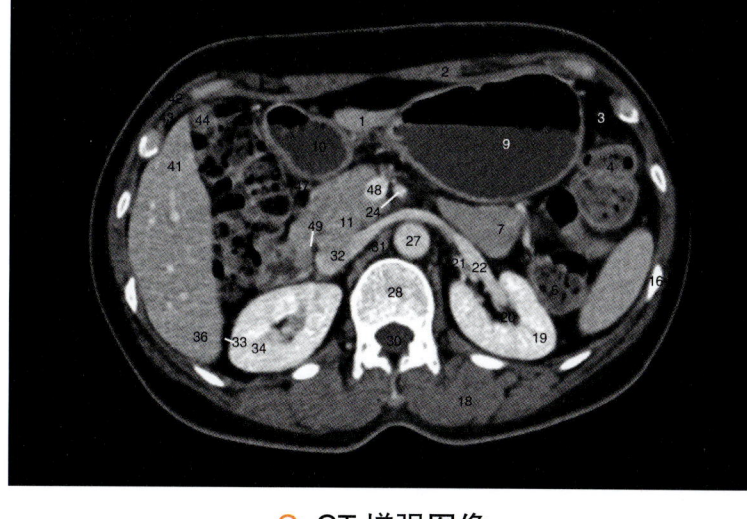

C. CT 增强图像

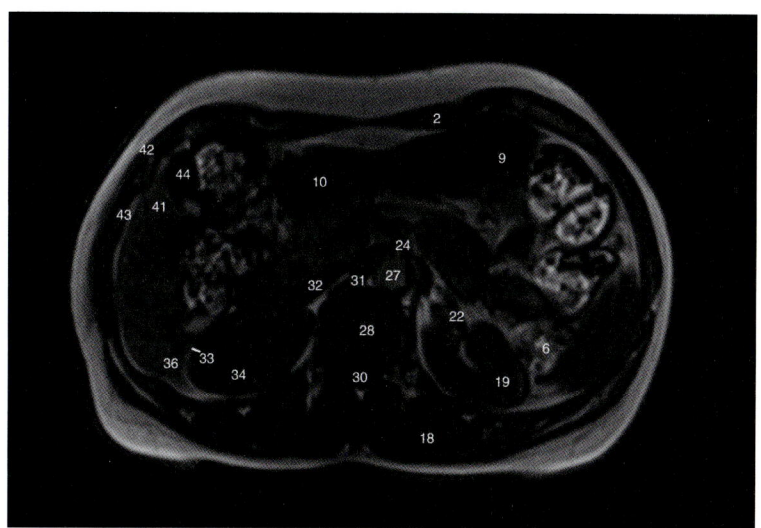

D. MR T1WI

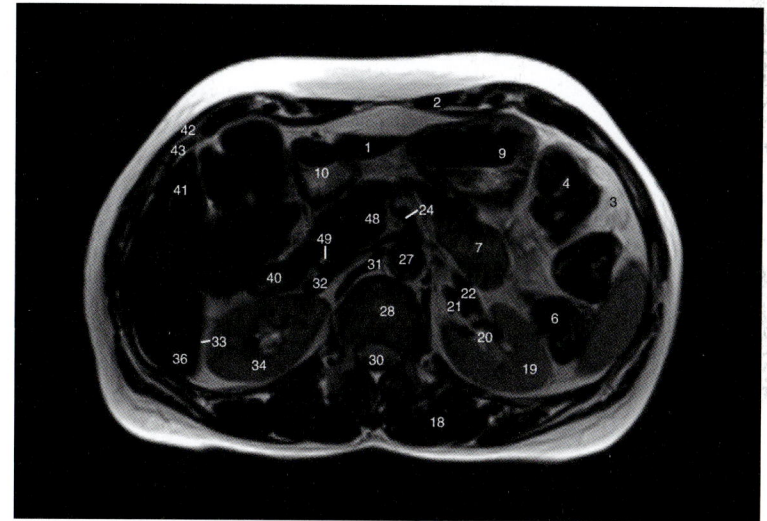

E. MR T2WI

关键结构：左肾静脉，十二指肠降部。

此断面经过第 1 腰椎椎体。

肝右叶和胆囊左侧可见十二指肠上部延伸至十二指肠降部，肠系膜上动脉与腹主动脉之间为左肾静脉。腹腔左侧为横结肠、降结肠及空肠。左肾静脉向右行经胰体和脾静脉的后方，继而在肠系膜上动脉起始处下方越过腹主动脉前缘汇入下腔静脉。胡桃夹综合征，即左肾静脉受压综合征，又称胡桃夹现象，是指走行于腹主动脉和肠系膜上动脉之间的左肾静脉受压导致血液回流障碍而引起血尿、蛋白尿等临床综合征。好发于青春期至 40 岁左右，儿童发病分布在 4~7 岁，青少年好发年龄为 13~16 岁。CT 肠系膜上动脉与腹主动脉之间的夹角大小，当夹角小于正常范围时，可见左肾静脉受压，并与下腔静脉和远侧扩张的左肾静脉共同形成哑铃样改变。左肾静脉造影是确诊的金标准，可直接观察到左肾静脉受压而出现对比剂充盈中断和远段及其属支的扩张，重者可见同侧卵巢静脉逆行显影、盆腔静脉粗迂曲[53]。还可通过测量左肾静脉内压力来诊断该病，一般认为左肾静脉与下腔静脉压力差 >5 cmH$_2$O 可高度提示该病[54]。

腹部连续横断层 56（FH.10810）

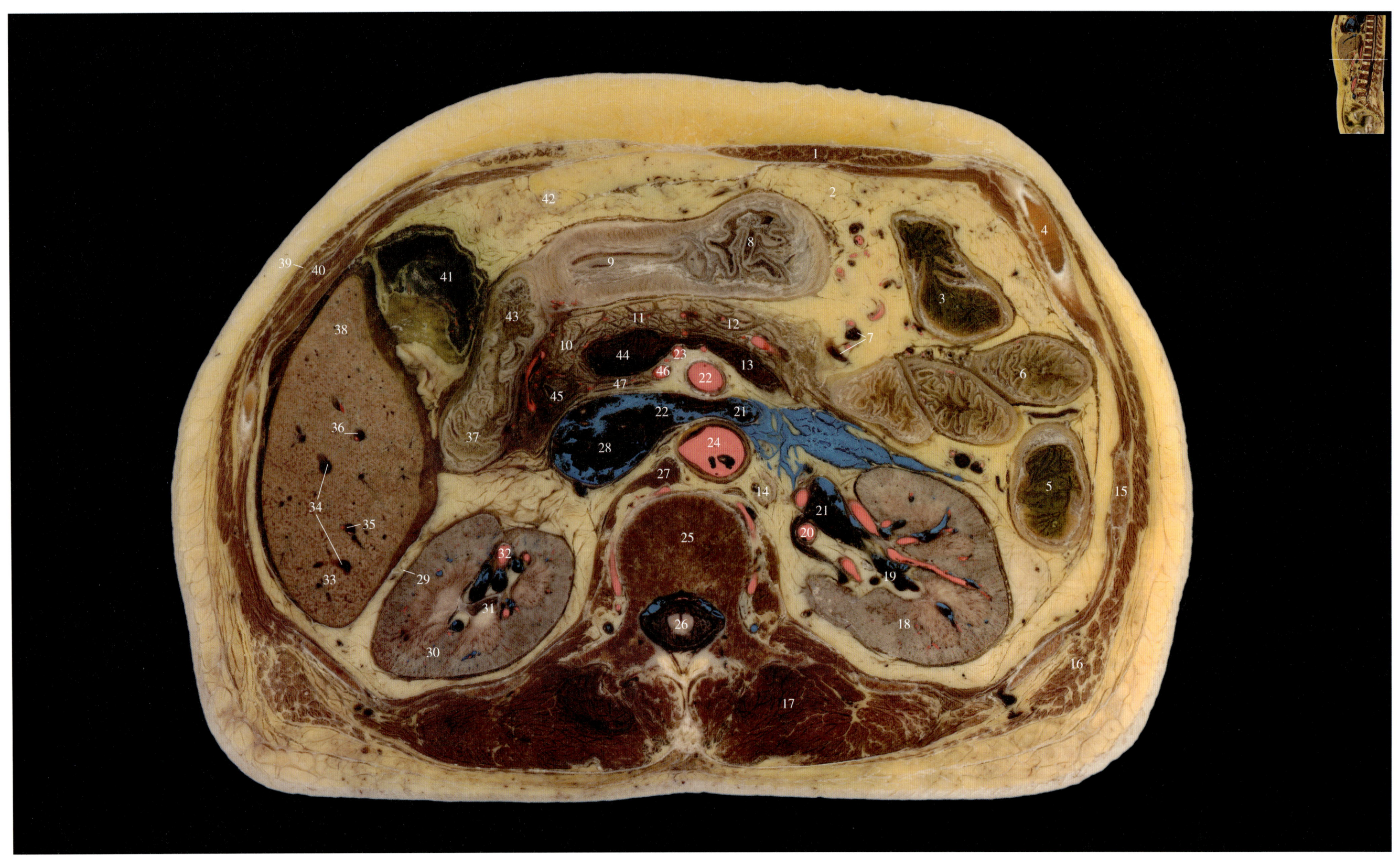

A. 断层标本图像

1. 腹直肌 rectus abdominis
2. 大网膜 greater omentum
3. 横结肠 transverse colon
4. 第10肋软骨 10th costal cartilage
5. 降结肠 descending colon
6. 空肠 jejunum
7. 空肠动、静脉 jejunal artery and vein
8. 胃体 body of stomach
9. 胃幽门部 pyloric part of stomach
10. 胰头 head of pancreas
11. 胰颈 neck of pancreas
12. 胰体 body of pancreas
13. 脾静脉 splenic vein
14. 左交感干 left sympathetic trunk
15. 第10肋骨 10th costal bone
16. 背阔肌 latissimus dorsi
17. 竖脊肌 erector spinae
18. 左肾 left kidney
19. 左肾盂 left renal pelvis
20. 左肾动脉 left renal artery
21. 左肾静脉 left renal vein
22. 肠系膜上动脉 superior mesenteric artery
23. 肝总动脉 common hepatic artery
24. 腹主动脉 abdominal aorta
25. 第1腰椎椎体 body of 1st lumbar vertebra
26. 脊髓 spinal cord
27. 右膈脚 right crus of diaphragm
28. 下腔静脉 inferior vena cava
29. 肝肾隐窝 hepatorenal recess
30. 右肾 right kidney
31. 肾小盏 minor renal calices
32. 右肾动脉 right renal artery
33. 肝右后叶下段 inferior segment of right posterior lobe of liver
34. 肝右静脉属支 tributary of right hepatic vein
35. 肝门静脉右后下支 right posteroinferior branch of hepatic portal vein
36. 肝门静脉右前下支 right anteroinferior branch of hepatic portal vein
37. 十二指肠降部 descending part of duodenum
38. 肝右前叶下段 inferior segment of right anterior lobe of liver
39. 腹外斜肌 obliquus externus abdominis
40. 腹内斜肌 obliquus internus abdominis
41. 胆囊 gallbladder
42. 肝圆韧带 ligamentum teres hepatis
43. 十二指肠上部 superior part of duodenum
44. 肠系膜上静脉 superior mesenteric vein
45. 胆总管 common bile duct
46. 肝右动脉 right hepatic artery
47. 胰钩突 uncinate process of pancreas

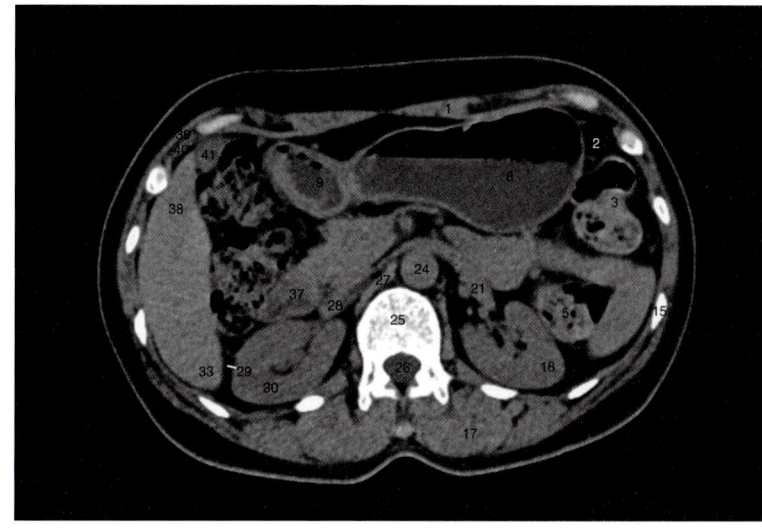

B. CT 平扫图像

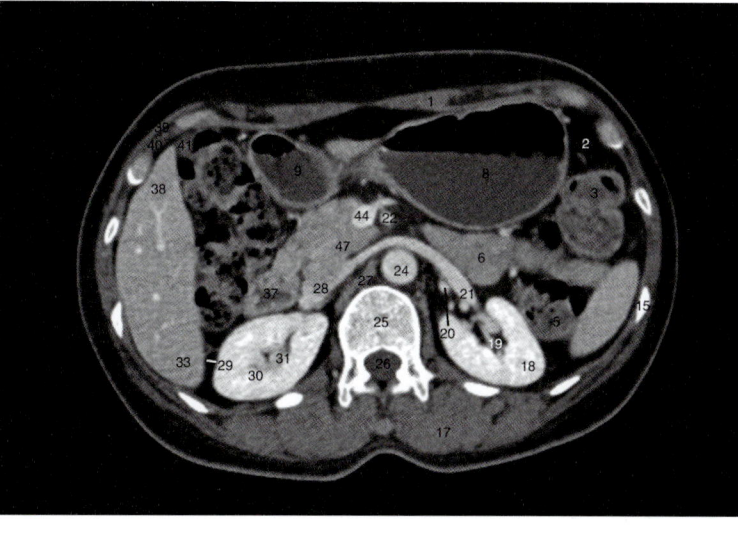

C. CT 增强图像

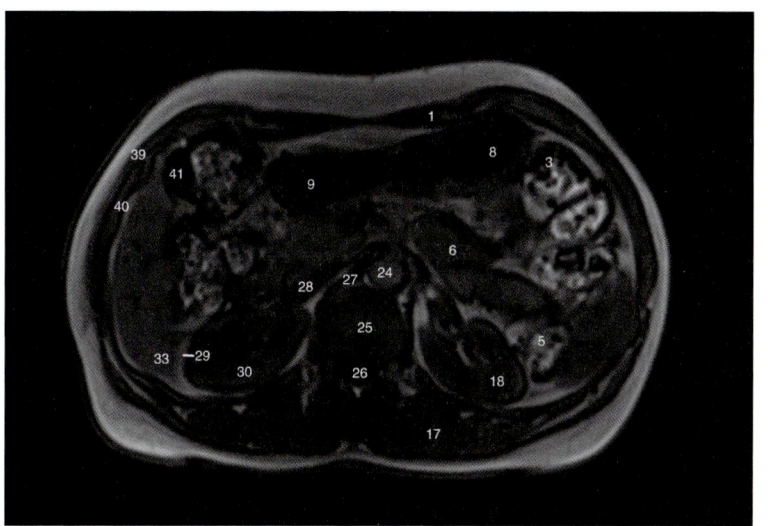

D. MR T1WI

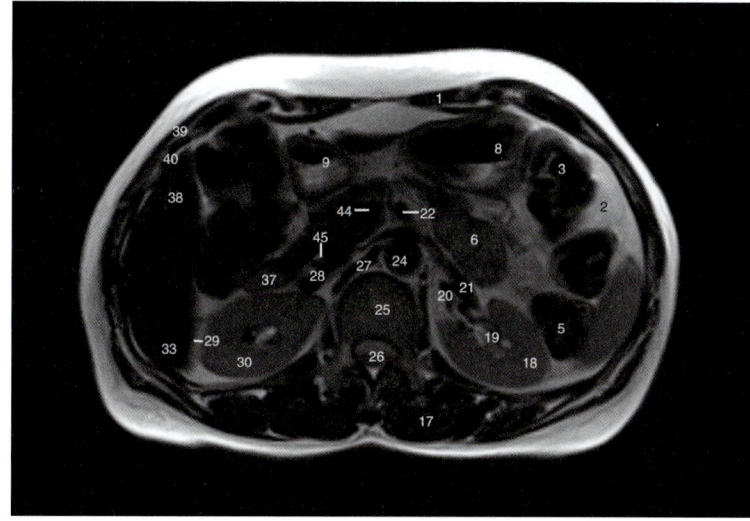

E. MR T2WI

关键结构：胰头，胰钩突，胆总管。

此断面经过第1腰椎椎体。

肝左叶消失，剩余的肝右叶位于腹腔最右侧，左侧可见十二指肠降部和胆总管。胰钩突位于肠系膜上静脉和下腔静脉之间。胰头为胰右端的膨大部分[55]，被十二指肠"C"形包绕，其下份有向左突出的钩突。胰头的上方是门静脉和肝动脉，前方及右侧为肝，右前方为胆囊，后方为下腔静脉。钩突的前方为肠系膜上静脉，后方为下腔静脉。胰腺导管癌是最常见的胰原发性恶性肿瘤，常表现为低强化的肿块。胰岛素瘤是最常见的胰腺神经内分泌肿瘤，

约50%发生在胰头部位[56]，动态增强CT扫描获得的动脉期图像可显著提高病变的检出率[57,58]。钩突在横断面上位于肠系膜上动、静脉与下腔静脉之间，约有80%的钩突与肾静脉在同一层面上。因钩突的下方是十二指肠水平部，故于断面识别时，易将十二指肠水平部误认为是钩突。在影像学上，肾静脉是钩突与十二指肠水平部的重要区分标志。钩突向左侧不超过肠系膜上动脉横径的1/2。由于钩突的特殊位置，该区的肿瘤往往不会造成胆管的阻塞，但会因为和十二指肠的密切关系而造成十二指肠第三段的压迫[43]。

腹部连续横断层 57（FH.10790）

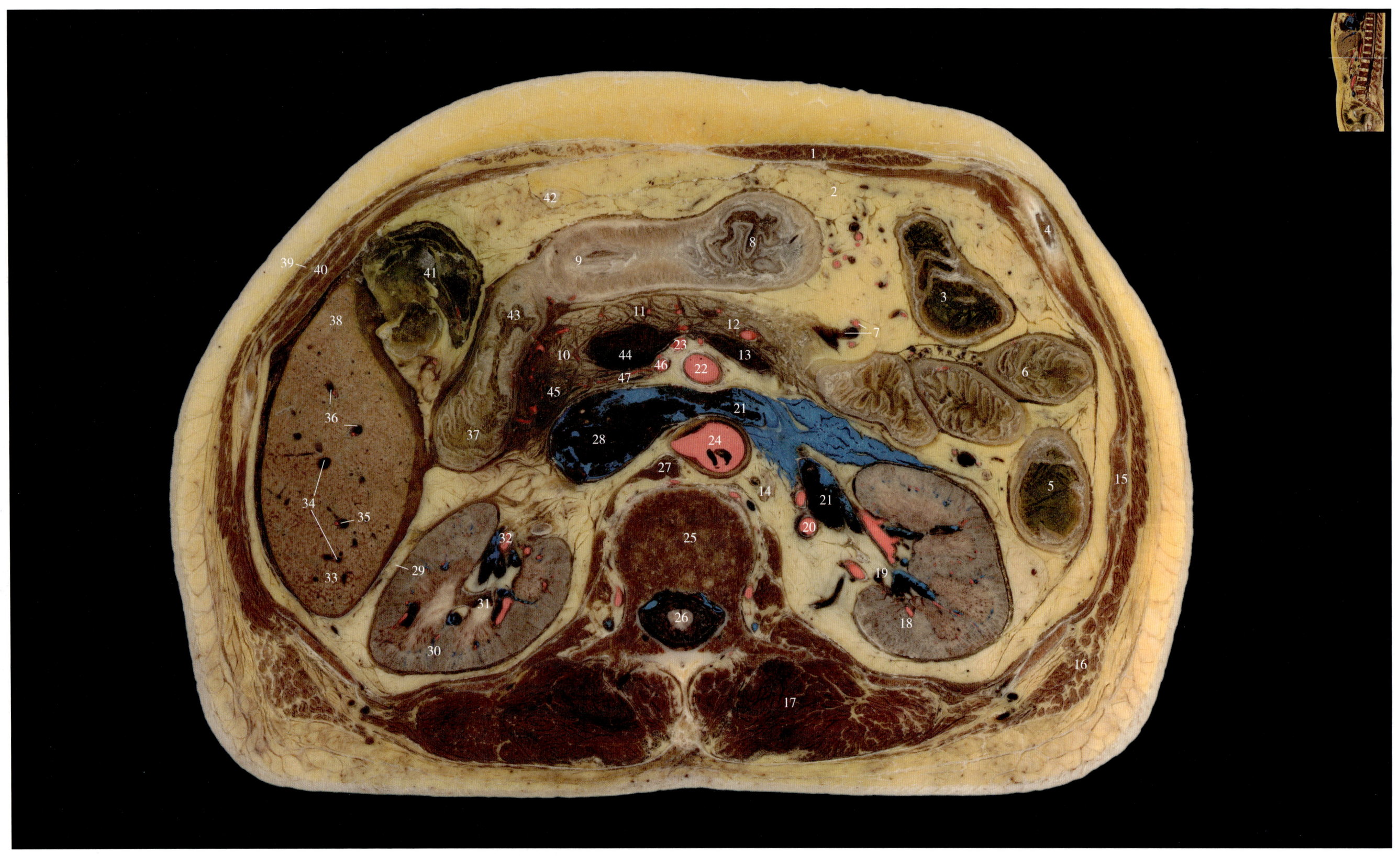

A. 断层标本图像

1. 腹直肌 rectus abdominis
2. 大网膜 greater omentum
3. 横结肠 transverse colon
4. 第10肋软骨 10th costal cartilage
5. 降结肠 descending colon
6. 空肠 jejunum
7. 空肠动、静脉 jejunal artery and vein
8. 胃体 body of stomach
9. 胃幽门部 pyloric part of stomach
10. 胰头 head of pancreas
11. 胰颈 neck of pancreas
12. 胰体 body of pancreas
13. 脾静脉 splenic vein
14. 左交感干 left sympathetic trunk
15. 第10肋骨 10th costal bone
16. 背阔肌 latissimus dorsi
17. 竖脊肌 erector spinae
18. 左肾 left kidney
19. 左肾盂 left renal pelvis
20. 左肾动脉 left renal artery
21. 左肾静脉 left renal vein
22. 肠系膜上动脉 superior mesenteric artery
23. 肝总动脉 common hepatic artery
24. 腹主动脉 abdominal aorta
25. 第1腰椎椎体 body of 1st lumbar vertebra
26. 脊髓 spinal cord
27. 右膈脚 right crus of diaphragm
28. 下腔静脉 inferior vena cava
29. 肝肾隐窝 hepatorenal recess
30. 右肾 right kidney
31. 肾小盏 minor renal calices
32. 右肾动脉 right renal artery
33. 肝右后叶下段 inferior segment of right posterior lobe of liver
34. 肝右静脉属支 tributary of right hepatic vein
35. 肝门静脉右后下支 right posteroinferior branch of hepatic portal vein
36. 肝门静脉右前下支 right anteroinferior branch of hepatic portal vein
37. 十二指肠降部 descending part of duodenum
38. 肝右前叶下段 inferior segment of right anterior lobe of liver
39. 腹外斜肌 obliquus externus abdominis
40. 腹内斜肌 obliquus internus abdominis
41. 胆囊 gallbladder
42. 肝圆韧带 ligamentum teres hepatis
43. 十二指肠上部 superior part of duodenum
44. 肠系膜上静脉 superior mesenteric vein
45. 胆总管 common bile duct
46. 肝右动脉 right hepatic artery
47. 胰钩突 uncinate process of pancreas

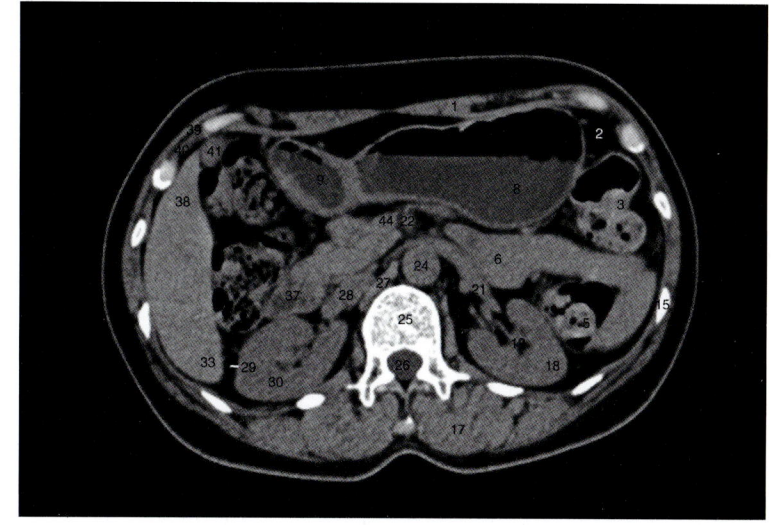

B. CT 平扫图像

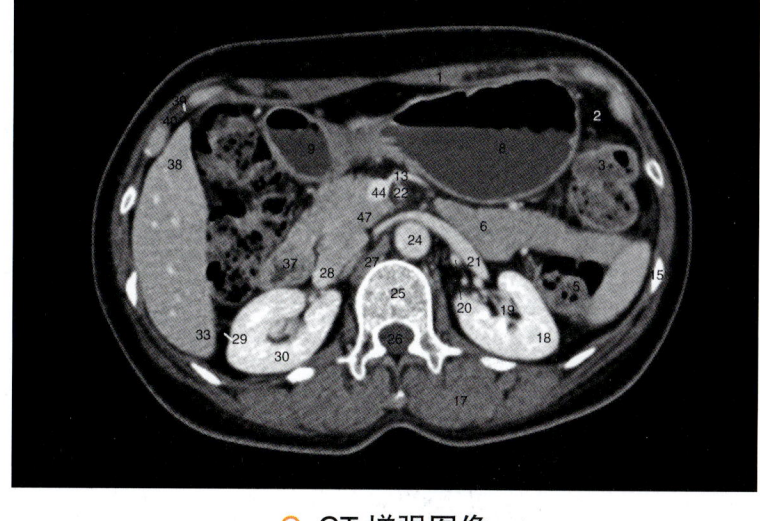

C. CT 增强图像

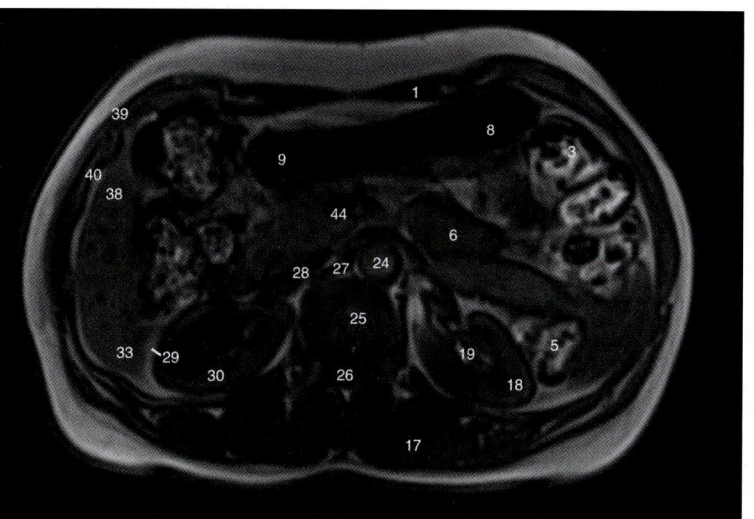

D. MR T1WI

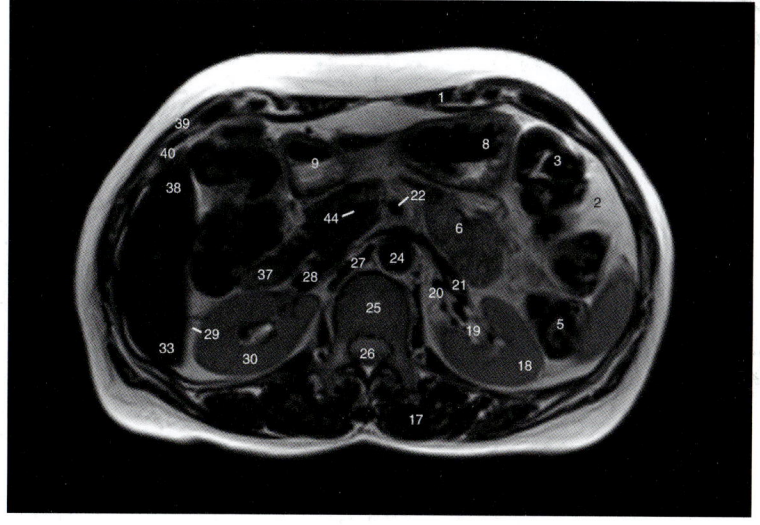

E. MR T2WI

关键结构：肝右叶，肾小盏。

此断面经过第1腰椎椎体。

脊柱前方由后向前依次为：腹主动脉、左肾静脉、肠系膜上动脉、脾静脉、胰、胃体。双肾位于脊柱两侧，脊柱后方为竖脊肌。脊柱左前方为左交感干，沿脊柱走行，肝仅剩很小的右叶。在增强CT增强图像上，可见强化的肝右动脉、门静脉右支和肝右静脉的属支，须结合毗邻关系和连续追踪进行鉴别。肝右叶是肝脏疾病的好发部位，肝硬化时右叶常常变形、萎缩，肝裂增宽；肝囊肿、血管瘤、肝转移瘤和肝癌也常发生于右叶。肾小盏是位于肾髓质深面、包绕肾乳头的漏斗形膜性管。肾小盏向内接肾乳头，有时1个肾小盏可包绕2~3个肾乳头，故肾小盏的数目比肾乳头的数目少。尿液经筛区进入肾小盏，由肾小盏再进入肾大盏。肾排泄性尿路造影或逆行造影可观察肾小盏的形状，对于诊断肾盂、输尿管疾病具有重要的价值。

腹部连续横断层 58（FH.10770）

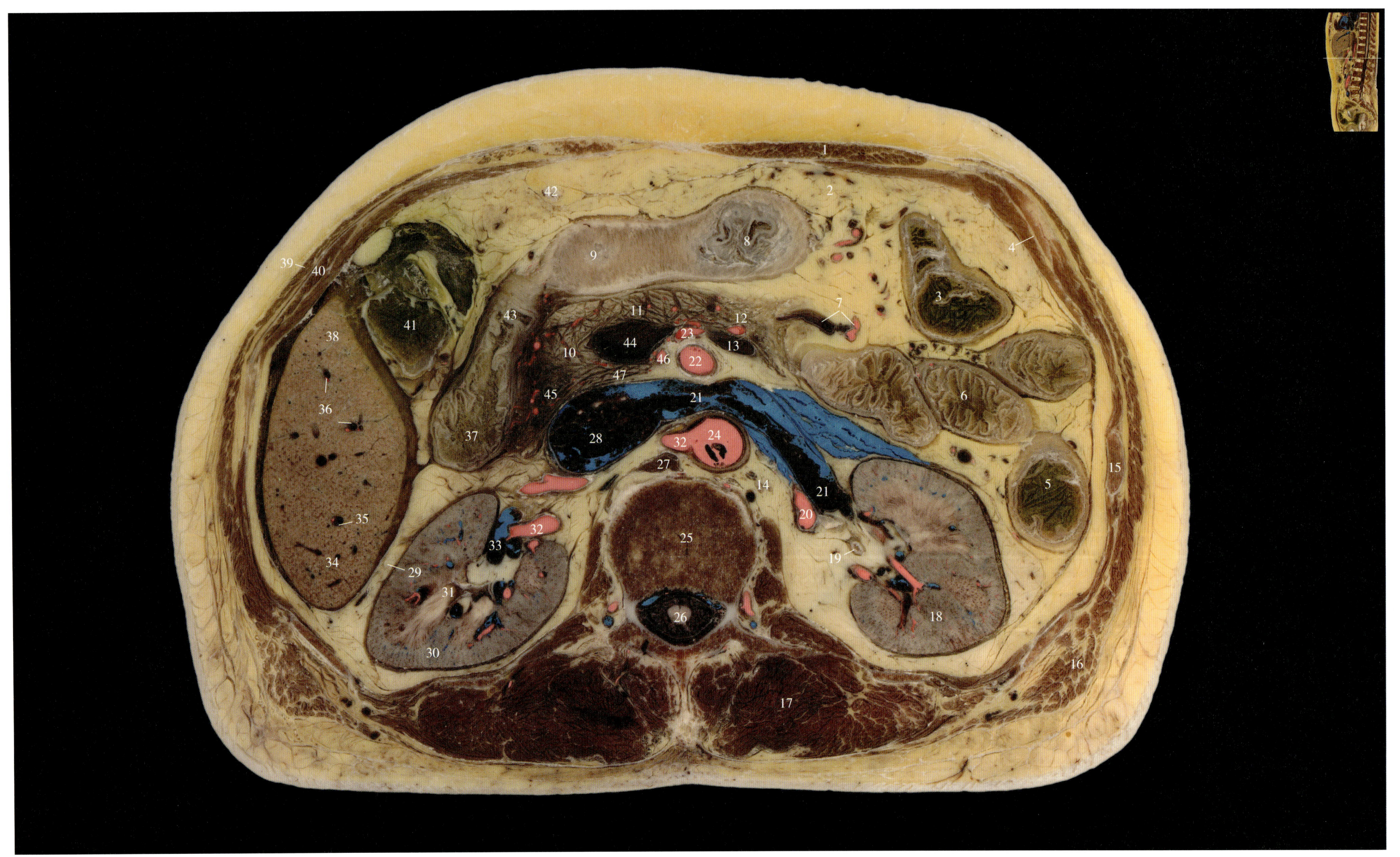

A. 断层标本图像

1. 腹直肌 rectus abdominis
2. 大网膜 greater omentum
3. 横结肠 transverse colon
4. 腹横肌 transversus abdominis
5. 降结肠 descending colon
6. 空肠 jejunum
7. 空肠动、静脉 jejunal artery and vein
8. 胃体 body of stomach
9. 胃幽门部 pyloric part of stomach
10. 胰头 head of pancreas
11. 胰颈 neck of pancreas
12. 胰体 body of pancreas
13. 脾静脉 splenic vein
14. 左交感干 left sympathetic trunk
15. 第 10 肋骨 10th costal bone
16. 背阔肌 latissimus dorsi
17. 竖脊肌 erector spinae
18. 左肾 left kidney
19. 左肾盂 left renal pelvis
20. 左肾动脉 left renal artery
21. 左肾静脉 left renal vein
22. 肠系膜上动脉 superior mesenteric artery
23. 肝总动脉 common hepatic artery
24. 腹主动脉 abdominal aorta
25. 第 1 腰椎椎体 body of 1st lumbar vertebra
26. 脊髓 spinal cord
27. 右膈脚 right crus of diaphragm
28. 下腔静脉 inferior vena cava
29. 肝肾隐窝 hepatorenal recess
30. 右肾 right kidney
31. 肾小盏 minor renal calices
32. 右肾动脉 right renal artery
33. 右肾静脉 right renal vein
34. 肝右后叶下段 inferior segment of right posterior lobe of liver
35. 肝门静脉右后下支 right posteroinferior branch of hepatic portal vein
36. 肝门静脉右前下支 right anteroinferior branch of hepatic portal vein
37. 十二指肠降部 descending part of duodenum
38. 肝右前叶下段 inferior segment of right anterior lobe of liver
39. 腹外斜肌 obliquus externus abdominis
40. 腹内斜肌 obliquus internus abdominis
41. 胆囊 gallbladder
42. 肝圆韧带 ligamentum teres hepatis
43. 十二指肠上部 superior part of duodenum
44. 肠系膜上静脉 superior mesenteric vein
45. 胆总管 common bile duct
46. 肝右动脉 right hepatic artery
47. 胰钩突 uncinate process of pancreas

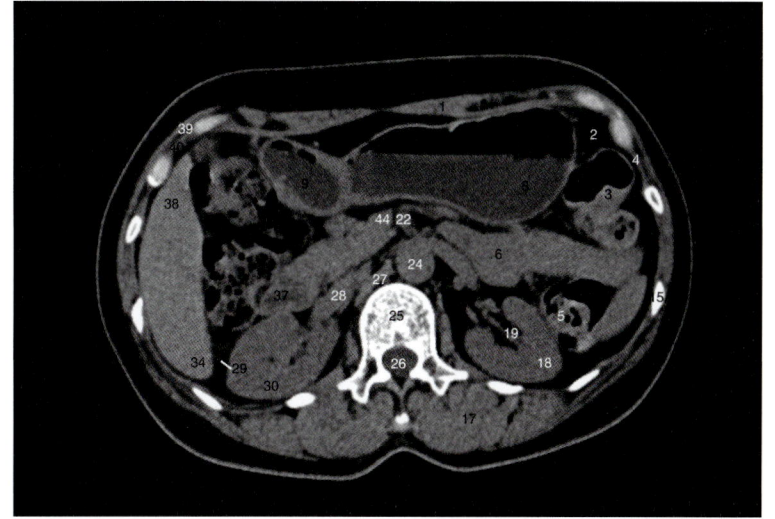

B. CT 平扫图像

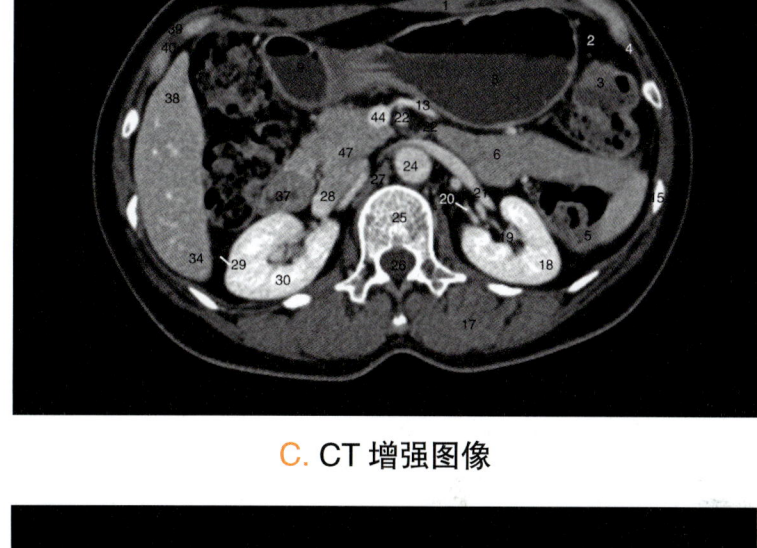

C. CT 增强图像

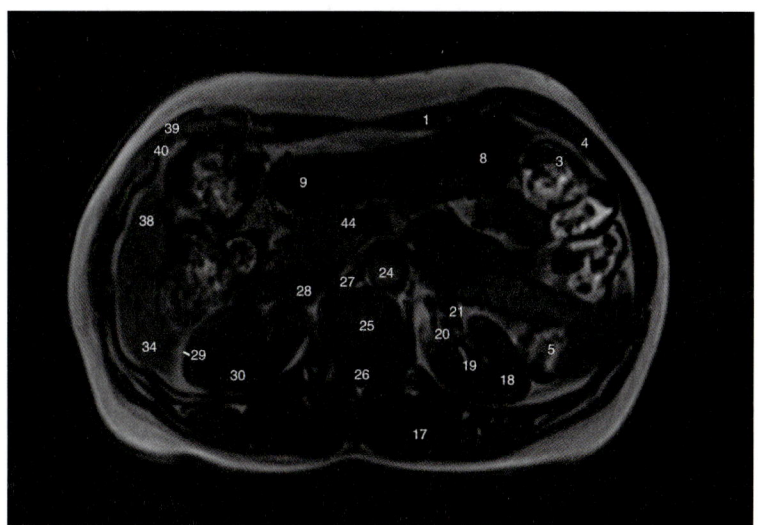

D. MR T1WI

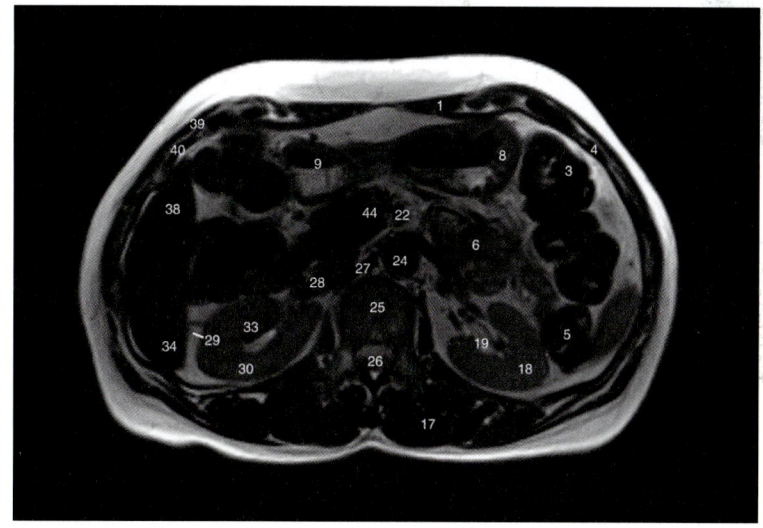

E. MR T2WI

关键结构：肠系膜上动、静脉，胰，空肠。

此断面经过第 1 腰椎椎体下份。

断面中部可见左肾静脉向左汇入下腔静脉，其前方为相互伴行的肠系膜上静脉和肠系膜上动脉，后方见腹主动脉向右发出右肾动脉，与右肾静脉伴行进入右肾。腹腔右侧为剩余的肝右叶，左侧为横、降结肠及空肠。胰腺位于腹膜后肾旁前间隙内，该断面可见头、颈、体 3 部分显示，胰腺横跨第 1、2 腰椎之前的区域，左侧胰尾端伸达脾门，右侧胰头端位于十二指肠环内，前面被构成网膜囊后壁的后腹膜所覆盖，后壁为腹膜后大血管中线区域结构，如腹主动脉、下腔静脉、双肾静脉及左肾上腺、腹腔神经丛、胸导管起始端等。儿童及青壮年胰腺形态饱满，边缘光滑，老年人因胰腺萎缩而呈边缘不规则的羽毛状改变，胰腺实质因脂肪沉积而密度降低。胰腺导管腺癌是胰腺最常见的恶性肿瘤，也是目前最致命的癌症之一，居癌症死亡的第四大原因。目前对比剂增强 CT 是检测和评估胰腺癌的首选方法[55,59]，动脉期肿块呈轻中度强化，边缘不清，静脉及延迟期呈渐进式强化，病灶中心易坏死。如病变位于胰头部，可压迫或侵犯胆总管下端，致上游胆总管和胰管扩张而呈现典型的"双管征"。

腹部连续横断层 59（FH.10750）

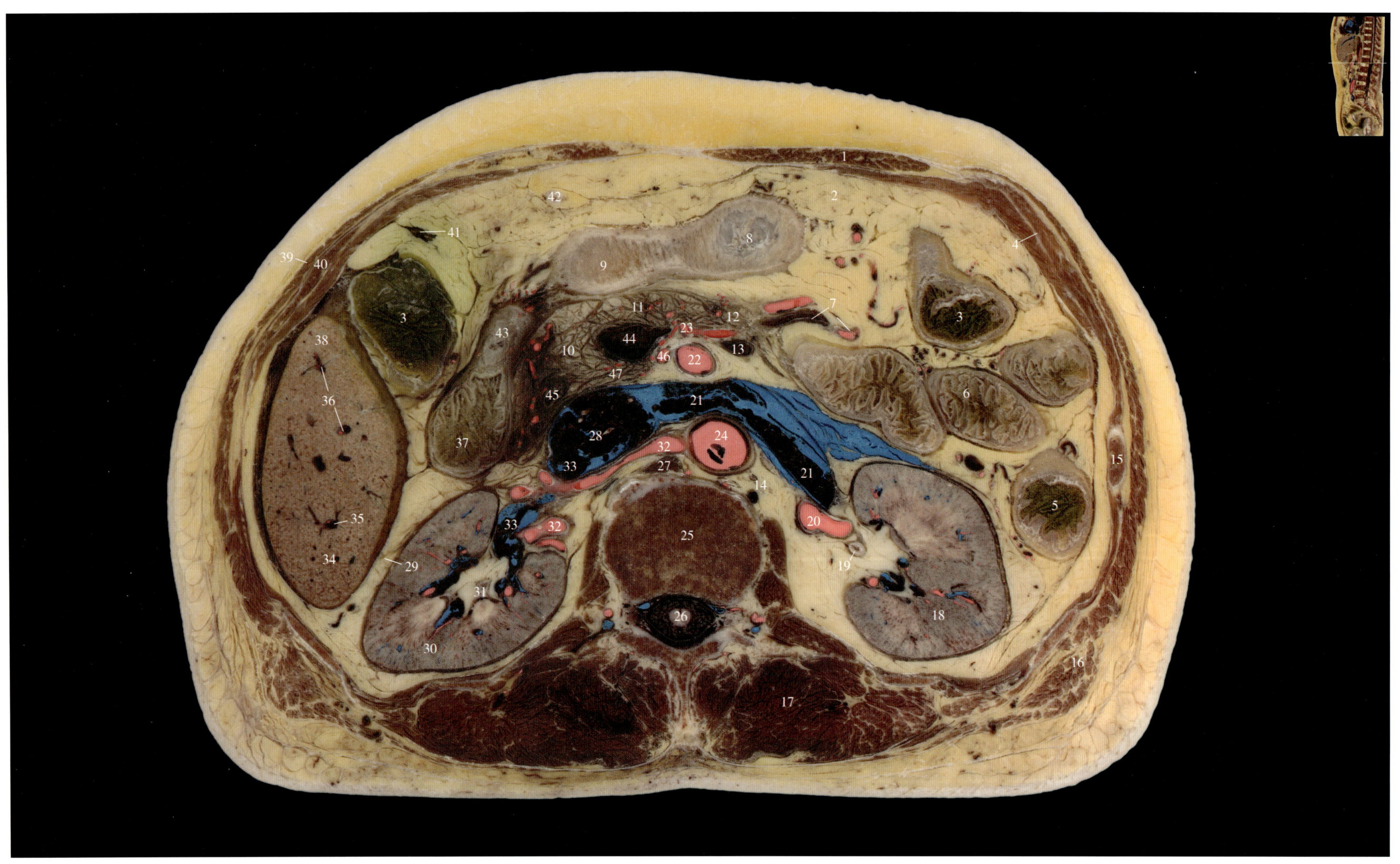

A. 断层标本图像

1. 腹直肌 rectus abdominis
2. 大网膜 greater omentum
3. 横结肠 transverse colon
4. 腹横肌 transversus abdominis
5. 降结肠 descending colon
6. 空肠 jejunum
7. 空肠动、静脉 jejunal artery and vein
8. 胃体 body of stomach
9. 胃幽门部 pyloric part of stomach
10. 胰头 head of pancreas
11. 胰颈 neck of pancreas
12. 胰体 body of pancreas
13. 肠系膜下静脉 inferior mesenteric vein
14. 左交感干 left sympathetic trunk
15. 第 10 肋骨 10th costal bone
16. 背阔肌 latissimus dorsi
17. 竖脊肌 erector spinae
18. 左肾 left kidney
19. 左肾盂 left renal pelvis
20. 左肾动脉 left renal artery
21. 左肾静脉 left renal vein
22. 肠系膜上动脉 superior mesenteric artery
23. 肝总动脉 common hepatic artery
24. 腹主动脉 abdominal aorta
25. 第 1 腰椎椎体 body of 1st lumbar vertebra
26. 脊髓 spinal cord
27. 右膈脚 right crus of diaphragm
28. 下腔静脉 inferior vena cava
29. 肝肾隐窝 hepatorenal recess
30. 右肾 right kidney
31. 肾小盏 minor renal calices
32. 右肾动脉 right renal artery
33. 右肾静脉 right renal vein
34. 肝右后叶下段 inferior segment of right posterior lobe of liver
35. 肝门静脉右后下支 right posteroinferior branch of hepatic portal vein
36. 肝门静脉右前下支 right anteroinferior branch of hepatic portal vein
37. 十二指肠降部 descending part of duodenum
38. 肝右前叶下段 inferior segment of right anterior lobe of liver
39. 腹外斜肌 obliquus externus abdominis
40. 腹内斜肌 obliquus internus abdominis
41. 胆囊 gallbladder
42. 肝圆韧带 ligamentum teres hepatis
43. 十二指肠上部 superior part of duodenum
44. 肠系膜上静脉 superior mesenteric vein
45. 胆总管 common bile duct
46. 肝右动脉 right hepatic artery
47. 胰钩突 uncinate process of pancreas

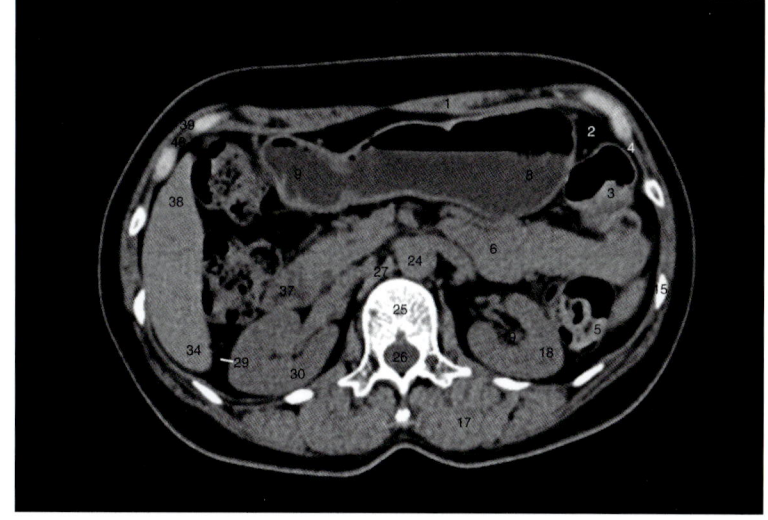

B. CT 平扫图像

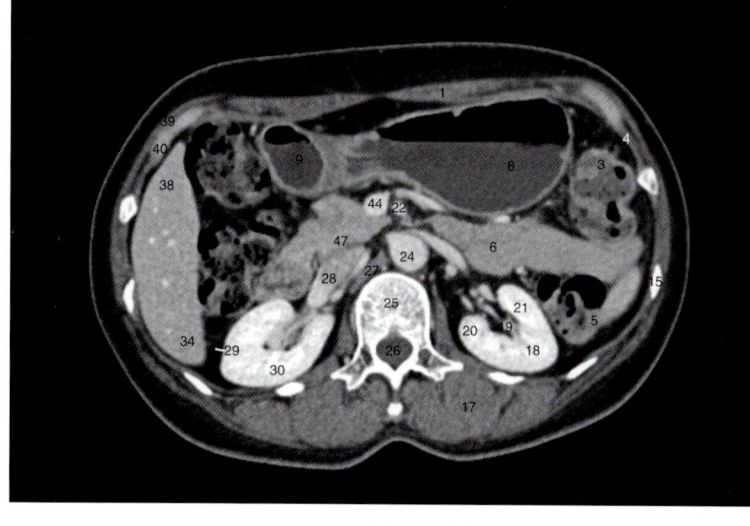

C. CT 增强图像

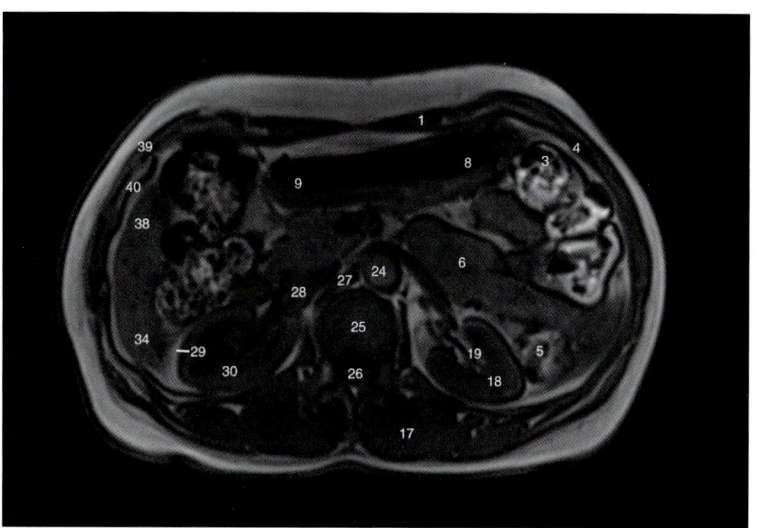

D. MR T1WI

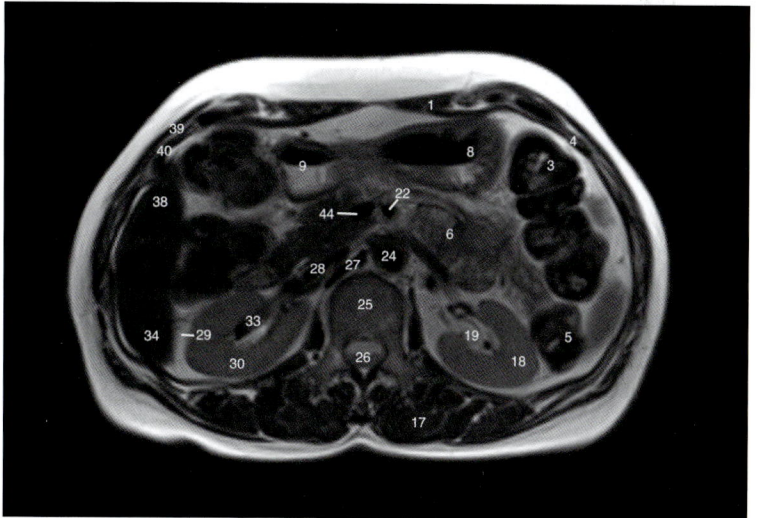

E. MR T2WI

关键结构：右肾动脉，肝圆韧带，横结肠。

此断面经过第 1 腰椎椎体下份。

腹腔前部为肝圆韧带，其在右下方与胆囊相邻，右部为小部分肝右叶，在肝右叶、十二指肠降部及胆囊间可见部分横结肠显示。腹腔左侧有横、降结肠及空肠，胰腺居中位于腹膜后。腹主动脉在肠系膜上动脉下方 1~2 cm 处，约 L1-2 椎间盘水平发出左、右两支肾动脉，左肾动脉起始部常高于右肾动脉。肾动脉横行向外，至肾门附近分为前后两干，经肾门入肾，在肾内再分为肾段动脉至各个肾段组织。肾动脉变异较多见，当一侧肾有 1 支以上的额外动脉，起源于腹主动脉或其分支，成为副肾动脉，其出现率 48.5%~69.3%。肾动脉在入肾门之前发出肾上腺下动脉至肾上腺，在腺体内与肾上腺上、中动脉吻合。肾动脉狭窄临床较常见，临床上主要表现为肾血管性高血压和缺血性肾病。肾动脉 CTA 和 MRA 可清晰地显示肾动脉管腔的程度和范围，结合图像后处理重组技术，可以为治疗提供准确的信息[48,60,61]。

腹部连续横断层 61（FH.10710）

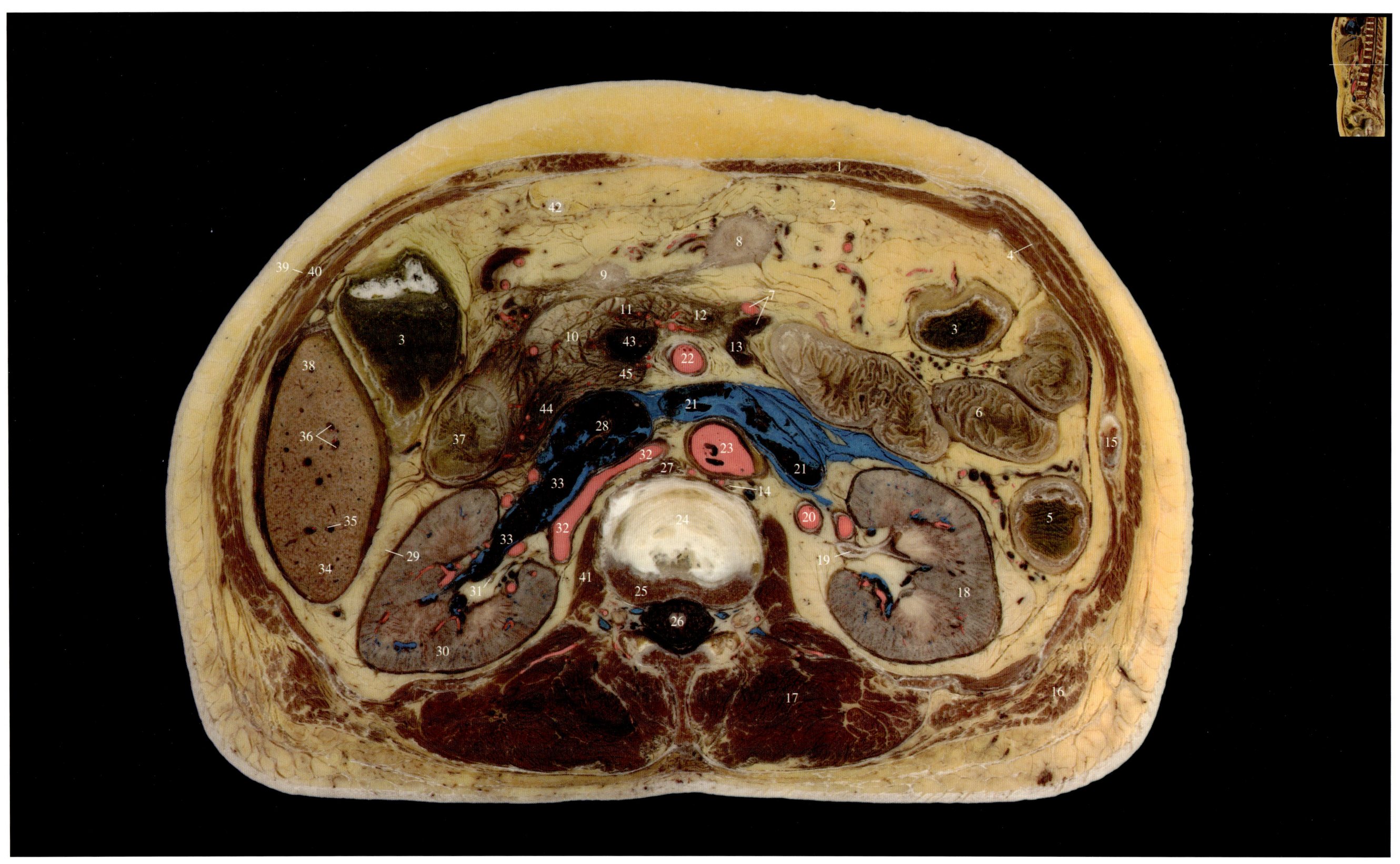

A. 断层标本图像

1. 腹直肌 rectus abdominis
2. 大网膜 greater omentum
3. 横结肠 transverse colon
4. 腹横肌 transversus abdominis
5. 降结肠 descending colon
6. 空肠 jejunum
7. 空肠动、静脉 jejunal artery and vein
8. 胃 stomach
9. 胃幽门部 pyloric part of stomach
10. 胰头 head of pancreas
11. 胰颈 neck of pancreas
12. 胰体 body of pancreas
13. 肠系膜下静脉 inferior mesenteric vein
14. 左交感干 left sympathetic trunk
15. 第 10 肋骨 10th costal bone
16. 背阔肌 latissimus dorsi
17. 竖脊肌 erector spinae
18. 左肾 left kidney
19. 左肾盂 left renal pelvis
20. 左肾动脉 left renal artery
21. 左肾静脉 left renal vein
22. 肠系膜上动脉 superior mesenteric artery
23. 腹主动脉 abdominal aorta
24. L1-2 椎间盘 L1-2 intervertebral disc
25. 第 1 腰椎椎体 body of 1st lumbar vertebra
26. 脊髓 spinal cord
27. 右膈脚 right crus of diaphragm
28. 下腔静脉 inferior vena cava
29. 肝肾隐窝 hepatorenal recess
30. 右肾 right kidney
31. 右肾盂 right renal pelvis
32. 右肾动脉 right renal artery
33. 右肾静脉 right renal vein
34. 肝右后叶下段 inferior segment of right posterior lobe of liver
35. 肝门静脉右后下支 right posteroinferior branch of hepatic portal vein
36. 肝门静脉右前下支 right anteroinferior branch of hepatic portal vein
37. 十二指肠降部 descending part of duodenum
38. 肝右前叶下段 inferior segment of right anterior lobe of liver
39. 腹外斜肌 obliquus externus abdominis
40. 腹内斜肌 obliquus internus abdominis
41. 腰大肌 psoas major
42. 肝圆韧带 ligamentum teres hepatis
43. 肠系膜上静脉 superior mesenteric vein
44. 胆总管 common bile duct
45. 胰钩突 uncinate process of pancreas

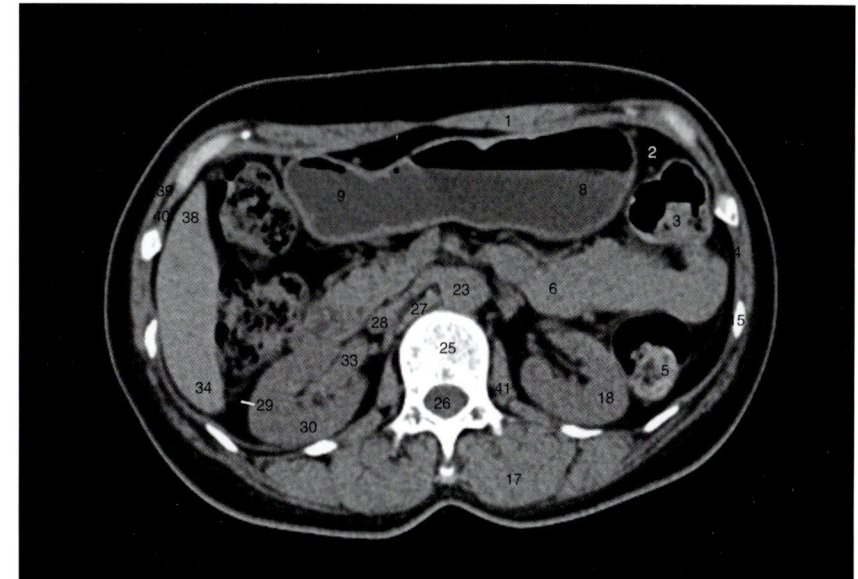

B. CT 平扫图像

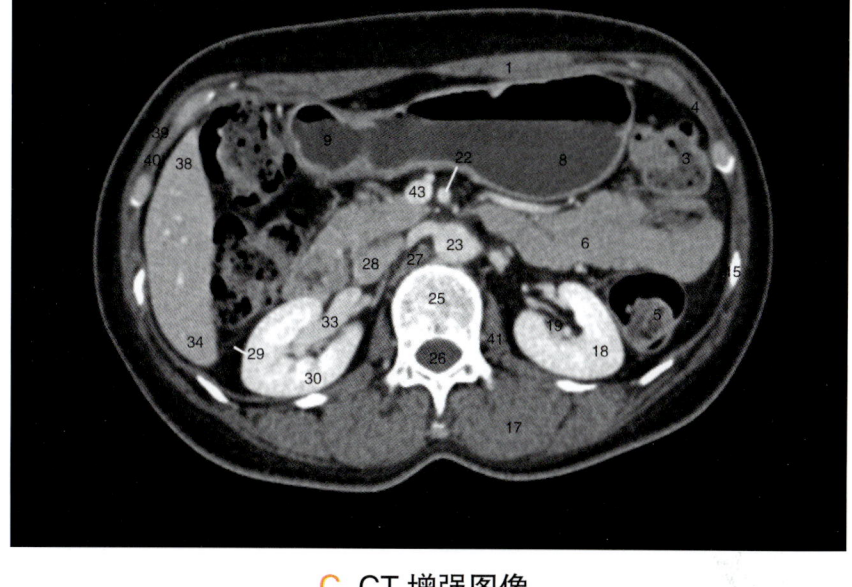

C. CT 增强图像

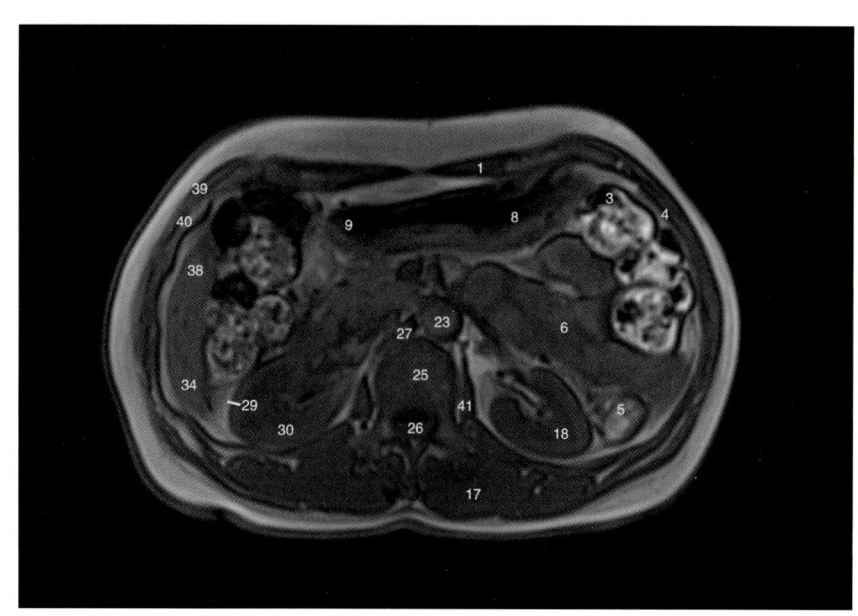

D. MR T1WI

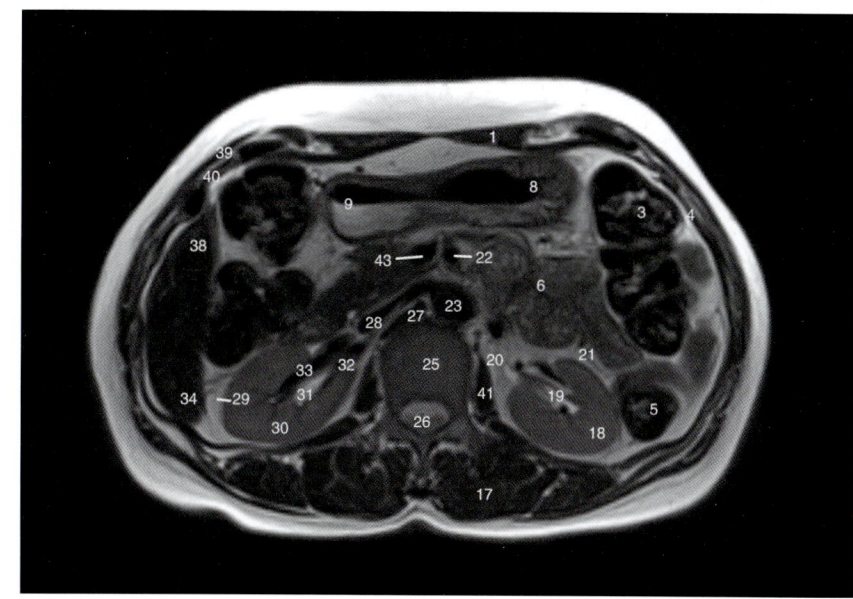

E. MR T2WI

关键结构：肠系膜下静脉，肾门，胰钩突。

此断面经过第 1 腰椎椎体和 L1-2 椎间盘。

胃大部分消失，仅剩余少许胃体及幽门，在胃的后方为逐渐缩小的胰腺，并可见胰头、胰体及胰钩突围绕肠系膜上静脉起始段，左侧依次为肠系膜上动脉、肠系膜下静脉。在动脉期 CT 或 MR 图像上，与强化的胰头实质相比，肠系膜上静脉呈低密度或混杂密度，易误诊为胰头肿块。肠系膜下静脉起自直肠上静脉，左侧与空肠相隔，跨过小骨盆上行，在左侧输尿管内侧跨过髂总血管，伴行于同名动脉的左侧，在腹膜壁层深面上行，越过左侧腰大肌后，逐渐离开同名动脉，行于十二指肠旁皱襞内，继而经十二指肠空肠曲和 Treitz 韧带左侧上行，达胰体后方并注入脾静脉，再经脾静脉汇入门静脉，或注入肠系膜上静脉，或注入肠系膜上静脉与脾静脉汇合处。腹部结核常累及肠系膜淋巴结，CT 是检测肿大淋巴结的首选检查技术。

腹部连续横断层 62（FH.10690）

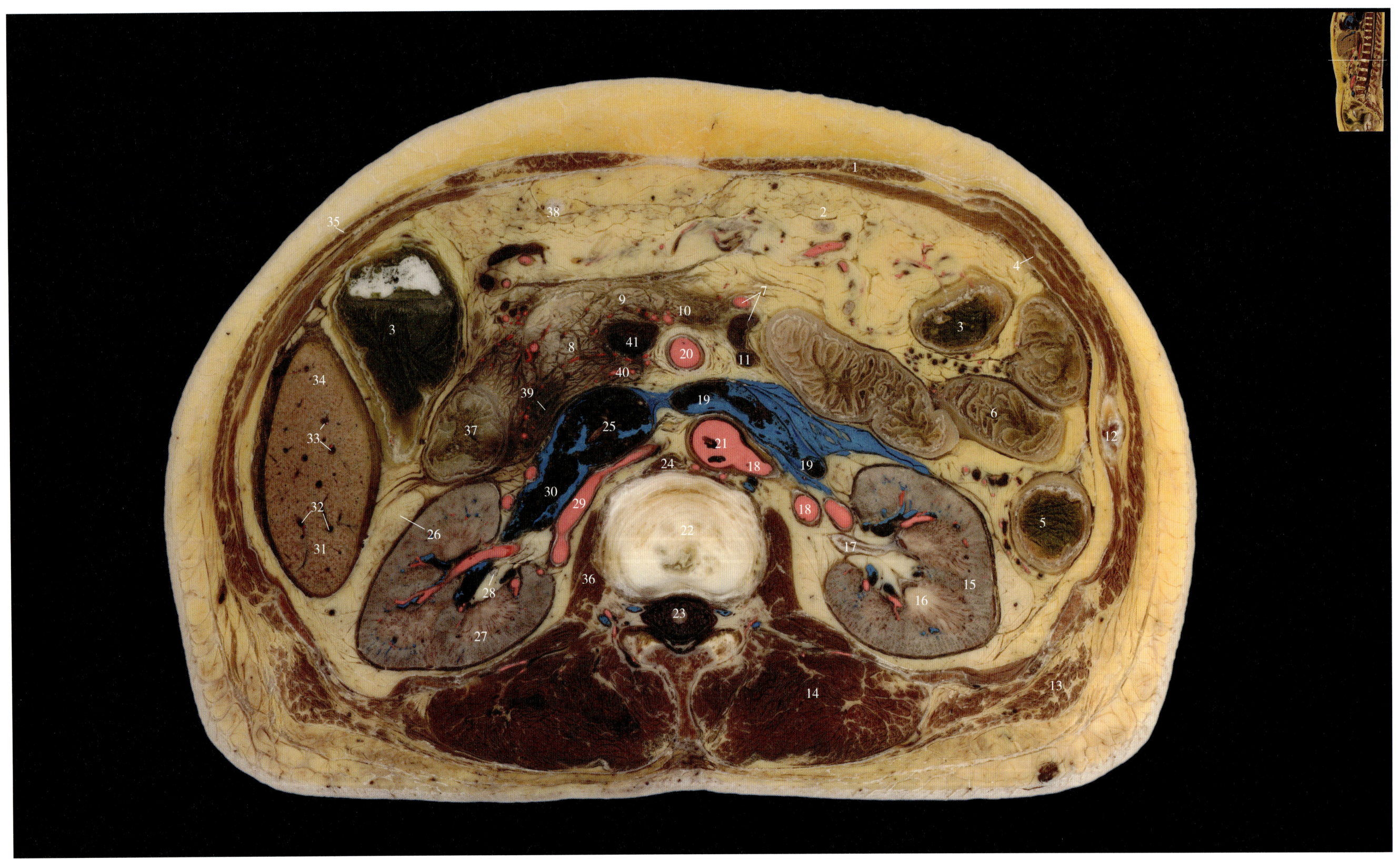

A. 断层标本图像

1. 腹直肌 rectus abdominis
2. 大网膜 greater omentum
3. 横结肠 transverse colon
4. 腹横肌 transversus abdominis
5. 降结肠 descending colon
6. 空肠 jejunum
7. 空肠动、静脉 jejunal artery and vein
8. 胰头 head of pancreas
9. 胰颈 neck of pancreas
10. 胰体 body of pancreas
11. 肠系膜下静脉 inferior mesenteric vein
12. 第10肋骨 10th costal bone
13. 背阔肌 latissimus dorsi
14. 竖脊肌 erector spinae
15. 左肾 left kidney
16. 肾锥体 renal pyramid
17. 左肾盂 left renal pelvis
18. 左肾动脉 left renal artery
19. 左肾静脉 left renal vein
20. 肠系膜上动脉 superior mesenteric artery
21. 腹主动脉 abdominal aorta
22. L1-2椎间盘 L1-2 intervertebral disc
23. 脊髓 spinal cord
24. 右膈脚 right crus of diaphragm
25. 下腔静脉 inferior vena cava
26. 肝肾隐窝 hepatorenal recess
27. 右肾 right kidney
28. 右肾盂 right renal pelvis
29. 右肾动脉 right renal artery
30. 右肾静脉 right renal vein
31. 肝右后叶下段 inferior segment of right posterior lobe of liver
32. 肝门静脉右后下支 right posteroinferior branch of hepatic portal vein
33. 肝门静脉右前下支 right anteroinferior branch of hepatic portal vein
34. 肝右前叶下段 inferior segment of right anterior lobe of liver
35. 腹外斜肌 obliquus externus abdominis
36. 腰大肌 psoas major
37. 十二指肠降部 descending part of duodenum
38. 肝圆韧带 ligamentum teres hepatis
39. 胆总管 common bile duct
40. 胰钩突 uncinate process of pancreas
41. 肠系膜上静脉 superior mesenteric vein

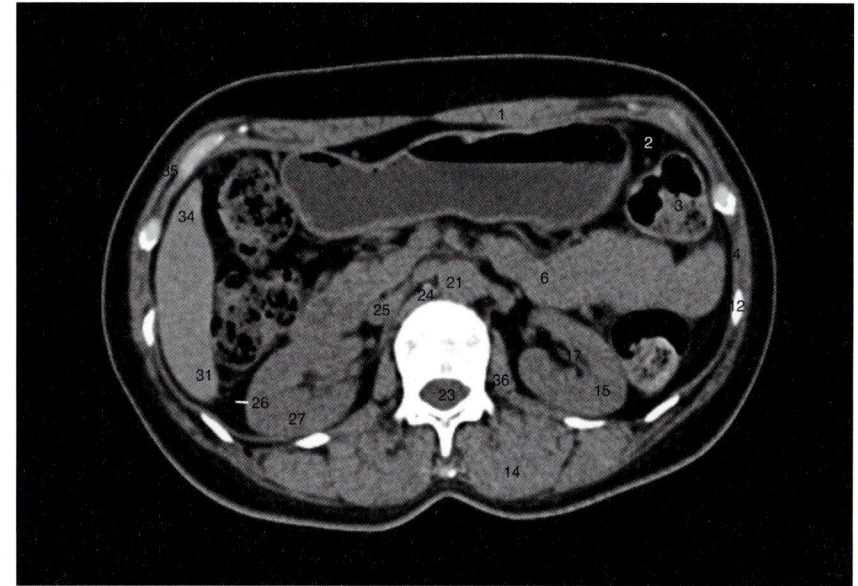

B. CT 平扫图像

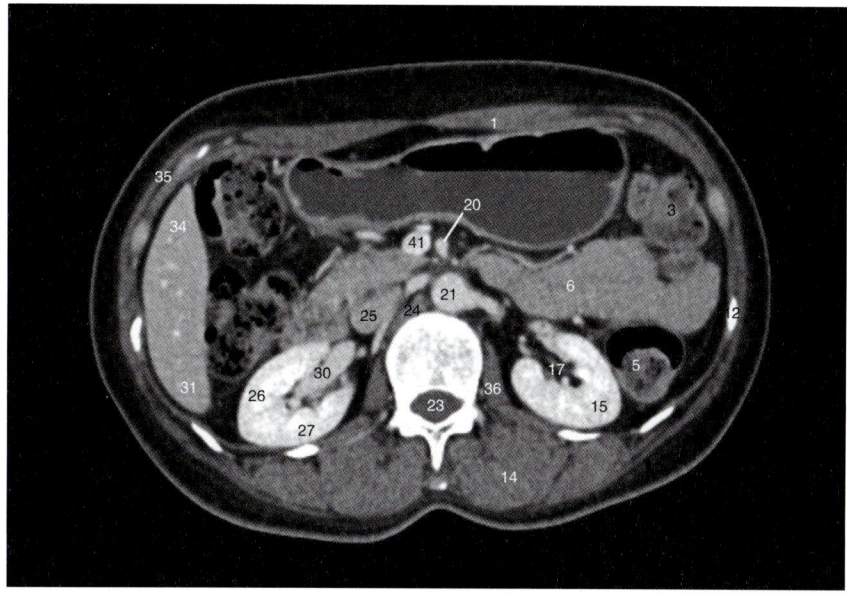

C. CT 增强图像

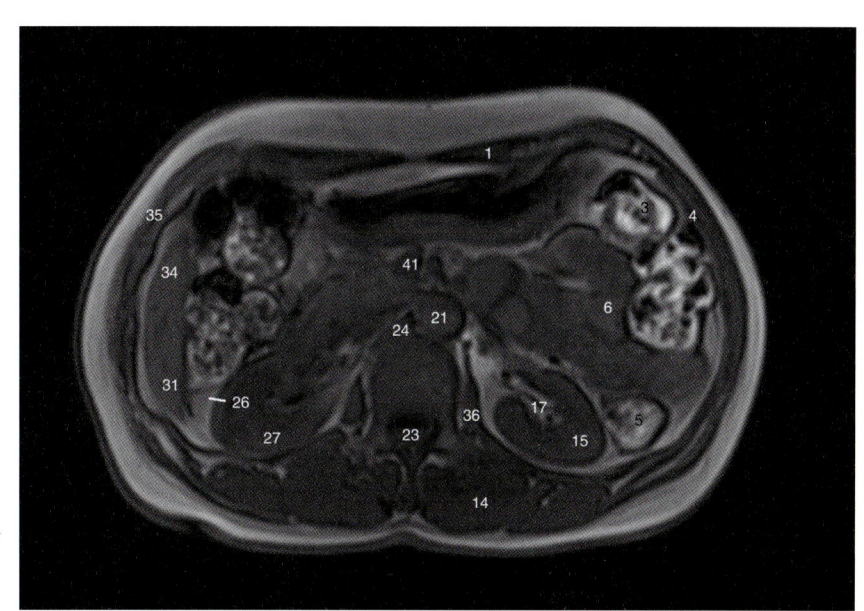

D. MR T1WI

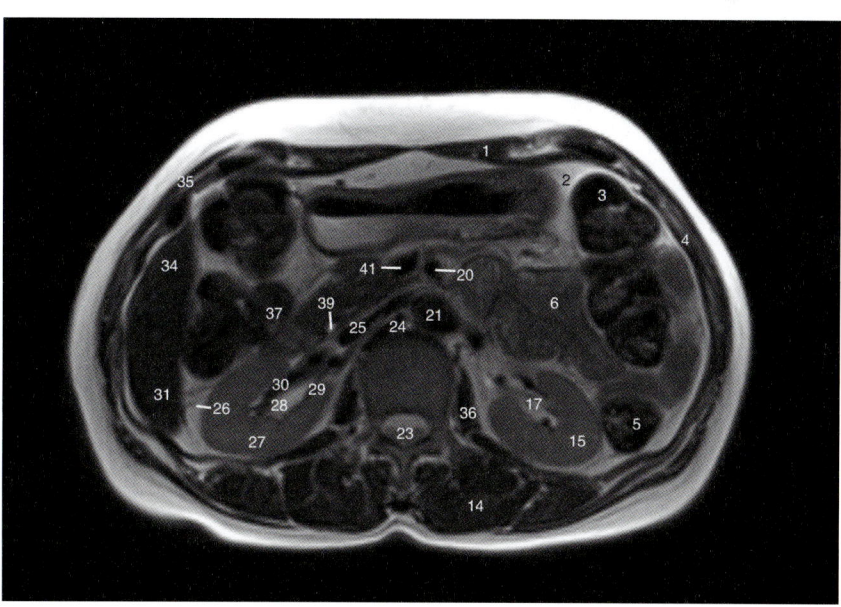

E. MR T2WI

关键结构：右肾盂，L1-2椎间盘，腹膜后间隙。

此断面经过 L1-2 椎间盘。

腹主动脉及下腔静脉继续在脊柱前方走行，分别向两侧发出肾动脉及肾静脉。腹腔右侧为肝右叶及横结肠，左侧为横、降结肠及空肠。肾盂是由肾大盏合并成的漏斗状扁囊，它位于肾窦内，出肾门后移行于输尿管。腹膜后间隙是壁腹膜和腹横筋膜之间的解剖间隙及其解剖结构的总称，是充满脂肪、结缔组织和筋膜的潜在间隙。其前界为壁腹膜，后界为腰大肌和腰方肌筋膜，上界为横膈，下达盆底筋膜，两侧为侧锥筋膜。以肾前筋膜（Gemta's 筋膜）和肾后筋膜（Zuekerkandle's 筋膜）为分界线，将腹膜后间隙分为肾旁前间隙、肾周间隙和肾旁后间隙：① 肾旁前间隙是后腹膜与肾前筋膜之间的区域，内有升、降结肠、十二指肠和胰腺；② 肾周间隙为肾前筋膜与肾后筋膜之间的区域，内包括肾、输尿管、肾上腺及其周围脂肪（脂肪囊）；③ 肾旁后间隙是位于肾后筋膜与覆盖腰大肌和腰方肌前面的髂腰筋膜之间的区域，内部为脂肪组织、腰交感神经干、乳糜池和淋巴结等。

椎间盘是由纤维环和髓核两部分组成。髓核位于椎间盘的中央，它是一种含水分、呈胶冻状的弹性蛋白。在髓核的周围是纤维环，CT 和 MRI 是显示椎间盘的主要成像技术。

腹部连续横断层 63（FH.10670）

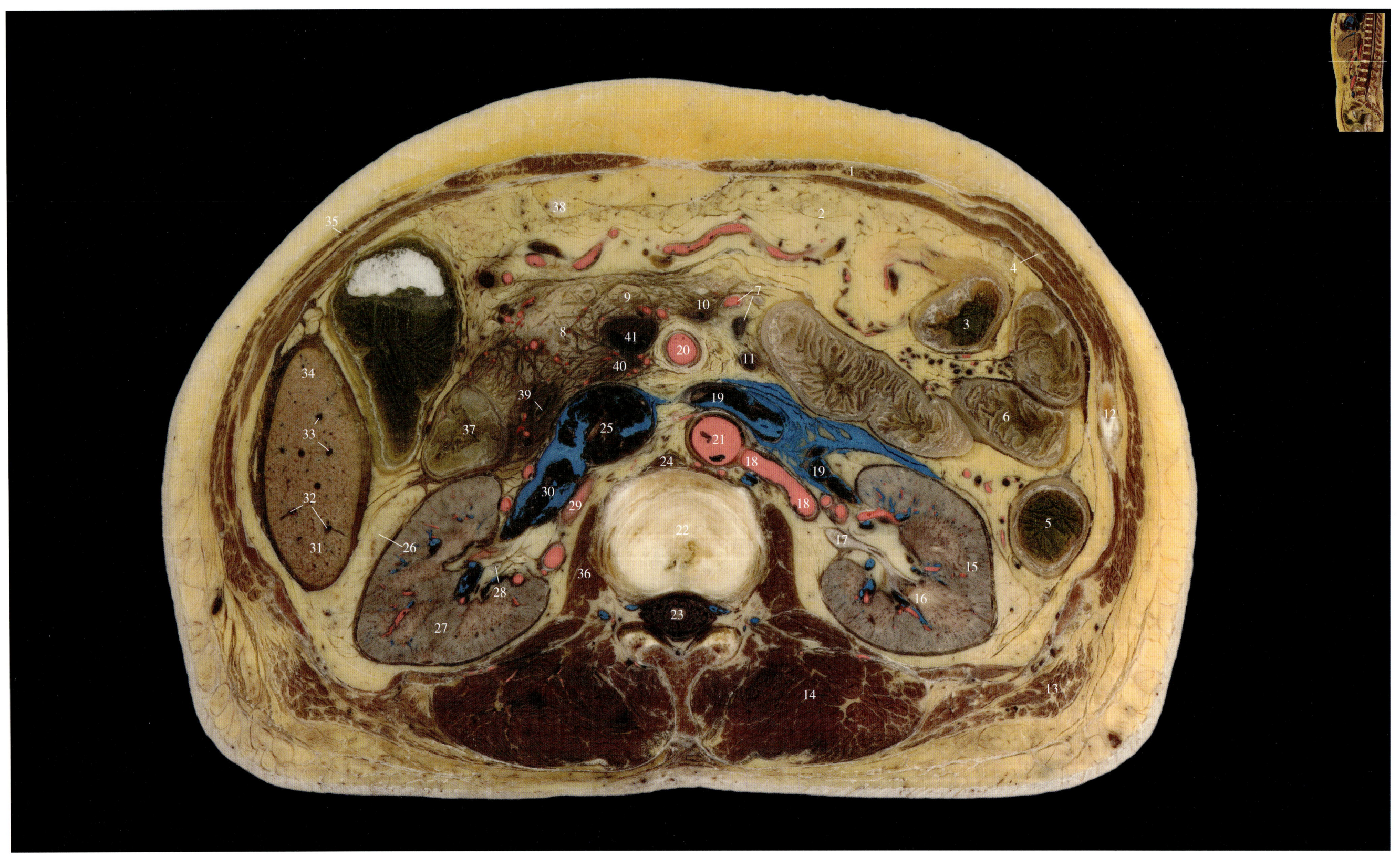

A. 断层标本图像

1. 腹直肌 rectus abdominis
2. 大网膜 greater omentum
3. 横结肠 transverse colon
4. 腹横肌 transversus abdominis
5. 降结肠 descending colon
6. 空肠 jejunum
7. 空肠动、静脉 jejunal artery and vein
8. 胰头 head of pancreas
9. 胰颈 neck of pancreas
10. 胰体 body of pancreas
11. 肠系膜下静脉 inferior mesenteric vein
12. 第 10 肋骨 10th costal bone
13. 背阔肌 latissimus dorsi
14. 竖脊肌 erector spinae
15. 左肾 left kidney
16. 肾锥体 renal pyramid
17. 左肾盂 left renal pelvis
18. 左肾动脉 left renal artery
19. 左肾静脉 left renal vein
20. 肠系膜上动脉 superior mesenteric artery
21. 腹主动脉 abdominal aorta
22. L1-2 椎间盘 L1-2 intervertebral disc
23. 脊髓 spinal cord
24. 右膈脚 right crus of diaphragm
25. 下腔静脉 inferior vena cava
26. 肝肾隐窝 hepatorenal recess
27. 右肾 right kidney
28. 右肾盂 right renal pelvis
29. 右肾动脉 right renal artery
30. 右肾静脉 right renal vein
31. 肝右后叶下段 inferior segment of right posterior lobe of liver
32. 肝门静脉右后下支 right posteroinferior branch of hepatic portal vein
33. 肝门静脉右前下支 right anteroinferior branch of hepatic portal vein
34. 肝右前叶下段 inferior segment of right anterior lobe of liver
35. 腹外斜肌 obliquus externus abdominis
36. 腰大肌 psoas major
37. 十二指肠降部 descending part of duodenum
38. 肝圆韧带 ligamentum teres hepatis
39. 胆总管 common bile duct
40. 胰钩突 uncinate process of pancreas
41. 肠系膜上静脉 superior mesenteric vein

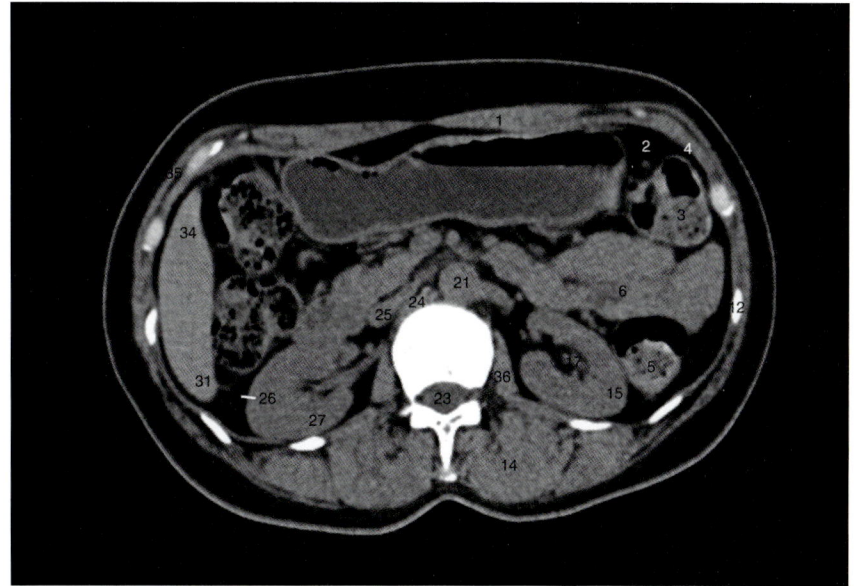

B. CT 平扫图像

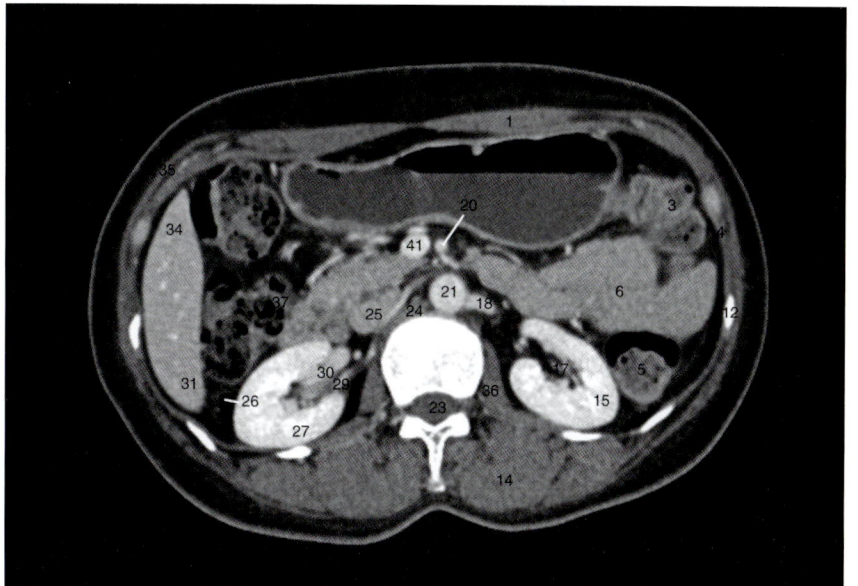

C. CT 增强图像

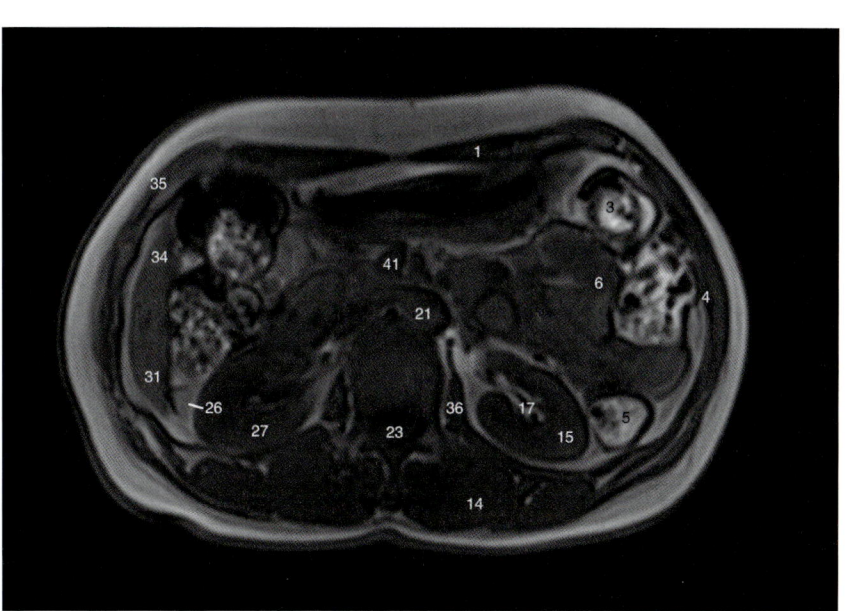

D. MR T1WI

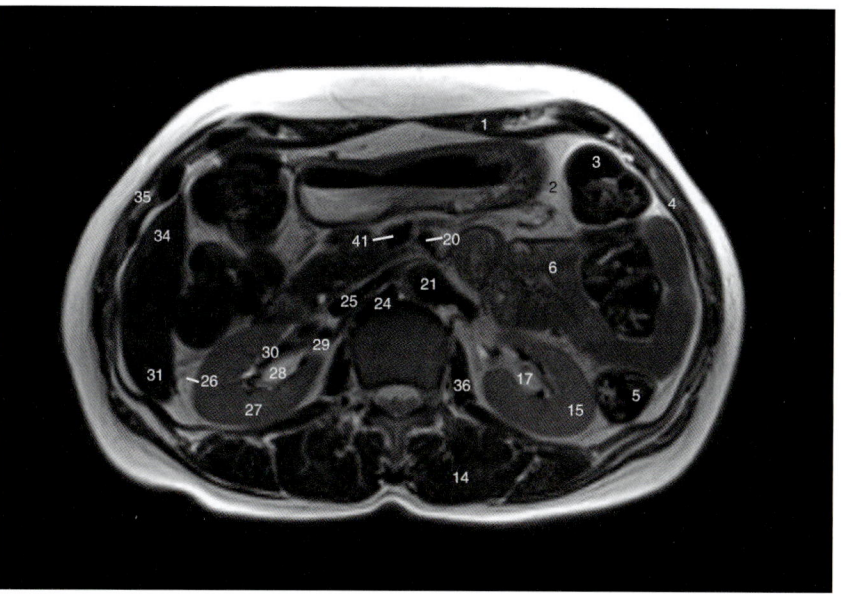

E. MR T2WI

关键结构：左肾动脉，空肠。

此断面经过 L1-2 椎间盘。

右肾与剩余肝右叶相对应处可见肝肾隐窝，仰卧时为腹腔最低的位置，腹腔积液易积聚于此。该间隙紧邻肝脏、右肾和右肾上腺，上界邻近胆囊，下界为横结肠及其系膜、结肠肝曲，因此邻近脏器的病变很容易占据该间隙，分界不清，导致定位困难。国人成人女性左肾动脉平均长度为 1.93 cm ± 1.11 cm，右侧为 3.25 cm ± 1.88 cm；左肾静脉为 3.50 cm ± 1.66 cm，右侧为 1.41 cm ± 0.66 cm。肾动脉在肾窦内分为叶间动脉，穿行于肾柱内；在肾锥体底部形成弓状动脉；弓状动脉又发出放射状分支小叶间动脉入皮质迷路，小叶间动脉沿途向两侧肾小叶发出入球小动脉，每条入球小动脉在肾小体内分成若干小支，形成肾小球。肾小球再集合成出球小动脉，离开肾小体后复成毛细血管网，这些毛细血管逐渐集合成与动脉平行的小叶间静脉、弓状静脉、叶间静脉，最后流入肾静脉经肾门出肾。因此，肾血流量丰富，且皮质大于髓质。因此，对比剂增强动脉期图像肾皮质的强化程度明显大于髓质，肾实质强化不均匀。如发生肾动脉栓塞，相应区域肾实质呈扇形的低或无强化区。当发生肾动脉瘤时，CTA 和 MRA 可清晰地显示动脉瘤的大小和形态。DSA 是诊断的金标准，还可同时进行介入治疗[50]。

腹部连续横断层 64（FH.10650）

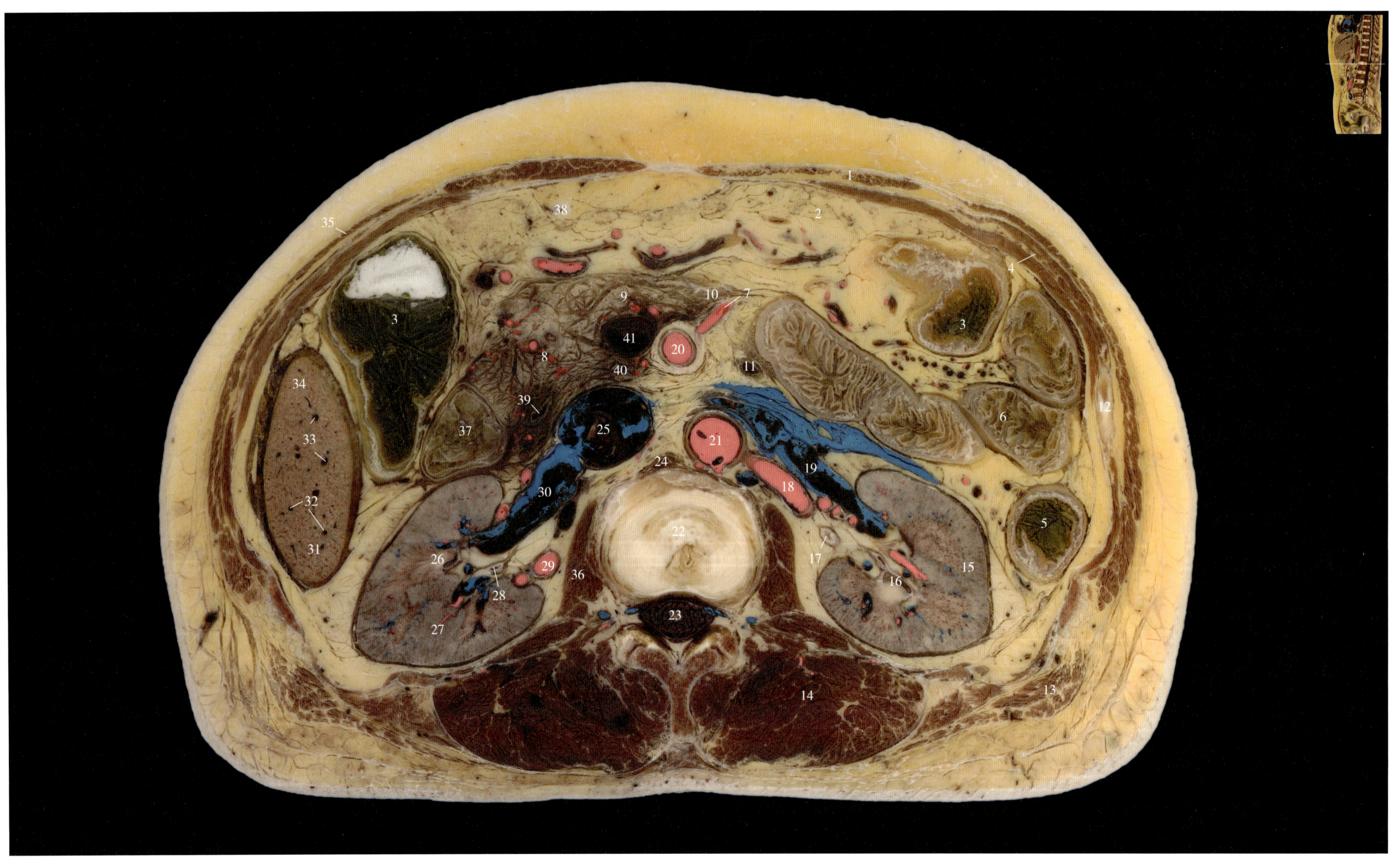

A. 断层标本图像

1. 腹直肌 rectus abdominis
2. 大网膜 greater omentum
3. 横结肠 transverse colon
4. 腹横肌 transversus abdominis
5. 降结肠 descending colon
6. 空肠 jejunum
7. 空肠动脉 jejunal artery
8. 胰头 head of pancreas
9. 胰颈 neck of pancreas
10. 胰体 body of pancreas
11. 肠系膜下静脉 inferior mesenteric vein
12. 第10肋软骨 10th costal cartilage
13. 背阔肌 latissimus dorsi
14. 竖脊肌 erector spinae
15. 左肾 left kidney
16. 肾大盏 major renal calices
17. 左肾盂 left renal pelvis
18. 左肾动脉 left renal artery
19. 左肾静脉 left renal vein
20. 肠系膜上动脉 superior mesenteric artery
21. 腹主动脉 abdominal aorta
22. L1-2 椎间盘 L1-2 intervertebral disc
23. 脊髓 spinal cord
24. 右膈脚 right crus of diaphragm
25. 下腔静脉 inferior vena cava
26. 肾锥体 renal pyramid
27. 右肾 right kidney
28. 右肾盂 right renal pelvis
29. 右肾动脉 right renal artery
30. 右肾静脉 right renal vein
31. 肝右后叶下段 inferior segment of right posterior lobe of liver
32. 肝门静脉右后下支 right posteroinferior branch of hepatic portal vein
33. 肝门静脉右前下支 right anteroinferior branch of hepatic portal vein
34. 肝右前叶下段 inferior segment of right anterior lobe of liver
35. 腹外斜肌 obliquus externus abdominis
36. 腰大肌 psoas major
37. 十二指肠降部 descending part of duodenum
38. 肝圆韧带 ligamentum teres hepatis
39. 胆总管 common bile duct
40. 胰钩突 uncinate process of pancreas
41. 肠系膜上静脉 superior mesenteric vein

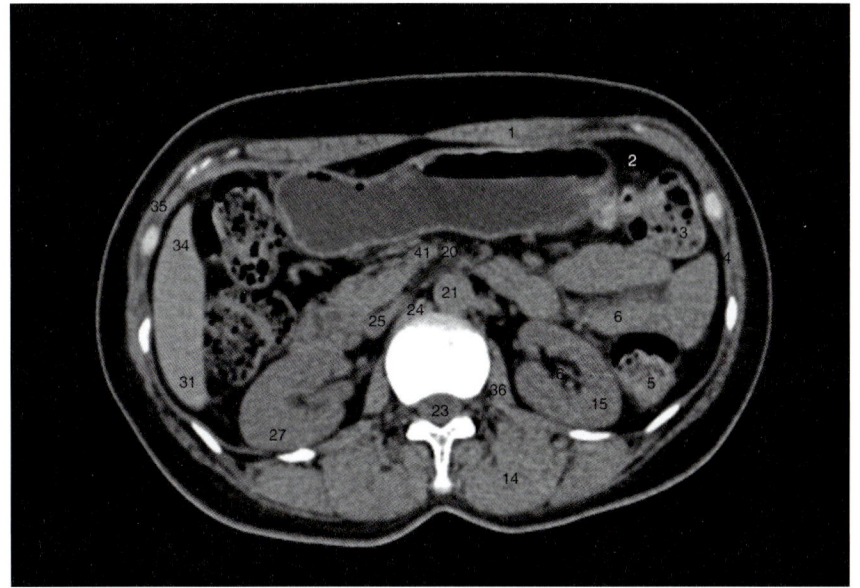

B. CT 平扫图像

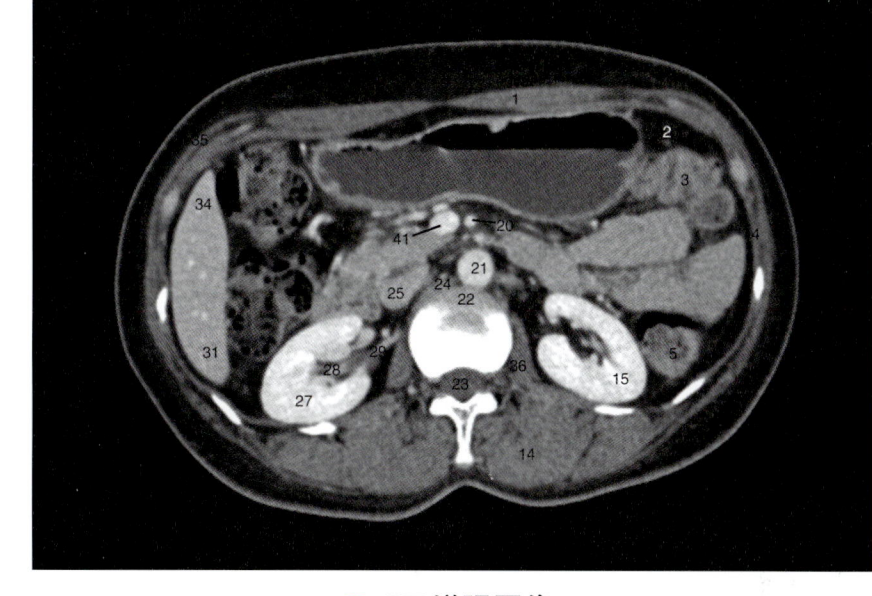

C. CT 增强图像

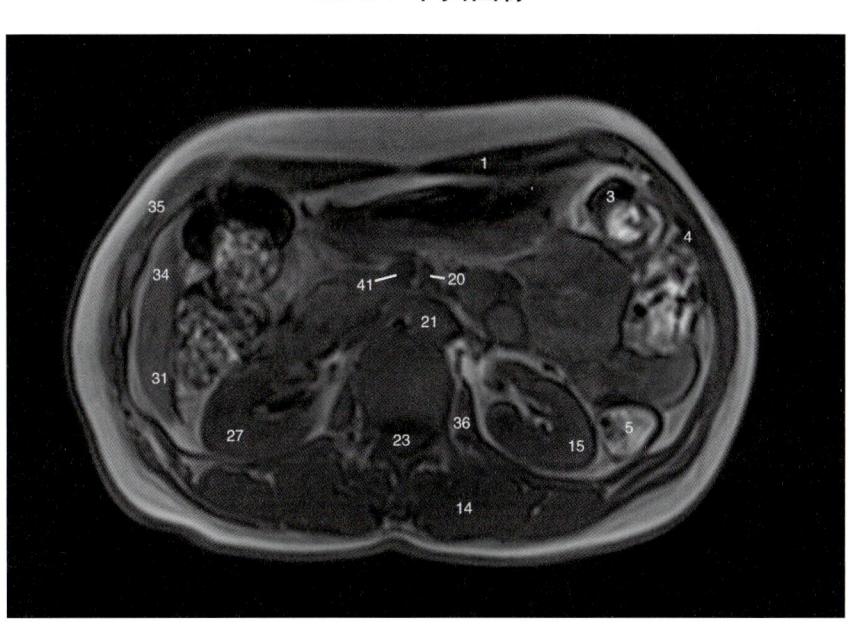

D. MR T1WI

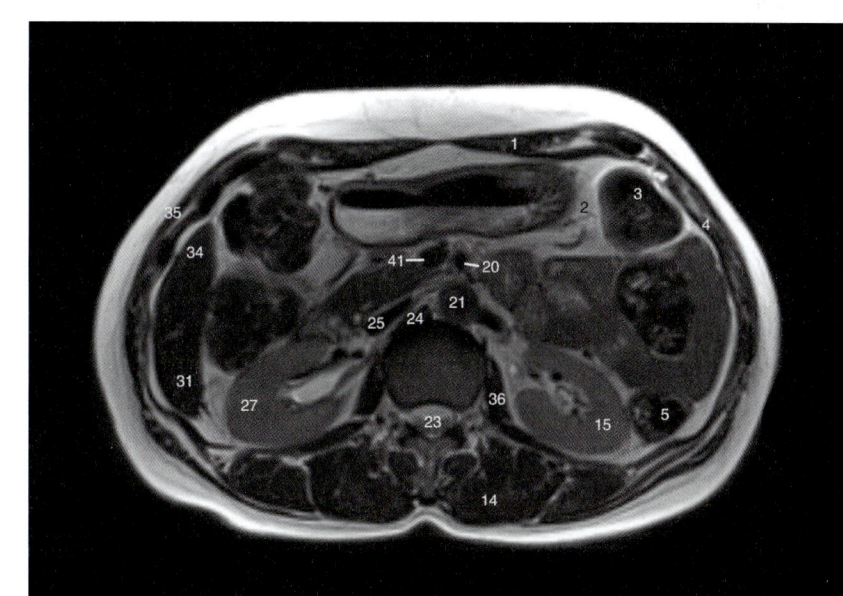

E. MR T2WI

关键结构：肾大盏，右肾静脉，胆总管。

此断面经过 L1-2 椎间盘。

下腔静脉及腹主动脉继续沿脊柱前方下行，其周围是由疏松组织构成的间隙，因此该间隙内出血或感染易扩散。此间隙内还含有交感神经和脊神经、淋巴管和淋巴结、脂肪、纤维结缔组织等，可发生相应的肿瘤，如神经源性肿瘤、淋巴管瘤、淋巴瘤、转移瘤、脂肪肉瘤、纤维肉瘤等。如肿瘤较大，可推压、包绕邻近的下腔静脉及腹主动脉，导致手术切除困难。

左肾静脉与肠系膜下静脉的前缘为空肠及其系膜。空肠位于腹腔的左上部，回肠位于右下部。空肠黏膜形成丰富的环状襞，且其上 1/3 段密度最高。进行小肠气钡双重造影或发生小肠梗阻时，可根据这些环形襞判断位置。空肠系膜连于腹后壁，活动度较大，其内含有大量脂肪，因此 CT 图像无法清晰地显示肠系膜，但可根据肠系膜血管的走行对其进行判断。

腹部连续横断层 65（FH.10630）

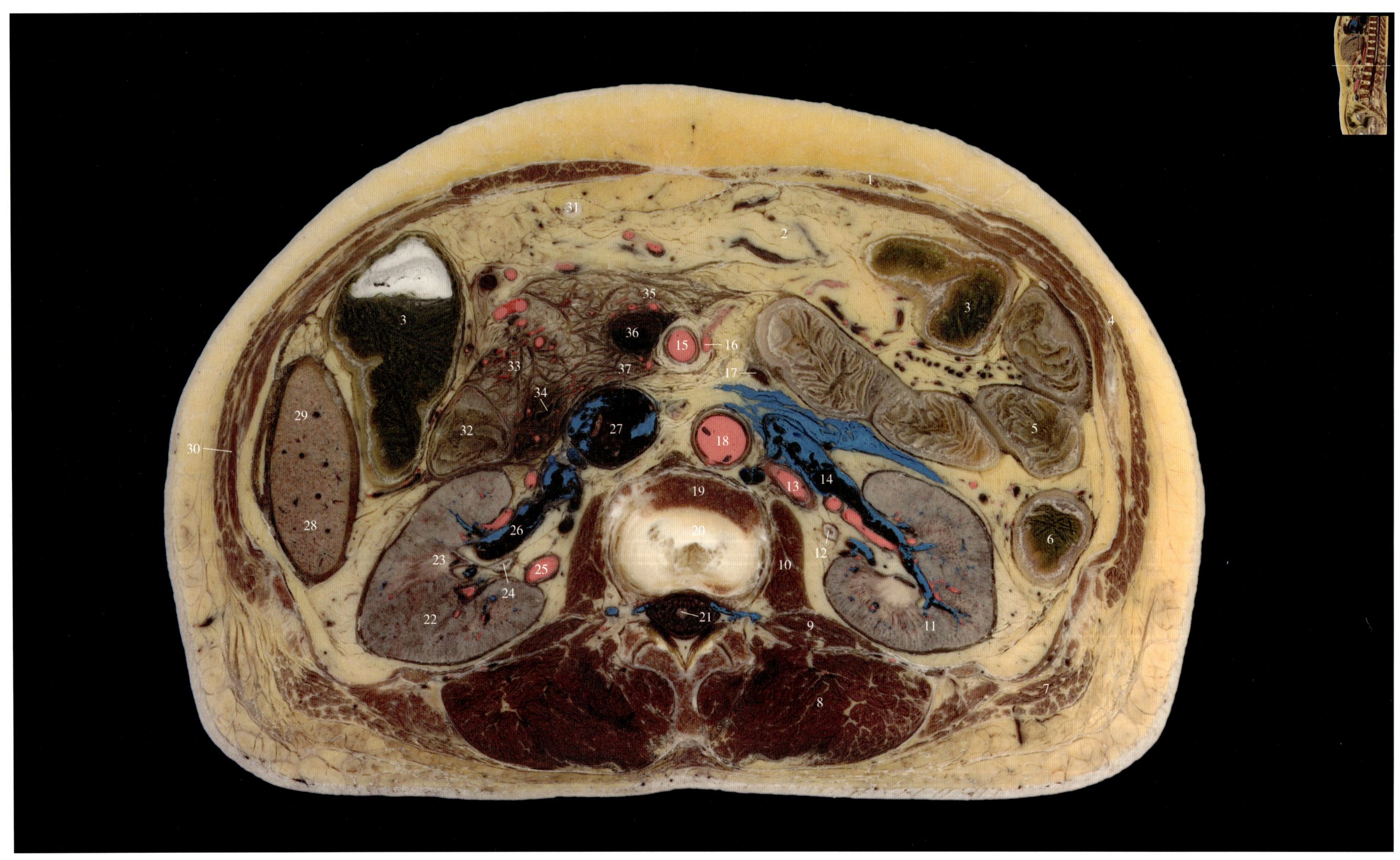

A. 断层标本图像

1. 腹直肌 rectus abdominis
2. 大网膜 greater omentum
3. 横结肠 transverse colon
4. 腹外斜肌 obliquus externus abdominis
5. 空肠 jejunum
6. 降结肠 descending colon
7. 背阔肌 latissimus dorsi
8. 竖脊肌 erector spinae
9. 腰方肌 quadratus lumborum
10. 腰大肌 psoas major
11. 左肾 left kidney
12. 左肾盂 left renal pelvis
13. 左肾动脉 left renal artery
14. 左肾静脉 left renal vein
15. 肠系膜上动脉 superior mesenteric artery
16. 空肠动脉 jejunal artery
17. 肠系膜下静脉 inferior mesenteric vein
18. 腹主动脉 abdominal aorta
19. 第2腰椎椎体 body of the 2nd lumbar vertebra
20. L1-2 椎间盘 L1-2 intervertebral disc
21. 脊髓 spinal cord
22. 右肾 right kidney
23. 肾锥体 renal pyramid
24. 右肾盂 right renal pelvis
25. 右肾动脉 right renal artery
26. 右肾静脉 right renal vein
27. 下腔静脉 inferior vena cava
28. 肝右后叶下段 inferior segment of right posterior lobe of liver
29. 肝右前叶下段 inferior segment of right anterior lobe of liver
30. 腹内斜肌 obliquus internus abdominis
31. 肝圆韧带 ligamentum teres hepatis
32. 十二指肠降部 descending part of duodenum
33. 胰头 head of pancreas
34. 胆总管 common bile duct
35. 胰颈 neck of pancreas
36. 肠系膜上静脉 superior mesenteric vein
37. 胰钩突 uncinate process of pancreas

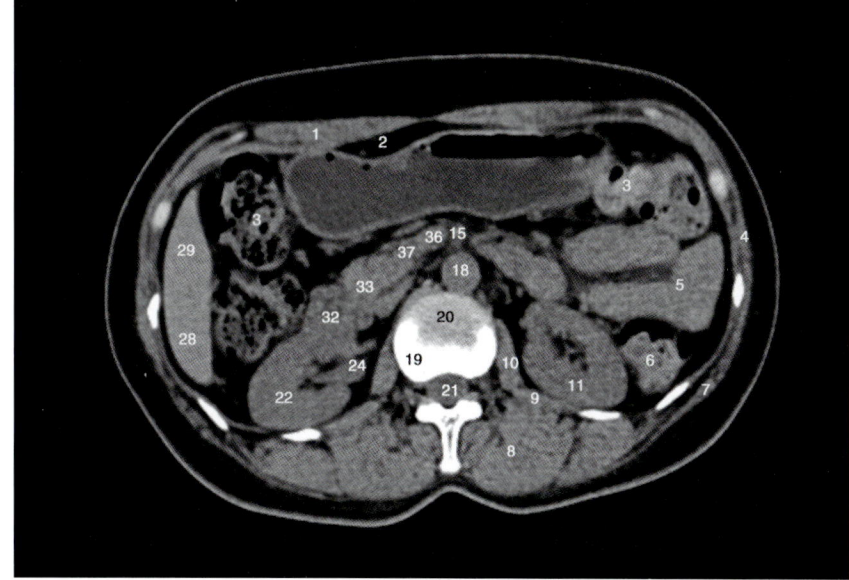

B. CT 平扫图像

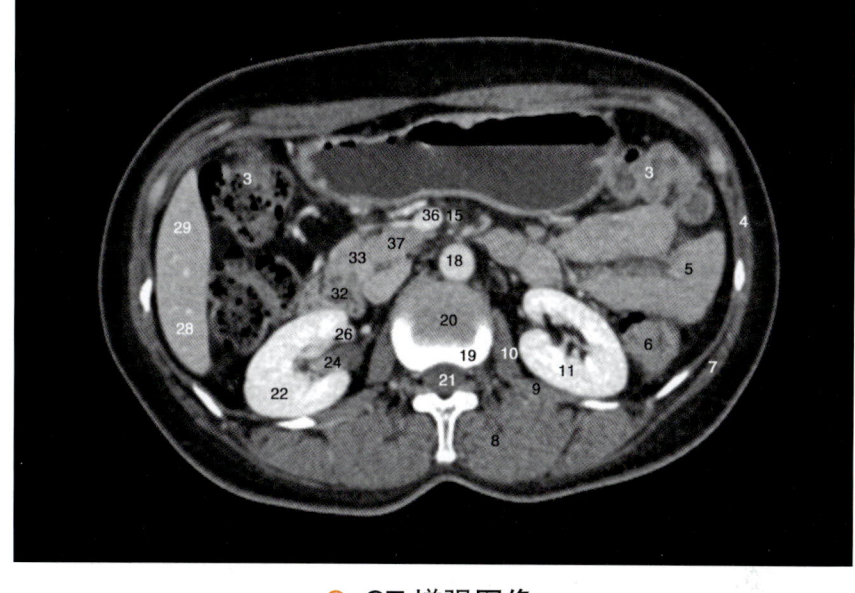

C. CT 增强图像

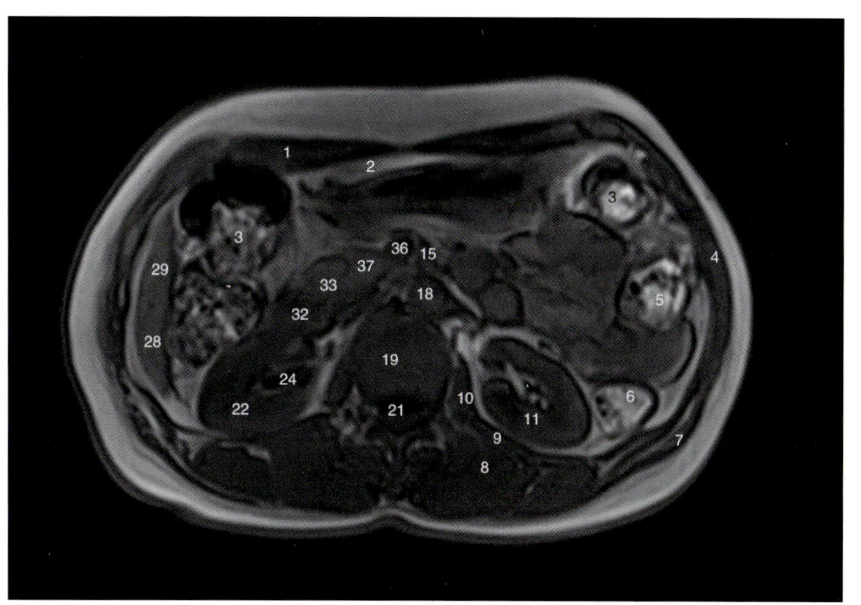

D. MR T1WI

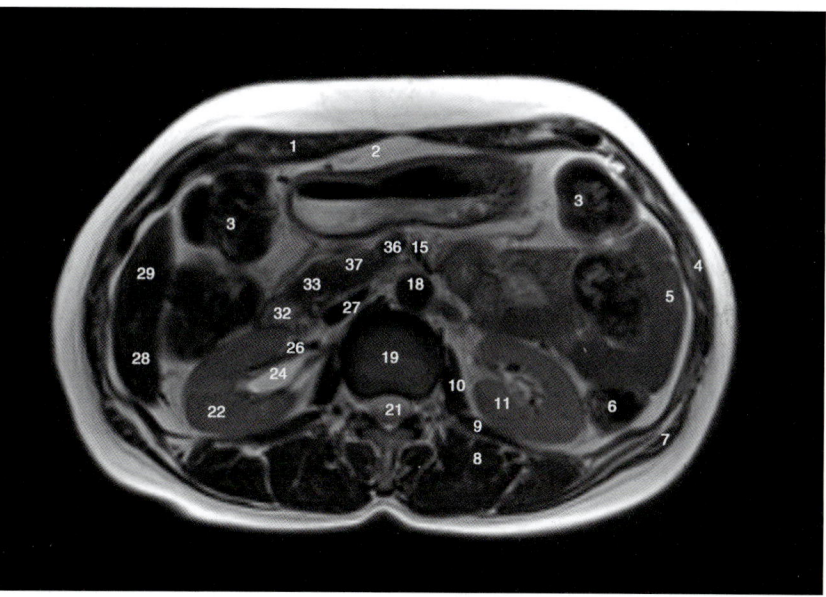

E. MR T2WI

关键结构：左、右肾门，竖脊肌。

此断面经过 L1-2 椎间盘和第 2 腰椎椎体。

胰体消失，肝脏体积进一步缩小。肾内侧缘中部凹陷，是肾血管、淋巴管、神经和肾盂出入部位，称为肾门。肾门约在腰背部第 1 腰椎体平面，相当于第 9 肋软骨前端高度，在正中线外侧约 5 cm。在横断面上，肾门断面通常出现于第 1 至第 2 腰椎平面。由肾门伸入肾实质的凹陷称肾窦。出入肾门诸结构为结缔组织所包裹称肾蒂，因下腔静脉靠近右肾故右肾蒂较左肾蒂短。肾蒂内各结构的排列关系，自前向后顺序为肾静脉、肾动脉和肾盂末端；自上向下顺序为：肾动脉、肾静脉和肾盂[62]。肾门在肾的手术中是结扎肾蒂各结构的标志。肾门内脂肪组织丰富，CT 表现为低密度，与肾盂和血管形成明显对比，利于病变的显示。

腹部连续横断层 66（FH.10610）

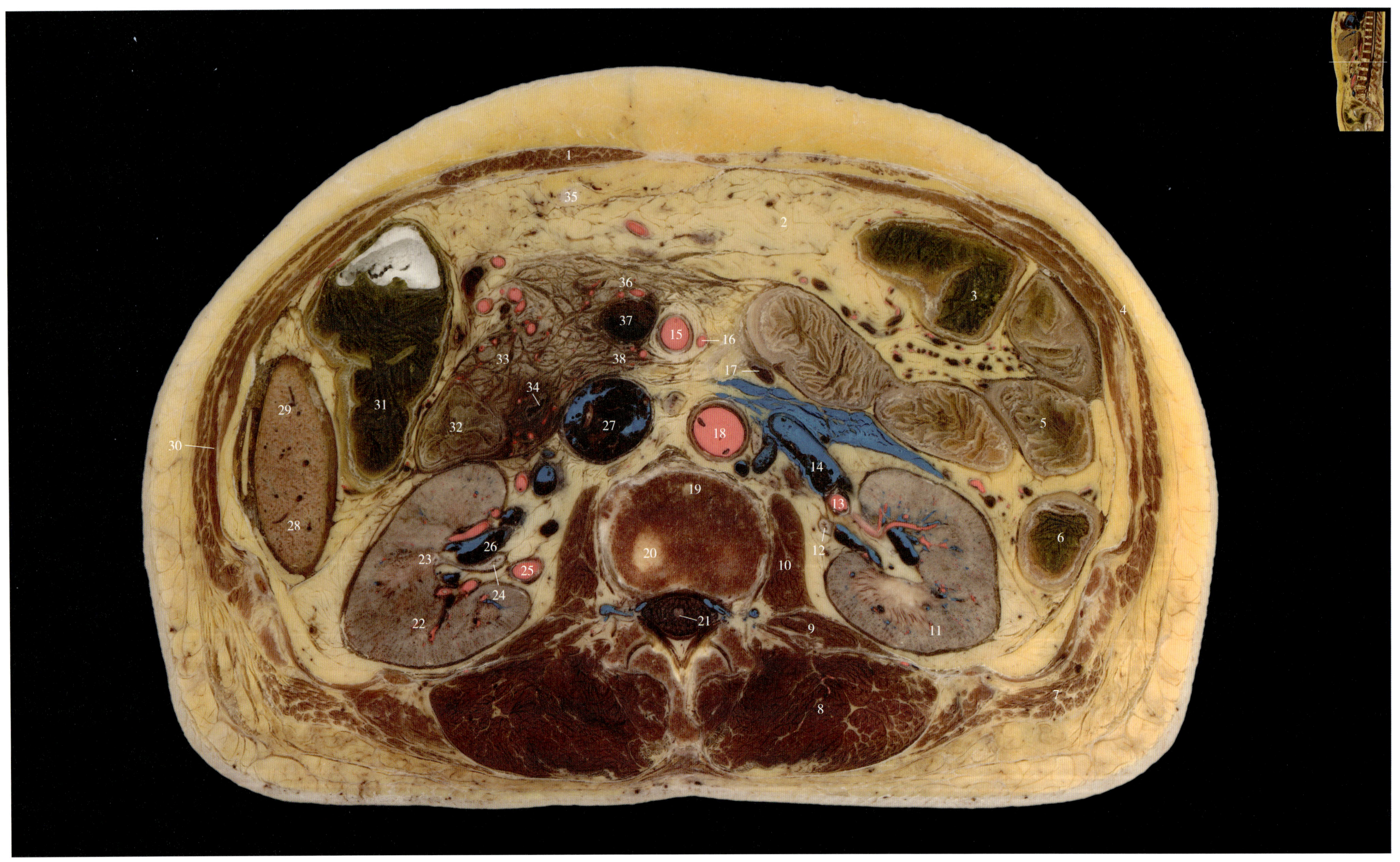

A. 断层标本图像

1. 腹直肌 rectus abdominis
2. 大网膜 greater omentum
3. 横结肠 transverse colon
4. 腹外斜肌 obliquus externus abdominis
5. 空肠 jejunum
6. 降结肠 descending colon
7. 背阔肌 latissimus dorsi
8. 竖脊肌 erector spinae
9. 腰方肌 quadratus lumborum
10. 腰大肌 psoas major
11. 左肾 left kidney
12. 左肾盂 left renal pelvis
13. 左肾动脉 left renal artery
14. 左肾静脉 left renal vein
15. 肠系膜上动脉 superior mesenteric artery
16. 空肠动脉 jejunal artery
17. 肠系膜下静脉 inferior mesenteric vein
18. 腹主动脉 abdominal aorta
19. 第2腰椎椎体 body of the 2nd lumbar vertebra
20. L1-2椎间盘 L1-2 intervertebral disc
21. 脊髓 spinal cord
22. 右肾 right kidney
23. 肾锥体 renal pyramid
24. 右肾盂 right renal pelvis
25. 右肾动脉 right renal artery
26. 右肾静脉 right renal vein
27. 下腔静脉 inferior vena cava
28. 肝右叶后段 inferior segment of right posterior lobe of liver
29. 肝右叶前段 inferior segment of right anterior lobe of liver
30. 腹内斜肌 obliquus internus abdominis
31. 升结肠 ascending colon
32. 十二指肠降部 descending part of duodenum
33. 胰头 head of pancreas
34. 胆总管 common bile duct
35. 肝圆韧带 ligamentum teres hepatis
36. 胰颈 neck of pancreas
37. 肠系膜上静脉 superior mesenteric vein
38. 胰钩突 uncinate process of pancreas

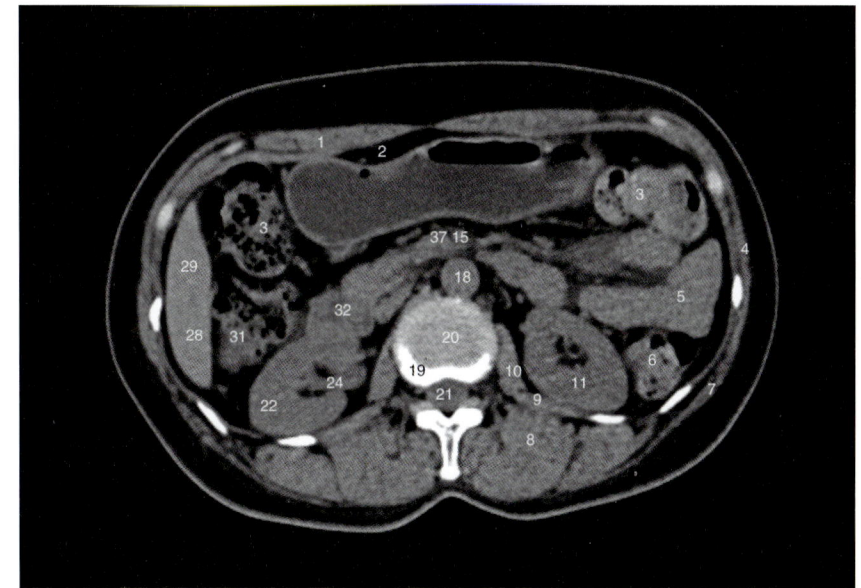

B. CT 平扫图像

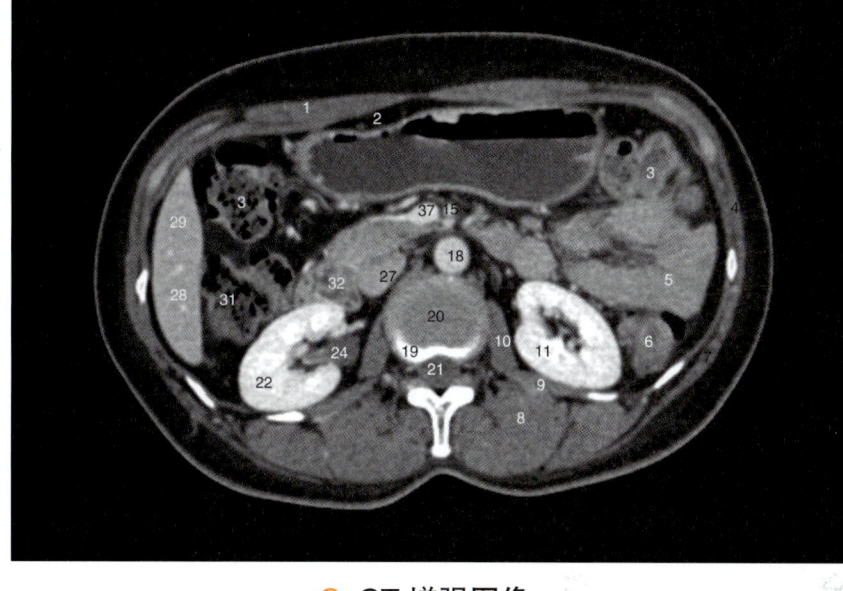

C. CT 增强图像

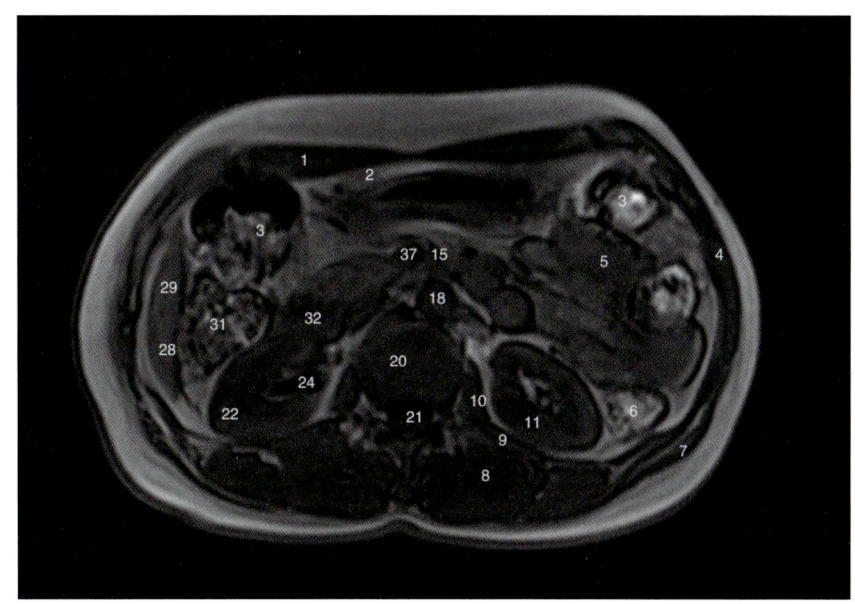

D. MR T1WI

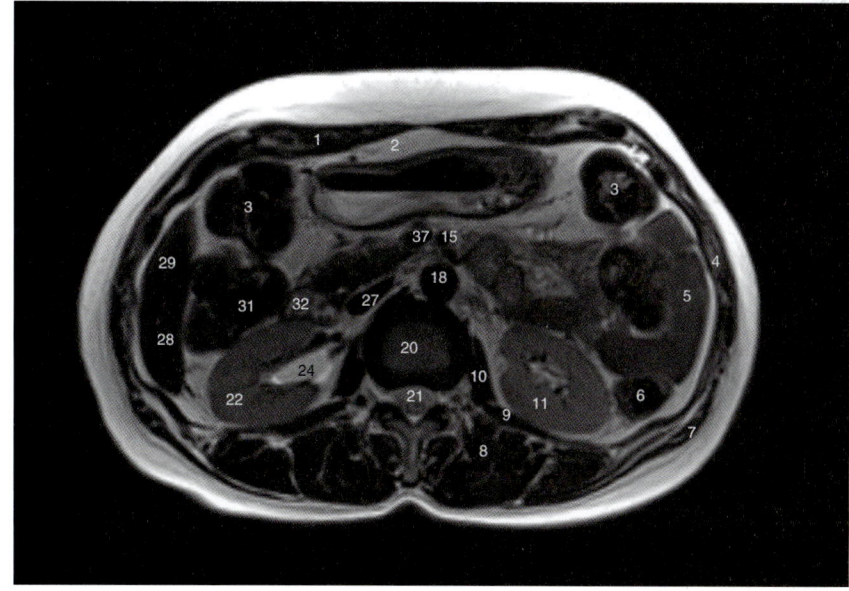

E. MR T2WI

关键结构：空肠，空肠动脉。

此断面经过 L1-2 椎间盘和第 2 腰椎椎体。

右侧升结肠初步显示。左侧腹腔大部被空肠、横结肠及降结肠占据。空、回肠动脉主干起源于肠系膜上动脉，该动脉向左分出 12~18 条空、回肠动脉，在肠系膜内呈放射状走向肠壁，途中分支吻合形成动脉弓。小肠近段只有 1~2 级动脉弓，远侧段弓数增多，可达 3~4 级，末级弓发出直动脉分布于肠壁，直动脉间缺少吻合[63]。因此，肠切除吻合术时应做扇形切除，以保证吻合口对系膜缘侧有充分血供，避免术后缺血坏死或愈合不良形成肠瘘。空肠与回肠肠系膜疾病少见，多为恶性肿瘤转移。空肠上 1/3 段的环状襞最密最高，向下逐渐减少，到回肠下部几乎消失。空肠梗阻时肠管扩张，内见气液平面，黏膜呈弹簧状。

腹部连续横断层 67 (FH.10590)

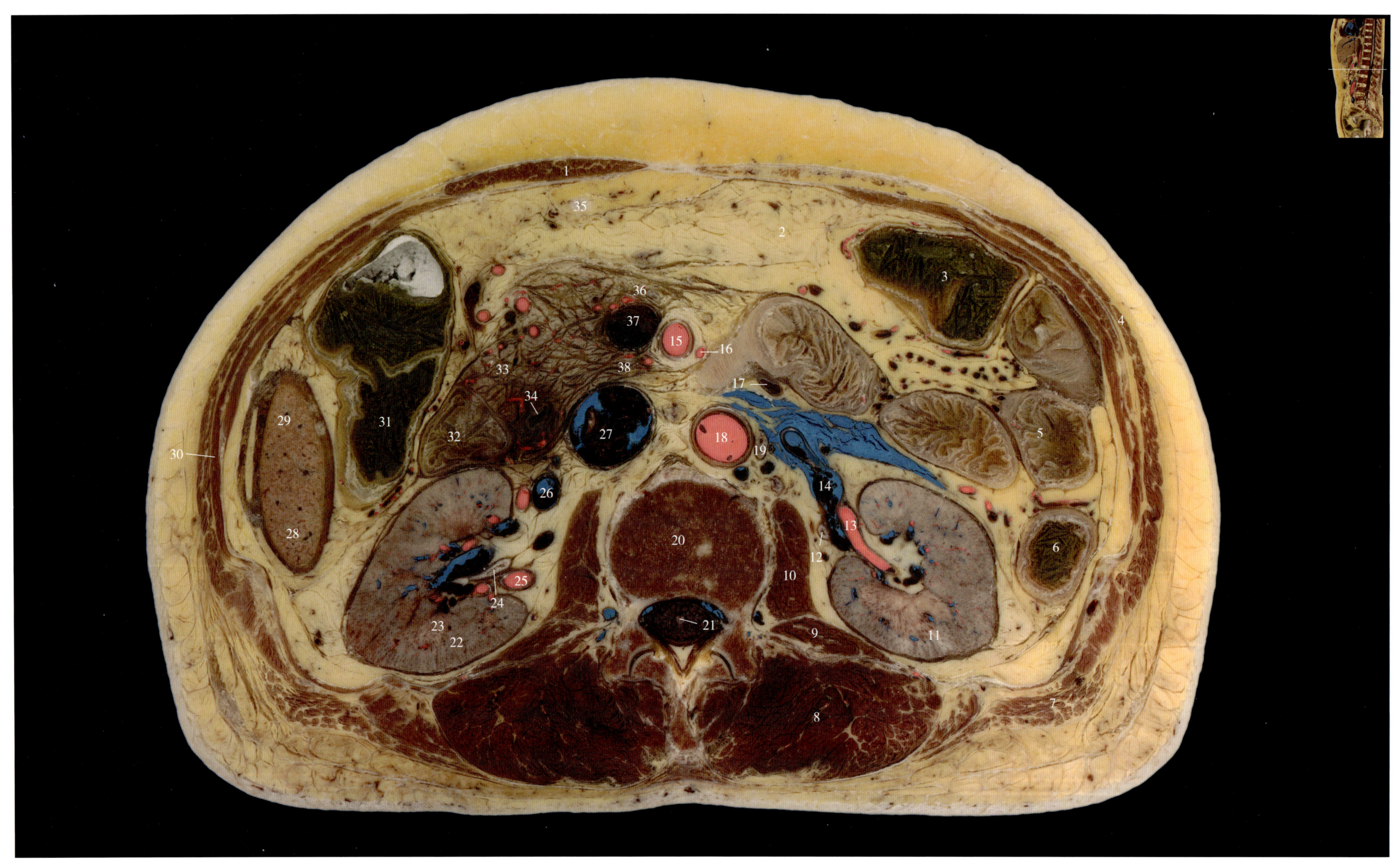

A. 断层标本图像

1. 腹直肌 rectus abdominis
2. 大网膜 greater omentum
3. 横结肠 transverse colon
4. 腹外斜肌 obliquus externus abdominis
5. 空肠 jejunum
6. 降结肠 descending colon
7. 背阔肌 latissimus dorsi
8. 竖脊肌 erector spinae
9. 腰方肌 quadratus lumborum
10. 腰大肌 psoas major
11. 左肾 left kidney
12. 左输尿管 left ureter
13. 左肾动脉 left renal artery
14. 左肾静脉 left renal vein
15. 肠系膜上动脉 superior mesenteric artery
16. 空肠动脉 jejunal artery
17. 肠系膜下静脉 inferior mesenteric vein
18. 腹主动脉 abdominal aorta
19. 淋巴结 lymph nodes
20. 第 2 腰椎椎体 body of the 2nd lumbar vertebra
21. 脊髓 spinal cord
22. 右肾 right kidney
23. 肾锥体 renal pyramid
24. 右肾盂 right renal pelvis
25. 右肾动脉 right renal artery
26. 右肾静脉 right renal vein
27. 下腔静脉 inferior vena cava
28. 肝右后叶下段 inferior segment of right posterior lobe of liver
29. 肝右前叶下段 inferior segment of right anterior lobe of liver
30. 腹内斜肌 obliquus internus abdominis
31. 升结肠 ascending colon
32. 十二指肠降部 descending part of duodenum
33. 胰头 head of pancreas
34. 胆总管 common bile duct
35. 肝圆韧带 ligamentum teres hepatis
36. 胰颈 neck of pancreas
37. 肠系膜上静脉 superior mesenteric vein
38. 胰钩突 uncinate process of pancreas

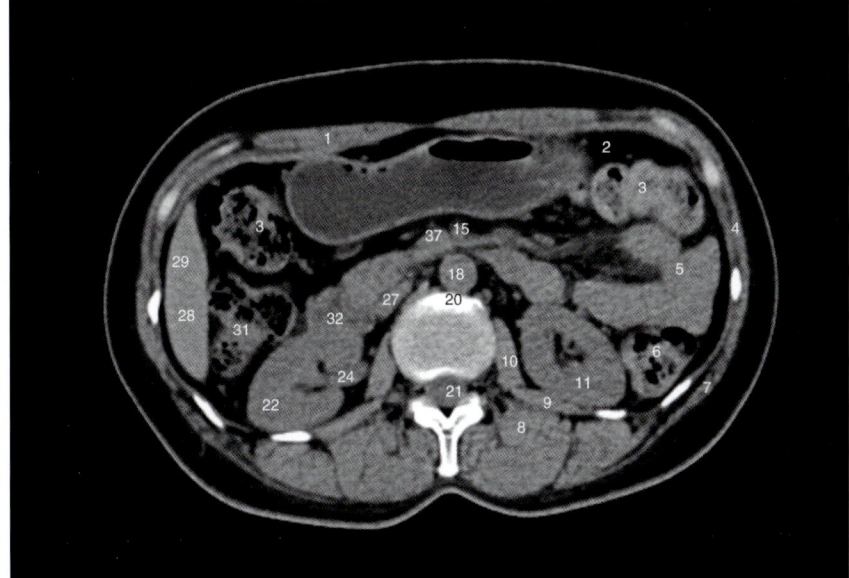

B. CT 平扫图像

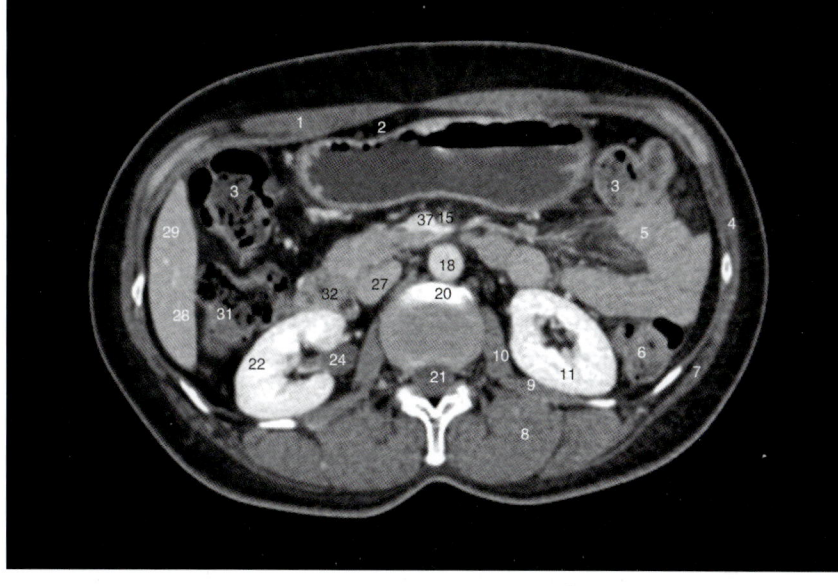

C. CT 增强图像

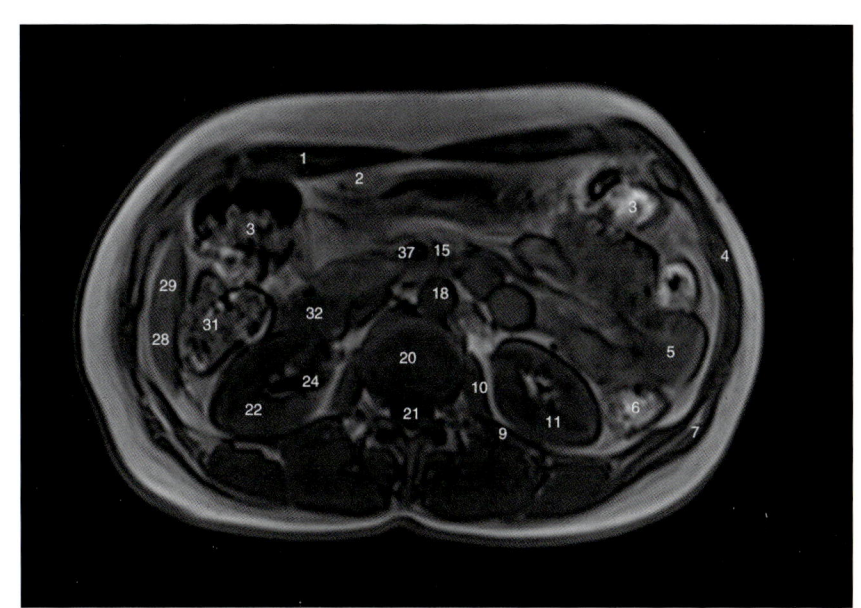

D. MR T1WI

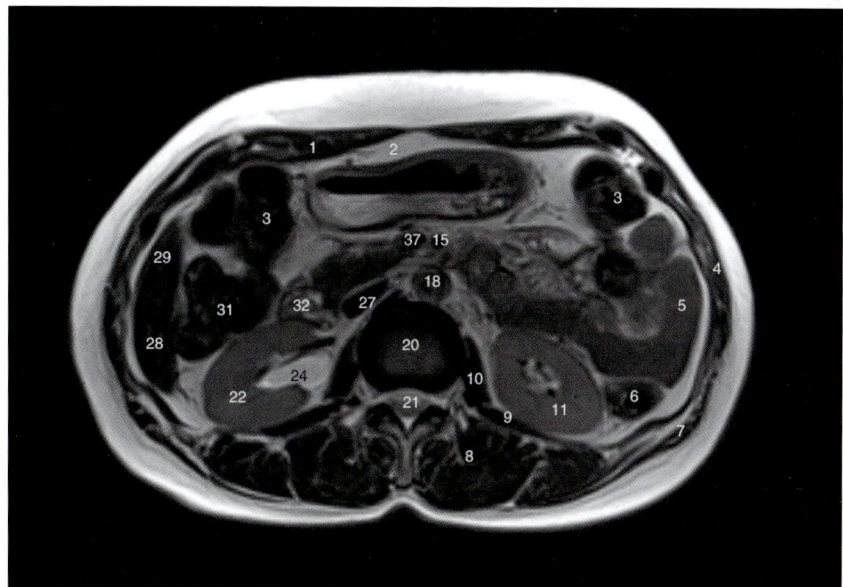

E. MR T2WI

关键结构：胰钩突，大网膜。

此断面经过第 2 腰椎椎体。

胰腺体积缩小明显，仅显示胰头、胰颈和胰钩突。胰头居肠系膜上静脉右壁的右侧和十二指肠降部之间，其中至肠系膜上静脉与下腔静脉之间的部分称钩突，胆总管下行于胰头后缘。胰颈位于肠系膜上静脉的前方，向左接续胰体。解剖学上胰头钩突部胰管为分支胰管，常汇集到副胰管。十二指肠乳头与主、副胰管汇合处距离 >23 mm 者，在正常人中约占 66.7%，因此只有当肿瘤较大累及胆总管下端时，才引起胆总管扩张[64]。

当钩突肿瘤较小且仅局限于分支胰管、尚未累及胆总管下端时，可不伴或仅伴有轻度胆胰管扩张。胰头钩突部癌时，正常胰头钩突部的三角形态消失，增强 MRI 显示胰钩突部出现边界不清的结节或肿块，呈轻中度强化，可伴有胰周血管侵犯，也可仅表现为胆总管或主胰管的扩张或二者均不扩张。而低位胆道梗阻可导致胆总管和胰管扩张[65]。该部位易与十二指肠的水平部相混淆，在疾病诊断上也易误诊，且肿瘤邻近的血管多，血性转移概率也多。

腹部连续横断层 68（FH.10570）

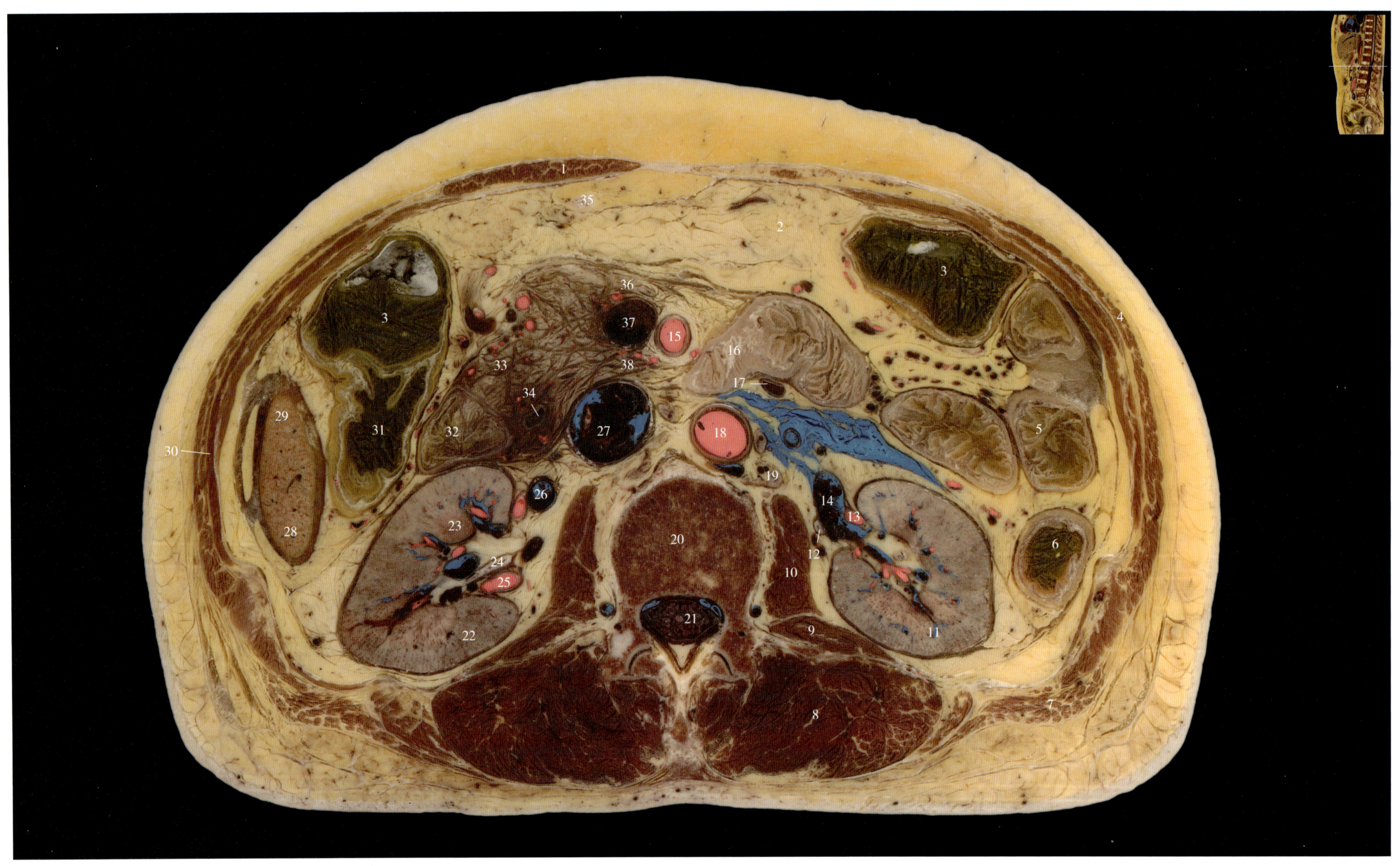

A. 断层标本图像

1. 腹直肌 rectus abdominis
2. 大网膜 greater omentum
3. 横结肠 transverse colon
4. 腹外斜肌 obliquus externus abdominis
5. 空肠 jejunum
6. 降结肠 descending colon
7. 背阔肌 latissimus dorsi
8. 竖脊肌 erector spinae
9. 腰方肌 quadratus lumborum
10. 腰大肌 psoas major
11. 左肾 left kidney
12. 左输尿管 left ureter
13. 左肾动脉 left renal artery
14. 左肾静脉 left renal vein
15. 肠系膜上动脉 superior mesenteric artery
16. 十二指肠升部 ascending part of duodenum
17. 肠系膜下静脉 inferior mesenteric vein
18. 腹主动脉 abdominal aorta
19. 淋巴结 lymph nodes
20. 第 2 腰椎椎体 body of the 2nd lumbar vertebra
21. 马尾 cauda equina
22. 右肾 right kidney
23. 肾锥体 renal pyramid
24. 右肾盂 right renal pelvis
25. 右肾动脉 right renal artery
26. 右肾静脉 right renal vein
27. 下腔静脉 inferior vena cava
28. 肝右后叶下段 inferior segment of right posterior lobe of liver
29. 肝右前叶下段 inferior segment of right anterior lobe of liver
30. 腹内斜肌 obliquus internus abdominis
31. 升结肠 ascending colon
32. 十二指肠降部 descending part of duodenum
33. 胰头 head of pancreas
34. 胆总管 common bile duct
35. 肝圆韧带 ligamentum teres hepatis
36. 胰颈 neck of pancreas
37. 肠系膜上静脉 superior mesenteric vein
38. 胰钩突 uncinate process of pancreas

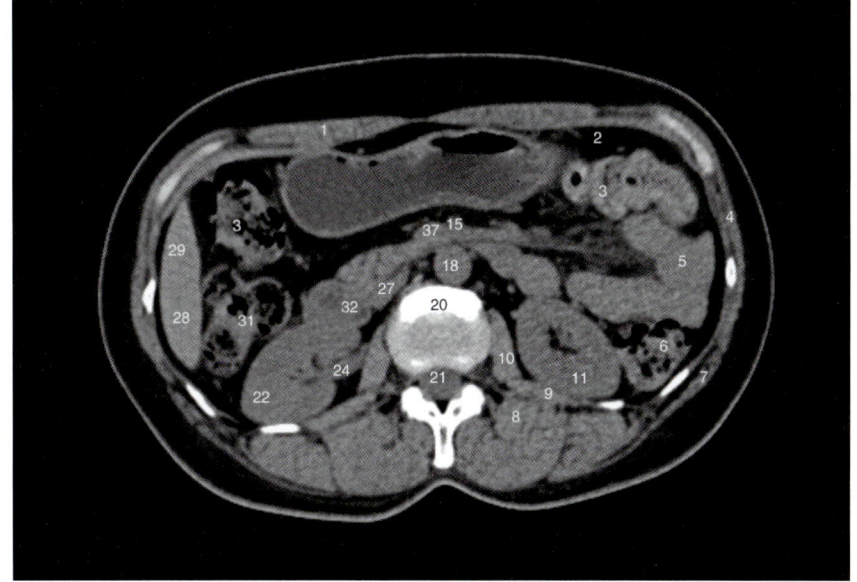

B. CT 平扫图像

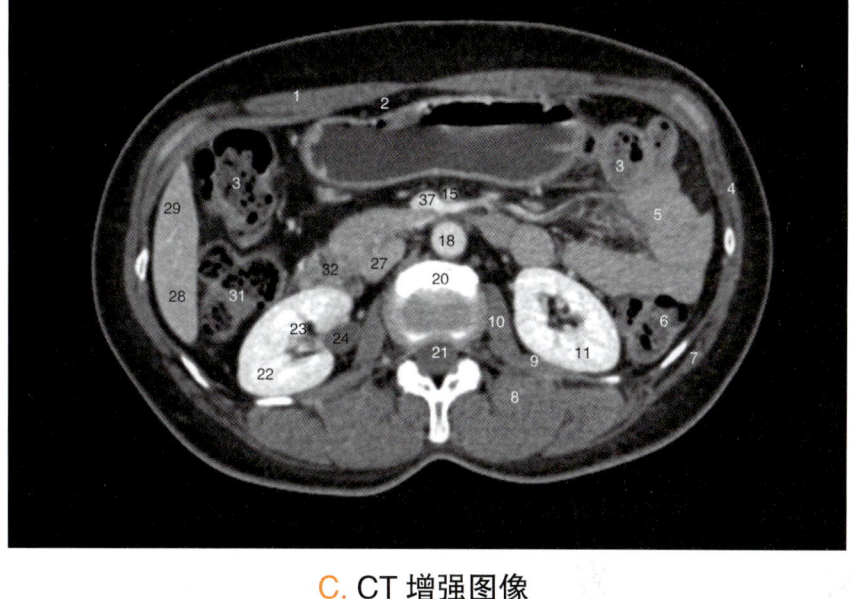

C. CT 增强图像

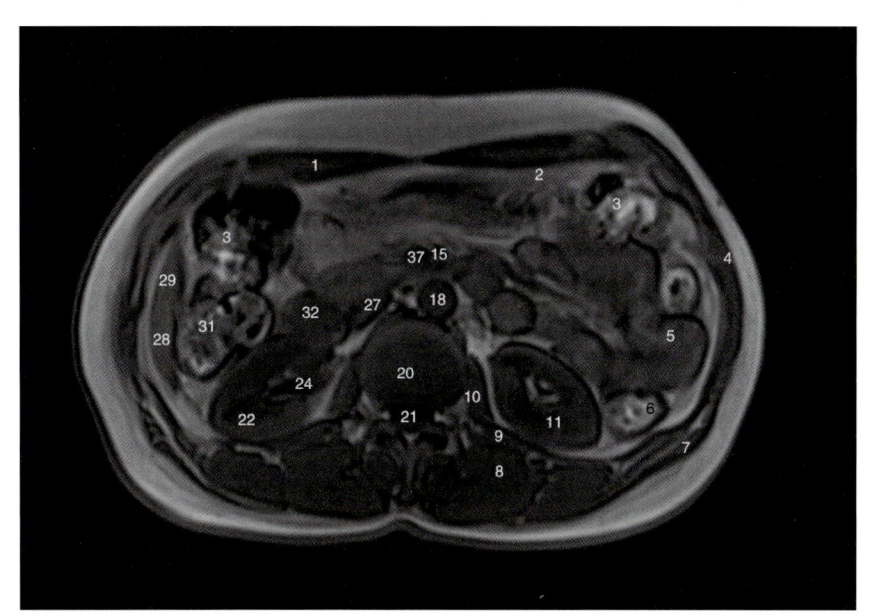

D. MR T1WI

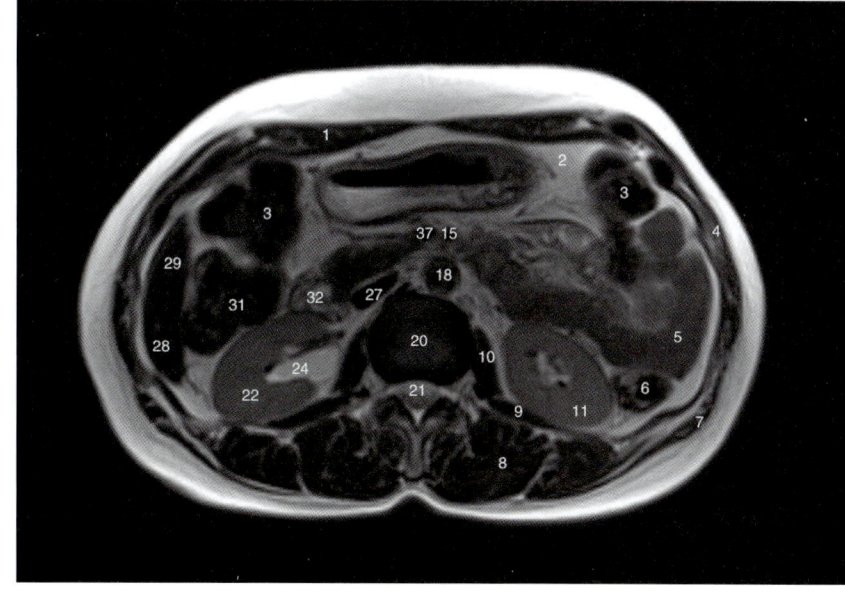

E. MR T2WI

关键结构：十二指肠升部，第 2 腰椎椎体。

此断面经过第 2 腰椎椎体。

空肠向右延伸，可见十二指肠升部初步显示。十二指肠升部是十二指肠的第 4 部分，长约 2.5 cm，起自腹主动脉的左侧，向上外侧走行到第 2 腰椎上缘水平，然后在十二指肠空肠曲处突然向前下反折，续于空肠，通过十二指肠悬韧带（或 Treitz 韧带）悬于腹膜后[66]。十二指肠悬韧带在临床上意义重大，它是外科手术时用以确定空肠的起点。十二指肠附近存在 5 个较重要的隐窝，分别是十二指肠上隐窝、十二指肠下隐窝、十二指肠旁隐窝（Landzert 隐窝）、结肠系膜间隐窝（Broesike 隐窝）和空肠旁隐窝（Waldeyer 隐窝）。其中 Landzert 隐窝位于十二指肠与空肠的交接处，尸检的检出率约 2%，该处降结肠系膜、横结肠系膜和小肠系膜发生融合，小肠会疝入这个肠系膜隐窝，引起左侧十二指肠旁疝。CT 表现为十二指肠悬韧带左侧，胰和胃之间囊状成簇扩张的小肠肠襻，供应疝囊内小肠的肠系膜血管在疝囊入口处群集、充盈和拉长。腰椎椎体较大，前高后低，横截面呈肾形。椎孔大，呈三角形，大于胸椎，小于颈椎。关节突为矢状位，上关节突的关节面凹向后内侧，下关节突的关节面凸向前外侧。乳突位于上关节的外侧，棘突为四方形的骨板，水平后突。横突短而薄，伸向后外方。第 1~3 腰椎的横突逐渐增长，以第 3 腰椎最长，第 4、5 腰椎的则逐渐变短，当第 5 腰椎与骶骨相接时，构成向前凸的岬。

腹部连续横断层 69（FH.10550）

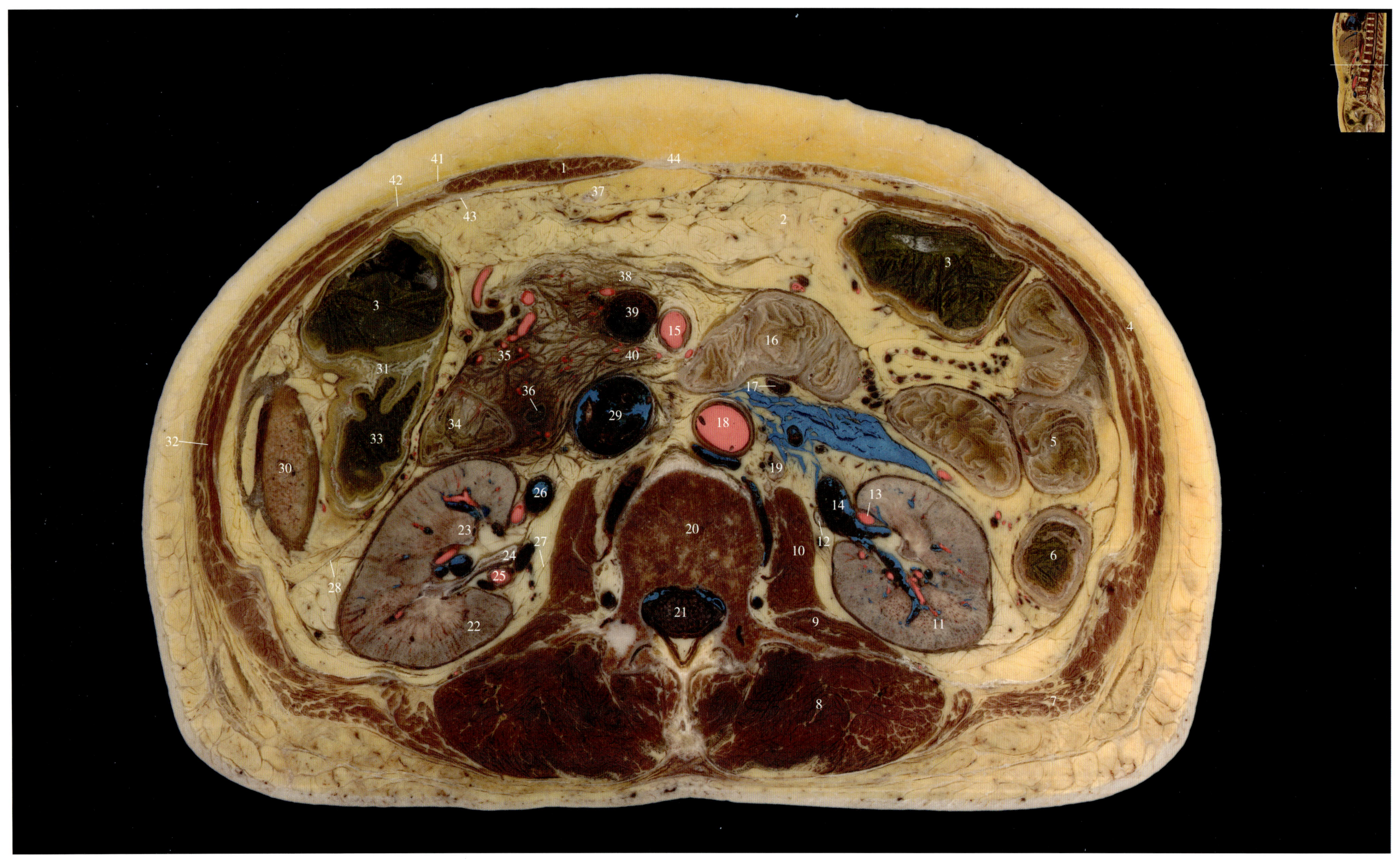

A. 断层标本图像

1. 腹直肌 rectus abdominis
2. 大网膜 greater omentum
3. 横结肠 transverse colon
4. 腹外斜肌 obliquus externus abdominis
5. 空肠 jejunum
6. 降结肠 descending colon
7. 背阔肌 latissimus dorsi
8. 竖脊肌 erector spinae
9. 腰方肌 quadratus lumborum
10. 腰大肌 psoas major
11. 左肾 left kidney
12. 左输尿管 left ureter
13. 左肾动脉 left renal artery
14. 左肾静脉 left renal vein
15. 肠系膜上动脉 superior mesenteric artery
16. 十二指肠升部 ascending part of duodenum
17. 肠系膜下静脉 inferior mesenteric vein
18. 腹主动脉 abdominal aorta
19. 淋巴结 lymph nodes
20. 第 2 腰椎椎体 body of the 2nd lumbar vertebra
21. 马尾 cauda equina
22. 右肾 right kidney
23. 肾锥体 renal pyramid
24. 右肾盂 right renal pelvis
25. 右肾动脉 right renal artery
26. 右肾静脉 right renal vein
27. 肾后筋膜 retrorenal fascia
28. 肾前筋膜 prerenal fascia
29. 下腔静脉 inferior vena cava
30. 肝右叶 right lobe of liver
31. 结肠右曲 right colic flexure
32. 腹内斜肌 obliquus internus abdominis
33. 升结肠 ascending colon
34. 十二指肠降部 descending part of duodenum
35. 胰头 head of pancreas
36. 胆总管 common bile duct
37. 肝圆韧带 ligamentum teres hepatis
38. 胰颈 neck of pancreas
39. 肠系膜上静脉 superior mesenteric vein
40. 胰钩突 uncinate process of pancreas
41. 腹外斜肌腱膜 aponeurosis of obliquus externus abdominis
42. 腹内斜肌腱膜 aponeurosis of obliquus internus abdominis
43. 腹横肌腱膜 aponeurosis of transversus abdominis
44. 白线 linea alba

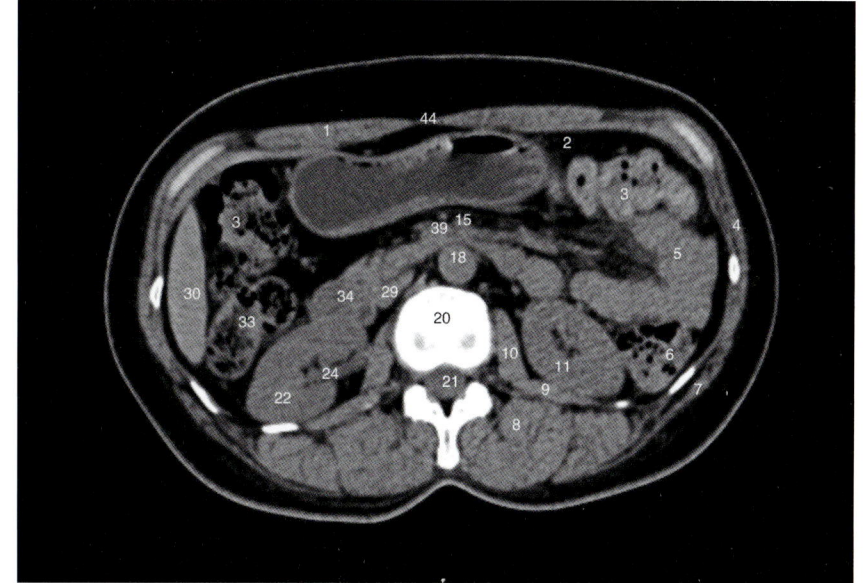

B. CT 平扫图像

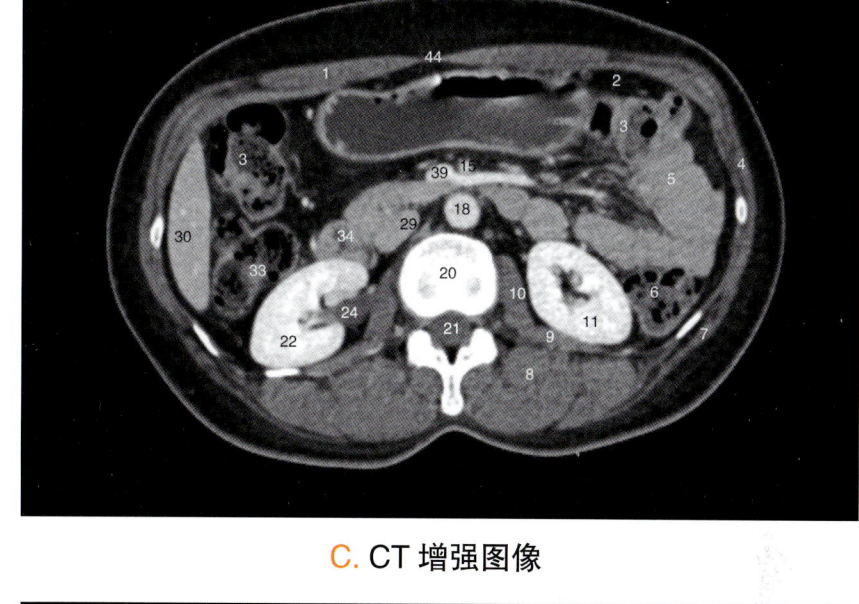

C. CT 增强图像

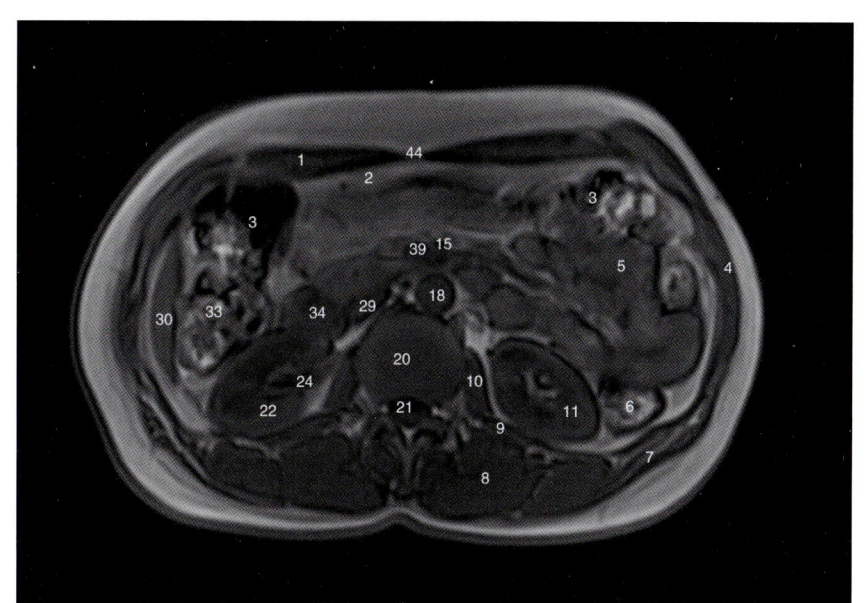

D. MR T1WI

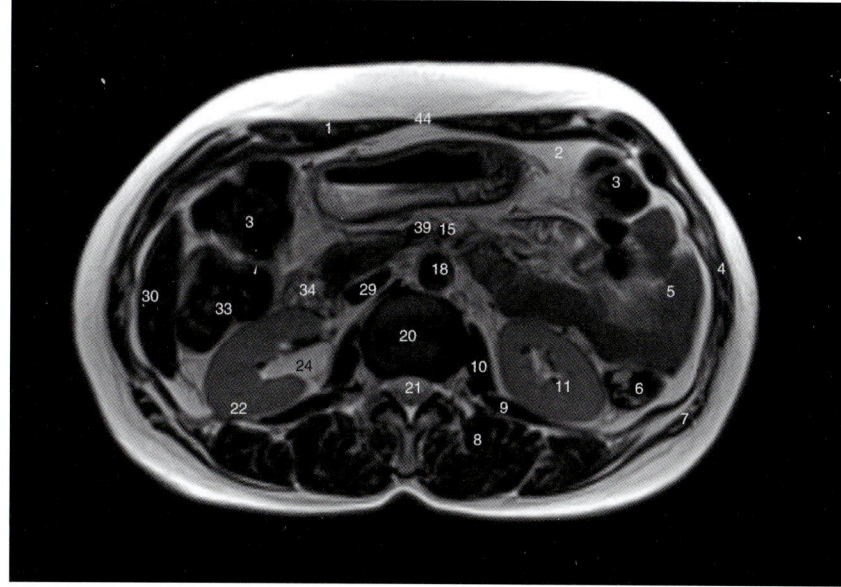

E. MR T2WI

关键结构：肾筋膜，空肠。

此断面经过第 2 腰椎椎体。

该断面为双肾中份断面水平，双肾前内侧可见肾窦，肾周纤维与脂肪组织构成致密有弹性的结缔组织鞘，被称作肾筋膜或 Gerota 筋膜，包被双肾及肾上腺及其血管。肾周脂肪在肾边界处最厚，在肾门处向肾窦延伸。肾筋膜并非由不同的筋膜融合而成，而是一个单独的多层结构，并向内侧与腰大肌、腰方肌的肌筋膜融合[67]。前后肾筋膜在中线上方融合并附着于各自侧的膈脚。在中线下方，肾前、后筋膜在肾的大部分是分离的，肾后筋膜与腰大肌筋膜融合，肾前筋膜则跨过中线延伸至大血管。前、后肾筋膜在下方融合形成一个尖端向盆腔开放的倒锥体。前、后筋膜的外侧与髂筋膜融合，内侧则与输尿管周围结缔组织融合[61]。一般单纯肾切除术仅将肾从肾筋膜中取出，而根治性肾切除术（用于治疗肾癌）则将肾周间隙的所有内容物，包括肾筋膜和肾上腺全部移除以完全清除肿瘤。当炎症、外伤或肾肿瘤侵犯时，CT 或 MR 图像上可表现为肾筋膜增厚、脂肪密度增高或积液[68]。

腹部连续横断层 70（FH.10530）

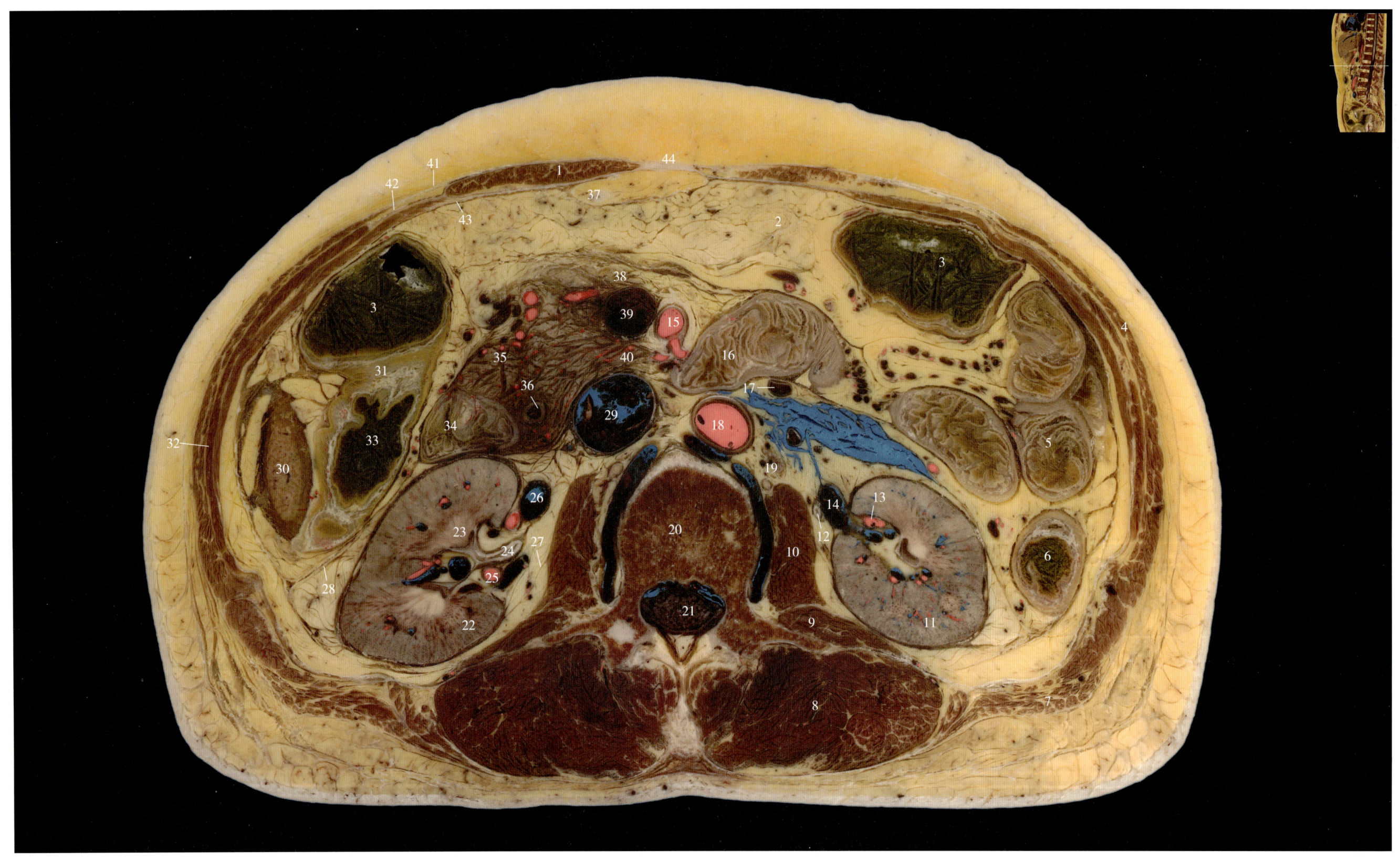

A. 断层标本图像

1. 腹直肌 rectus abdominis
2. 大网膜 greater omentum
3. 横结肠 transverse colon
4. 腹外斜肌 obliquus externus abdominis
5. 空肠 jejunum
6. 降结肠 descending colon
7. 背阔肌 latissimus dorsi
8. 竖脊肌 erector spinae
9. 腰方肌 quadratus lumborum
10. 腰大肌 psoas major
11. 左肾 left kidney
12. 左输尿管 left ureter
13. 左肾动脉 left renal artery
14. 左肾静脉 left renal vein
15. 肠系膜上动脉 superior mesenteric artery
16. 十二指肠升部 ascending part of duodenum
17. 肠系膜下静脉 inferior mesenteric vein
18. 腹主动脉 abdominal aorta
19. 淋巴结 lymph nodes
20. 第 2 腰椎椎体 body of the 2nd lumbar vertebra
21. 马尾 cauda equina
22. 右肾 right kidney
23. 肾锥体 renal pyramid
24. 右肾盂 right renal pelvis
25. 右肾动脉 right renal artery
26. 右肾静脉 right renal vein
27. 肾后筋膜 retrorenal fascia
28. 肾前筋膜 prerenal fascia
29. 下腔静脉 inferior vena cava
30. 肝右叶 right lobe of liver
31. 结肠右曲 right colic flexure
32. 腹内斜肌 obliquus internus abdominis
33. 升结肠 ascending colon
34. 十二指肠降部 descending part of duodenum
35. 胰头 head of pancreas
36. 胆总管 common bile duct
37. 肝圆韧带 ligamentum teres hepatis
38. 胰颈 neck of pancreas
39. 肠系膜上静脉 superior mesenteric vein
40. 胰钩突 uncinate process of pancreas
41. 腹外斜肌腱膜 aponeurosis of obliquus externus abdominis
42. 腹内斜肌腱膜 aponeurosis of obliquus internus abdominis
43. 腹横肌腱膜 aponeurosis of transversus abdominis
44. 白线 linea alba

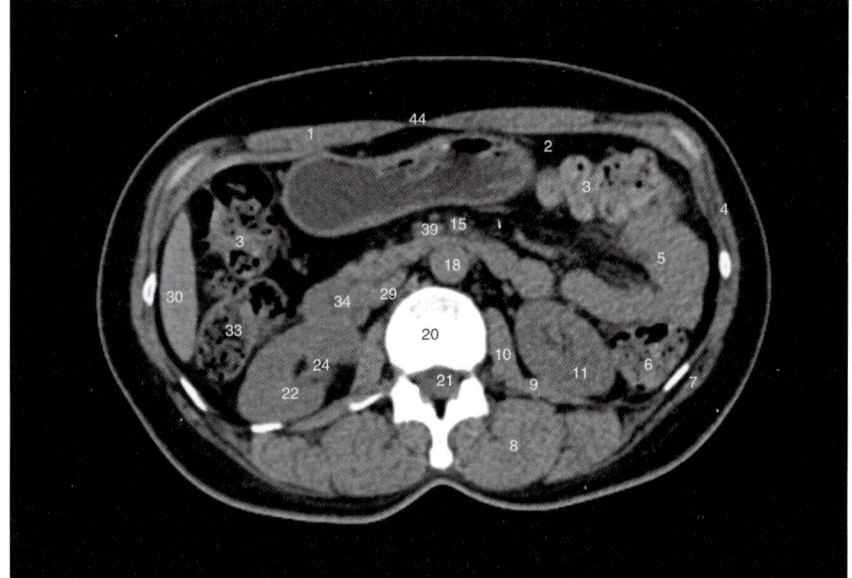

B. CT 平扫图像

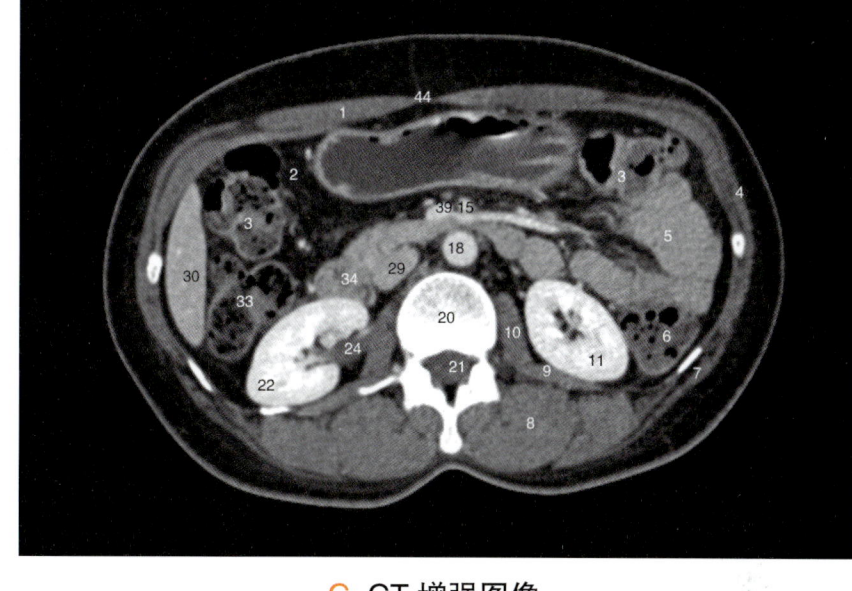

C. CT 增强图像

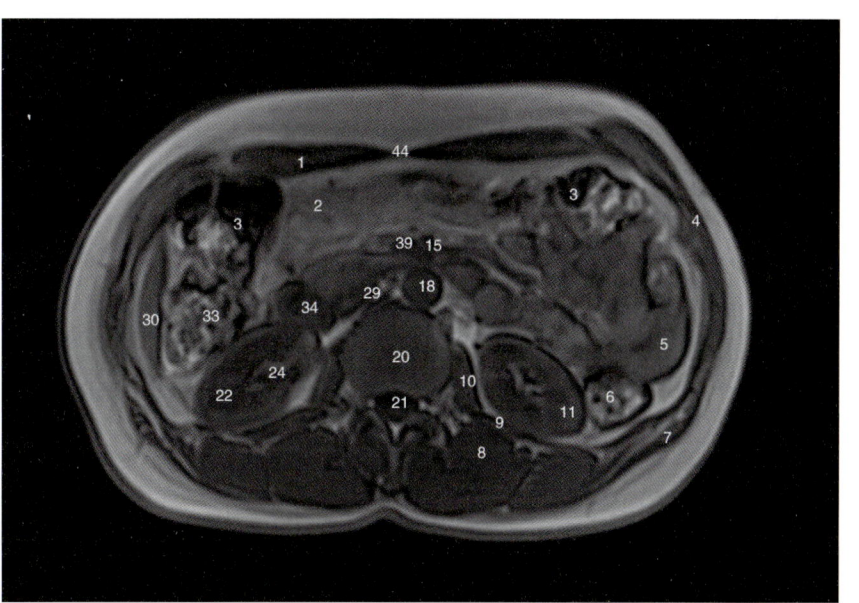

D. MR T1WI

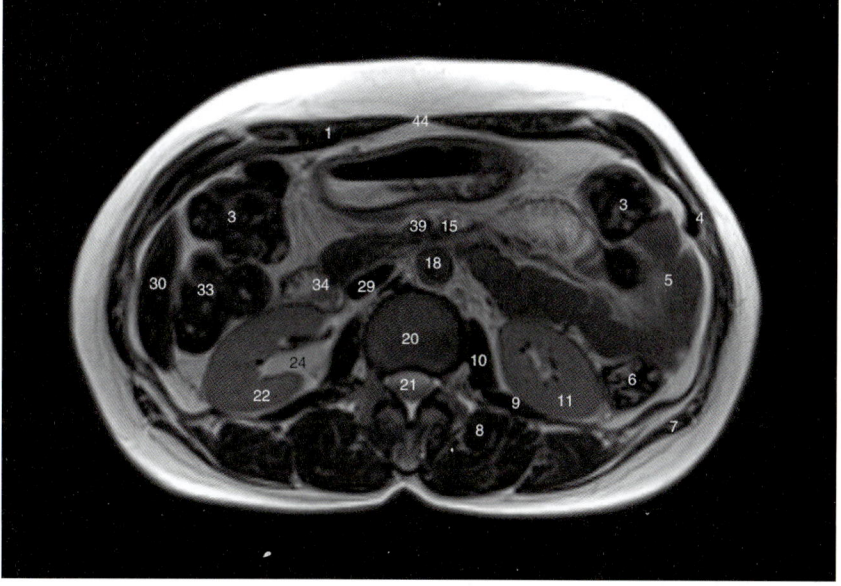

E. MR T2WI

关键结构：腹外斜肌，腹内斜肌，腹横肌腱膜。

此断面经过第 2 腰椎椎体。

腹直肌位居腹前壁中线两侧，腹前外侧壁上由内向外依次排列是腹外斜肌、腹内斜肌和腹横肌。腹外斜肌是腹前外侧壁 3 块扁肌中最大和最浅的一块。它弯曲走行在腹外侧部和前部，附着于下 8 位肋骨的外面和下缘。腹内斜肌大部分位于腹外斜肌的深面，比腹外斜肌深而小，起于腹股沟韧带沟状上缘的外 2/3，弓形向下，在内侧跨过子宫圆韧带，逐渐变为腱性，与腹横肌肌腱膜融合形成联合腱，止于髂嵴和耻骨梳的内侧份。腹横肌是腹前外侧肌中最内层的肌，起于腹股沟韧带的外 1/3 及相关的髂筋膜，止于前面的腹横肌腱膜。后者弓形向下外方，在脐平面离腹直肌鞘的外侧缘最远处，然后再弓形向下内到达腹股沟浅环，而下部止于联合腱。CT 图像可显示正常腹壁的肌肉和皮下组织，以及腹壁的一些疾病，如疝、血肿、脓肿、肿瘤等[69]。

腹部连续横断层 71（FH.10510）

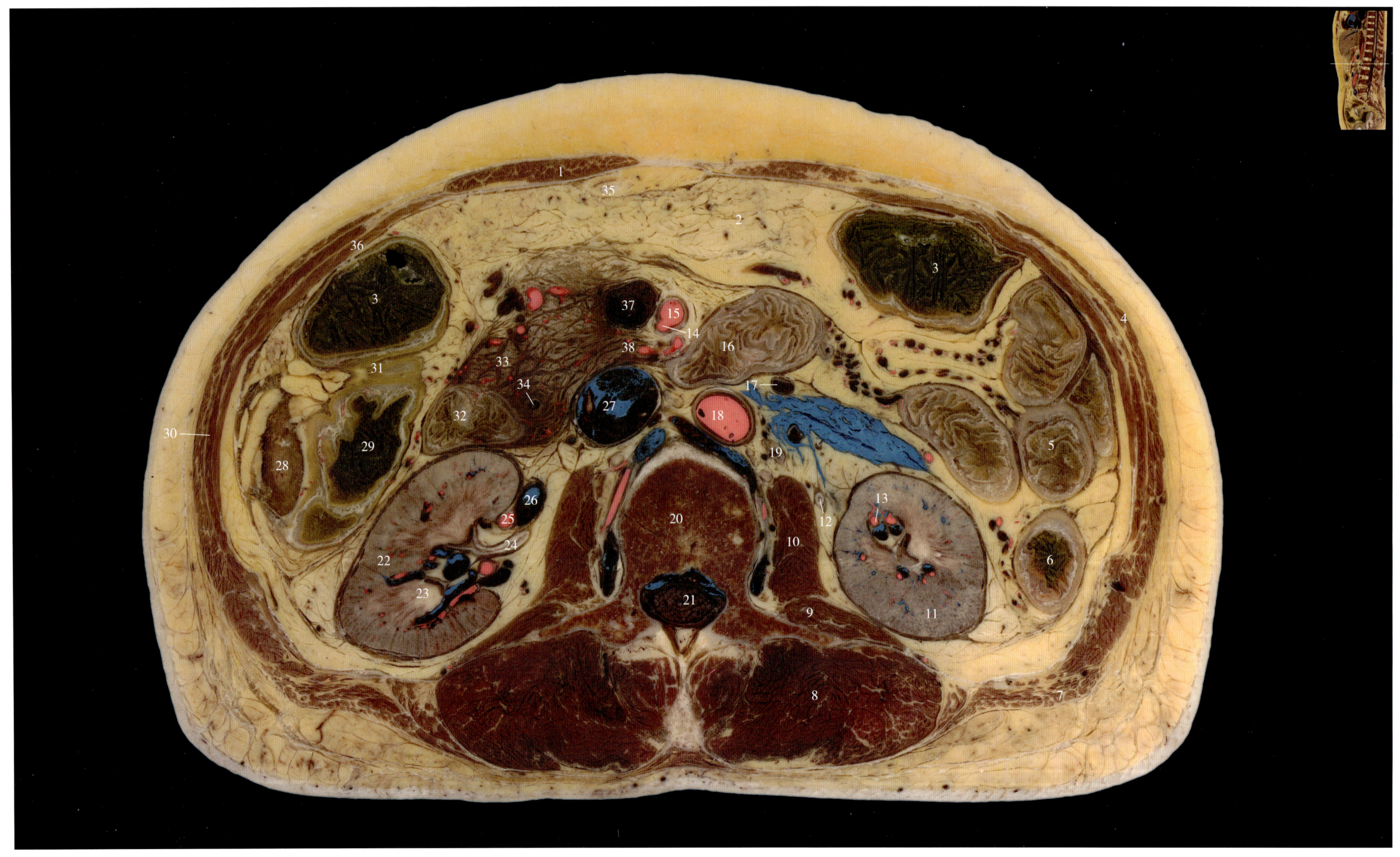

A. 断层标本图像

1. 腹直肌 rectus abdominis
2. 大网膜 greater omentum
3. 横结肠 transverse colon
4. 腹外斜肌 obliquus externus abdominis
5. 空肠 jejunum
6. 降结肠 descending colon
7. 背阔肌 latissimus dorsi
8. 竖脊肌 erector spinae
9. 腰方肌 quadratus lumborum
10. 腰大肌 psoas major
11. 左肾 left kidney
12. 左输尿管 left ureter
13. 左肾动脉 left renal artery
14. 胰十二指肠下动脉 inferior pancreaticoduodenal artery
15. 肠系膜上动脉 superior mesenteric artery
16. 十二指肠升部 ascending part of duodenum
17. 肠系膜下静脉 inferior mesenteric vein
18. 腹主动脉 abdominal aorta
19. 淋巴结 lymph nodes
20. 第2腰椎椎体 body of the 2nd lumbar vertebra
21. 马尾 cauda equina
22. 右肾 right kidney
23. 肾锥体 renal pyramid
24. 右肾盂 right renal pelvis
25. 右肾动脉 right renal artery
26. 右肾静脉 right renal vein
27. 下腔静脉 inferior vena cava
28. 肝右叶 right lobe of liver
29. 升结肠 ascending colon
30. 腹内斜肌 obliquus internus abdominis
31. 结肠右曲 right colic flexure
32. 十二指肠降部 descending part of duodenum
33. 胰头 head of pancreas
34. 胆总管 common bile duct
35. 肝圆韧带 ligamentum teres hepatis
36. 腹横肌 transversus abdominis
37. 肠系膜上静脉 superior mesenteric vein
38. 胰钩突 uncinate process of pancreas

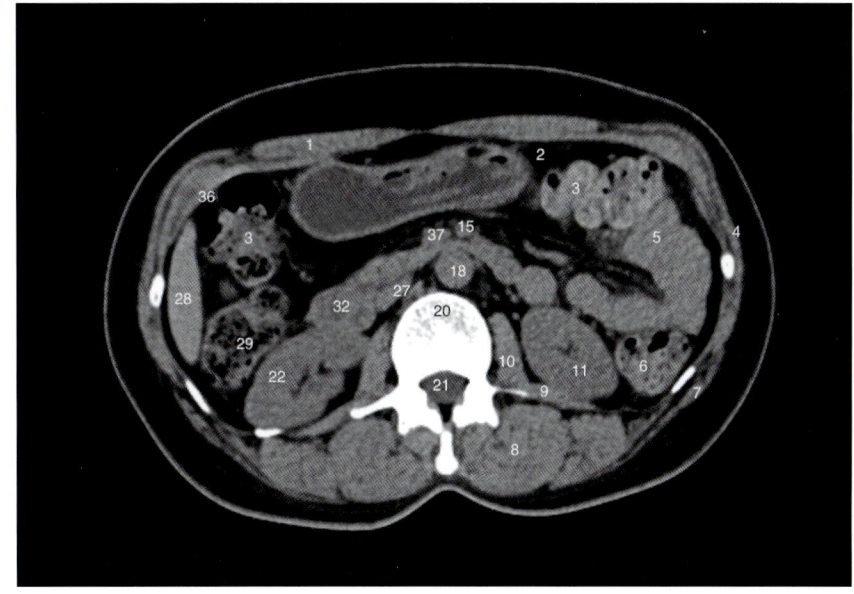

B. CT 平扫图像

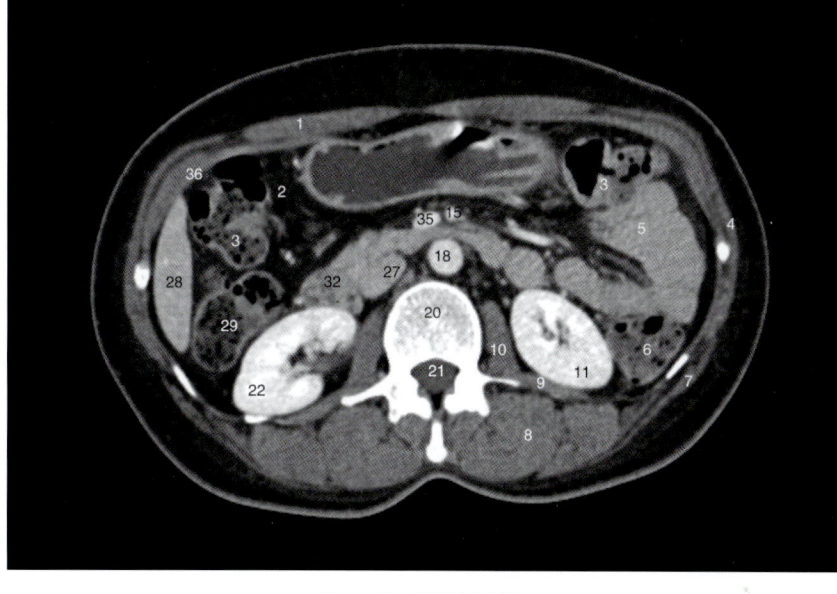

C. CT 增强图像

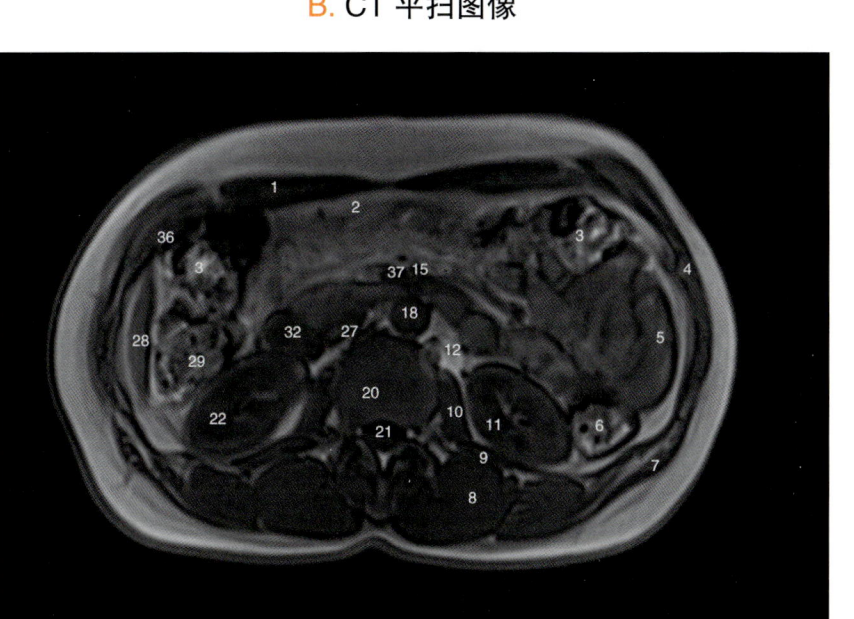

D. MR T1WI

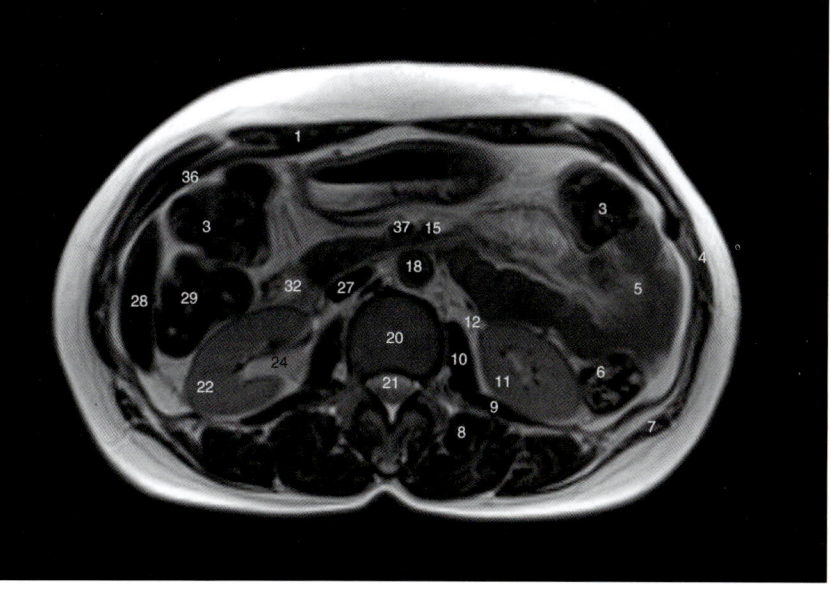

E. MR T2WI

关键结构：升结肠，结肠右曲。

此断面经过第2腰椎椎体。

右侧仅剩极小部分肝脏。十二指肠升部继续向右侧延伸。升结肠也叫上行结肠，下端接盲肠，上缘在肝下与横结肠相连（即结肠右曲），长12~20 cm；其前面及两侧有腹膜遮盖，使其固定于腹后壁及腹侧壁；前方有小肠及大网膜和腹前壁；后方借疏松结缔组织与腹后壁相连，由上向下有右肾、腰背筋膜，内侧有十二指肠降部、右输尿管，手术分离较困难。

升结肠侧后方可见结肠旁沟，少量腹腔积液可在此积聚。在断面图像上，升结肠位置固定，因结肠袋结构形态而常呈花环样，肠腔内存在气体或密度不等的粪块，浆膜层清晰，周围偶可见小淋巴结。升结肠癌可导致右半结肠的肠壁不规则增厚，肠腔扩张，肿瘤多为溃疡型或突向肠腔的菜花样肿块，较少有环状狭窄，故不常发生肠梗阻[70,71]。肿瘤侵及浆膜层时，邻近脂肪组织密度增高，可见大小不等的淋巴结。

腹部连续横断层 72（FH.10490）

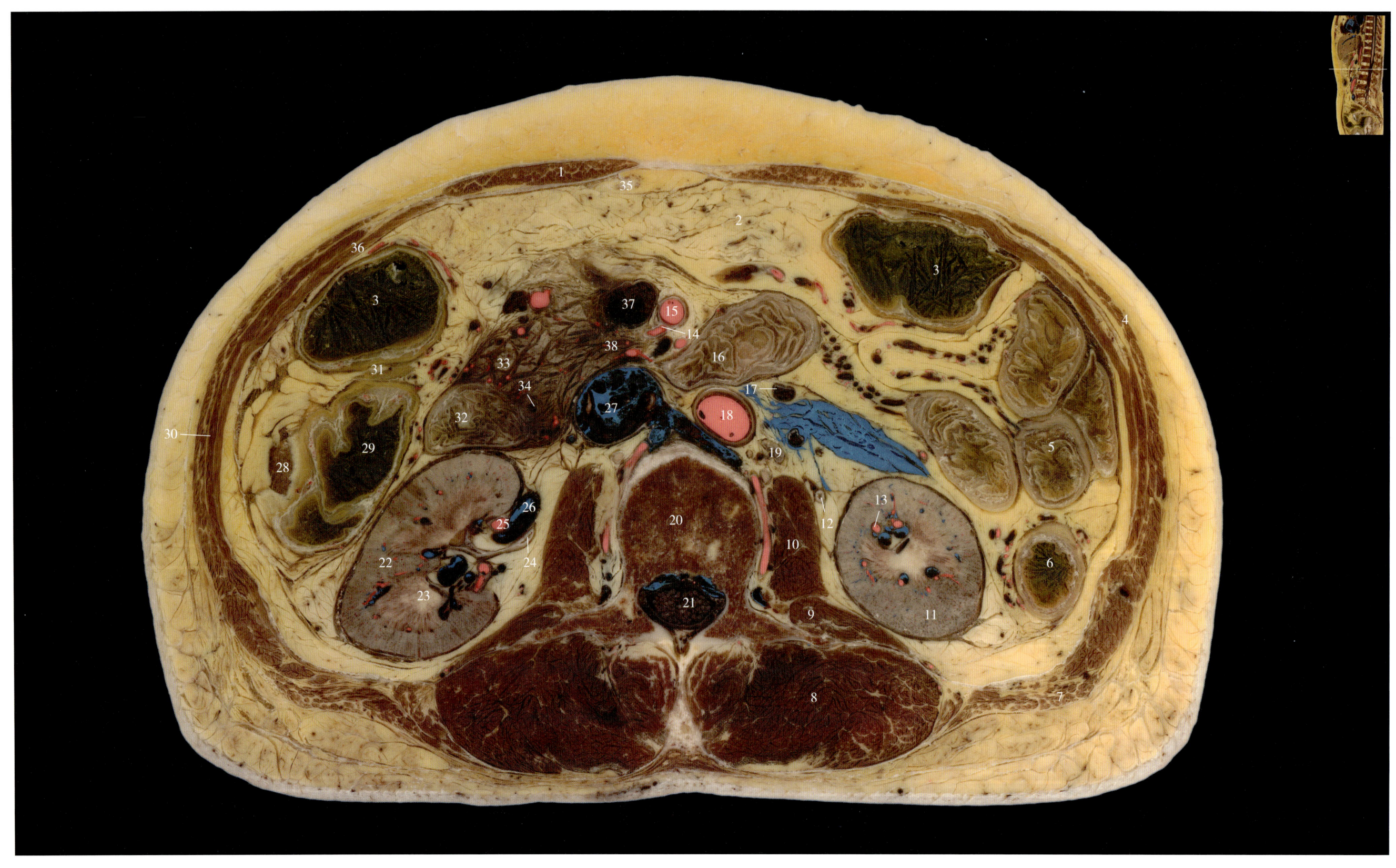

A. 断层标本图像

1. 腹直肌 rectus abdominis
2. 大网膜 greater omentum
3. 横结肠 transverse colon
4. 腹外斜肌 obliquus externus abdominis
5. 空肠 jejunum
6. 降结肠 descending colon
7. 背阔肌 latissimus dorsi
8. 竖脊肌 erector spinae
9. 腰方肌 quadratus lumborum
10. 腰大肌 psoas major
11. 左肾 left kidney
12. 左输尿管 left ureter
13. 左肾动脉 left renal artery
14. 胰十二指肠下动脉 inferior pancreaticoduodenal artery
15. 肠系膜上动脉 superior mesenteric artery
16. 十二指肠升部 ascending part of duodenum
17. 肠系膜下静脉 inferior mesenteric vein
18. 腹主动脉 abdominal aorta
19. 淋巴结 lymph nodes
20. 第2腰椎椎体 body of the 2nd lumbar vertebra
21. 马尾 cauda equina
22. 右肾 right kidney
23. 肾锥体 renal pyramid
24. 右肾盂 right renal pelvis
25. 右肾动脉 right renal artery
26. 右肾静脉 right renal vein
27. 下腔静脉 inferior vena cava
28. 肝右叶 right lobe of liver
29. 升结肠 ascending colon
30. 腹内斜肌 obliquus internus abdominis
31. 结肠右曲 right colic flexure
32. 十二指肠降部 descending part of duodenum
33. 胰头 head of pancreas
34. 胆总管 common bile duct
35. 肝圆韧带 ligamentum teres hepatis
36. 腹横肌 transversus abdominis
37. 肠系膜上静脉 superior mesenteric vein
38. 胰钩突 uncinate process of pancreas

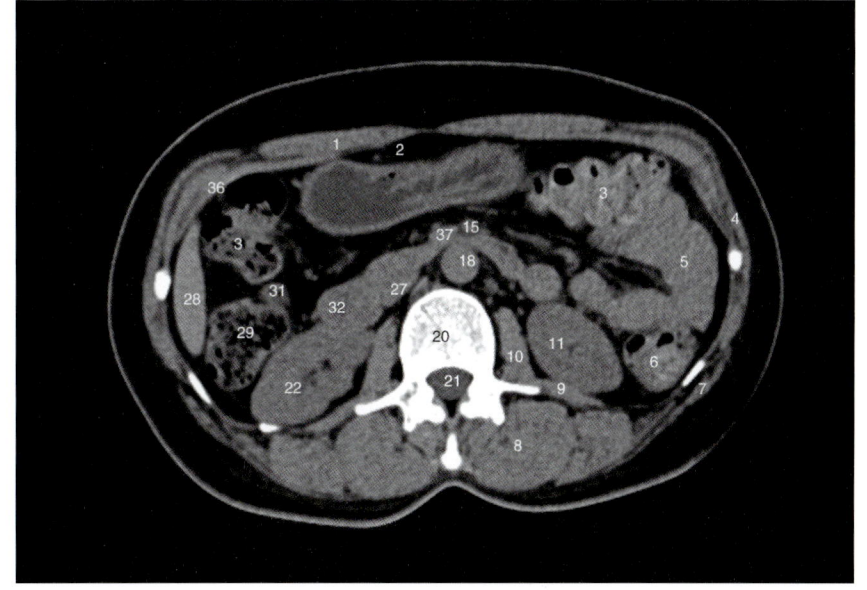

B. CT 平扫图像

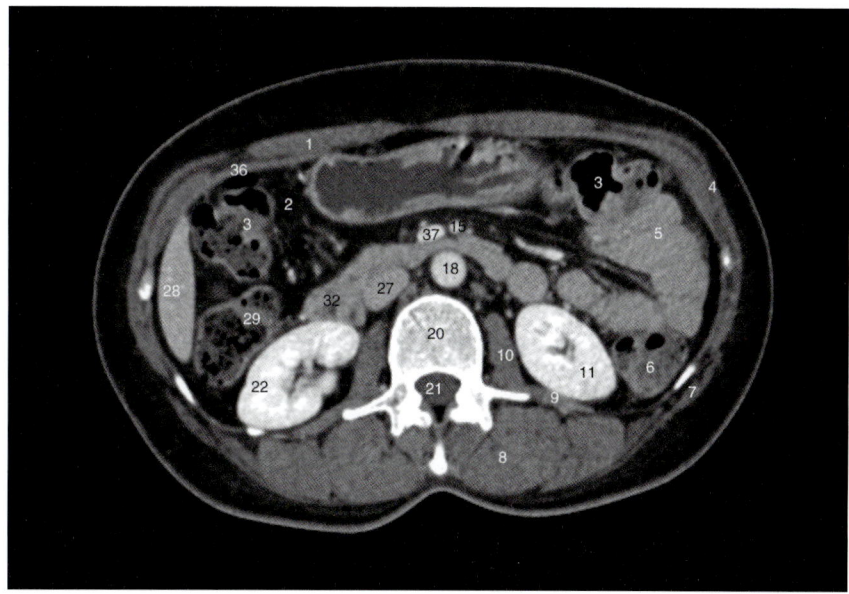

C. CT 增强图像

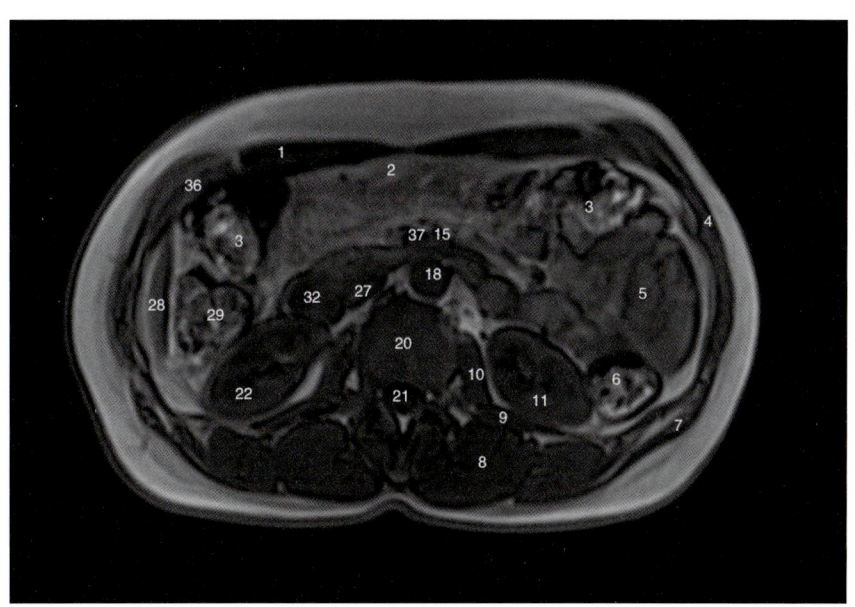

D. MR T1WI

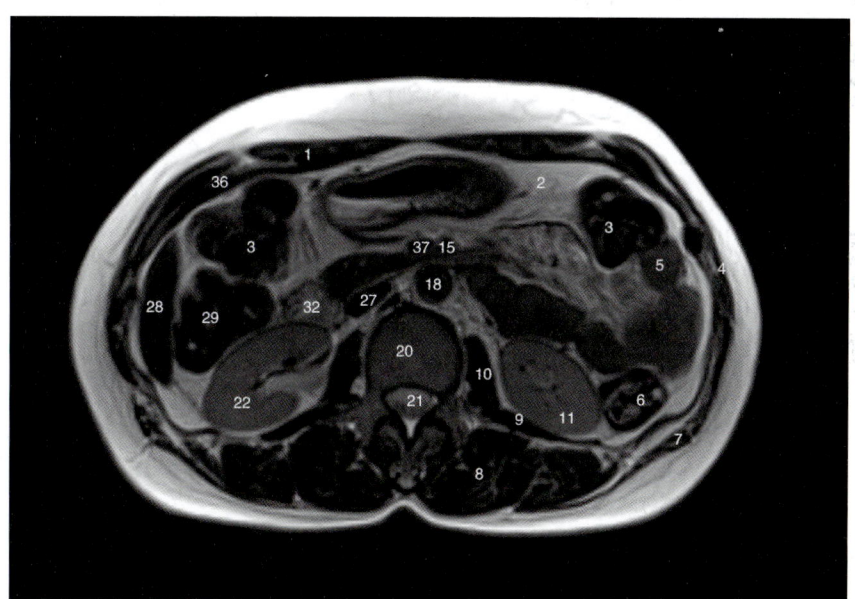

E. MR T2WI

关键结构：十二指肠降部，胰头，胆总管。

此断面经过第2腰椎椎体。

大网膜位于此断面前方，分为前叶与后叶，每叶含有两层腹膜，在横结肠下紧密附着。十二指肠降部是十二指肠的第2部，长5~7 cm，由十二指肠上曲沿右肾内侧缘下降，至第3腰椎水平，弯向左侧，转折处为十二指肠下曲。十二指肠降部断面内前方可见胰头断面，并见胆总管断面走行于胰头内并与十二指肠降部平行，致使黏膜呈略凸向肠腔的纵行隆起，称十二指肠纵襞。纵襞的下端为圆形隆起，称十二指肠大乳头，是胆总管和胰管的共同开口。胆总管居于胰头后缘右端和十二指肠降部之间，向下即穿入十二指肠壁内。大乳头稍上方，有时可见十二指肠小乳头，这是副胰管的开口之处。在断面图像上，十二指肠降部常表现为含气环状影，受邻近结构挤压，形态变化较大，但可根据胰头进行定位。临床多见十二指肠憩室，十二指肠憩室是黏膜、黏膜下层通过肠壁肌层薄弱处向肠腔外突出而形成的囊袋状结构，临床上多无明显症状，常在上消化道造影中偶然发现，憩室并发炎症时，可有上腹疼痛等症状[72]。憩室在CT和MR图像表现为十二指肠环内侧突出囊袋状气体或液体密度/信号填充，憩室体积较大时可悬垂于十二指肠外后侧，憩室口常表现为十二指肠黏膜相延续，CT对于憩室内气体和内容物显示较MRI敏感。

腹部连续横断层 73（FH.10470）

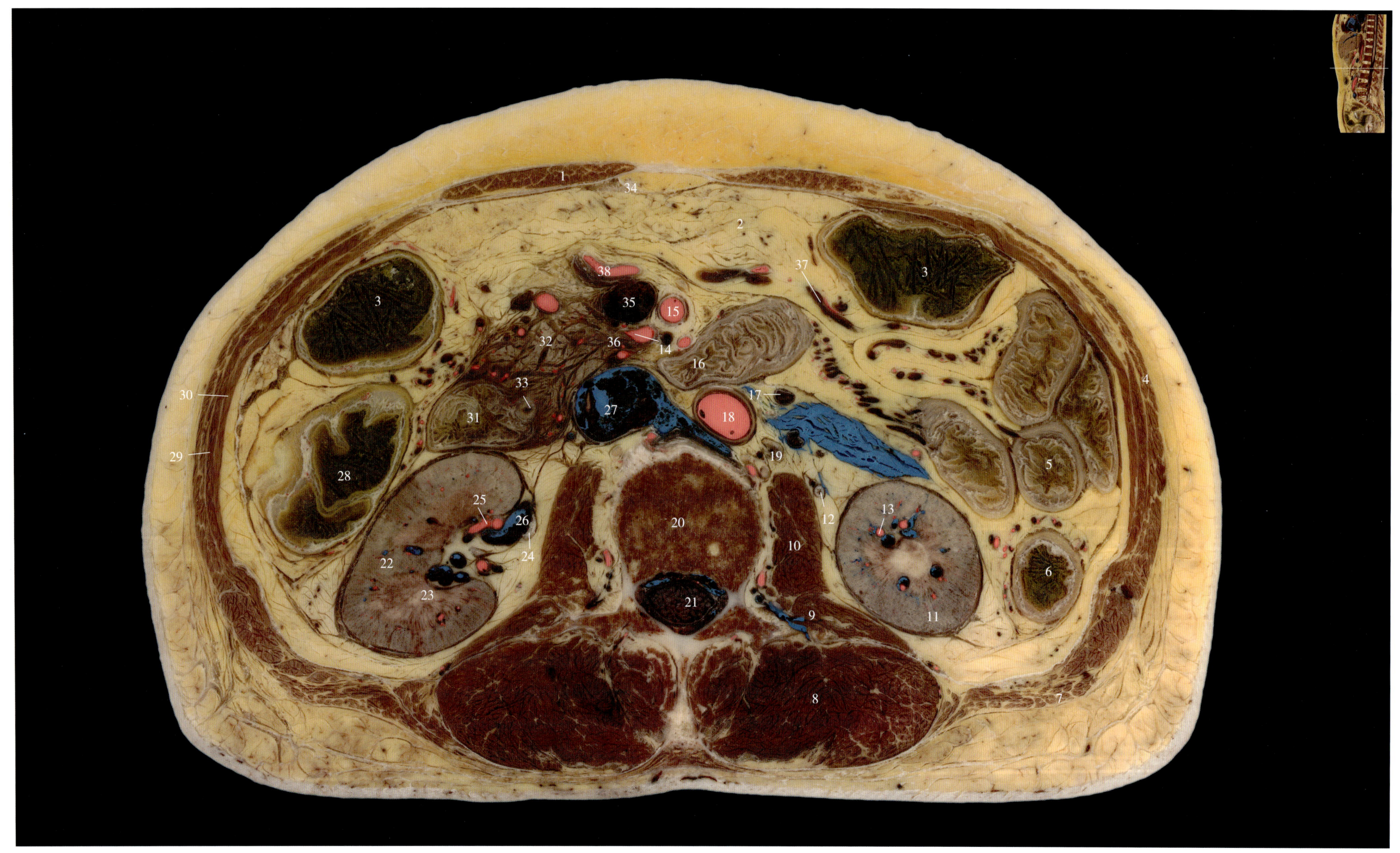

A. 断层标本图像

1. 腹直肌 rectus abdominis
2. 大网膜 greater omentum
3. 横结肠 transverse colon
4. 腹外斜肌 obliquus externus abdominis
5. 空肠 jejunum
6. 降结肠 descending colon
7. 背阔肌 latissimus dorsi
8. 竖脊肌 erector spinae
9. 腰方肌 quadratus lumborum
10. 腰大肌 psoas major
11. 左肾 left kidney
12. 左输尿管 left ureter
13. 左肾动脉 left renal artery
14. 胰十二指肠下动脉 inferior pancreaticoduodenal artery
15. 肠系膜上动脉 superior mesenteric artery
16. 十二指肠升部 ascending part of duodenum
17. 肠系膜下静脉 inferior mesenteric vein
18. 腹主动脉 abdominal aorta
19. 淋巴结 lymph nodes
20. 第2腰椎椎体 body of the 2nd lumbar vertebra
21. 马尾 cauda equina
22. 右肾 right kidney
23. 肾锥体 renal pyramid
24. 右肾盂 right renal pelvis
25. 右肾动脉 right renal artery
26. 右肾静脉 right renal vein
27. 下腔静脉 inferior vena cava
28. 升结肠 ascending colon
29. 腹内斜肌 obliquus internus abdominis
30. 腹横肌 transversus abdominis
31. 十二指肠降部 descending part of duodenum
32. 胰头 head of pancreas
33. 胆总管 common bile duct
34. 肝圆韧带 ligamentum teres hepatis
35. 肠系膜上静脉 superior mesenteric vein
36. 胰钩突 uncinate process of pancreas
37. 空肠动、静脉 jejunal artery and vein
38. 回肠动、静脉 ileal artery and vein

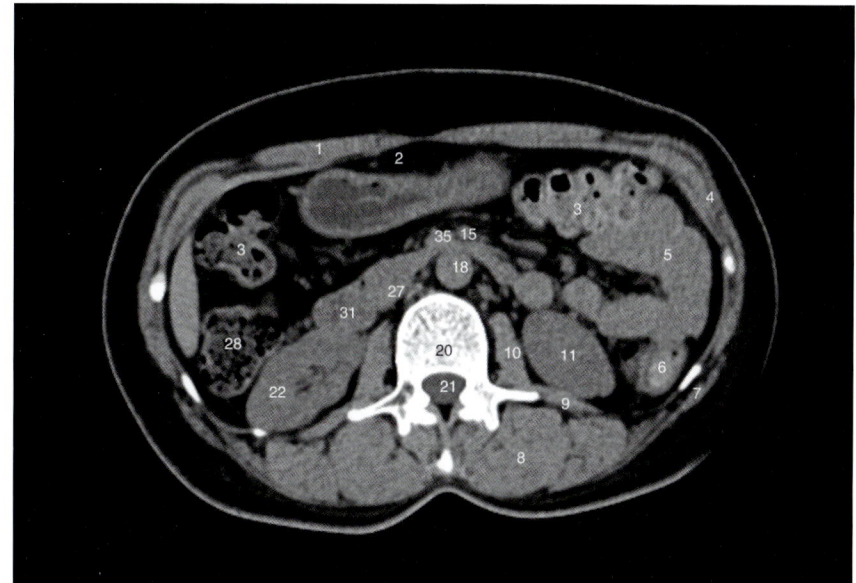

B. CT 平扫图像

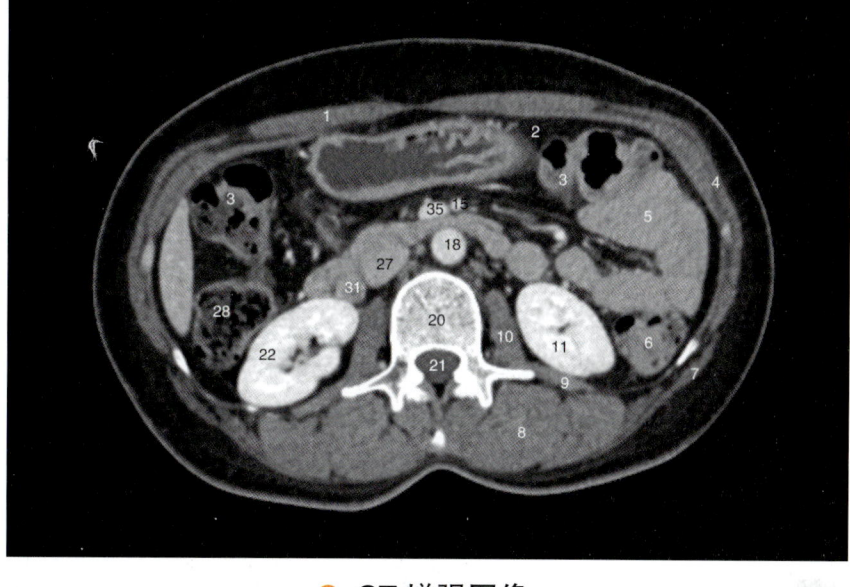

C. CT 增强图像

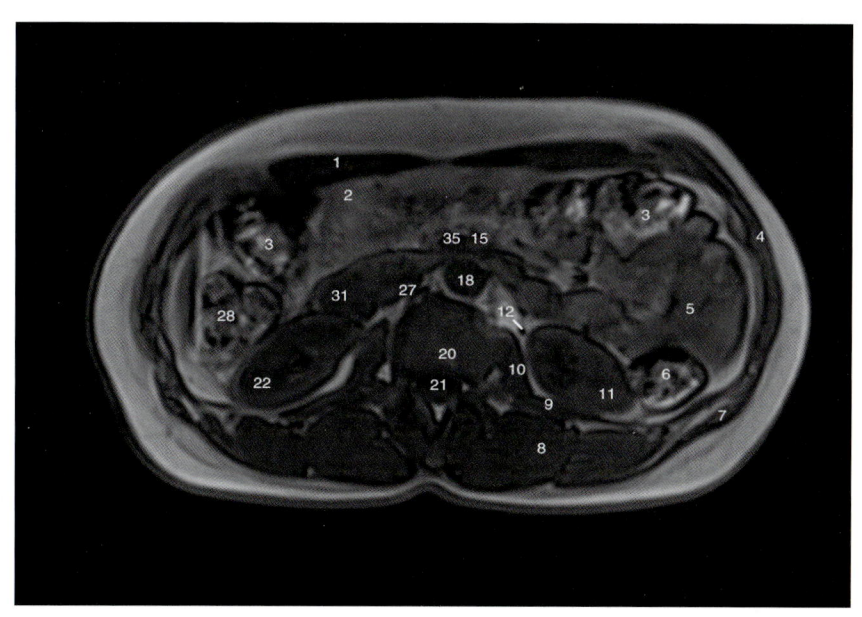

D. MR T1WI

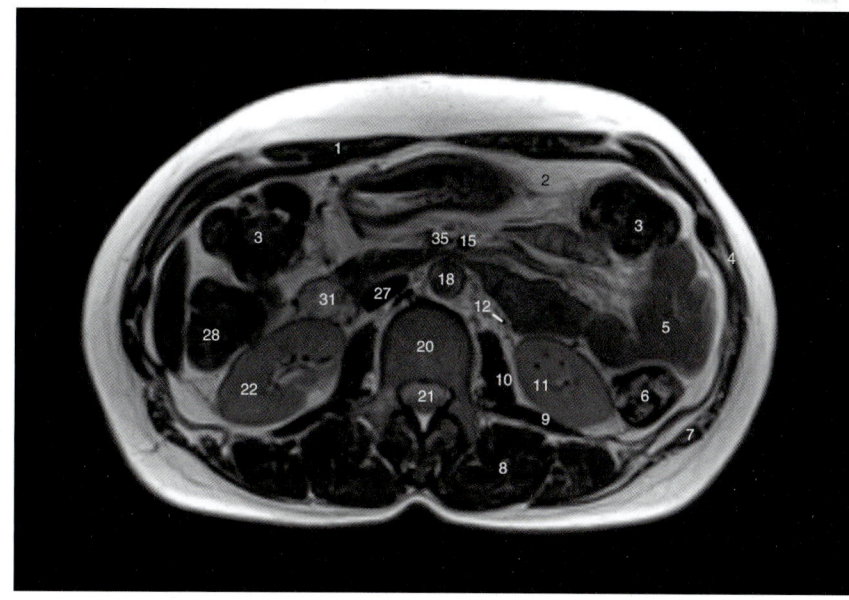

E. MR T2WI

关键结构：空、回肠动、静脉，大网膜。

此断面经过第2腰椎椎体。

肝右叶消失，空回肠的动脉和静脉分支相伴走行于肠系膜内，垂直于断面者呈环样，平行于断面者呈管样。空肠动脉来自肠系膜上动脉上半部分的左侧，通常为4~6条，通过1~3层动脉血管弓分布于空肠，直血管由最远端部位发出，几乎平行走行于肠系膜内。而回肠动脉支数比空肠动脉多，但管径比空肠动脉小。它们来源于肠系膜上动脉的左前方。回肠动脉形成2级和6级动脉弓，然后发出多条直动脉直接进入回肠壁。这些分支在肠系膜内平行走行，并交替分布于回肠。它们比相似的空肠动脉更短更薄，尤其在回肠末端更明显。终末回肠中弓形血管接受来自回结肠动脉发出的回肠支和肠系膜上动脉发出的末端回肠支[73]，而肠系膜上静脉接受空肠静脉、回肠静脉、回结肠静脉等的血液[74]。

腹部连续横断层 74（FH.10450）

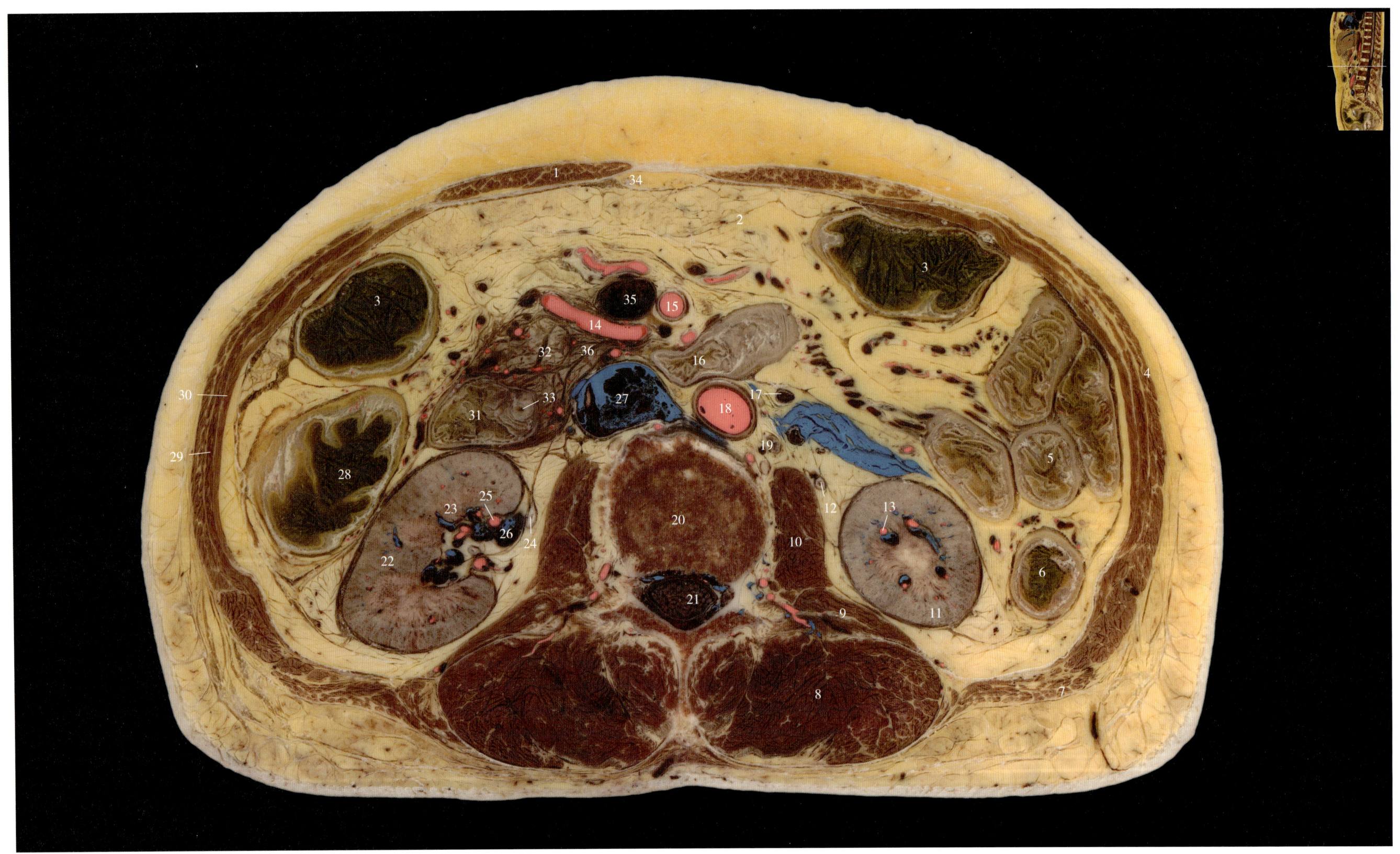

A. 断层标本图像

1. 腹直肌 rectus abdominis
2. 大网膜 greater omentum
3. 横结肠 transverse colon
4. 腹外斜肌 obliquus externus abdominis
5. 空肠 jejunum
6. 降结肠 descending colon
7. 背阔肌 latissimus dorsi
8. 竖脊肌 erector spinae
9. 腰方肌 quadratus lumborum
10. 腰大肌 psoas major
11. 左肾 left kidney
12. 左输尿管 left ureter
13. 左肾动脉 left renal artery
14. 胰十二指肠下动脉 inferior pancreaticoduodenal artery
15. 肠系膜上动脉 superior mesenteric artery
16. 十二指肠升部 ascending part of duodenum
17. 肠系膜下静脉 inferior mesenteric vein
18. 腹主动脉 abdominal aorta
19. 淋巴结 lymph nodes
20. 第 2 腰椎椎体 body of the 2nd lumbar vertebra
21. 马尾 cauda equina
22. 右肾 right kidney
23. 肾锥体 renal pyramid
24. 右肾盂 right renal pelvis
25. 右肾动脉 right renal artery
26. 右肾静脉 right renal vein
27. 下腔静脉 inferior vena cava
28. 升结肠 ascending colon
29. 腹内斜肌 obliquus internus abdominis
30. 腹横肌 transversus abdominis
31. 十二指肠降部 descending part of duodenum
32. 胰头 head of pancreas
33. 十二指肠大乳头 major duodenal papilla
34. 肝圆韧带 ligamentum teres hepatis
35. 肠系膜上静脉 superior mesenteric vein
36. 胰钩突 uncinate process of pancreas

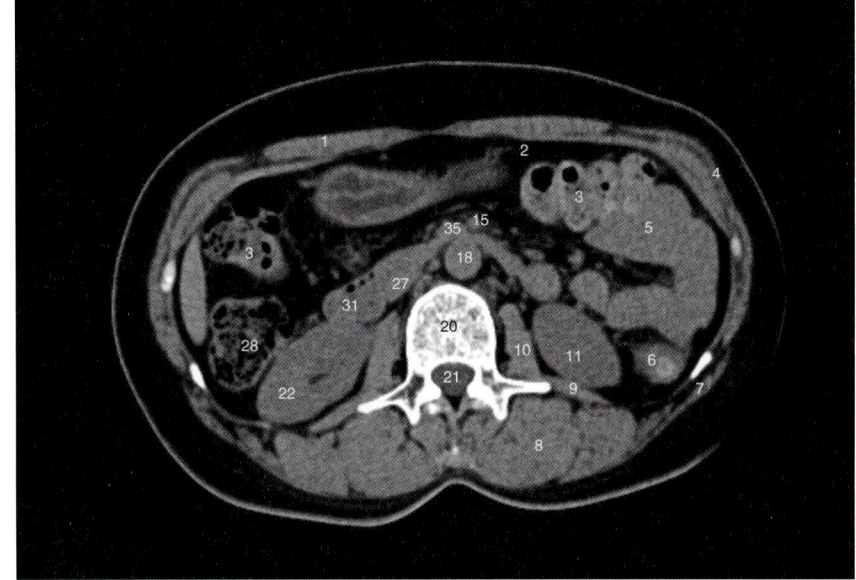

B. CT 平扫图像

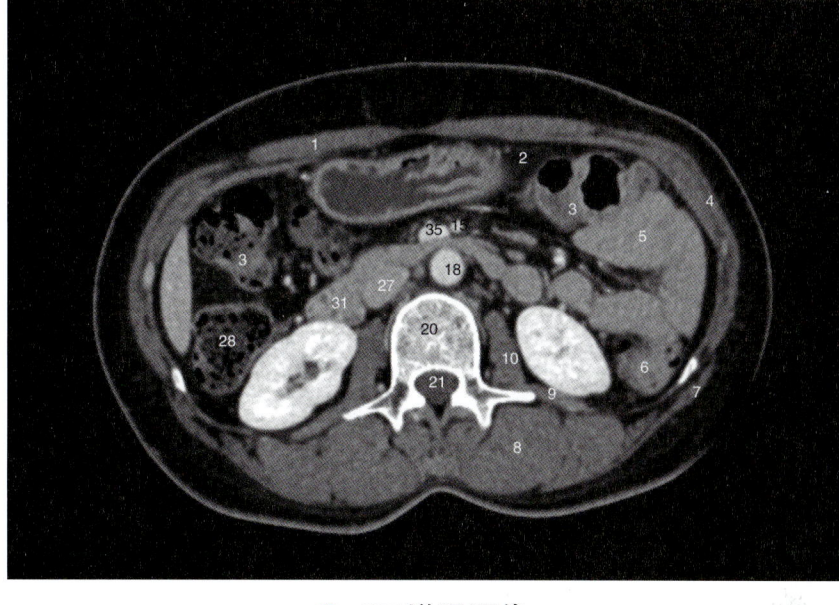

C. CT 增强图像

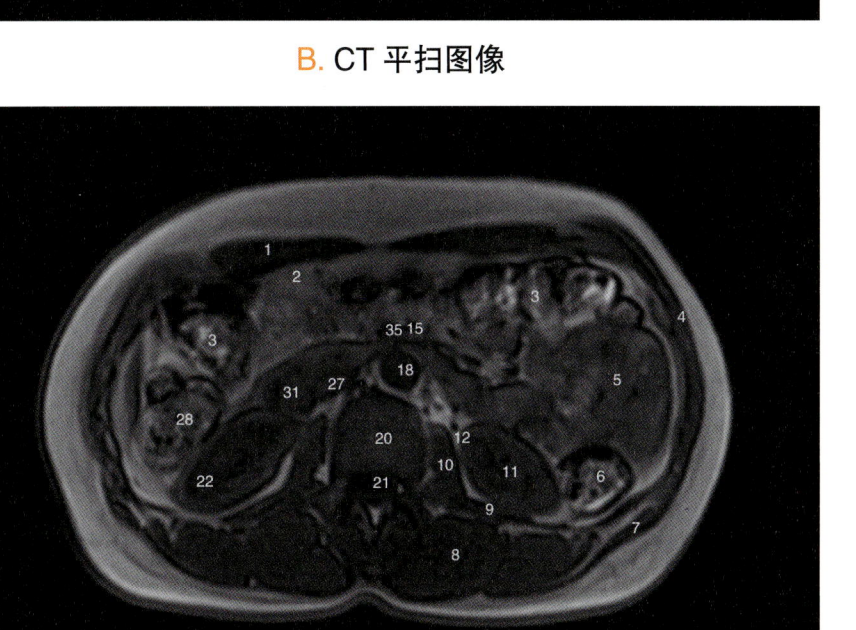

D. MR T1WI

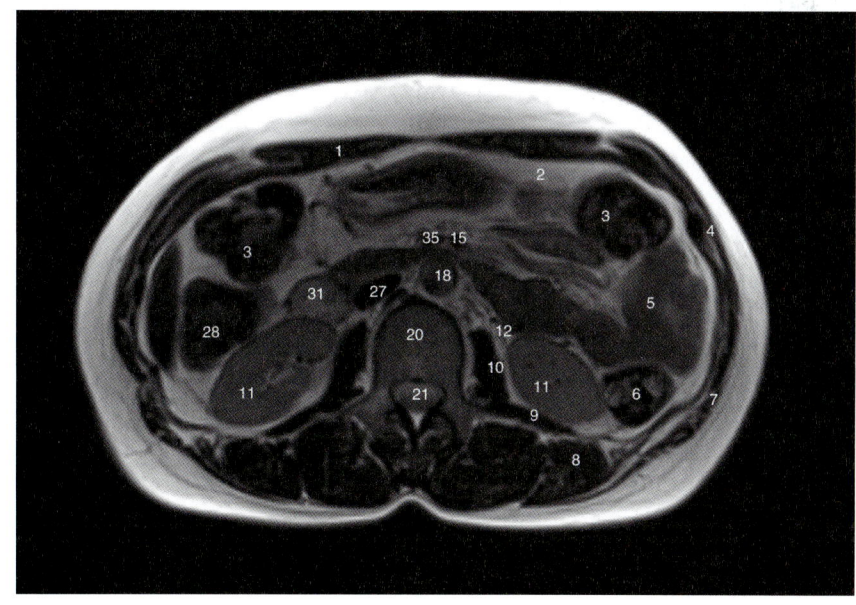

E. MR T2WI

关键结构：胰十二指肠下动脉，横结肠，空肠。

此断面经过第 2 腰椎椎体。

下腔静脉和腹主动脉仍走行在脊柱前方。左肾左前方可见输尿管断面，表现为小圆形低密度结构。在胰头与肠系膜上静脉之间可见胰十二指肠下动脉，该动脉常于十二指肠水平段的上缘起源于肠系膜上动脉或其第一个空肠分支，并走行在肠系膜上静脉的后方，向后至胰钩突，然后分成前、后支。前支向右向下走行，然后向前到达胰头下缘，再向上走行与胰十二指肠上动脉前支相吻合。后支向后上方向右走行，至胰头下缘的后方，与胰十二指肠上后动脉相吻合。两支都供应胰头及其钩突、十二指肠降段和水平段的血液[75]。极少的情况下，前支和后支从肠系膜上动脉或第一空肠动脉分开。CTA 图像可以显示胰十二指肠下动脉，有助于判断胰腺癌对胰腺外血管的侵犯[76]。

腹部连续横断层 75（FH.10430）

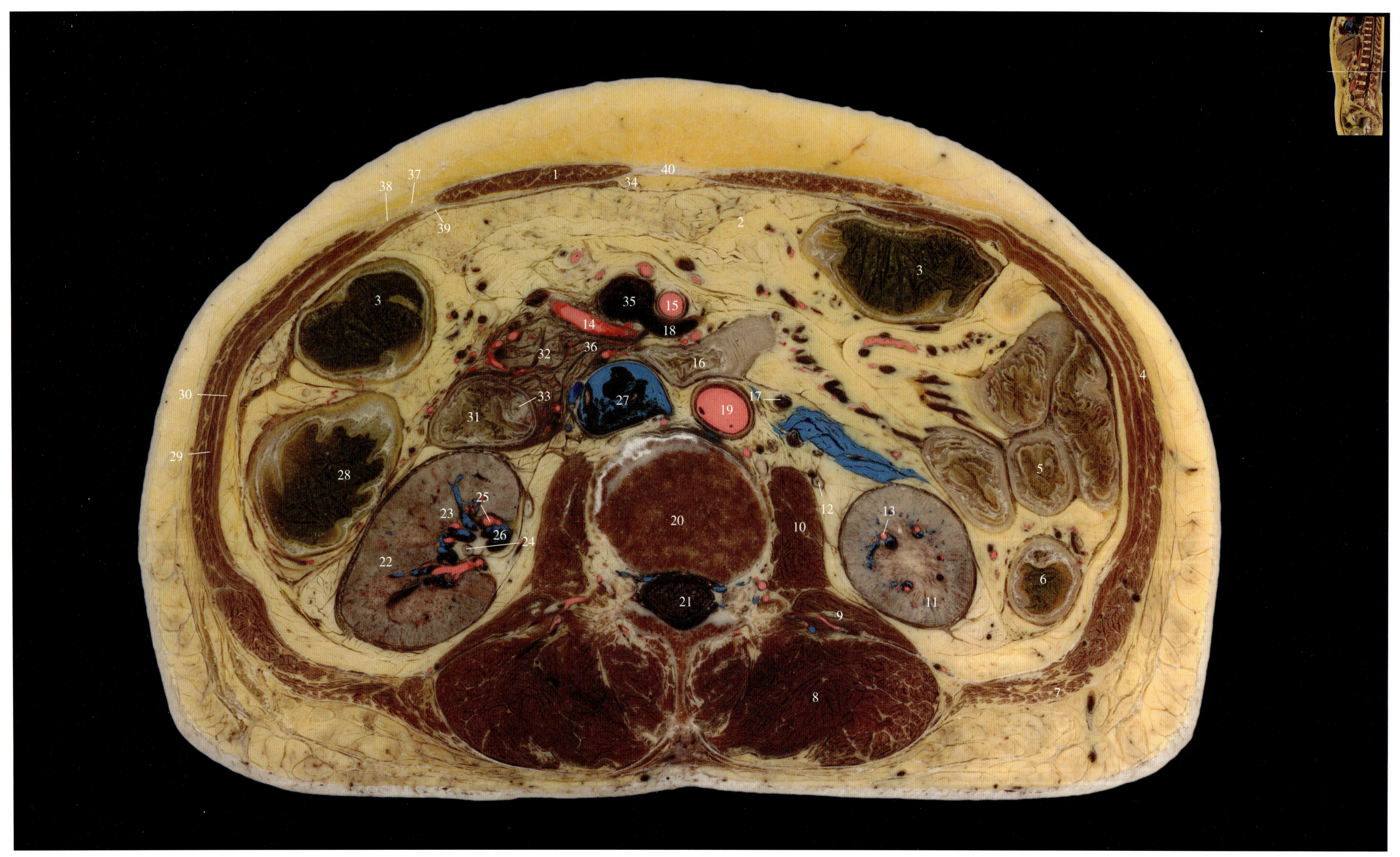

A. 断层标本图像

1. 腹直肌 rectus abdominis
2. 大网膜 greater omentum
3. 横结肠 transverse colon
4. 腹外斜肌 obliquus externus abdominis
5. 空肠 jejunum
6. 降结肠 descending colon
7. 背阔肌 latissimus dorsi
8. 竖脊肌 erector spinae
9. 腰方肌 quadratus lumborum
10. 腰大肌 psoas major
11. 左肾 left kidney
12. 左输尿管 left ureter
13. 左肾动脉 left renal artery
14. 胰十二指肠下动脉 inferior pancreaticoduodenal artery
15. 肠系膜上动脉 superior mesenteric artery
16. 十二指肠升部 ascending part of duodenum
17. 肠系膜下静脉 inferior mesenteric vein
18. 空肠静脉 jejunal vein
19. 腹主动脉 abdominal aorta
20. 第 2 腰椎椎体 body of the 2nd lumbar vertebra
21. 马尾 cauda equina
22. 右肾 right kidney
23. 肾锥体 renal pyramid
24. 右肾盂 right renal pelvis
25. 右肾动脉 right renal artery
26. 右肾静脉 right renal vein
27. 下腔静脉 inferior vena cava
28. 升结肠 ascending colon
29. 腹内斜肌 obliquus internus abdominis
30. 腹横肌 transversus abdominis
31. 十二指肠降部 descending part of duodenum
32. 胰头 head of pancreas
33. 十二指肠大乳头 major duodenal papilla
34. 肝圆韧带 ligamentum teres hepatis
35. 肠系膜上静脉 superior mesenteric vein
36. 胰钩突 uncinate process of pancreas
37. 腹外斜肌腱膜 aponeurosis of obliquus externus abdominis
38. 腹内斜肌腱膜 aponeurosis of obliquus internus abdominis
39. 腹横肌腱膜 aponeurosis of transversus abdominis
40. 白线 linea alba

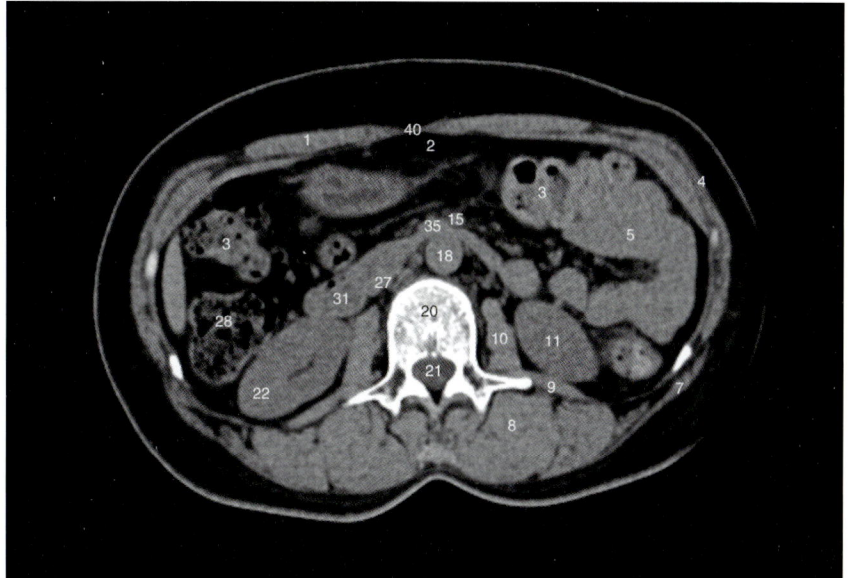

B. CT 平扫图像

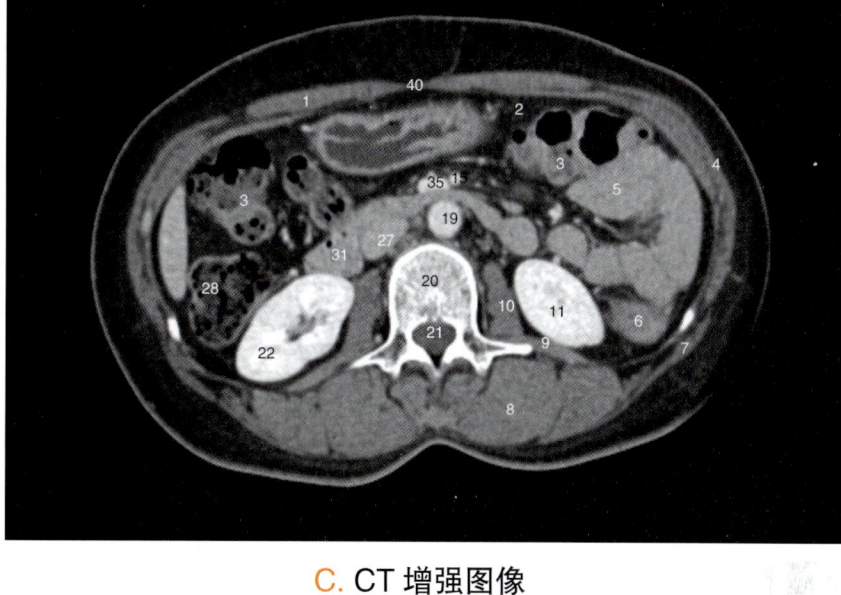

C. CT 增强图像

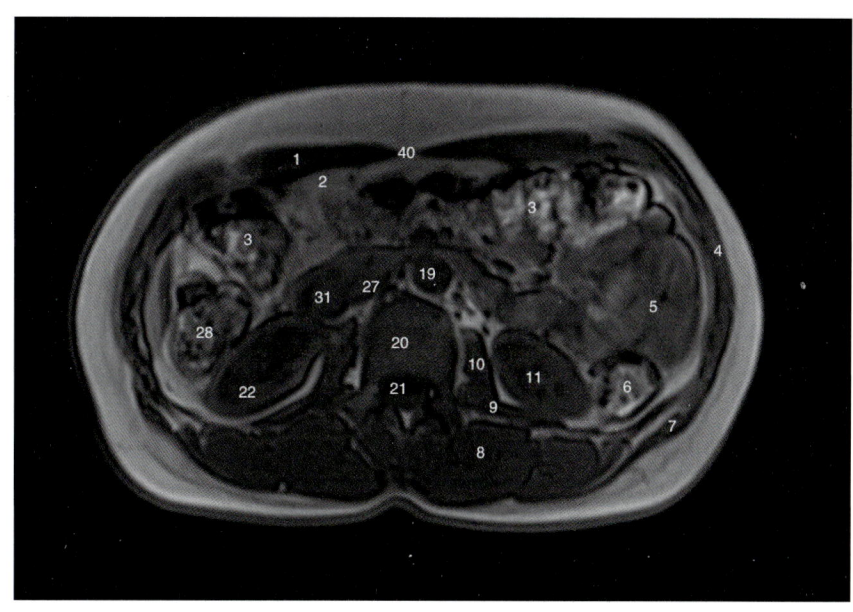

D. MR T1WI

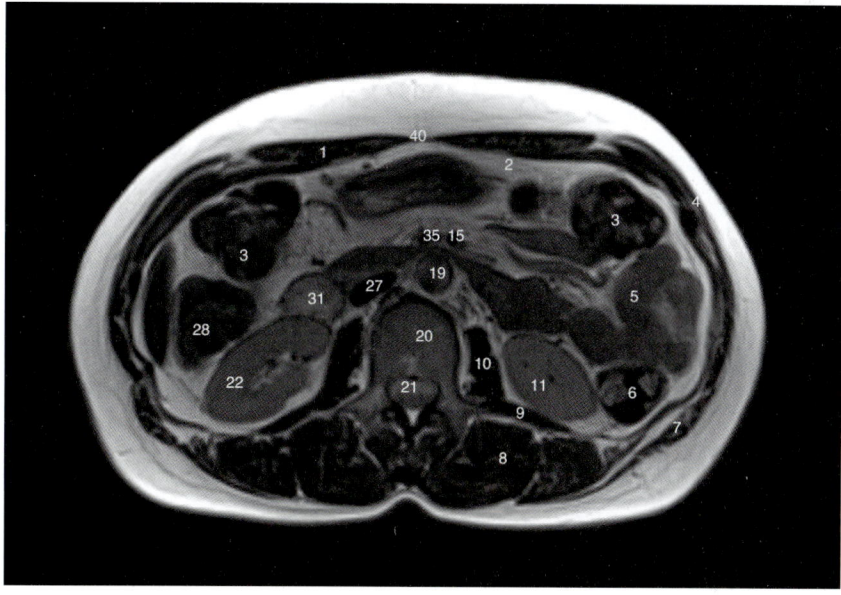

E. MR T2WI

关键结构：十二指肠大乳头，空肠静脉。

此断面经过第 2 腰椎椎体。

左肾体积明显缩小。腹腔前侧中份可见空肠静脉由肠系膜上静脉发出。成年人十二指肠长约 25 cm，在仰卧位的第 1 和第 3 腰椎水平之间形成一个 "C" 形，将胰头和钩突部包裹 "C" 形的凹面，当出现较大的胰头肿瘤时，钡餐造影该 "C" 形明显增大。十二指肠大乳头可伸入肠腔内 1 cm，距幽门 8~10 cm。胆总管开口在降部下 1/3 段者占 66%，中 1/3 者占 27%，上 1/3 者占 4%。十二指肠小乳头位于大乳头上方约 2 cm 处。胆总管位置开口的变异对于胆道外科手术及 ERCP 治疗须引起重视。当该部位发生结石、炎症或肿瘤时，往往导致上游胆管的扩张，临床表现为黄疸[77]。增强 CT 和 MR 动脉期图像有助于十二指肠乳头及其周围正常解剖结构的观察，从而为壶腹部疾病诊断和治疗提供有价值的信息[78]。十二指肠原发性肿瘤中，发生于降部的腺癌最为多见。

腹部连续横断层 76（FH.10410）

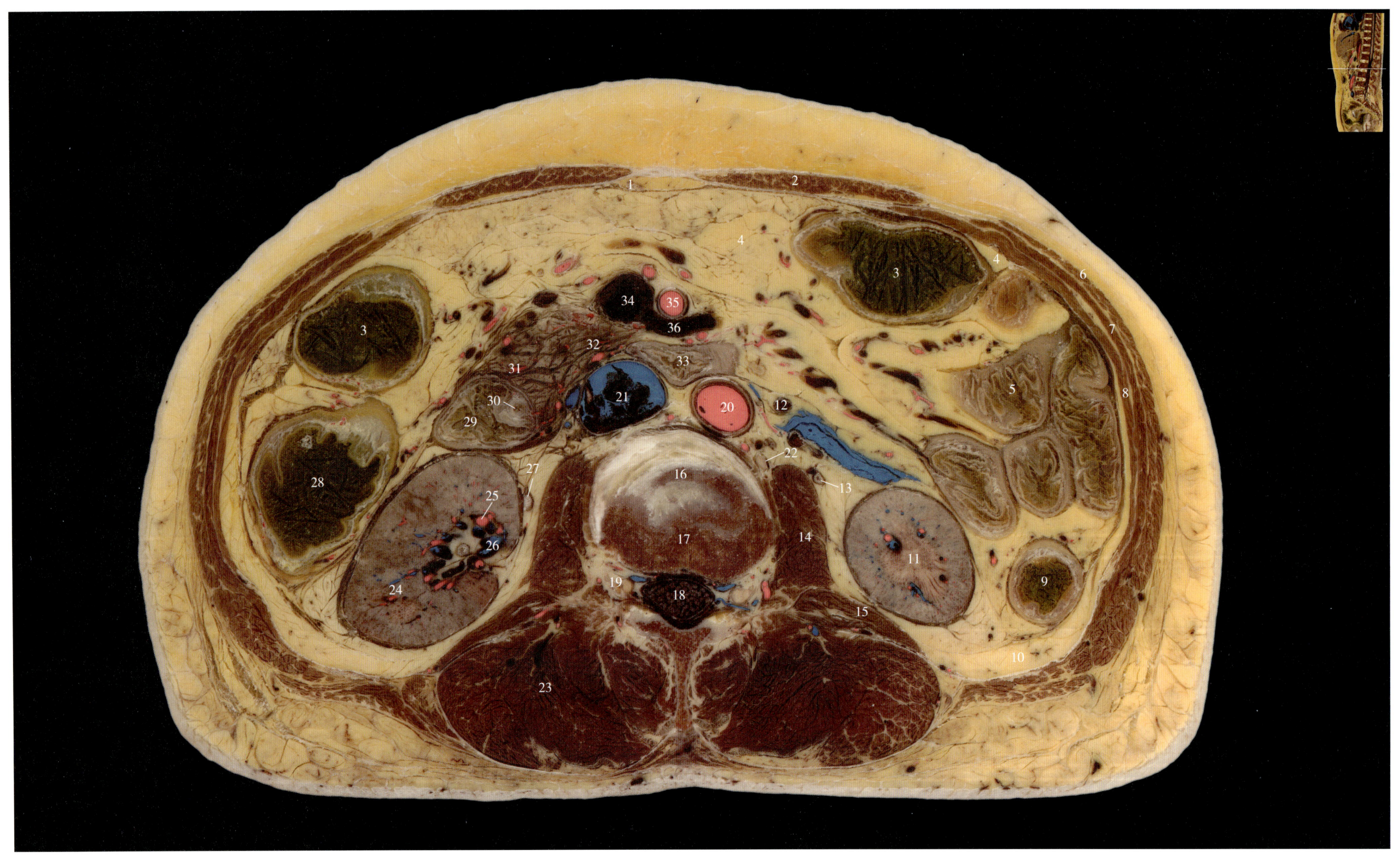

A. 断层标本图像

1. 肝圆韧带 ligamentum teres hepatis
2. 腹直肌 rectus abdominis
3. 横结肠 transverse colon
4. 大网膜 greater omentum
5. 空肠 jejunum
6. 腹外斜肌 obliquus externus abdominis
7. 腹内斜肌 obliquus internus abdominis
8. 腹横肌 transverses abdominis
9. 降结肠 descending colon
10. 腹膜外脂肪 extraperitoneal fat
11. 左肾 left kidney
12. 肠系膜下静脉 inferior mesenteric vein
13. 左输尿管 left ureter
14. 腰大肌 psoas major
15. 腰方肌 quadratus lumborum
16. L2-3 椎间盘 L2-3 intervertebral disc
17. 第 2 腰椎椎体 body of the 2nd lumbar vertebra
18. 马尾 cauda equina
19. 第 2 腰神经 2nd lumbar nerve
20. 腹主动脉 abdominal aorta
21. 下腔静脉 inferior vena cava
22. 左交感干 left sympathetic trunk
23. 竖脊肌 erector spinae
24. 右肾 right kidney
25. 右肾动脉 right renal artery
26. 右肾静脉 right renal vein
27. 右输尿管 right ureter
28. 升结肠 ascending colon
29. 十二指肠降部 descending part of duodenum
30. 十二指肠大乳头 major duodenal papilla
31. 胰头 head of pancreas
32. 胰钩突 uncinate process of pancreas
33. 十二指肠水平部 horizontal part of duodenum
34. 肠系膜上静脉 superior mesenteric vein
35. 肠系膜上动脉 superior mesenteric artery
36. 空肠静脉 jejunal vein

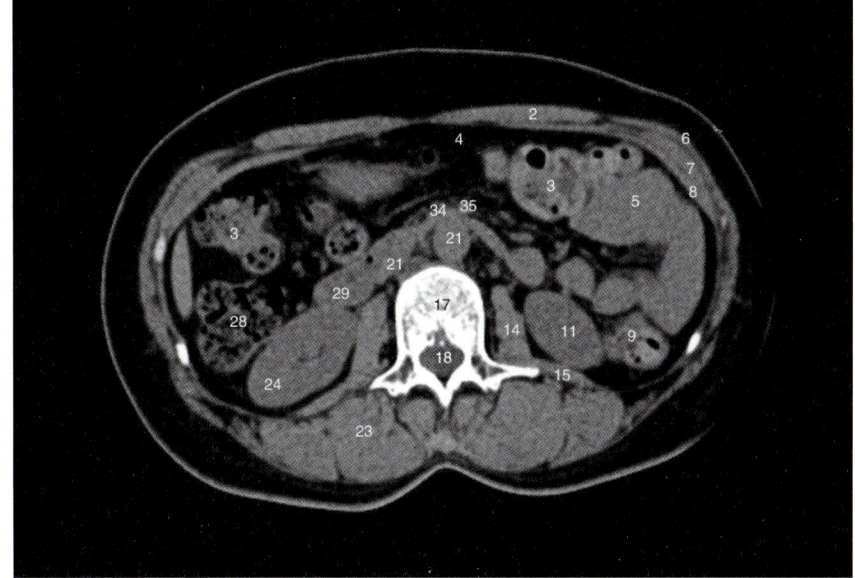

B. CT 平扫图像

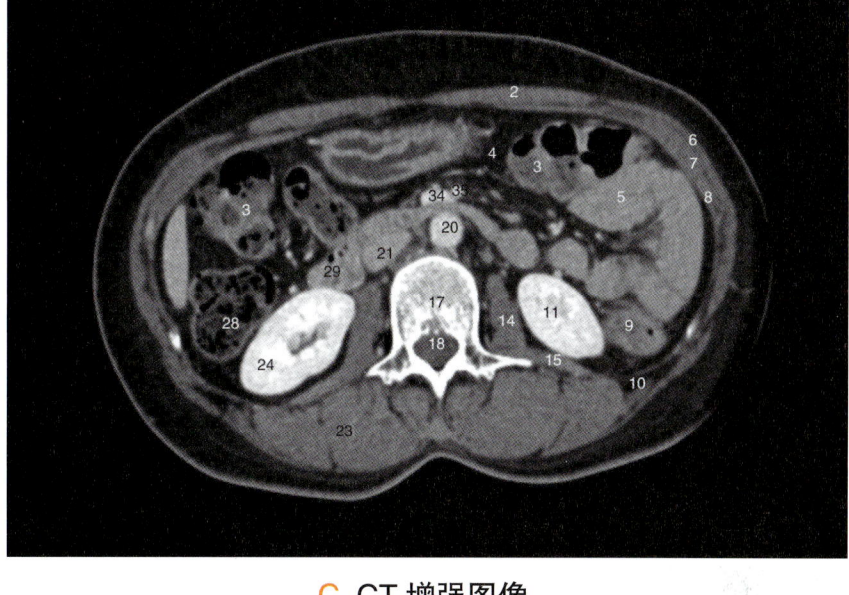

C. CT 增强图像

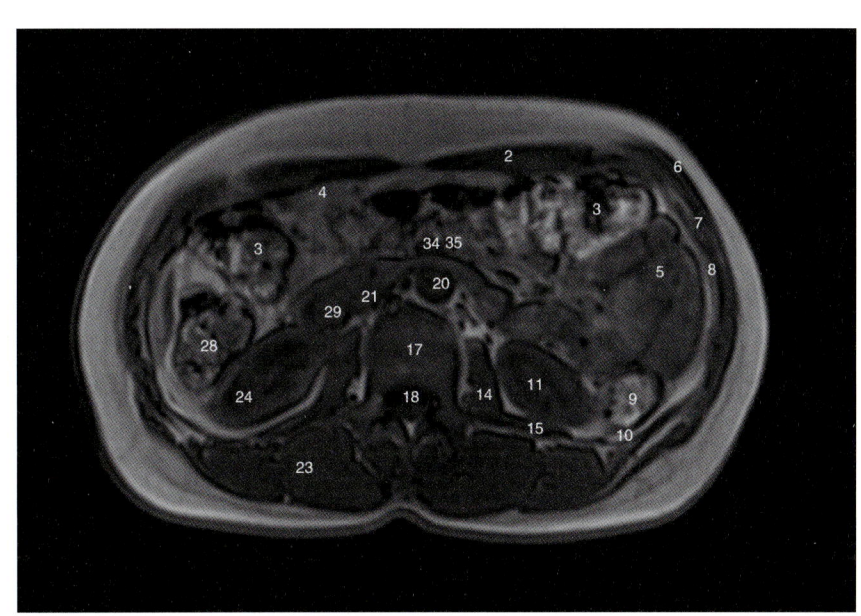

D. MR T1WI

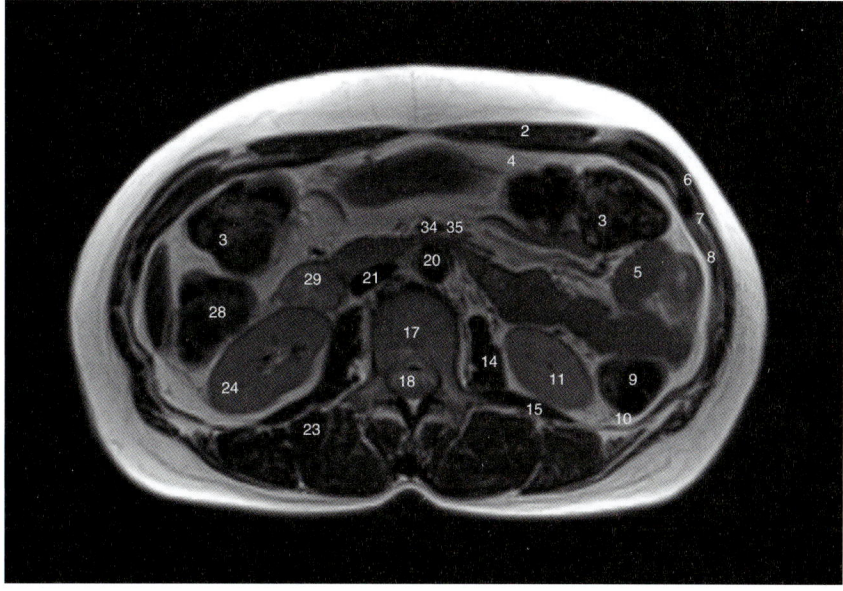

E. MR T2WI

关键结构：十二指肠水平部，空肠，输尿管。

此断面经过第 2 腰椎椎体和 L2-3 椎间盘。

右侧输尿管在该断面显示。十二指肠升部向右移行为十二指肠水平部，走行在下腔静脉与腹主动脉前方，十二指肠升部消失。十二指肠水平部又称十二指肠下部，长约 10 cm，起自十二指肠下曲，横过下腔静脉和第 3 腰椎椎体的前方，至腹主动脉前方和第 3 腰椎椎体左前方，移行为升部。肠系膜上动、静脉紧贴十二指肠水平部前面下行，在某些情况下，肠系膜上动脉可压迫该部引起十二指肠排泄延迟甚至梗阻。在 CT 平扫图像上，十二指肠水平部表现为位于腹主动脉和下腔静脉的管状结构，增强图像可较清晰地显示肠壁的分层。十二指肠水平部可根据前方的肠系膜上动脉及上方的胰头而进行定位。发生急性胰腺炎时，常可见十二指肠水平部及降段肠壁增厚、分层，邻近脂肪组织模糊。

腹部连续横断层 77（FH.10390）

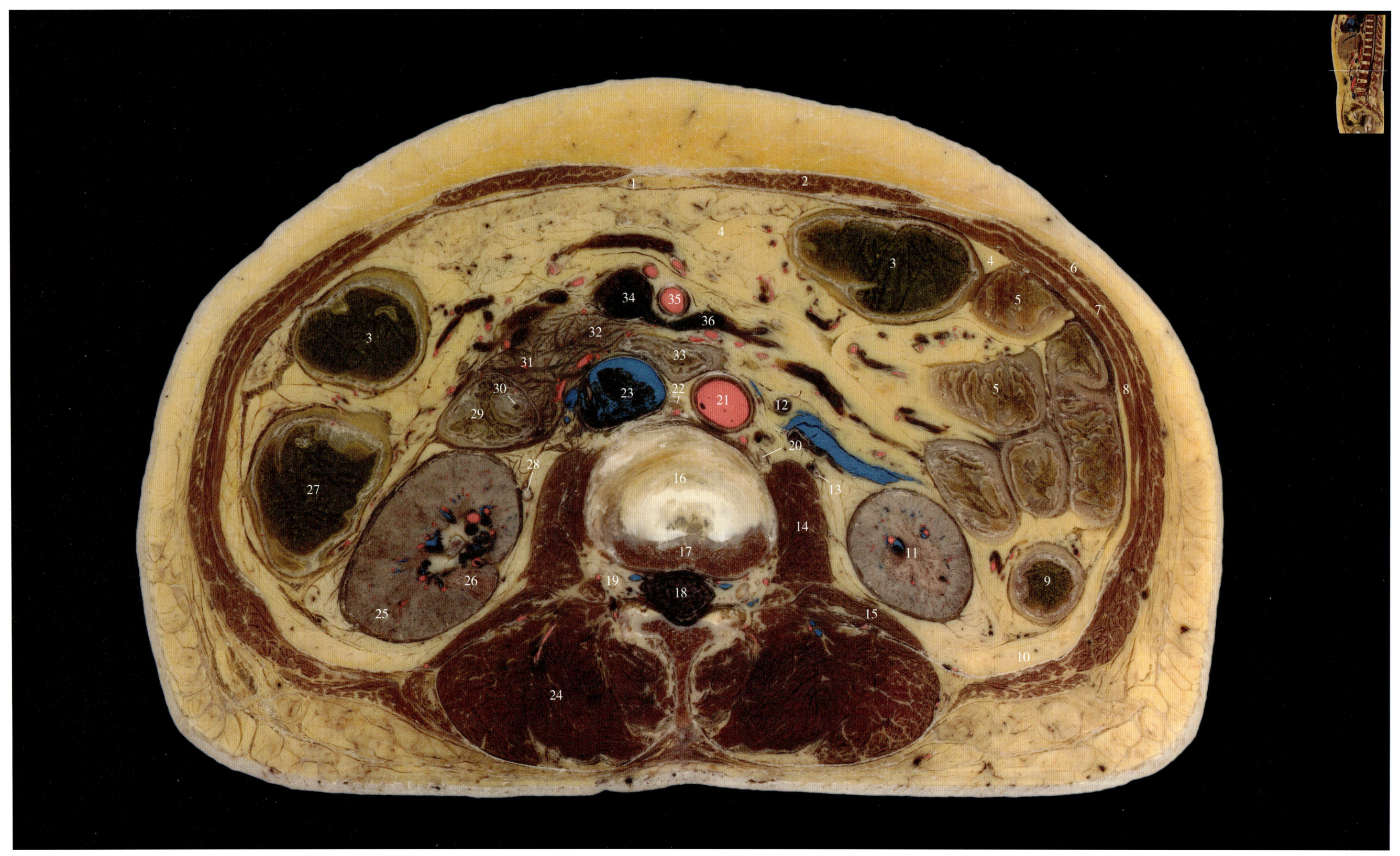

A. 断层标本图像

1. 肝圆韧带 ligamentum teres hepatis
2. 腹直肌 rectus abdominis
3. 横结肠 transverse colon
4. 大网膜 greater omentum
5. 空肠 jejunum
6. 腹外斜肌 obliquus externus abdominis
7. 腹内斜肌 obliquus internus abdominis
8. 腹横肌 transverses abdominis
9. 降结肠 descending colon
10. 腹膜外脂肪 extraperitoneal fat
11. 左肾 left kidney
12. 肠系膜下静脉 inferior mesenteric vein
13. 左输尿管 left ureter
14. 腰大肌 psoas major
15. 腰方肌 quadratus lumborum
16. L2-3 椎间盘 L2-3 intervertebral disc
17. 第 2 腰椎椎体 body of the 2nd lumbar vertebra
18. 马尾 cauda equina
19. 第 2 腰神经 2nd lumbar nerve
20. 左交感干 left sympathetic trunk
21. 腹主动脉 abdominal aorta
22. 中间腰淋巴结 intermediate lumbar lymph node
23. 下腔静脉 inferior vena cava
24. 竖脊肌 erector spinae
25. 右肾 right kidney
26. 肾锥体 renal pyramid
27. 升结肠 ascending colon
28. 右输尿管 right ureter
29. 十二指肠降部 descending part of duodenum
30. 十二指肠大乳头 major duodenal papilla
31. 胰头 head of pancreas
32. 胰钩突 uncinate process of pancreas
33. 十二指肠水平部 horizontal part of duodenum
34. 肠系膜上静脉 superior mesenteric vein
35. 肠系膜上动脉 superior mesenteric artery
36. 空肠静脉 jejunal vein

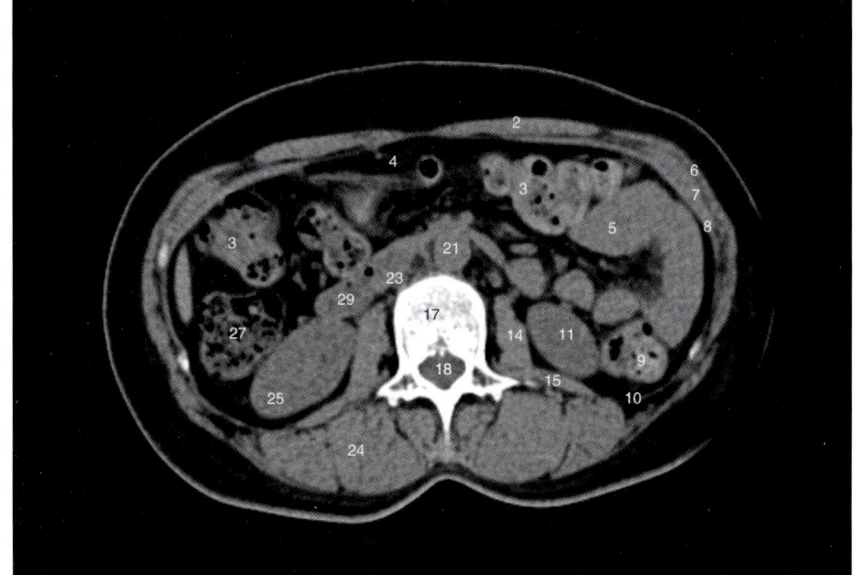

B. CT 平扫图像

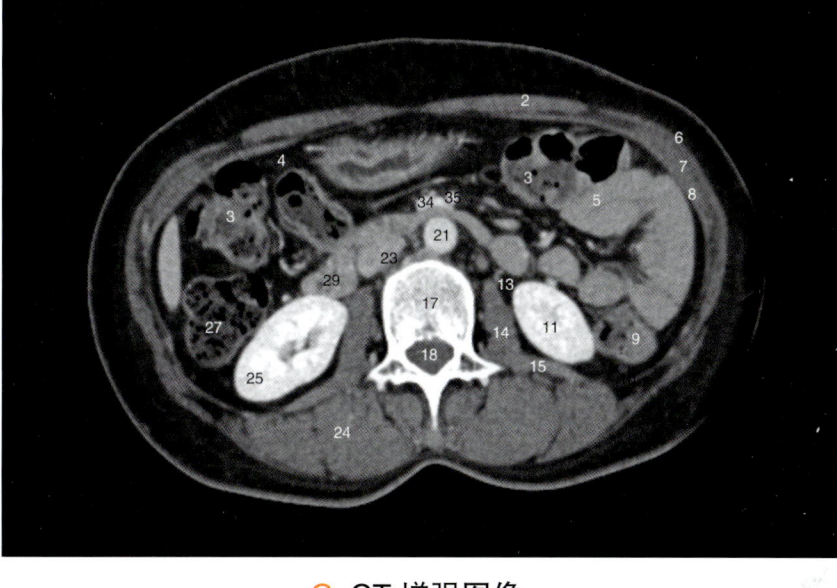

C. CT 增强图像

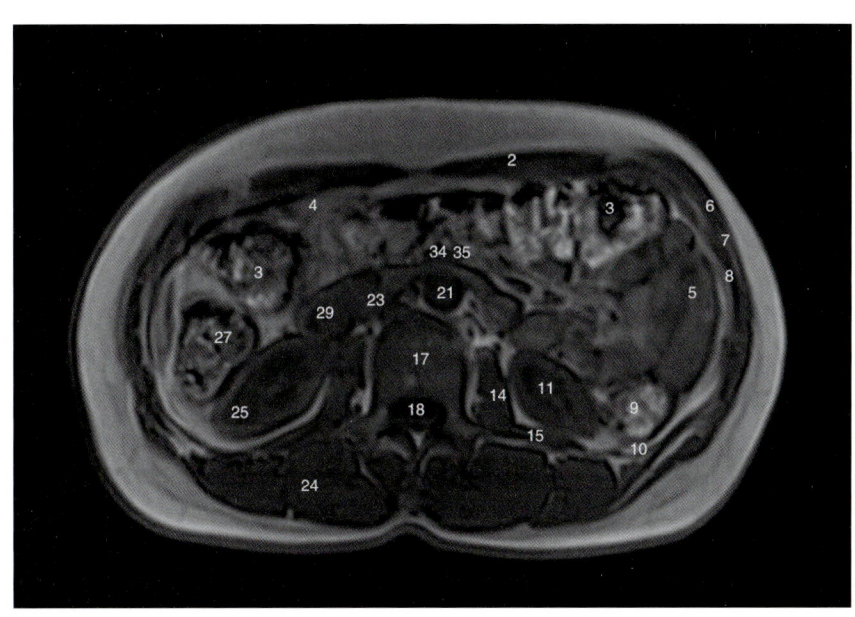

D. MR T1WI

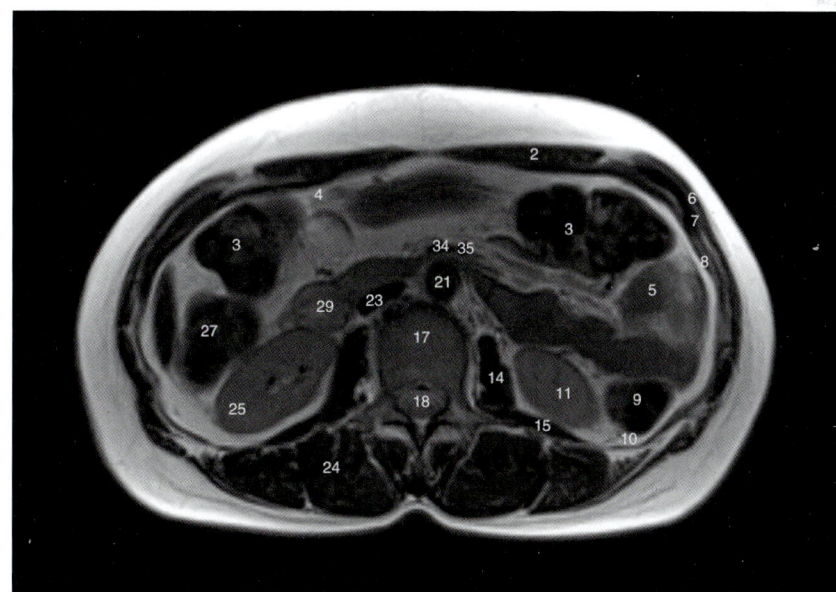

E. MR T2WI

关键结构：肠系膜上静脉，空肠静脉。

此断面经过第 2 腰椎椎体和 L2-3 椎间盘。

腰大肌附着在脊柱两侧，脊柱后方为竖脊肌，在竖脊肌与腰大肌间可见腰方肌。剩余的胰腺居腹后部中间，此断面仅剩胰头和胰钩突结构显示。在胰钩突的左前方可见肠系膜上静脉及由此发出的空肠静脉。肠系膜上静脉引流小肠、盲肠、部分升结肠和横结肠、部分胃和大网膜的血液。终末回肠、盲肠和阑尾的分支连合在小肠系膜内形成肠系膜上静脉。在肠系膜内，肠系膜上静脉向上至肠系膜上动脉的右侧，越过右输尿管、下腔静脉、十二指肠第 3 部和胰钩突的前方，在幽门水平面（第 1 腰椎下缘）胰颈的后方与脾静脉汇合形成门静脉。肠系膜上动、静脉是中腹部的重要血管，它既是胰颈、钩突和左肾静脉的识别标志，又有助于辨识肠系膜根的起始段，还在中肠扭转不良的诊断中具有重要意义。在影像断层图像上，可根据门静脉的延伸判断肠系膜上静脉。克罗恩病、腹腔感染或腹腔静脉回流受阻可引起肠系膜静脉血栓形成，CTA 后处理图像可清晰地显示肠系膜上静脉主干内的血栓，为诊断该病提供直接证据[79]。此外，CT 增强检查有助于显示引流肠管肠壁水肿与强化程度、有无坏死积气、肠腔积液及肠系膜脂肪密度的变化等[80,81]。

腹部连续横断层 78（FH.10370）

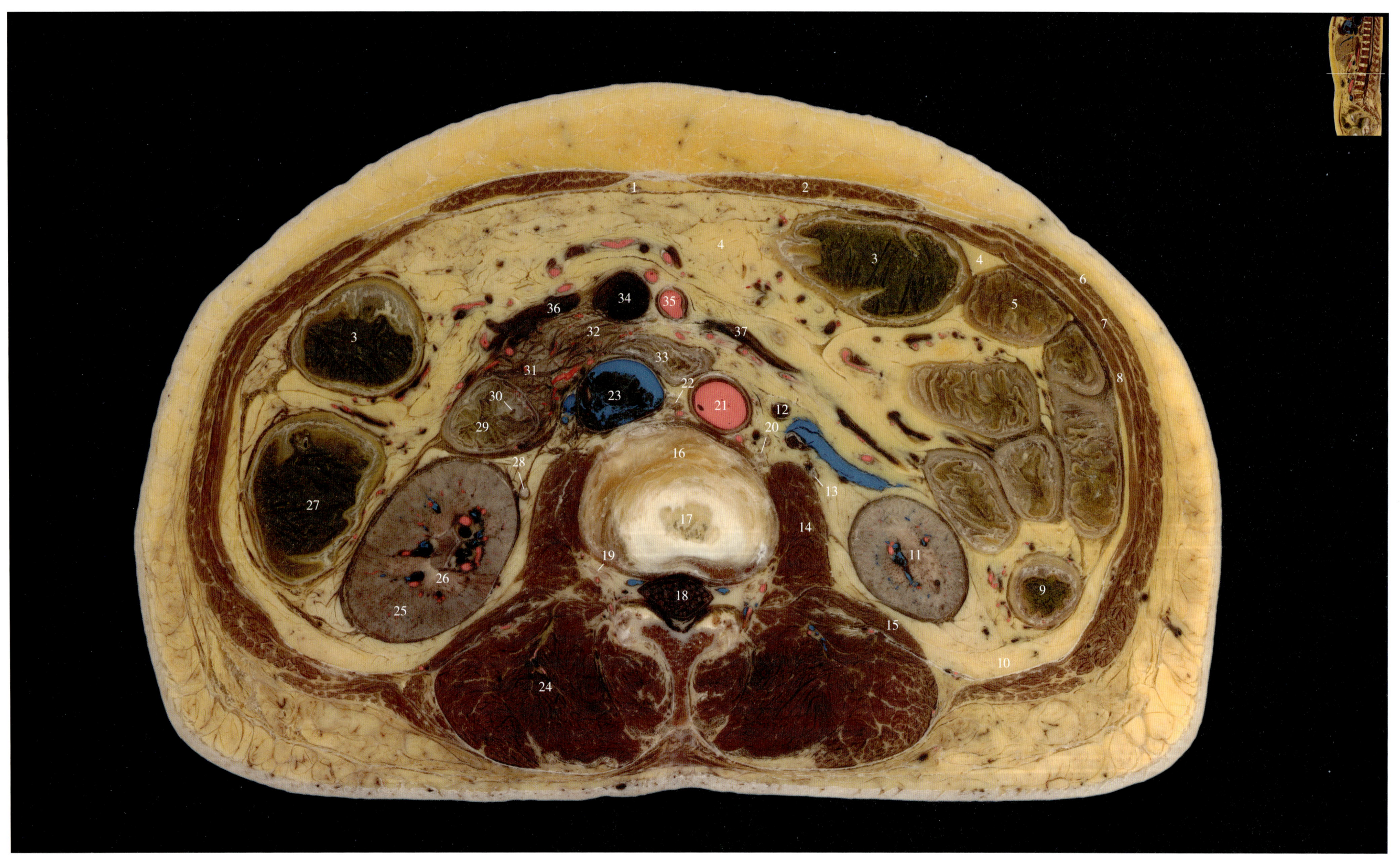

A. 断层标本图像

1. 肝圆韧带 ligamentum teres hepatis
2. 腹直肌 rectus abdominis
3. 横结肠 transverse colon
4. 大网膜 greater omentum
5. 空肠 jejunum
6. 腹外斜肌 obliquus externus abdominis
7. 腹内斜肌 obliquus internus abdominis
8. 腹横肌 transverses abdominis
9. 降结肠 descending colon
10. 腹膜外脂肪 extraperitoneal fat
11. 左肾 left kidney
12. 肠系膜下静脉 inferior mesenteric vein
13. 左输尿管 left ureter
14. 腰大肌 psoas major
15. 腰方肌 quadratus lumborum
16. L2-3 椎间盘 L2-3 intervertebral disc
17. 髓核 nucleus pulposus
18. 马尾 cauda equina
19. 第 2 腰神经 2nd lumbar nerve
20. 左交感干 left sympathetic trunk
21. 腹主动脉 abdominal aorta
22. 中间腰淋巴结 intermediate lumbar lymph node
23. 下腔静脉 inferior vena cava
24. 竖脊肌 erector spinae
25. 右肾 right kidney
26. 肾锥体 renal pyramid
27. 升结肠 ascending colon
28. 右输尿管 right ureter
29. 十二指肠降部 descending part of duodenum
30. 十二指肠大乳头 major duodenal papilla
31. 胰头 head of pancreas
32. 胰钩突 uncinate process of pancreas
33. 十二指肠水平部 horizontal part of duodenum
34. 肠系膜上静脉 superior mesenteric vein
35. 肠系膜上动脉 superior mesenteric artery
36. 结肠静脉 colic vein
37. 空肠静脉 jejunal vein

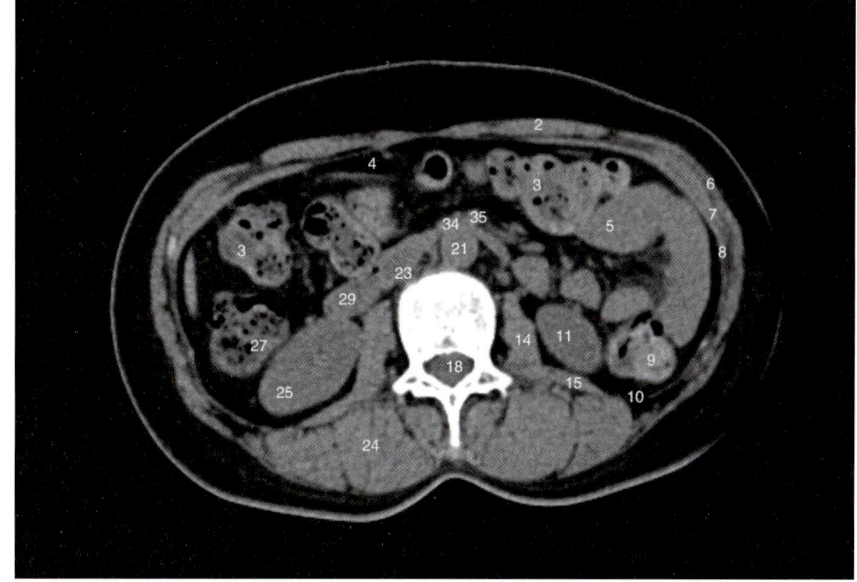

B. CT 平扫图像

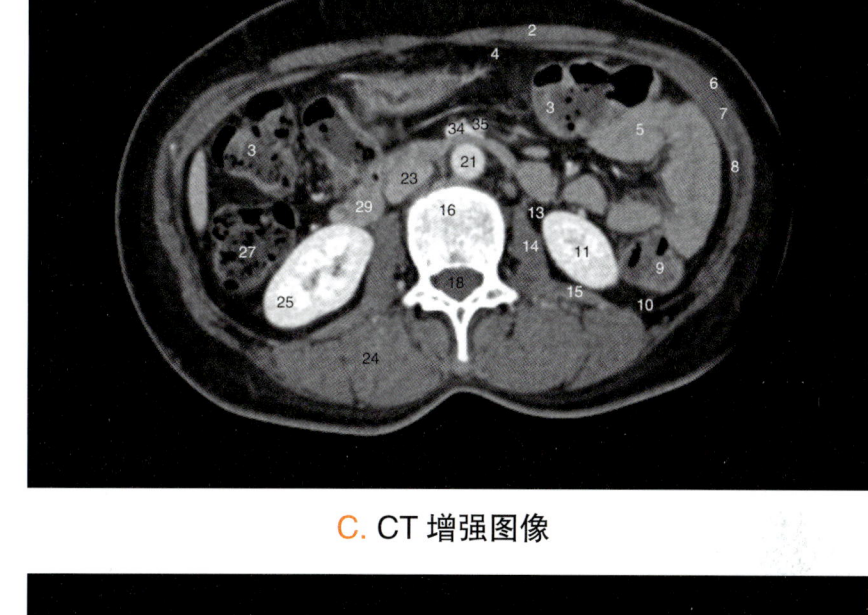

C. CT 增强图像

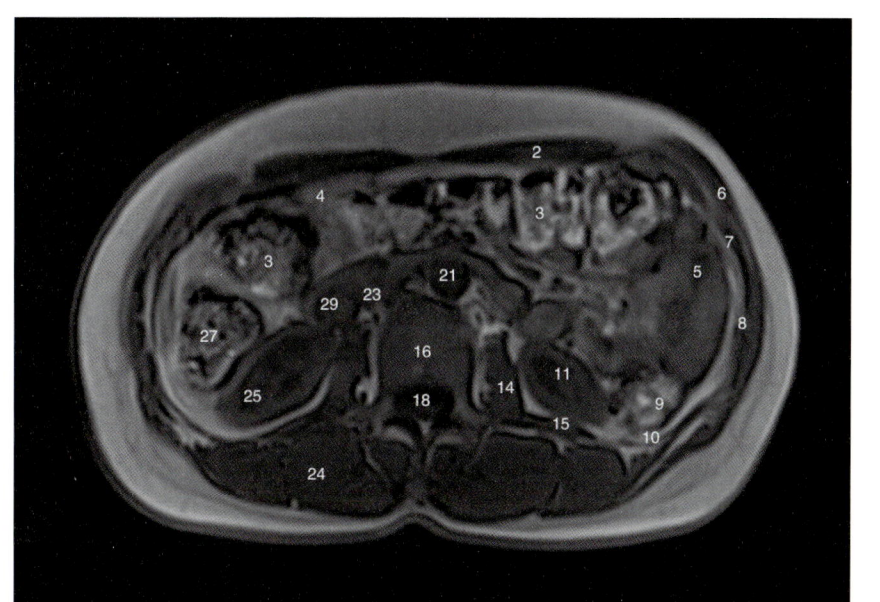

D. MR T1WI

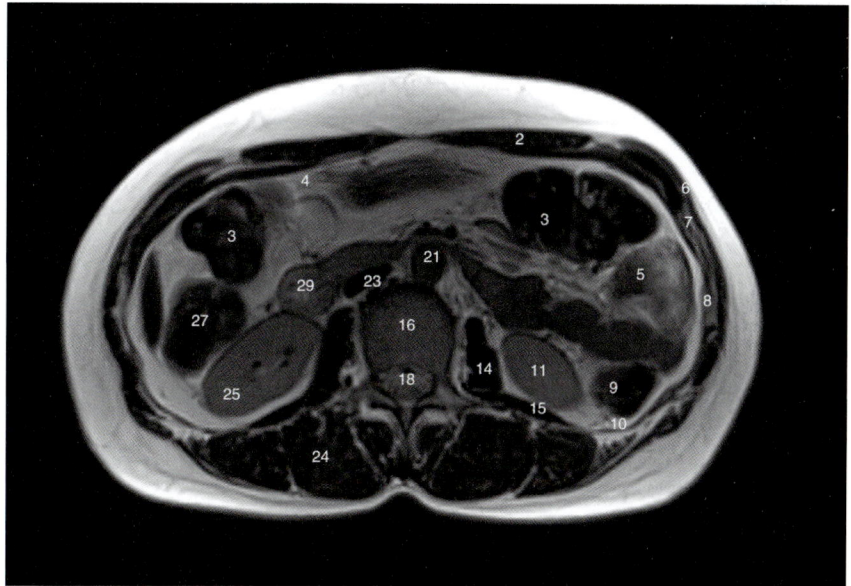

E. MR T2WI

关键结构：L2-3 椎间盘，第 2 腰神经。

此断面经过 L2-3 椎间盘。

后方正中可见 L2-3 椎间盘，中心为髓核，外周为环形的纤维环和软骨板。腰椎间盘位于两个椎体之间，由髓核、纤维环和软骨板三部分构成，是一个具有流体力学特性的结构。其中，髓核为中央部分，纤维环为周围部分，包绕髓核、软骨板直接与椎体骨组织相连，整个腰椎间盘的厚度 8~10 mm。CT 和 MRI 是显示椎间盘及其病变的主要方式，以后者更为敏感。腰椎间盘感染时，MRI 显示椎间盘充血水肿呈高信号，可有小的脓肿形成，相邻椎体呈现以长 T2 为主的混杂高信号，椎旁及椎管内硬膜外间隙可形成脓肿[82]。腰神经根共 5 对，在椎间孔内由前根和后根组成腰神经，L1~4 的椎间神经节位于椎间孔内，L5 间神经节位于骶管内。腰神经发出脊膜支组成脊膜丛，支配相应节段的脊髓膜。发出交通支至椎旁交感神经干。高位的腰椎间盘突出症，突出的椎间盘可压迫 L1、L2 和 L3 神经根，出现相应的神经根支配的腹股沟区疼痛或大腿内侧疼痛。目前，MRI 可对腰神经根进行显示，从而进行疾病的诊断和评估。

腹部连续横断层 79（FH.10350）

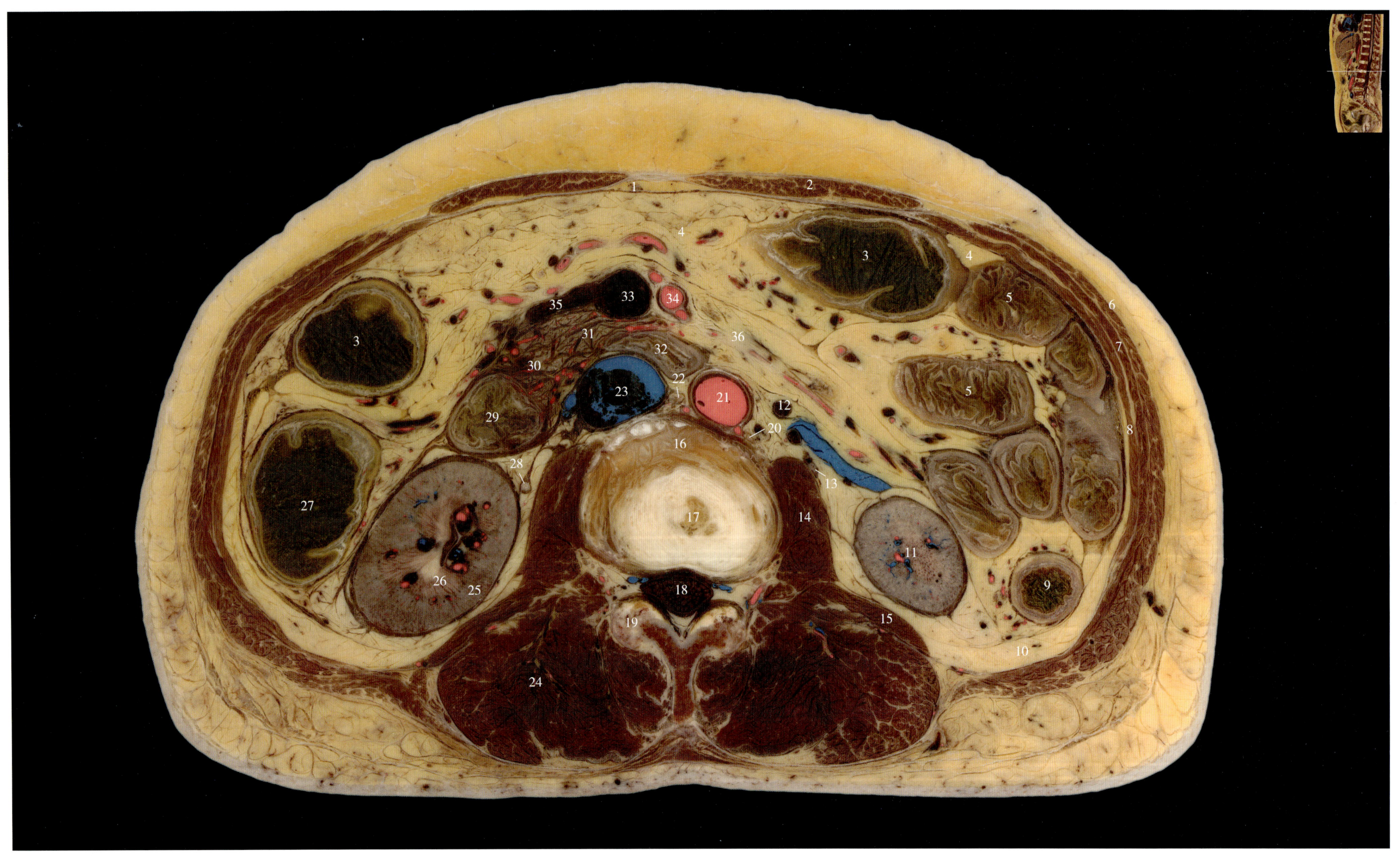

A. 断层标本图像

1. 肝圆韧带 ligamentum teres hepatis
2. 腹直肌 rectus abdominis
3. 横结肠 transverse colon
4. 大网膜 greater omentum
5. 空肠 jejunum
6. 腹外斜肌 obliquus externus abdominis
7. 腹内斜肌 obliquus internus abdominis
8. 腹横肌 transverses abdominis
9. 降结肠 descending colon
10. 腹膜外脂肪 extraperitoneal fat
11. 左肾 left kidney
12. 肠系膜下静脉 inferior mesenteric vein
13. 左输尿管 left ureter
14. 腰大肌 psoas major
15. 腰方肌 quadratus lumborum
16. L2-3 椎间盘 L2-3 intervertebral disc
17. 髓核 nucleus pulposus
18. 马尾 cauda equina
19. 关节突关节 zygapophysial joint
20. 左交感干 left sympathetic trunk
21. 腹主动脉 abdominal aorta
22. 中间腰淋巴结 intermediate lumbar lymph node
23. 下腔静脉 inferior vena cava
24. 竖脊肌 erector spinae
25. 右肾 right kidney
26. 肾锥体 renal pyramid
27. 升结肠 ascending colon
28. 右输尿管 right ureter
29. 十二指肠降部 descending part of duodenum
30. 胰头 head of pancreas
31. 胰钩突 uncinate process of pancreas
32. 十二指肠水平部 horizontal part of duodenum
33. 肠系膜上静脉 superior mesenteric vein
34. 肠系膜上动脉 superior mesenteric artery
35. 结肠静脉 colic vein
36. 肠系膜 mesentery

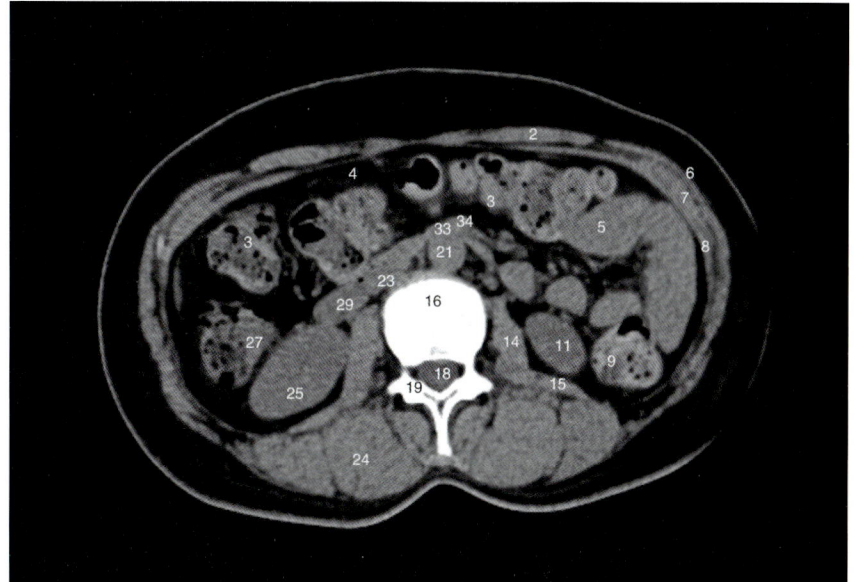

B. CT 平扫图像

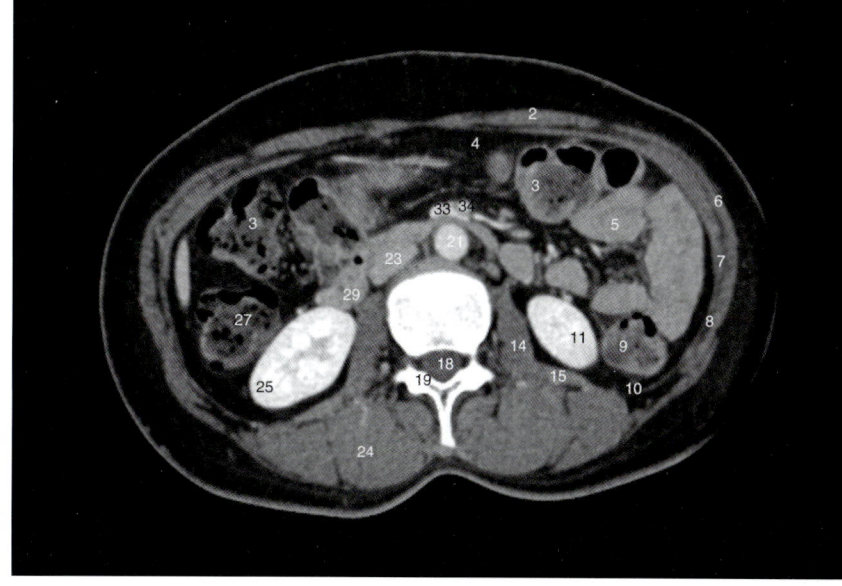

C. CT 增强图像

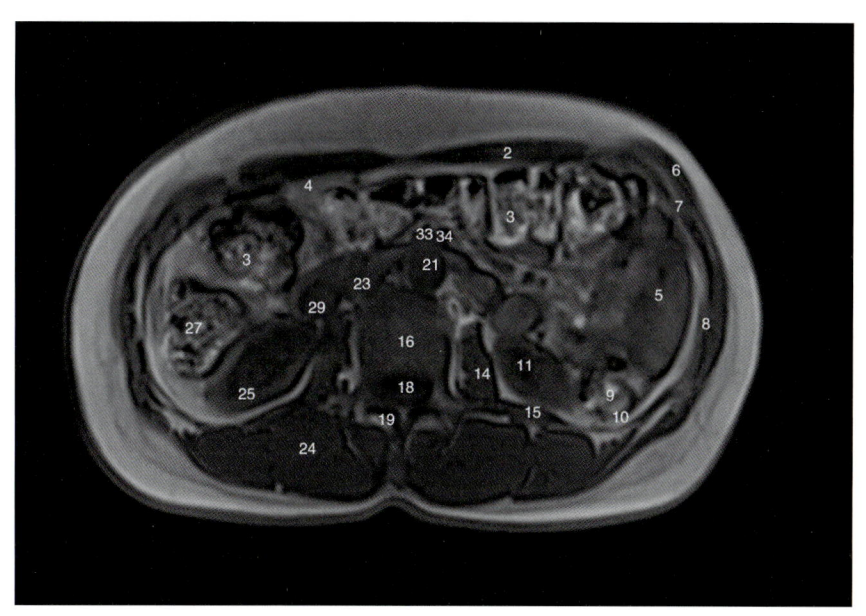

D. MR T1WI

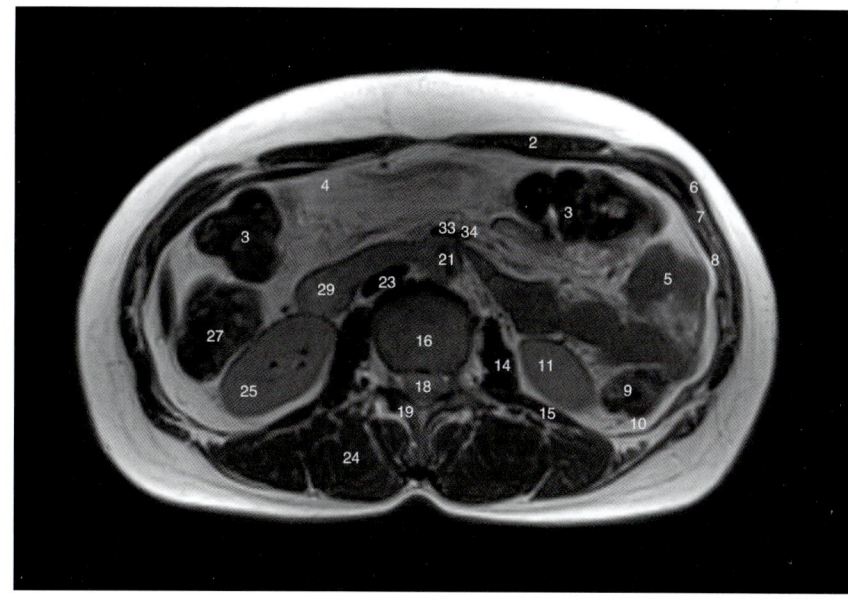

E. MR T2WI

关键结构：结肠静脉，髓核，左肾下极。

此断面经过 L2-3 椎间盘。

结肠静脉主干在此断面出现，并可见汇入肠系膜上静脉。十二指肠水平部继续向右移行，居肠系膜上静脉与下腔静脉之间。结肠静脉主要汇入肠系膜上静脉和肠系膜下静脉，直肠有部分静脉血经直肠中静脉汇入髂内静脉或阴部内静脉。肠系膜上静脉的结肠支收集中肠（盲肠、阑尾、升结肠和横结肠近端 2/3）的血液，肠系膜下静脉收集后肠（横结肠远端 1/3、降结肠、乙状结肠、直肠和肛管上段）的血液[62]。髓核为椎间盘的中间组成部分，富含水分，在 20 岁以前构成髓核的主要物质是大量蛋白多糖复合体、胶原纤维和纤维软骨，随着年龄的增长，髓核中的蛋白多糖解聚增多，水分逐渐减少，胶原增粗并逐渐被纤维软骨所替代，故老年人发生椎间盘突出的机会明显高于青壮年。

腹部连续横断层 80（FH.10330）

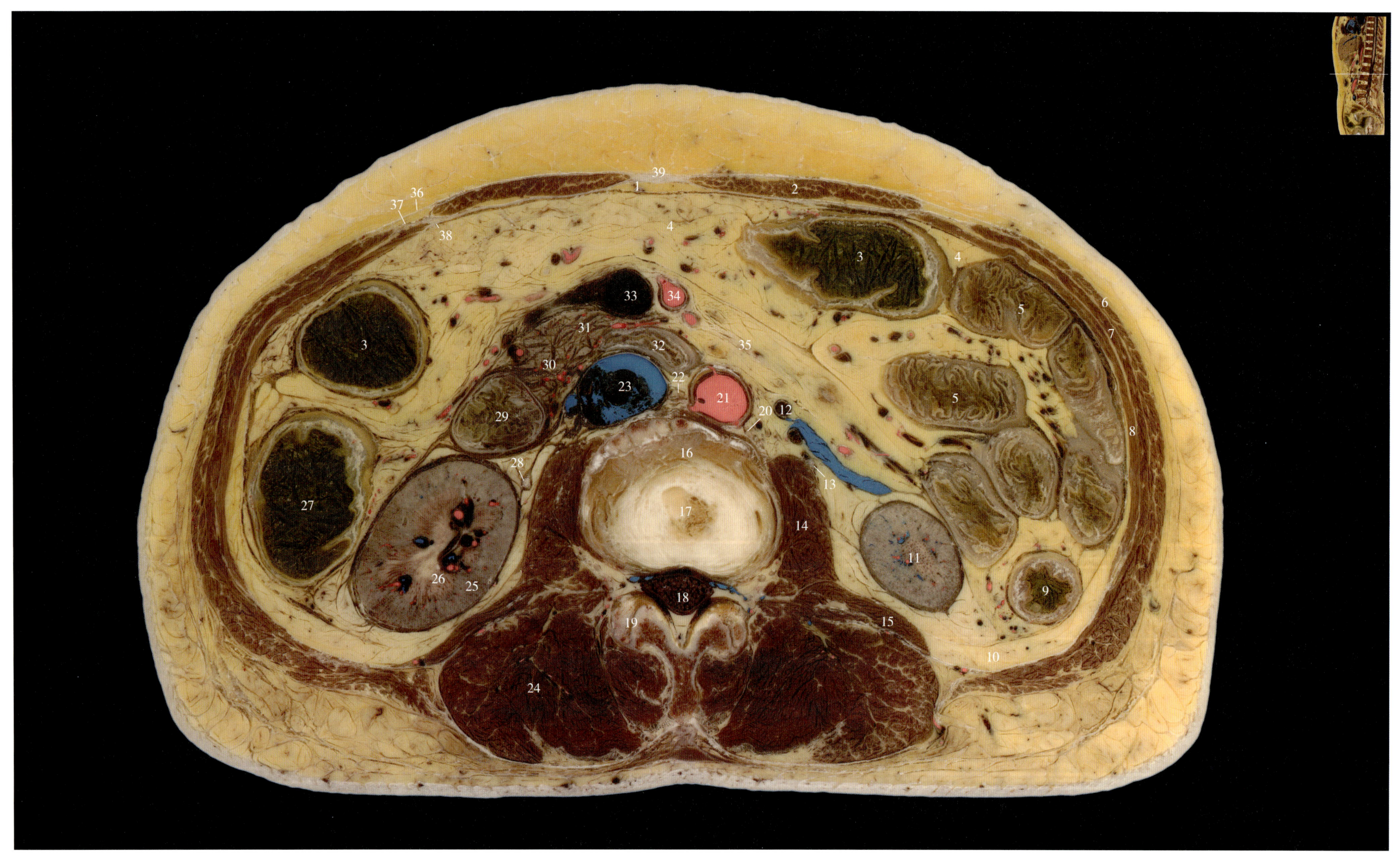

A. 断层标本图像

1. 肝圆韧带 ligamentum teres hepatis
2. 腹直肌 rectus abdominis
3. 横结肠 transverse colon
4. 大网膜 greater omentum
5. 空肠 jejunum
6. 腹外斜肌 obliquus externus abdominis
7. 腹内斜肌 obliquus internus abdominis
8. 腹横肌 transverses abdominis
9. 降结肠 descending colon
10. 腹膜外脂肪 extraperitoneal fat
11. 左肾 left kidney
12. 肠系膜下静脉 inferior mesenteric vein
13. 左输尿管 left ureter
14. 腰大肌 psoas major
15. 腰方肌 quadratus lumborum
16. L2-3 椎间盘 L2-3 intervertebral disc
17. 髓核 nucleus pulposus
18. 马尾 cauda equina
19. 关节突关节 zygapophysial joint
20. 左交感干 left sympathetic trunk
21. 腹主动脉 abdominal aorta
22. 中间腰淋巴结 intermediate lumbar lymph node
23. 下腔静脉 inferior vena cava
24. 竖脊肌 erector spinae
25. 右肾 right kidney
26. 肾锥体 renal pyramid
27. 升结肠 ascending colon
28. 右输尿管 right ureter
29. 十二指肠降部 descending part of duodenum
30. 胰头 head of pancreas
31. 胰钩突 uncinate process of pancreas
32. 十二指肠水平部 horizontal part of duodenum
33. 肠系膜上静脉 superior mesenteric vein
34. 肠系膜上动脉 superior mesenteric artery
35. 肠系膜 mesentery
36. 腹外斜肌腱膜 aponeurosis of obliquus externus abdominis
37. 腹内斜肌腱膜 aponeurosis of obliquus internus abdominis
38. 腹横肌腱膜 aponeurosis of transversus abdominis
39. 白线 linea alba

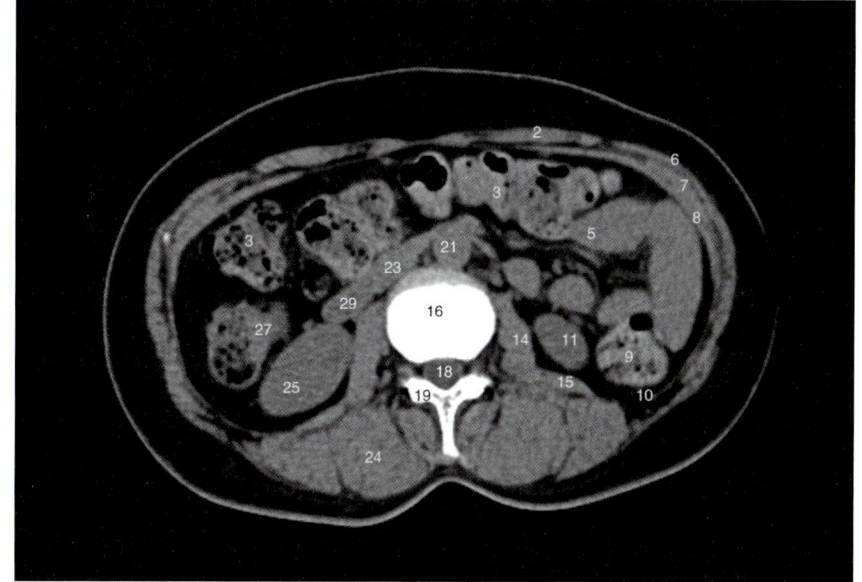

B. CT 平扫图像

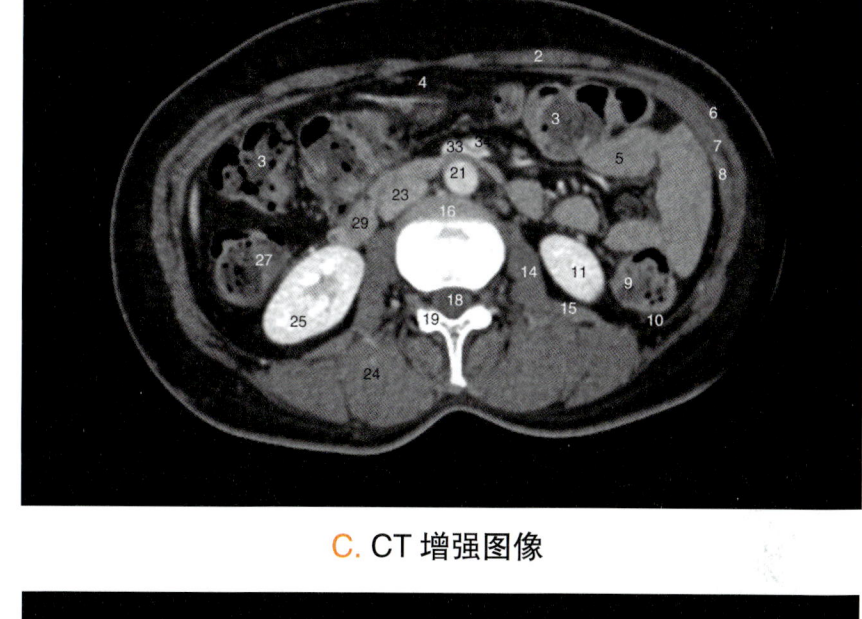

C. CT 增强图像

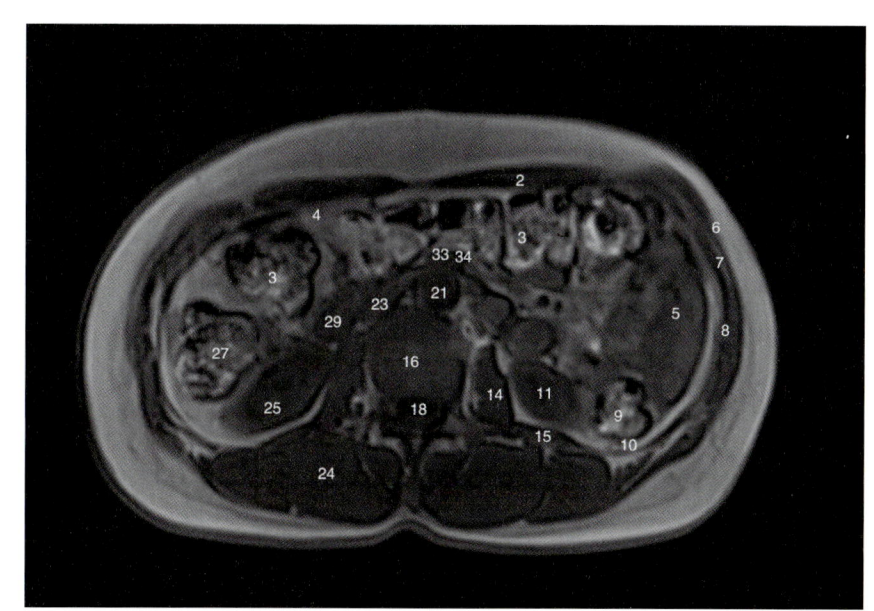

D. MR T1WI

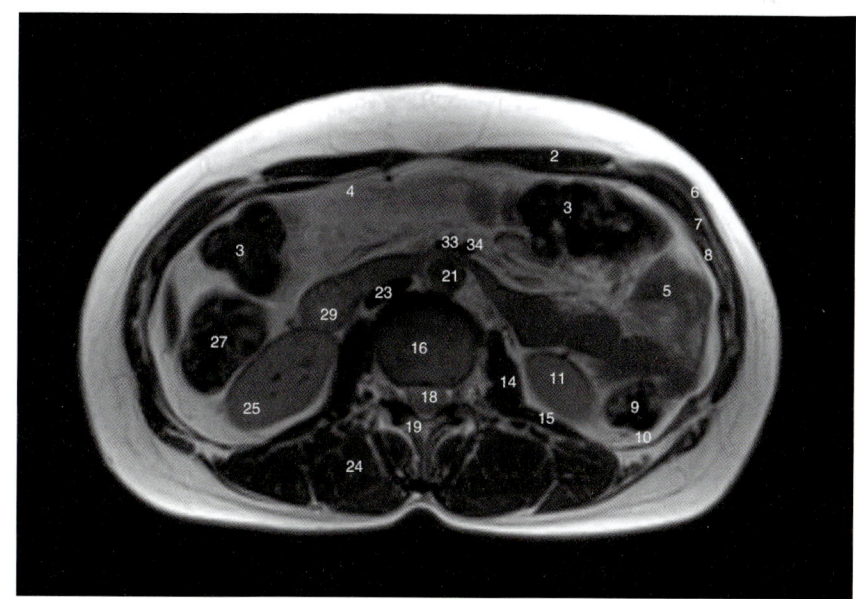

E. MR T2WI

关键结构：肠系膜上动、静脉，胰头。

此断面经过 L2-3 椎间盘。

胰头和胰钩突被肠系膜上静脉、下腔静脉、十二指肠水平部和十二指肠降部包绕。肠系膜上动静脉相伴而行，并呈辐射状走行于扇形的肠系膜内。肠系膜上动脉周围的脂肪、淋巴管和神经组织有助于增大其与主动脉之间的角度和距离，防止压迫十二指肠与其交叉的部位。肠系膜动脉栓塞多发生于肠系膜上动脉，常引起腹痛、便血、呼吸困难三联征[62]。结合病史、症状和体征，CTA 或血管造影利于该病的确诊，CTA 增强扫描或造影图像表现为管腔突然消失，出现截断征或充盈缺损，此征象对诊断肠系膜上动脉栓塞具有重要的意义；同时伴有肠壁水肿增厚或变薄，肠腔扩张，则更有助于诊断[83]。肠系膜上动脉偶可见夹层动脉瘤和真性动脉瘤形成，CTA 是敏感的检测方法。肠系膜血管周围间隙也是感染和肿瘤蔓延的重要解剖基础，相关疾病并不少见。

腹部连续横断层 81（FH.10310）

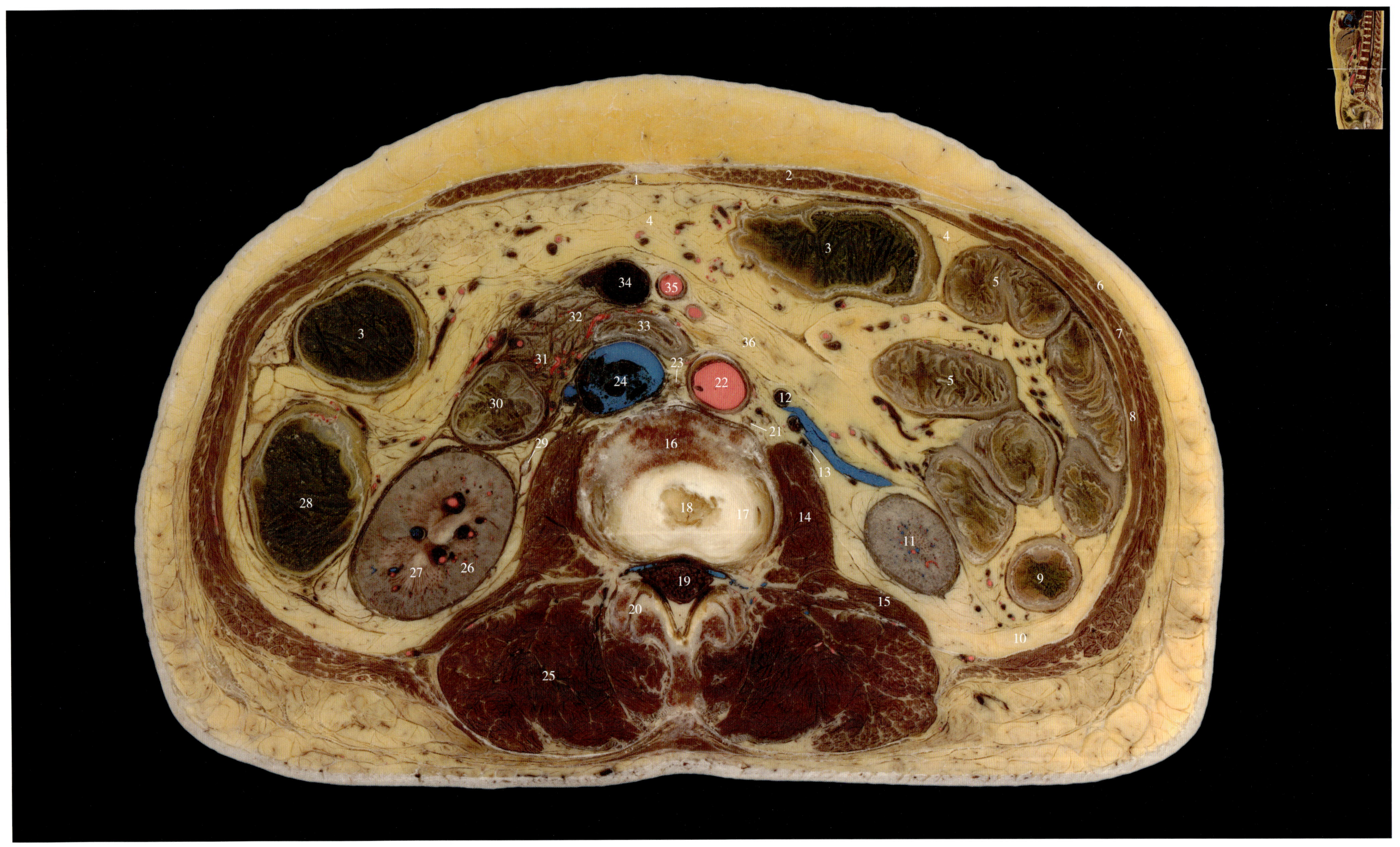

A. 断层标本图像

1. 肝圆韧带 ligamentum teres hepatis
2. 腹直肌 rectus abdominis
3. 横结肠 transverse colon
4. 大网膜 greater omentum
5. 空肠 jejunum
6. 腹外斜肌 obliquus externus abdominis
7. 腹内斜肌 obliquus internus abdominis
8. 腹横肌 transverses abdominis
9. 降结肠 descending colon
10. 腹膜外脂肪 extraperitoneal fat
11. 左肾 left kidney
12. 肠系膜下静脉 inferior mesenteric vein
13. 左输尿管 left ureter
14. 腰大肌 psoas major
15. 腰方肌 quadratus lumborum
16. 第 3 腰椎椎体 body of 3rd lumbar vertebra
17. L2-3 椎间盘 L2-3 intervertebral disc
18. 髓核 nucleus pulposus
19. 马尾 cauda equina
20. 关节突关节 zygapophysial joint
21. 左交感干 left sympathetic trunk
22. 腹主动脉 abdominal aorta
23. 中间腰淋巴结 intermediate lumbar lymph node
24. 下腔静脉 inferior vena cava
25. 竖脊肌 erector spinae
26. 右肾 right kidney
27. 肾锥体 renal pyramid
28. 升结肠 ascending colon
29. 右输尿管 right ureter
30. 十二指肠降部 descending part of duodenum
31. 胰头 head of pancreas
32. 胰钩突 uncinate process of pancreas
33. 十二指肠水平部 horizontal part of duodenum
34. 肠系膜上静脉 superior mesenteric vein
35. 肠系膜上动脉 superior mesenteric artery
36. 肠系膜 mesentery

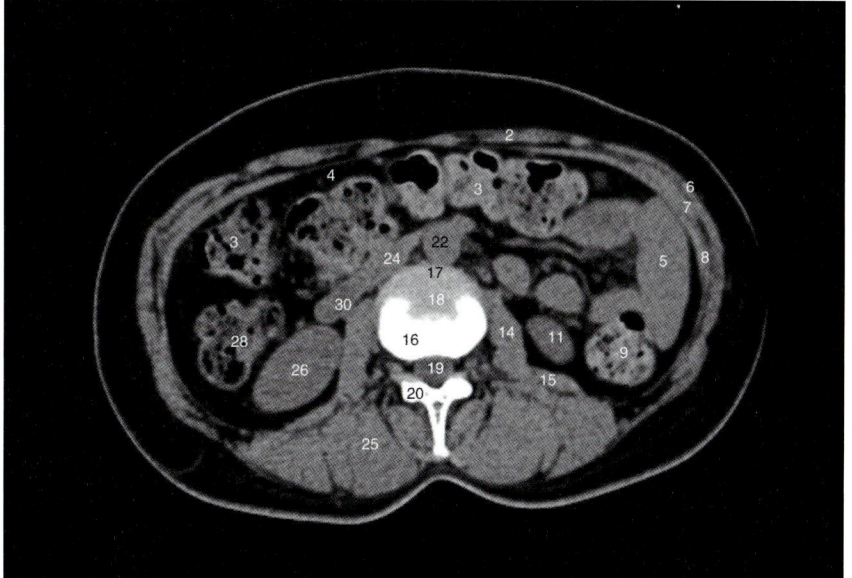

B. CT 平扫图像

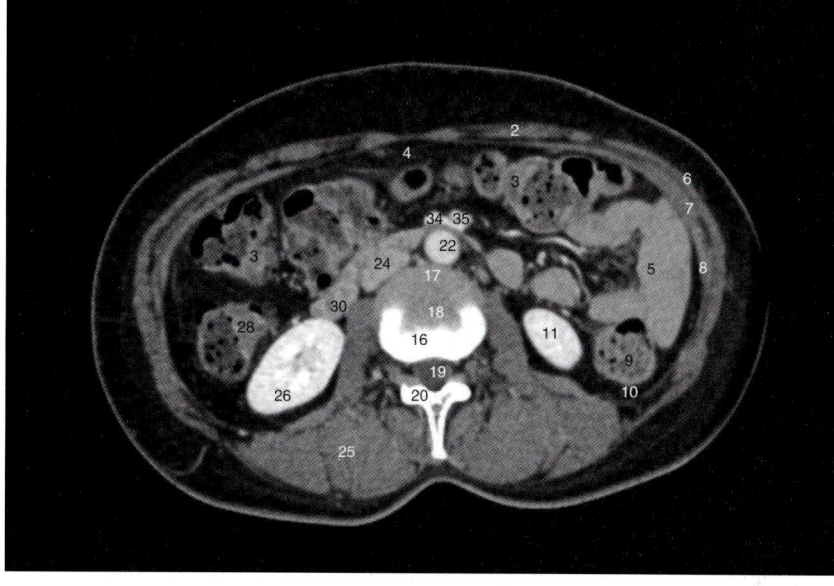

C. CT 增强图像

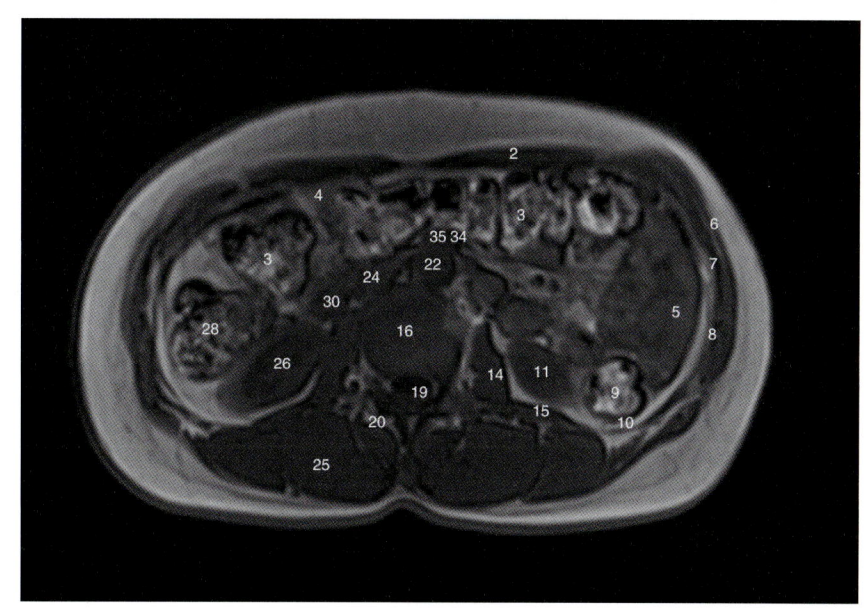

D. MR T1WI

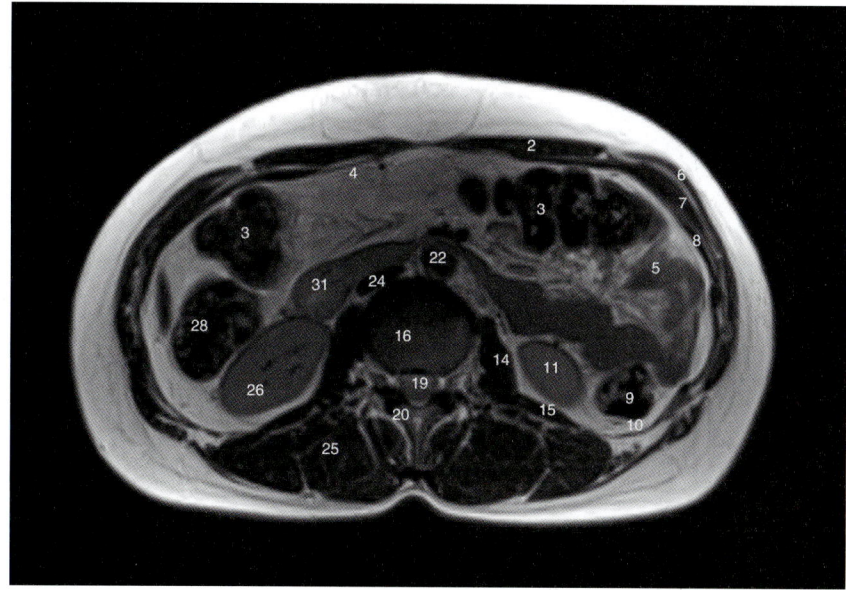

E. MR T2WI

关键结构：结肠，空肠。

此断面经过 L2-3 椎间盘和第 3 腰椎椎体。

左肾体积进一步缩小。此断面腹腔内肠道的配布特点是：空肠与肠系膜居断面左侧部及中份，两侧为横结肠、升结肠、降结肠，脊柱右前方为十二指肠降部与水平部移行部。结肠起始于右髂窝内的盲肠和阑尾，延伸至肛门。升结肠或右结肠上行于腹部右侧，至右季肋区向左弯曲形成结肠肝曲（或结肠右曲），续为横结肠。横结肠肠祥凸向前下方，横跨腹部，直至左季肋区弯曲向下形成结肠脾曲，续为降结肠，降结肠沿腹壁左侧下降，延续为乙状结肠。CT 和 MR 横断面图像上，结肠可能被肠腔内粪便颗粒或空气填充，易于显示。正常人的结肠壁很薄。盲肠和升结肠常含有残留的粪便，位于右侧腹膜后隙；而横结肠因系膜悬吊而位置不固定；降结肠含有的粪便常常较少，位于右左侧腹膜后隙；乙状结肠位置较固定。清洁肠道后，CT 结肠造影或下消化道气钡双重造影可用于结肠病变检出[84]。

腹部连续横断层 82（FH.10290）

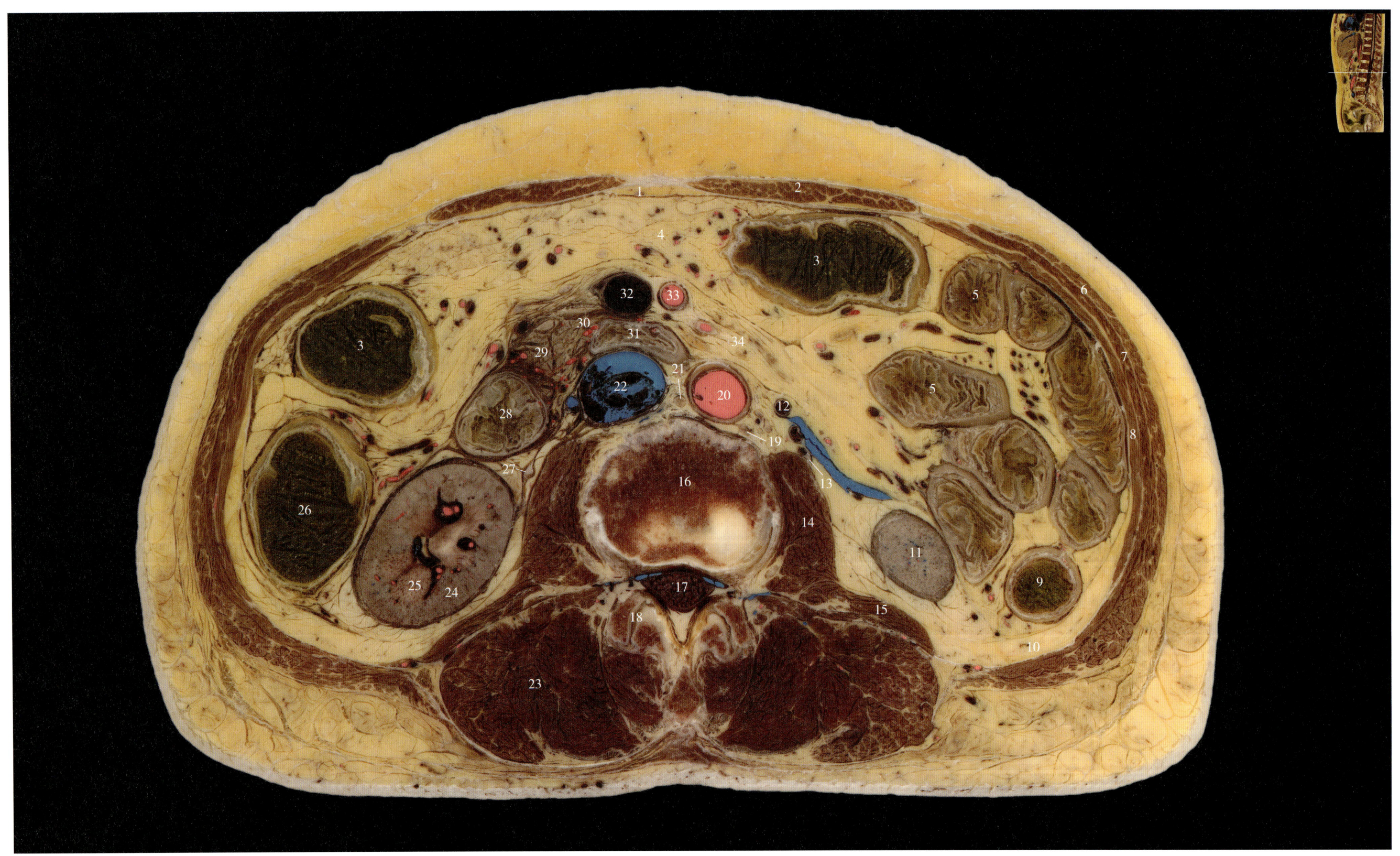

A. 断层标本图像

1. 肝圆韧带 ligamentum teres hepatis
2. 腹直肌 rectus abdominis
3. 横结肠 transverse colon
4. 大网膜 greater omentum
5. 空肠 jejunum
6. 腹外斜肌 obliquus externus abdominis
7. 腹内斜肌 obliquus internus abdominis
8. 腹横肌 transverses abdominis
9. 降结肠 descending colon
10. 腹膜外脂肪 extraperitoneal fat
11. 左肾 left kidney
12. 肠系膜下静脉 inferior mesenteric vein
13. 左输尿管 left ureter
14. 腰大肌 psoas major
15. 腰方肌 quadratus lumborum
16. 第 3 腰椎椎体 body of 3rd lumbar vertebra
17. 马尾 cauda equina
18. 关节突关节 zygapophysial joint
19. 左交感干 left sympathetic trunk
20. 腹主动脉 abdominal aorta
21. 中间腰淋巴结 intermediate lumbar lymph node
22. 下腔静脉 inferior vena cava
23. 竖脊肌 erector spinae
24. 右肾 right kidney
25. 肾锥体 renal pyramid
26. 升结肠 ascending colon
27. 右输尿管 right ureter
28. 十二指肠降部 descending part of duodenum
29. 胰头 head of pancreas
30. 胰钩突 uncinate process of pancreas
31. 十二指肠水平部 horizontal part of duodenum
32. 肠系膜上静脉 superior mesenteric vein
33. 肠系膜上动脉 superior mesenteric artery
34. 肠系膜 mesentery

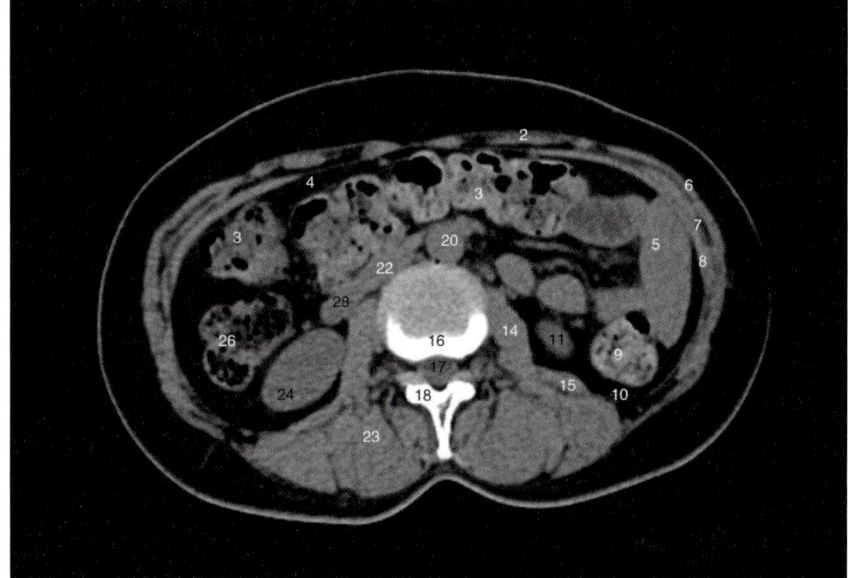

B. CT 平扫图像

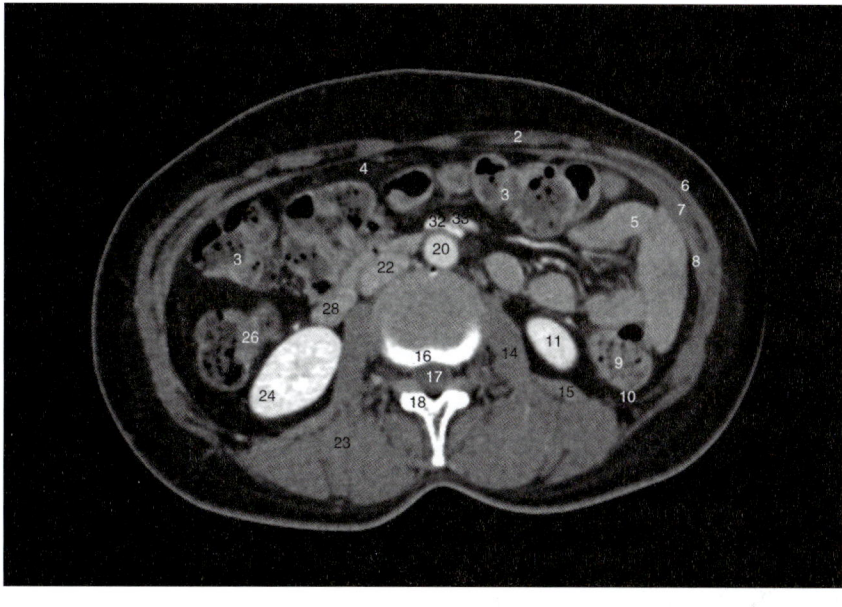

C. CT 增强图像

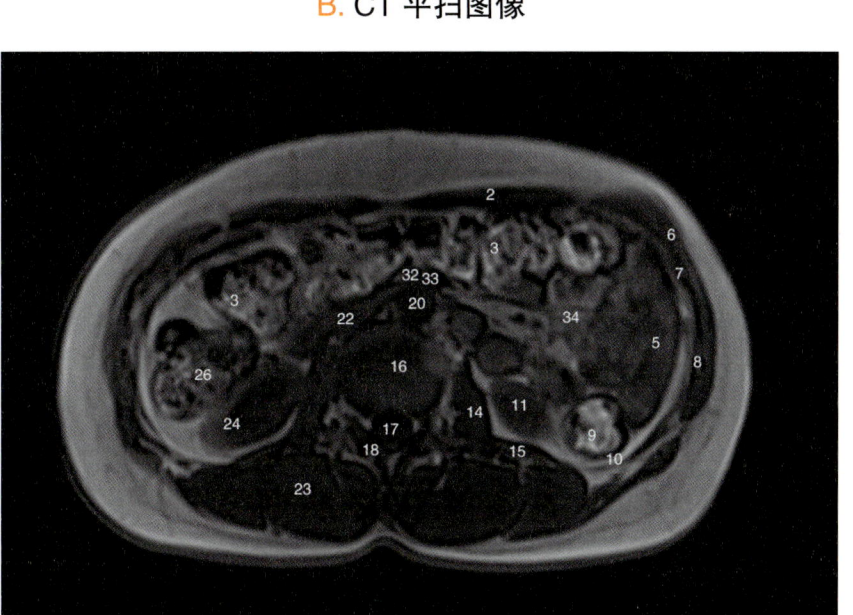

D. MR T1WI

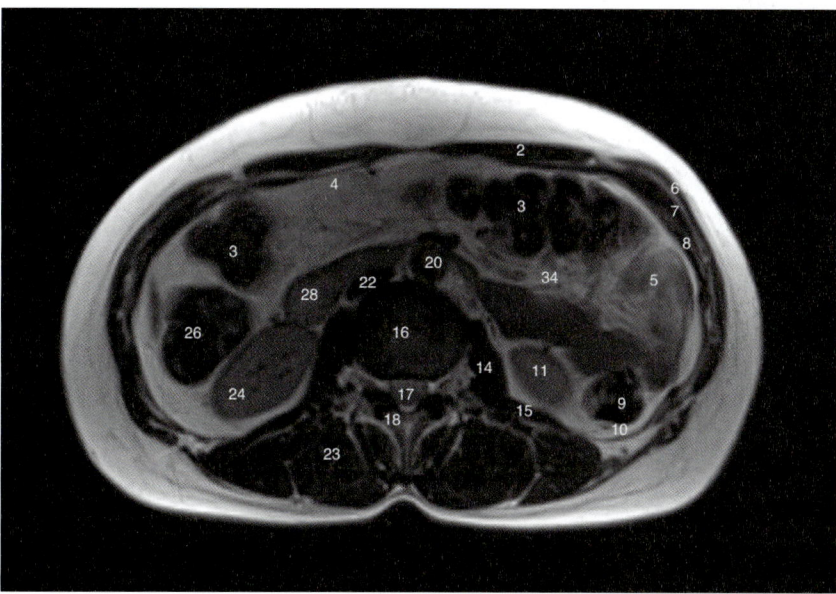

E. MR T2WI

关键结构：腰交感干，输尿管。

此断面经过第 3 腰椎椎体。

大网膜占据腹腔前大部，在脊柱前方，下腔静脉与腹主动脉间可见中间腰淋巴结。在脊柱与腰大肌之间可见腰交感干。腰交感干由 3 个或 4 个神经节和节间支构成，并被椎前筋膜所覆盖，上方连于胸交感干，下方延续为骶交感干。左腰交感干与腹主动脉左缘相邻，干的下端位于左髂总静脉的后方。在正常人解剖上腰交感干通常位于脊柱与腰大肌之间，并被椎前筋膜所覆盖，但有时它藏于腰大肌与脊柱之间，被腰大肌起点部分覆盖。腰交感干分裂的出现率为 73%，在不同腰椎平面可分为两条或多条。腰交感干附近常有小的淋巴结，在影像诊断中应注意鉴别。

腹部连续横断层83（FH.10270）

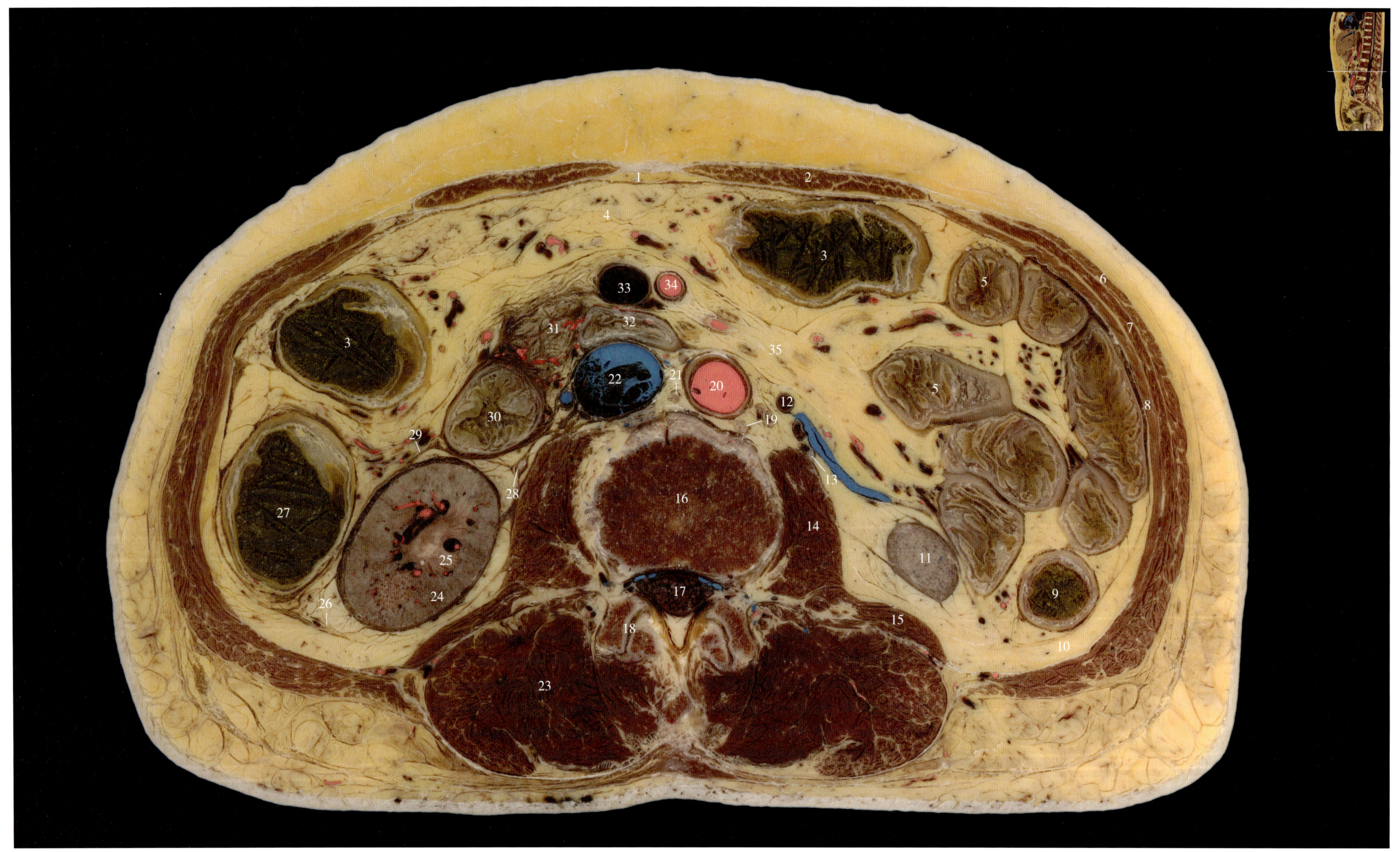

A. 断层标本图像

1. 肝圆韧带 ligamentum teres hepatis
2. 腹直肌 rectus abdominis
3. 横结肠 transverse colon
4. 大网膜 greater omentum
5. 空肠 jejunum
6. 腹外斜肌 obliquus externus abdominis
7. 腹内斜肌 obliquus internus abdominis
8. 腹横肌 transverses abdominis
9. 降结肠 descending colon
10. 腹膜外脂肪 extraperitoneal fat
11. 左肾 left kidney
12. 肠系膜下静脉 inferior mesenteric vein
13. 左输尿管 left ureter
14. 腰大肌 psoas major
15. 腰方肌 quadratus lumborum
16. 第 3 腰椎椎体 body of 3rd lumbar vertebra
17. 马尾 cauda equina
18. 关节突关节 zygapophysial joint
19. 左交感干 left sympathetic trunk
20. 腹主动脉 abdominal aorta
21. 中间腰淋巴结 intermediate lumbar lymph node
22. 下腔静脉 inferior vena cava
23. 竖脊肌 erector spinae
24. 右肾 right kidney
25. 肾锥体 renal pyramid
26. 肾后筋膜 retrorenal fascia
27. 升结肠 ascending colon
28. 右输尿管 right ureter
29. 肾前筋膜 prerenal fascia
30. 十二指肠降部 descending part of duodenum
31. 胰头 head of pancreas
32. 十二指肠水平部 horizontal part of duodenum
33. 肠系膜上静脉 superior mesenteric vein
34. 肠系膜上动脉 superior mesenteric artery
35. 肠系膜 mesentery

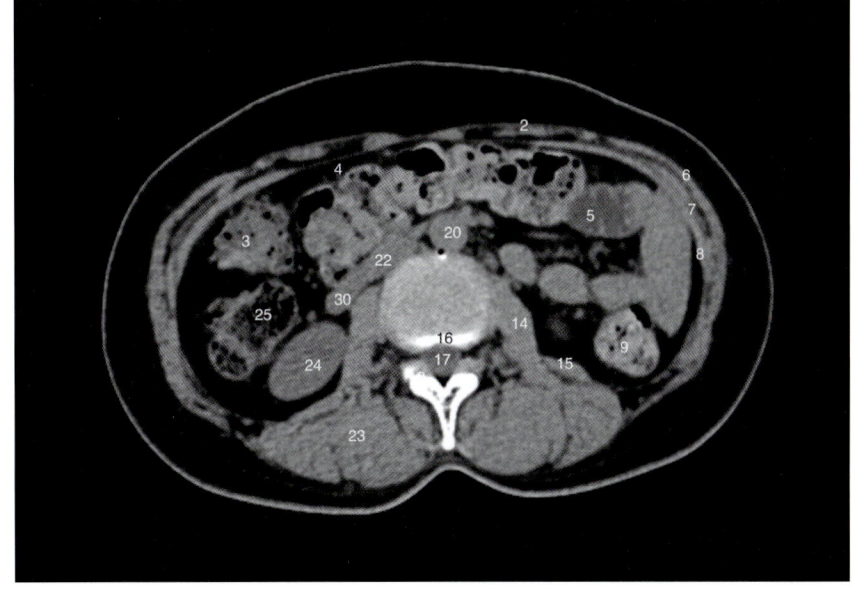

B. CT 平扫图像

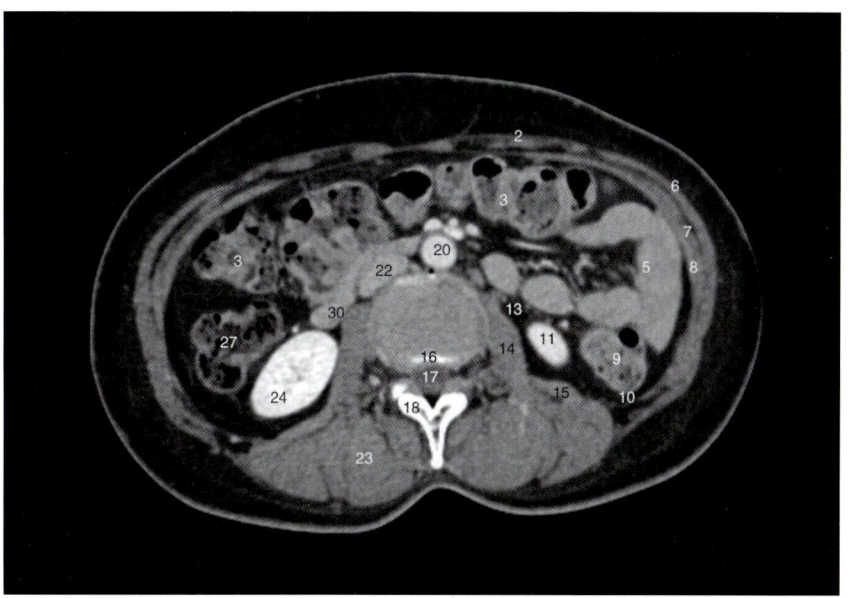

C. CT 增强图像

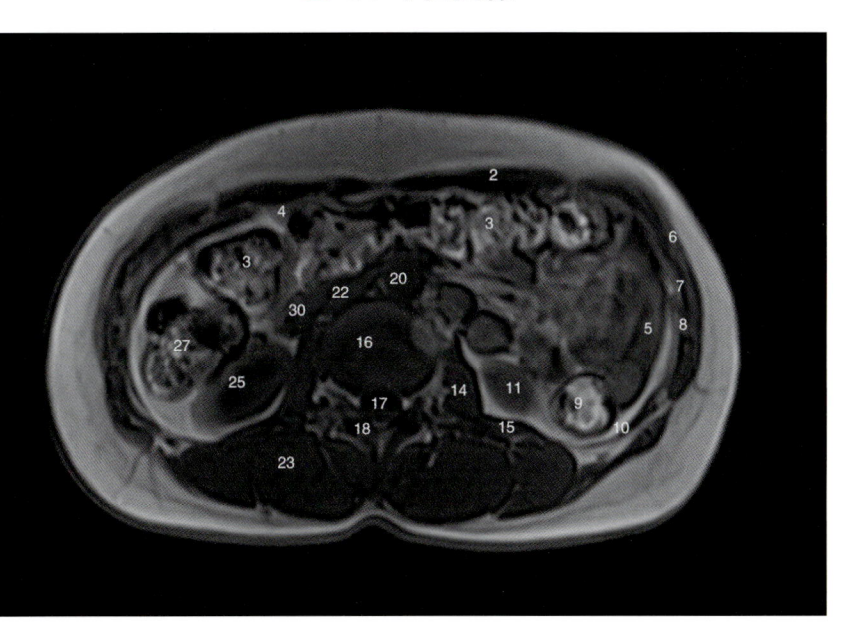

D. MR T1WI

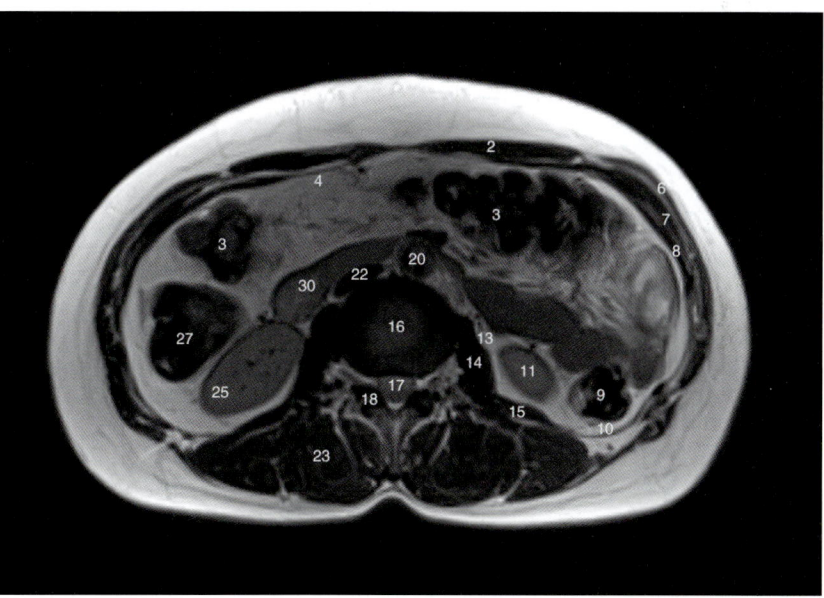

E. MR T2WI

关键结构：腹膜后淋巴结，第 3 腰椎。

此断面经过第 3 腰椎椎体。

胰钩突消失，胰腺仅剩胰头存在。在此断面，左肾明显变小。升降结肠分列于右侧部和左侧部，横结肠和肠系膜居断面的中份，腹主动脉与下腔静脉位于腹膜后，腹主动脉旁有多个小淋巴结。腹主动脉旁腹膜后淋巴结可分为主动脉前淋巴结、主动脉旁和主动脉后淋巴结组。主动脉前淋巴结在腹部不成对脏器前聚集，引流包括胰、肝和脾等胃肠脏器，可以被分为腹腔淋巴结、肠系膜上淋巴结和肠系膜下淋巴结。主动脉外侧（或主动脉旁）淋巴结位于腹主动脉和下腔静脉的一侧，腰大肌、膈脚和交感干的前面，包括膈后脚淋巴结（主动脉裂孔膈脚的后面）、左肾门或右肾门淋巴结、主动脉腔静脉淋巴结、腔静脉旁淋巴结、腔静脉后淋巴结和腔静脉前淋巴结。主动脉后淋巴结也是主动脉旁淋巴结组成部分。CT 或 MRI 可显示腹膜后小淋巴结，尤其是 MRI 的血管流空现象可用于鉴别血管断面与淋巴结[62]。当腹膜后淋巴结因肿瘤、转移或炎性反应而增大时，CT 或 MRI 更易于显示[85]，但需要对淋巴结肿大的原因进行鉴别。

腹部连续横断层 84（FH.10250）

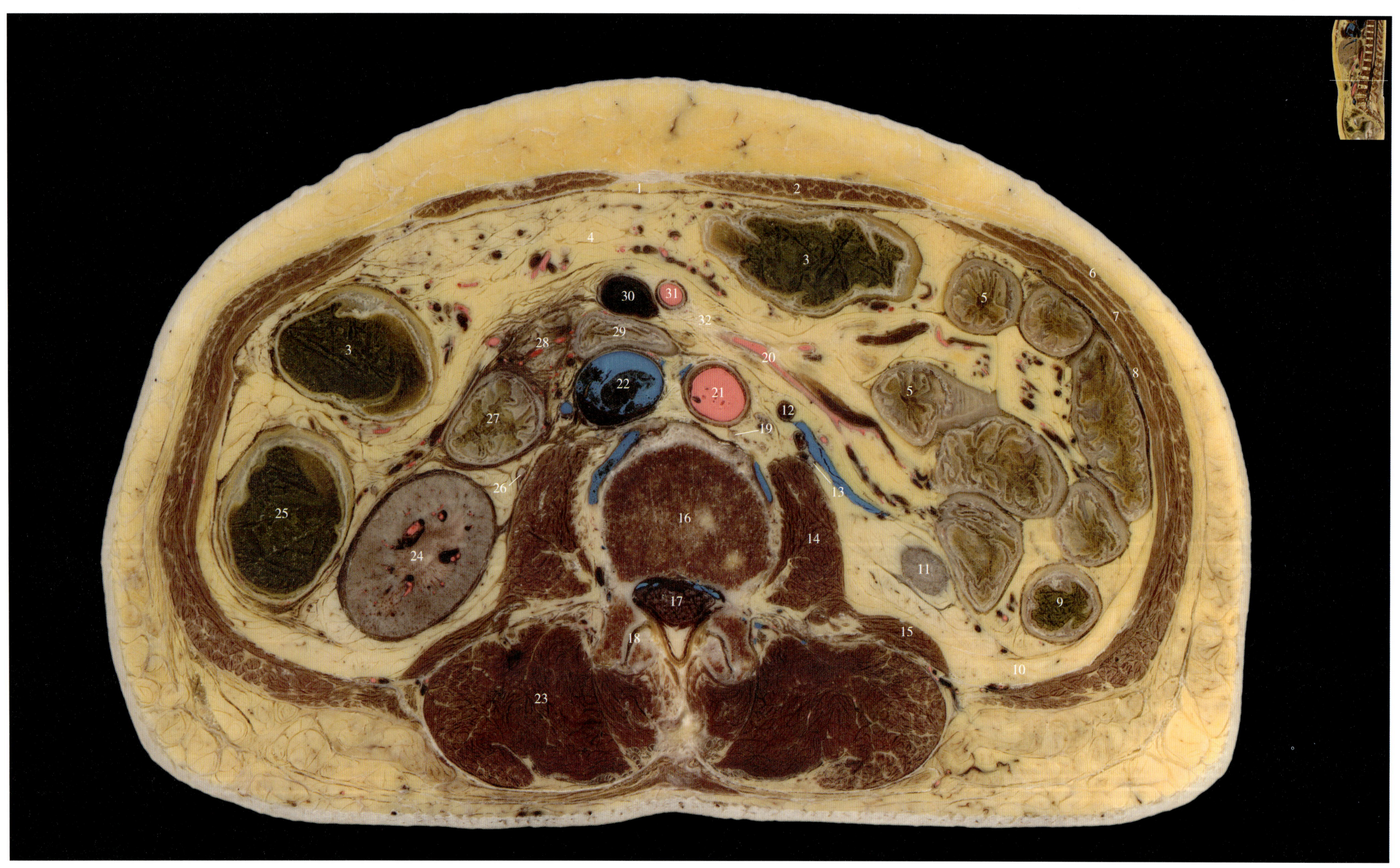

A. 断层标本图像

1. 肝圆韧带 ligamentum teres hepatis
2. 腹直肌 rectus abdominis
3. 横结肠 transverse colon
4. 大网膜 greater omentum
5. 空肠 jejunum
6. 腹外斜肌 obliquus externus abdominis
7. 腹内斜肌 obliquus internus abdominis
8. 腹横肌 transverses abdominis
9. 降结肠 descending colon
10. 腹膜外脂肪 extraperitoneal fat
11. 左肾 left kidney
12. 肠系膜下静脉 inferior mesenteric vein
13. 左输尿管 left ureter
14. 腰大肌 psoas major
15. 腰方肌 quadratus lumborum
16. 第 3 腰椎椎体 body of 3rd lumbar vertebra
17. 马尾 cauda equina
18. 关节突关节 zygapophysial joint
19. 左交感干 left sympathetic trunk
20. 空肠动脉 jejunal artery
21. 腹主动脉 abdominal aorta
22. 下腔静脉 inferior vena cava
23. 竖脊肌 erector spinae
24. 右肾 right kidney
25. 升结肠 ascending colon
26. 右输尿管 right ureter
27. 十二指肠降部 descending part of duodenum
28. 胰头 head of pancreas
29. 十二指肠水平部 horizontal part of duodenum
30. 肠系膜上静脉 superior mesenteric vein
31. 肠系膜上动脉 superior mesenteric artery
32. 肠系膜 mesentery

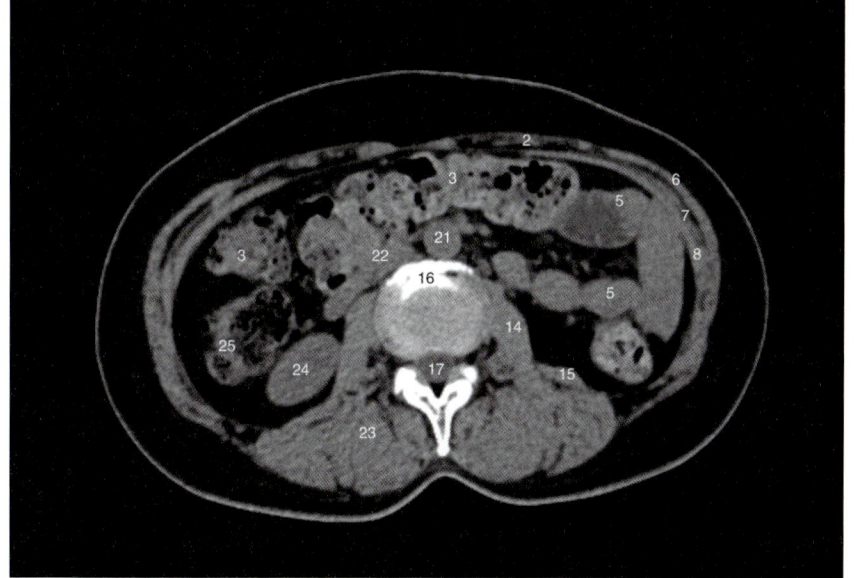

B. CT 平扫图像

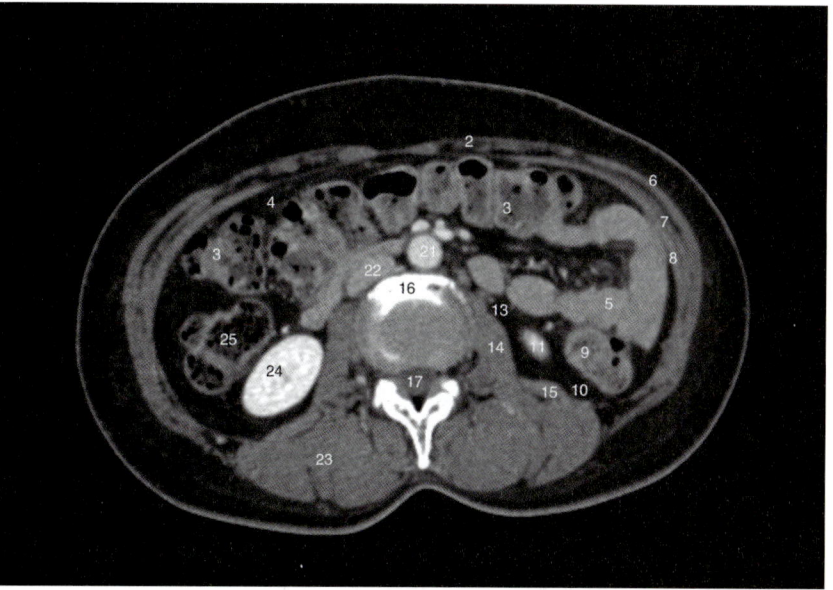

C. CT 增强图像

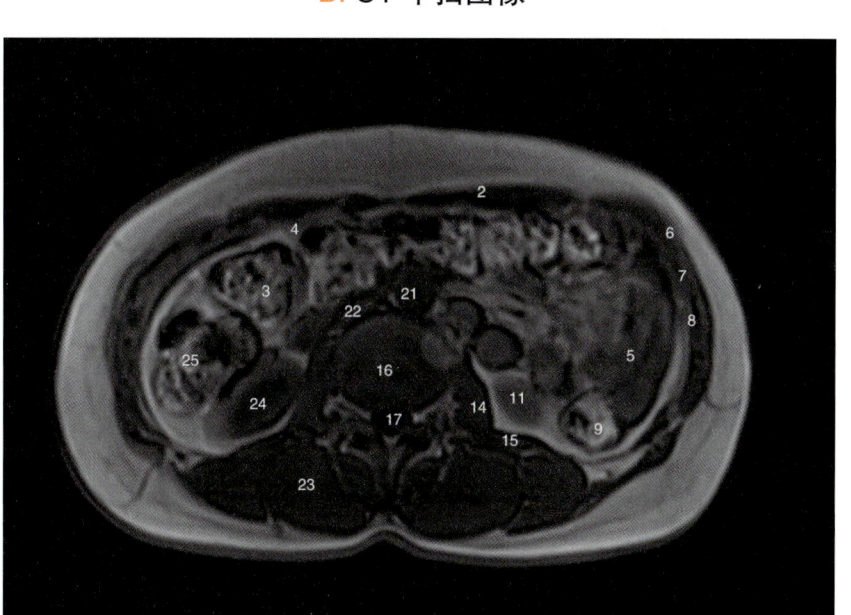

D. MR T1WI

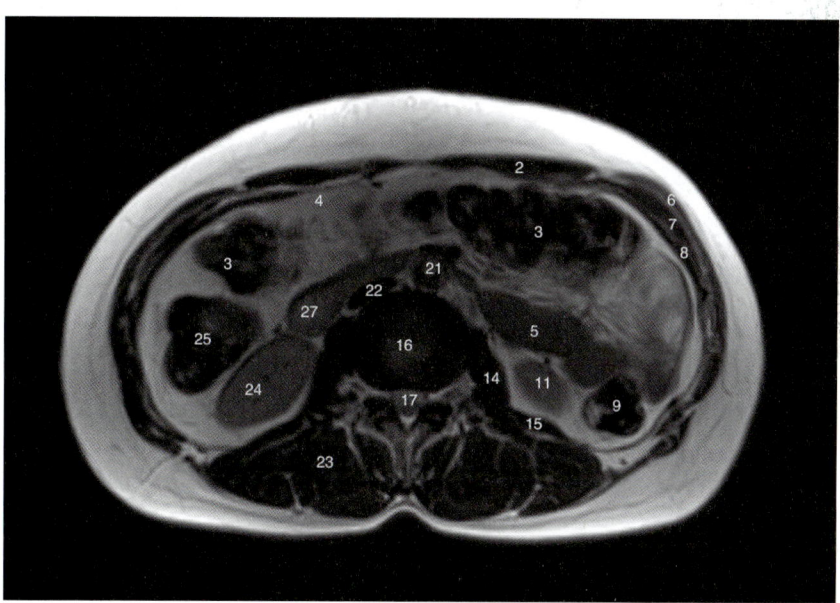

E. MR T2WI

关键结构：左肾下极，输尿管，肠系膜。

此断面经过第 3 腰椎椎体。

双肾体积明显缩小，左肾仅剩极小部分，肠道结构的配布大致同上一断层。肾位于腹膜背面后方，脊柱两侧各一，为脂肪组织所包绕。上抵第 12 胸椎上缘平面，下至第 3 腰椎平面。左肾位置通常比右肾略高，左肾比右肾稍长而窄，且距正中矢状面更近。双肾的长轴均指向外下方，横轴指向后内侧。成年人肾长约 11 cm，宽约 6 cm，前后径约 3 cm，左肾可比右肾长 1.5 cm[79]。由于左右肾上下位置并不一致，在断面图像上一侧肾下极会出现类似孤立的肿块，此时须结合上方的层面进行判读。肾脏可表现为形态异常，常见的是马蹄肾，发生率 0.01%~0.1%，表现为两肾的上极或下极相互融合，以下极融合多见，融合部位称峡部，多为肾实质，常横跨腹部大血管前方。CT 或 MRI 均可显示马蹄肾，表现为横跨于脊柱前方的肾实质连接两肾下极或上极（少见），其密度、信号强度及强化表现均同于正常肾实质[86]。

腹部连续横断层 85（FH.10230）

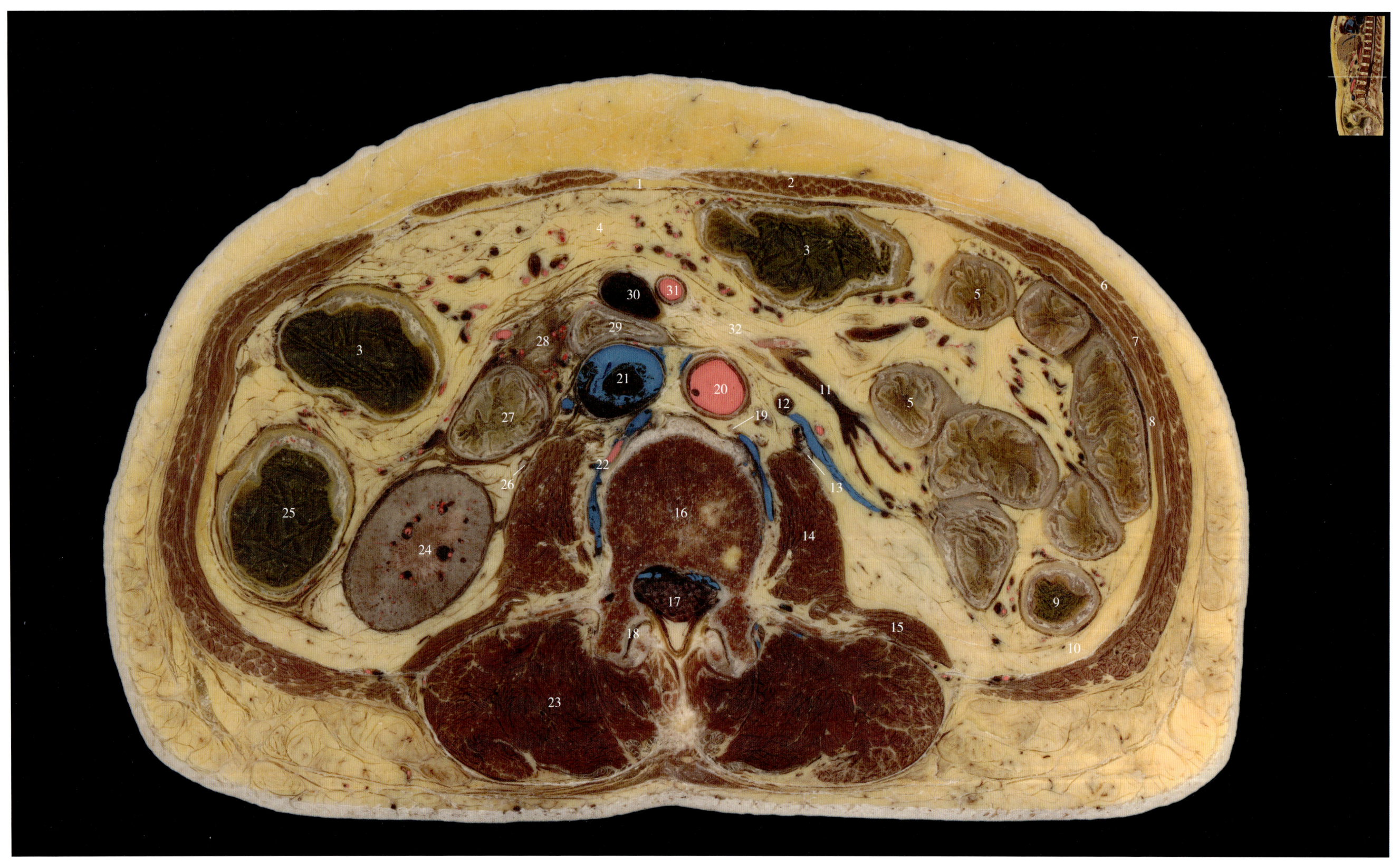

A. 断层标本图像

1. 肝圆韧带 ligamentum teres hepatis
2. 腹直肌 rectus abdominis
3. 横结肠 transverse colon
4. 大网膜 greater omentum
5. 空肠 jejunum
6. 腹外斜肌 obliquus externus abdominis
7. 腹内斜肌 obliquus internus abdominis
8. 腹横肌 transverses abdominis
9. 降结肠 descending colon
10. 腹膜外脂肪 extraperitoneal fat
11. 空肠静脉 jejunal vein
12. 肠系膜下静脉 inferior mesenteric vein
13. 左输尿管 left ureter
14. 腰大肌 psoas major
15. 腰方肌 quadratus lumborum
16. 第 3 腰椎椎体 body of 3rd lumbar vertebra
17. 马尾 cauda equina
18. 关节突关节 zygapophysial joint
19. 左交感干 left sympathetic trunk
20. 腹主动脉 abdominal aorta
21. 下腔静脉 inferior vena cava
22. 腰动、静脉 lumbar artery and vein
23. 竖脊肌 erector spinae
24. 右肾 right kidney
25. 升结肠 ascending colon
26. 右输尿管 right ureter
27. 十二指肠降部 descending part of duodenum
28. 胰头 head of pancreas
29. 十二指肠水平部 horizontal part of duodenum
30. 肠系膜上静脉 superior mesenteric vein
31. 肠系膜上动脉 superior mesenteric artery
32. 肠系膜 mesentery

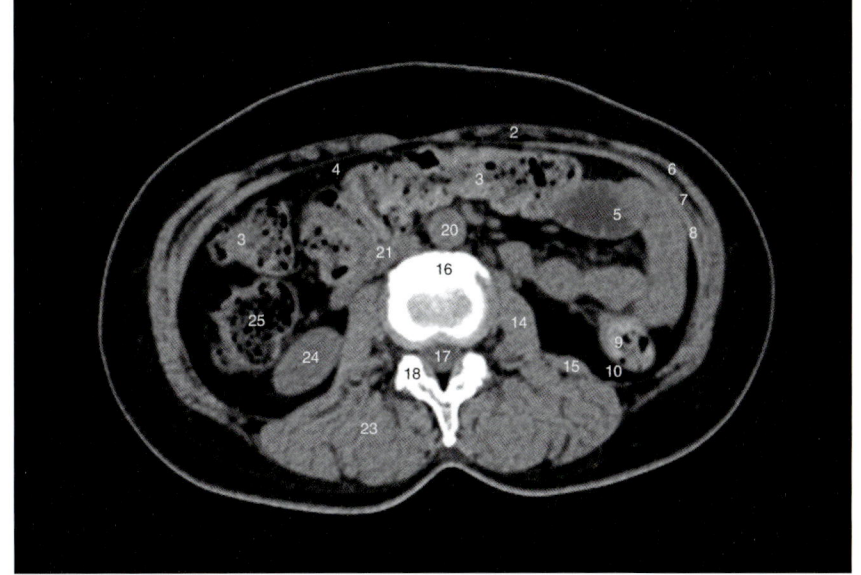

B. CT 平扫图像

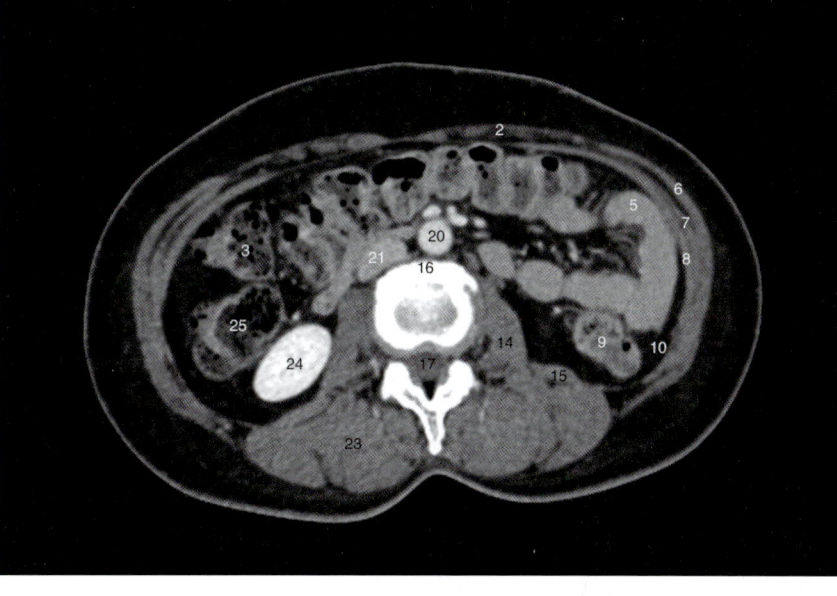

C. CT 增强图像

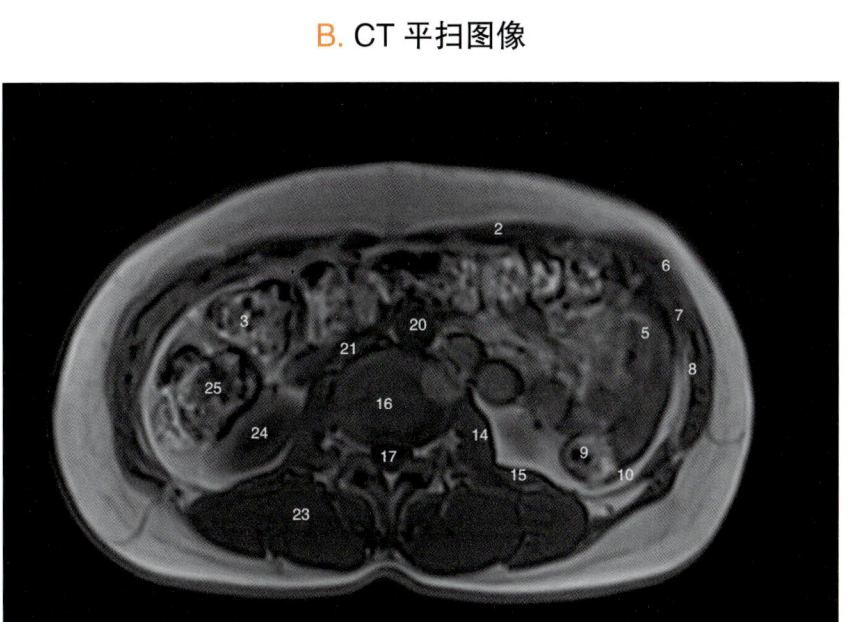

D. MR T1WI

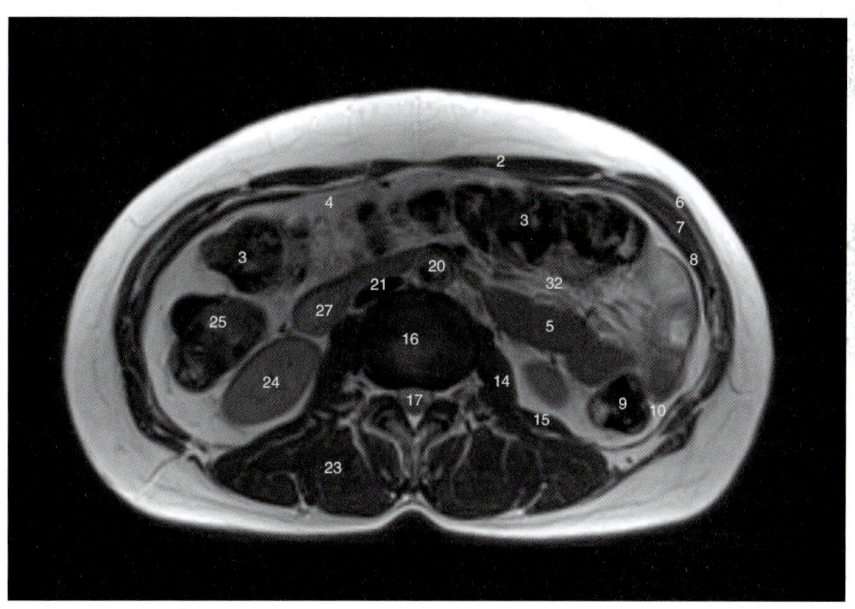

E. MR T2WI

关键结构：第 3 腰椎椎体，右肾下极，输尿管。

此断面经过第 3 腰椎椎体。

左肾在该断面消失。在脊柱两侧，腰大肌的内侧可见腰动、静脉。第 3 腰椎处于腰椎生理前凸弧度的顶点，为承受力学传递的重要部位，因此易受外力作用的影响导致损伤从而引起该处附着肌肉撕裂、出血、瘢痕粘连、筋膜增厚挛缩，使得血管神经束受摩擦、刺激和压迫而产生症状。第 3 腰椎横突特别长，且水平位伸出，附近有很多血管、神经束经过，有较多的肌筋膜附着。腰部多发生腰椎间盘突出，其次是颈部，胸部极少[80]。腰椎间盘突出 90% 发生在 L4-5 和 L5-S1 椎间盘。腰椎 CT 或 MRI 有助于腰椎间盘突出的显示，在影像学上表现为椎间盘后缘向后局限性突起，大多数呈丘状、新月形或半圆形突入椎管内。同时可伴有硬脊膜囊受压、变形、移位，神经根肿胀、受压移位，神经根湮没，碎块形成、滑移，以及钙化等间接表现[87,88]。

腹部连续横断层 86（FH.10210）

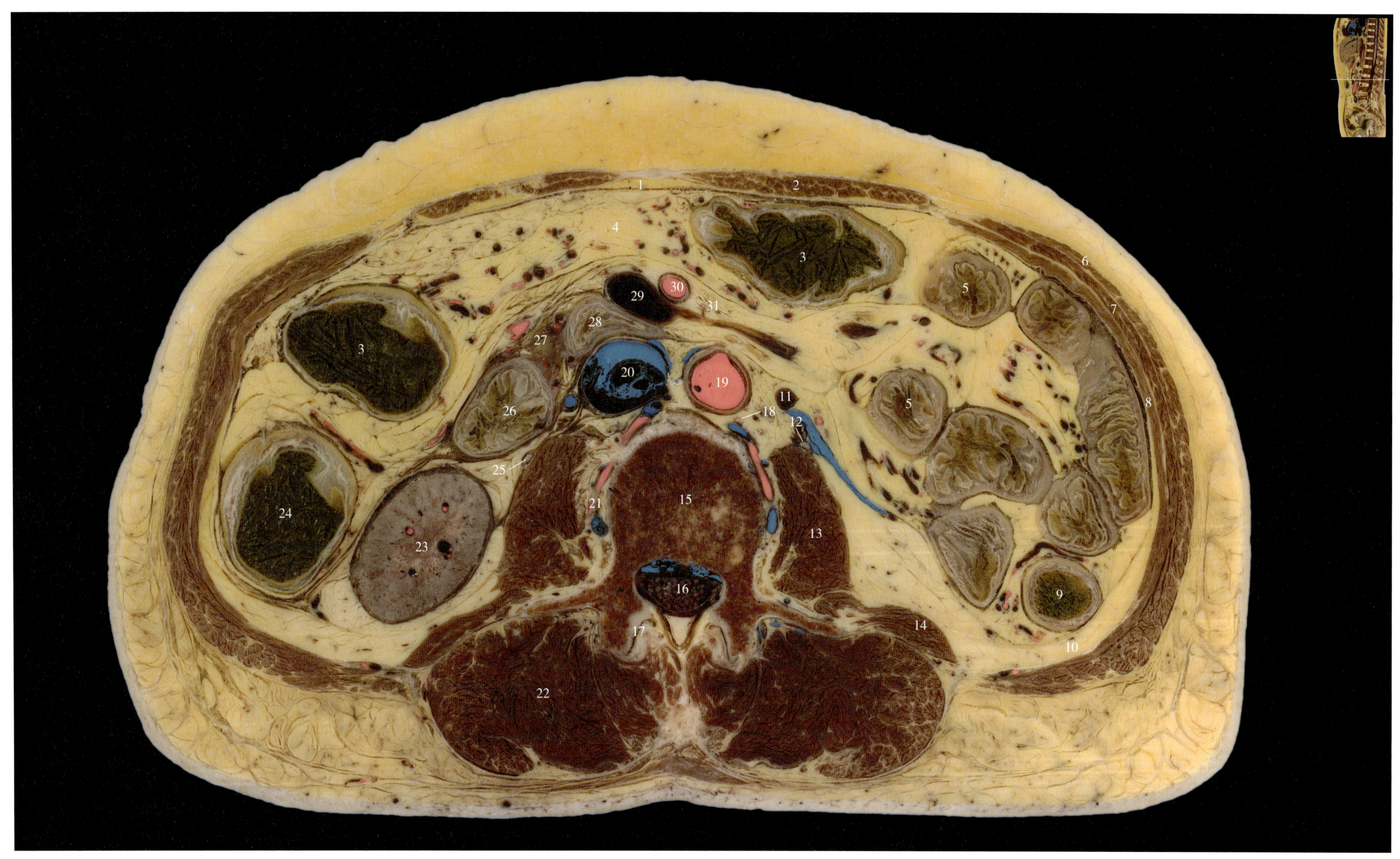

A. 断层标本图像

1. 肝圆韧带 ligamentum teres hepatis
2. 腹直肌 rectus abdominis
3. 横结肠 transverse colon
4. 大网膜 greater omentum
5. 空肠 jejunum
6. 腹外斜肌 obliquus externus abdominis
7. 腹内斜肌 obliquus internus abdominis
8. 腹横肌 transverses abdominis
9. 降结肠 descending colon
10. 腹膜外脂肪 extraperitoneal fat
11. 肠系膜下静脉 inferior mesenteric vein
12. 左输尿管 left ureter
13. 腰大肌 psoas major
14. 腰方肌 quadratus lumborum
15. 第 3 腰椎椎体 body of 3rd lumbar vertebra
16. 马尾 cauda equina
17. 关节突关节 zygapophysial joint
18. 左交感干 left sympathetic trunk
19 腹主动脉 abdominal aorta
20. 下腔静脉 inferior vena cava
21. 腰动、静脉 lumbar artery and vein
22. 竖脊肌 erector spinae
23. 右肾 right kidney
24. 升结肠 ascending colon
25. 右输尿管 right ureter
26. 十二指肠降部 descending part of duodenum
27. 胰头 head of pancreas
28. 十二指肠水平部 horizontal part of duodenum
29. 肠系膜上静脉 superior mesenteric vein
30. 肠系膜上动脉 superior mesenteric artery
31. 肠系膜 mesentery

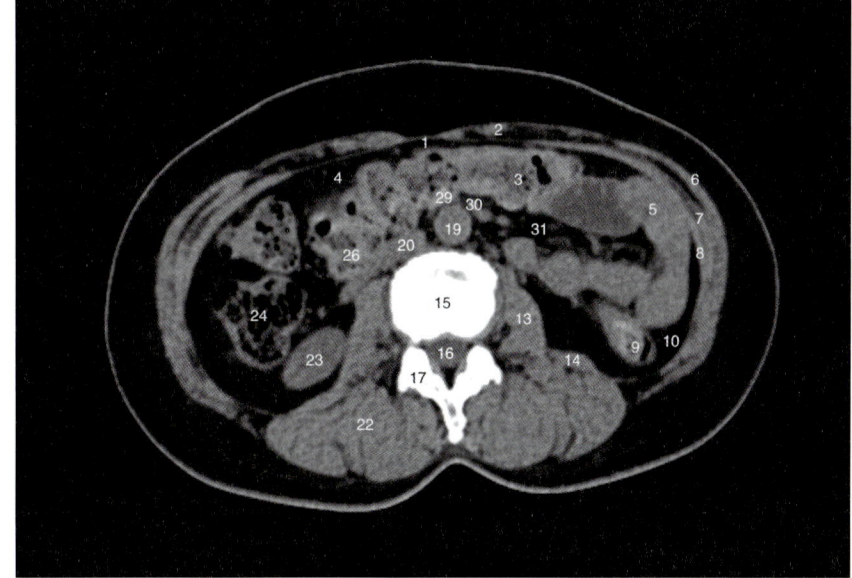

B. CT 平扫图像

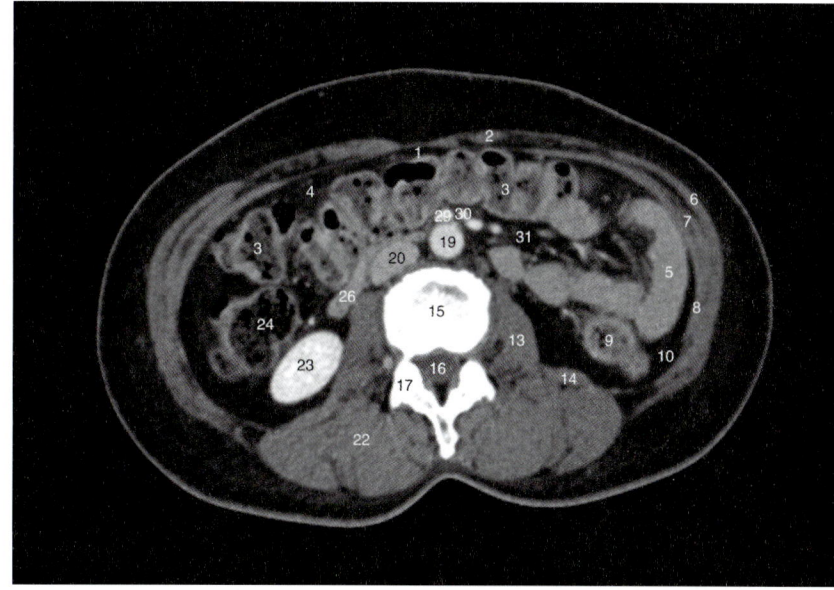

C. CT 增强图像

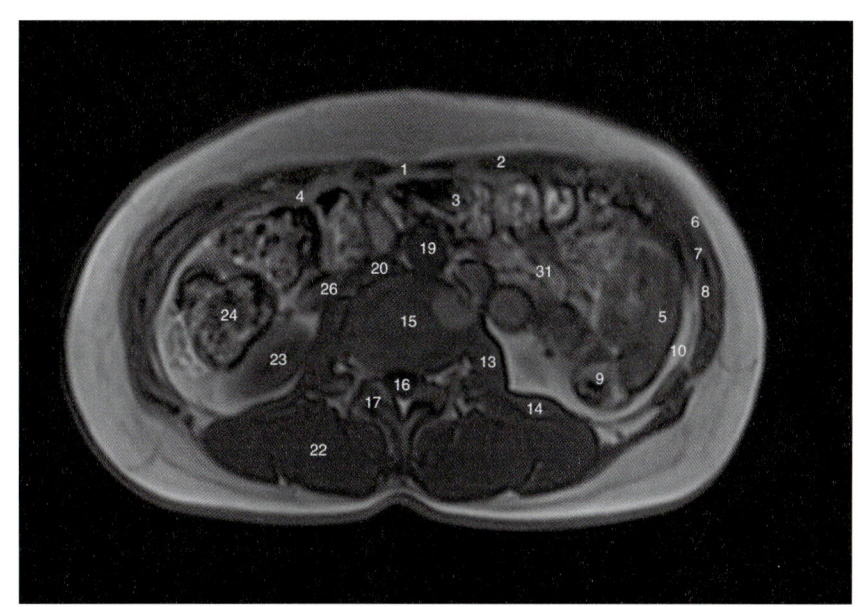

D. MR T1WI

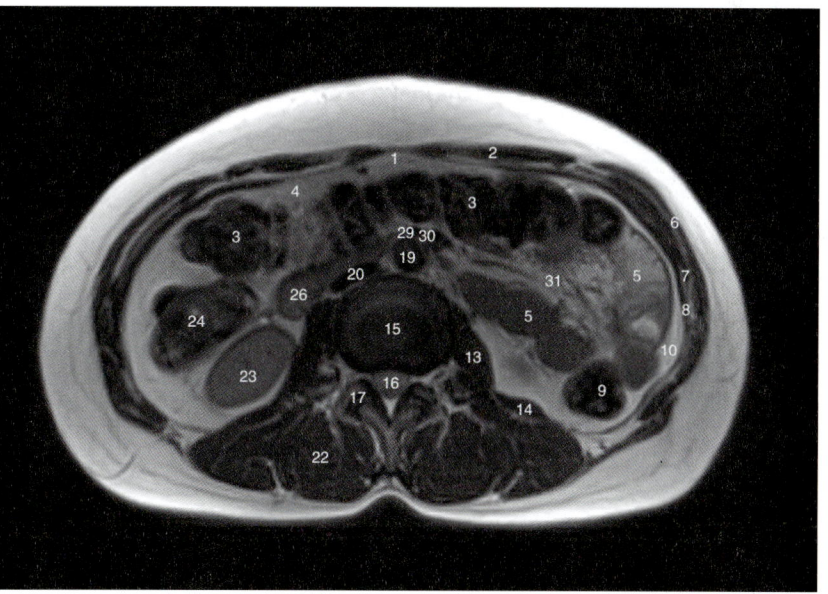

E. MR T2WI

关键结构：空肠，肠系膜，肠系膜上动脉，肠系膜上静脉。

此断面经过第 3 腰椎椎体。

脊柱前方有下腔静脉和腹主动脉走行，下腔静脉前方有十二指肠水平部经过，右侧有十二指肠降部，二者之间可见即将消失的胰头。肠系膜上静脉和肠系膜上动脉伴行居十二指肠水平部前方。脊柱的右侧为右肾下端，其与十二指肠水平部右侧分别为升结肠和横结肠。脊柱左前方空肠占据较大区域，向右接十二指肠空肠曲，向右下方延续为回肠。空肠和回肠分界不明显，空肠管径较粗，管壁较厚，动脉弓级数较少，直血管较长，血供更丰富。空、回肠有肠系膜包绕，借肠系膜根固定于腹后壁，肠系膜内可见大量的小血管。小肠系膜是双层腹膜结构，面积较大且呈扇形，由于其宽而长，故空、回肠活动度较大，当肠蠕动失调时，容易发生系膜和肠袢的扭转。硬化性肠系膜炎是一种肠系膜脂肪组织非特异性感染和纤维化，好发于 60~70 岁老年人，多见于男性，有腹痛、发热、恶心及呕吐等症状，多数患者有自限性且预后良好。硬化性肠系膜炎分为肠系膜脂膜炎及肠系膜脂质营养不良，前者以慢性感染为主，后者以脂肪坏死占优势[89]。

173

腹部连续横断层 87 (FH.10190)

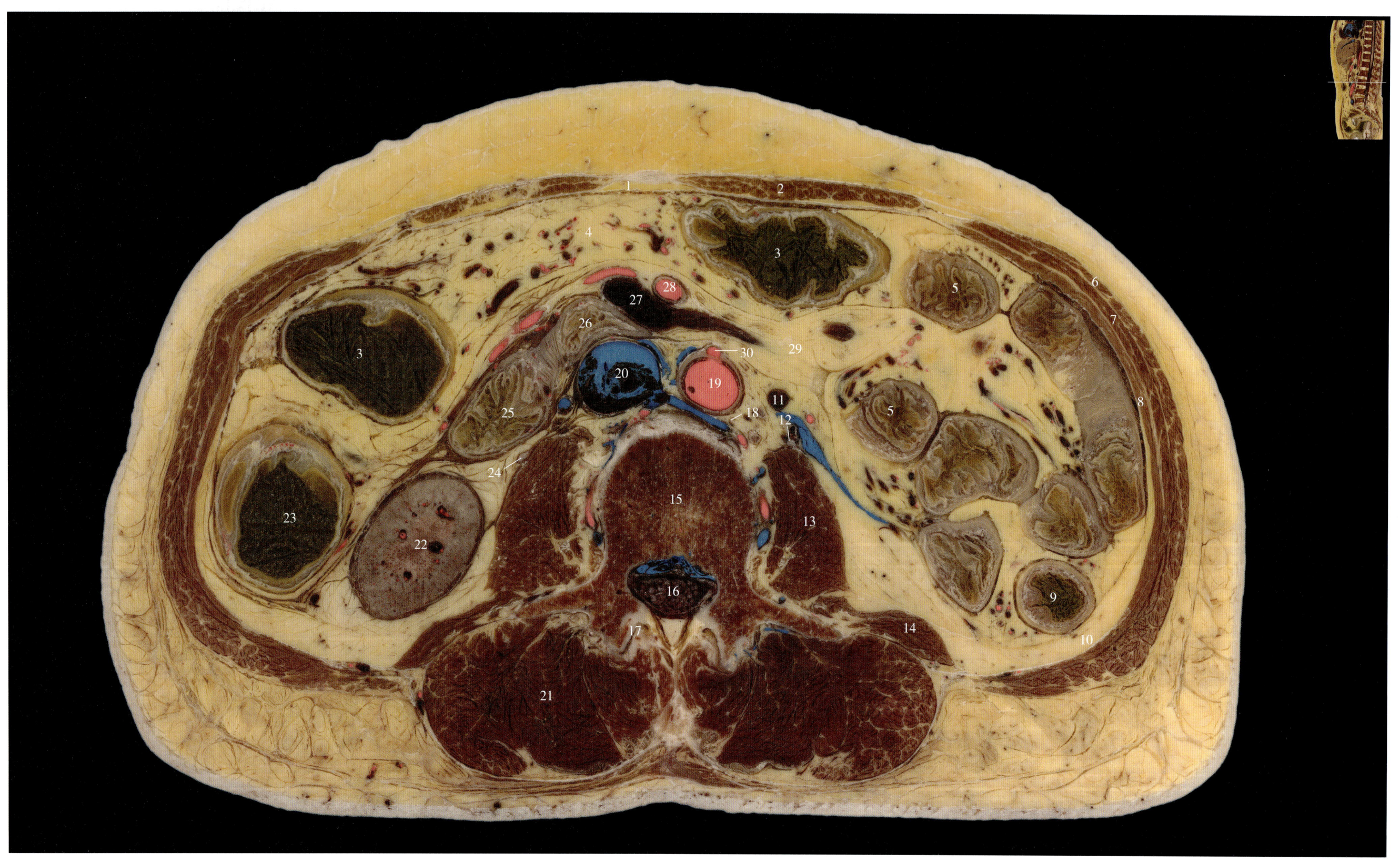

A. 断层标本图像

1. 肝圆韧带 ligamentum teres hepatis
2. 腹直肌 rectus abdominis
3. 横结肠 transverse colon
4. 大网膜 greater omentum
5. 空肠 jejunum
6. 腹外斜肌 obliquus externus abdominis
7. 腹内斜肌 obliquus internus abdominis
8. 腹横肌 transverses abdominis
9. 降结肠 descending colon
10. 腹膜外脂肪 extraperitoneal fat
11. 肠系膜下静脉 inferior mesenteric vein
12. 左输尿管 left ureter
13. 腰大肌 psoas major
14. 腰方肌 quadratus lumborum
15. 第 3 腰椎椎体 body of 3rd lumbar vertebra
16. 马尾 cauda equina
17. 关节突关节 zygapophysial joint
18. 左交感干 left sympathetic trunk
19. 腹主动脉 abdominal aorta
20. 下腔静脉 inferior vena cava
21. 竖脊肌 erector spinae
22. 右肾 right kidney
23. 升结肠 ascending colon
24. 右输尿管 right ureter
25. 十二指肠降部 descending part of duodenum
26. 十二指肠水平部 horizontal part of duodenum
27. 肠系膜上静脉 superior mesenteric vein
28. 肠系膜上动脉 superior mesenteric artery
29. 肠系膜 mesentery
30. 肠系膜下动脉 inferior mesenteric artery

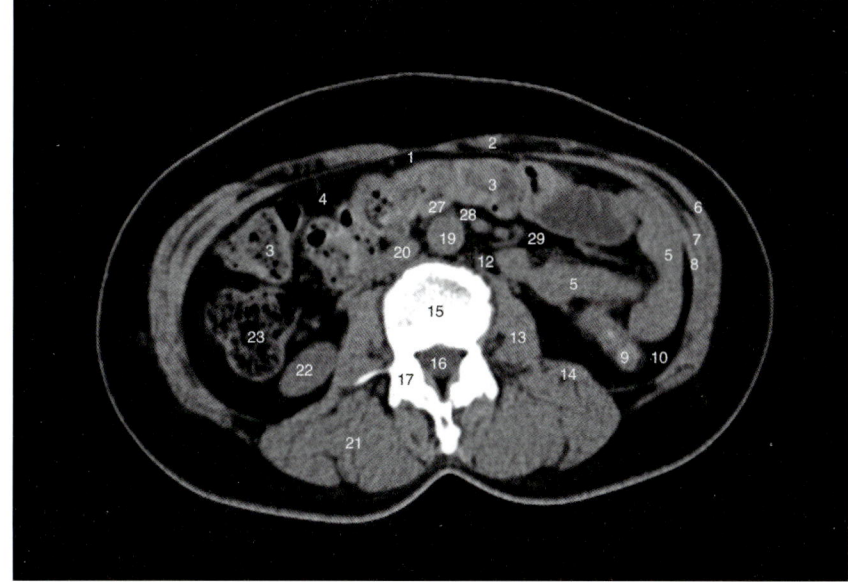

B. CT 平扫图像

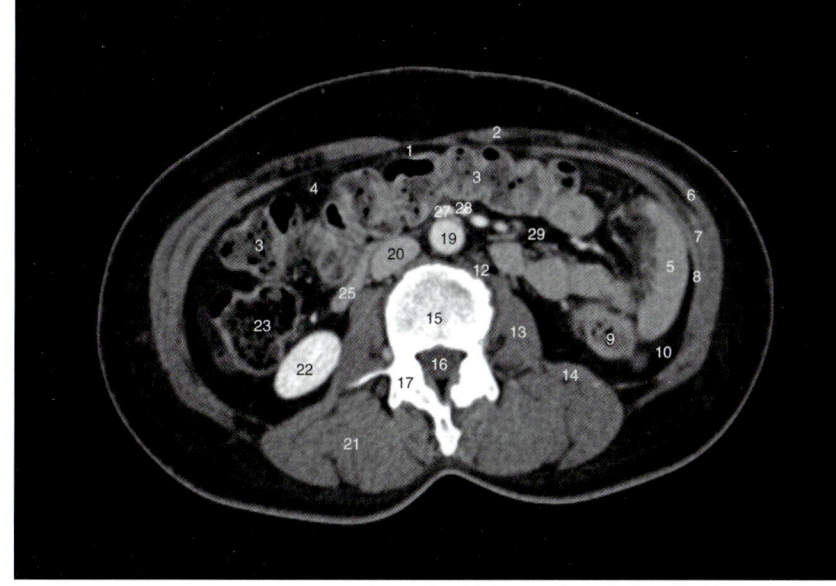

C. CT 增强图像

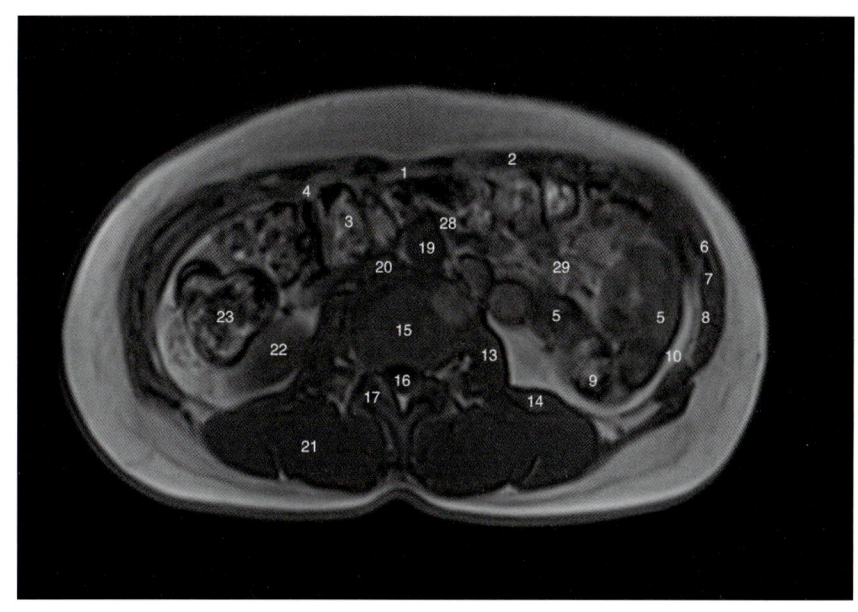

D. MR T1WI

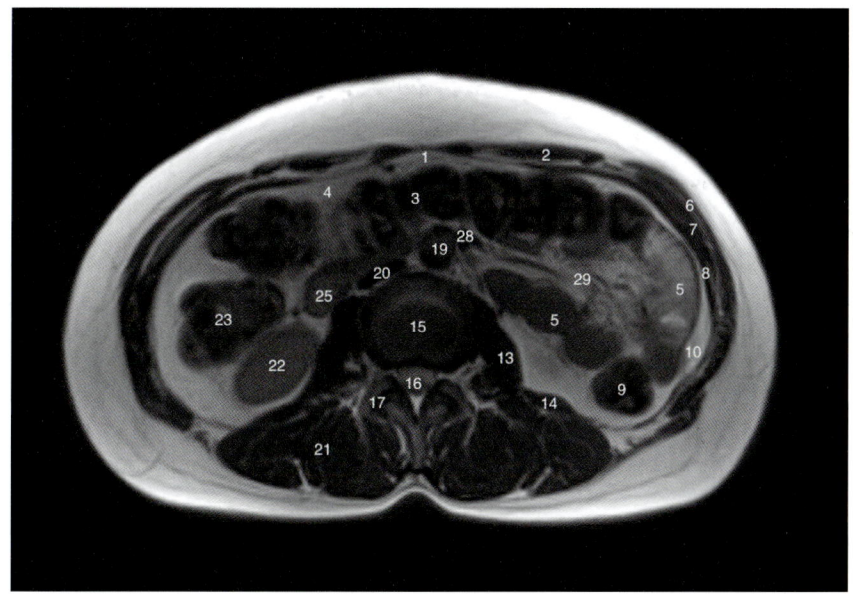

E. MR T2WI

关键结构：十二指肠降部、水平部，下腔静脉。

此断面经过第 3 腰椎椎体。

腹主动脉与下腔静脉于脊柱前方走行，十二指肠水平部在下腔静脉右前方接续十二指肠降部，水平向左走行，移行为十二结肠升部。两侧腰大肌的侧前方均有输尿管通行，脊柱左前方，腹主动脉已发出肠系膜下动脉。十二指肠降部属腹膜外位器官，成人降部长度为 5~10 cm，内侧紧贴胰头，降部黏膜形成发达的环形皱襞，其中份后内侧壁上有一纵行的皱襞称十二指肠纵襞，其下端的圆形隆起称十二指肠大乳头，是胆总管和胰管的共同开口，该处距幽门为 8~10 cm[37]。十二指肠降部和水平部的移行处可见肝胰壶腹，水平部位于有肠系膜上动、静脉和下腔静脉与腹主动脉之间，如肠系膜上动脉起点过低，可能引起肠系膜上动脉压迫综合征。十二指肠憩室是常见的十二指肠降部病变，可压迫胆总管和胰管引起胆道梗阻或胰腺炎，也可发生出血或穿孔，引起急腹症。病变多为单发，大小不一，绝大多数憩室位于十二指肠内侧，距肝胰壶腹约 2.5 cm。憩室一般呈囊袋状，有时囊内见造影剂、液体及空气，如憩室炎波及乳头，可见因乳头水肿造成的十二指肠黏膜压迹，严重者可造成胆总管压迫形成梗阻，临床上常将此称为"十二指肠乳头旁憩室综合征"[90]。

腹部连续横断层 88（FH.10170）

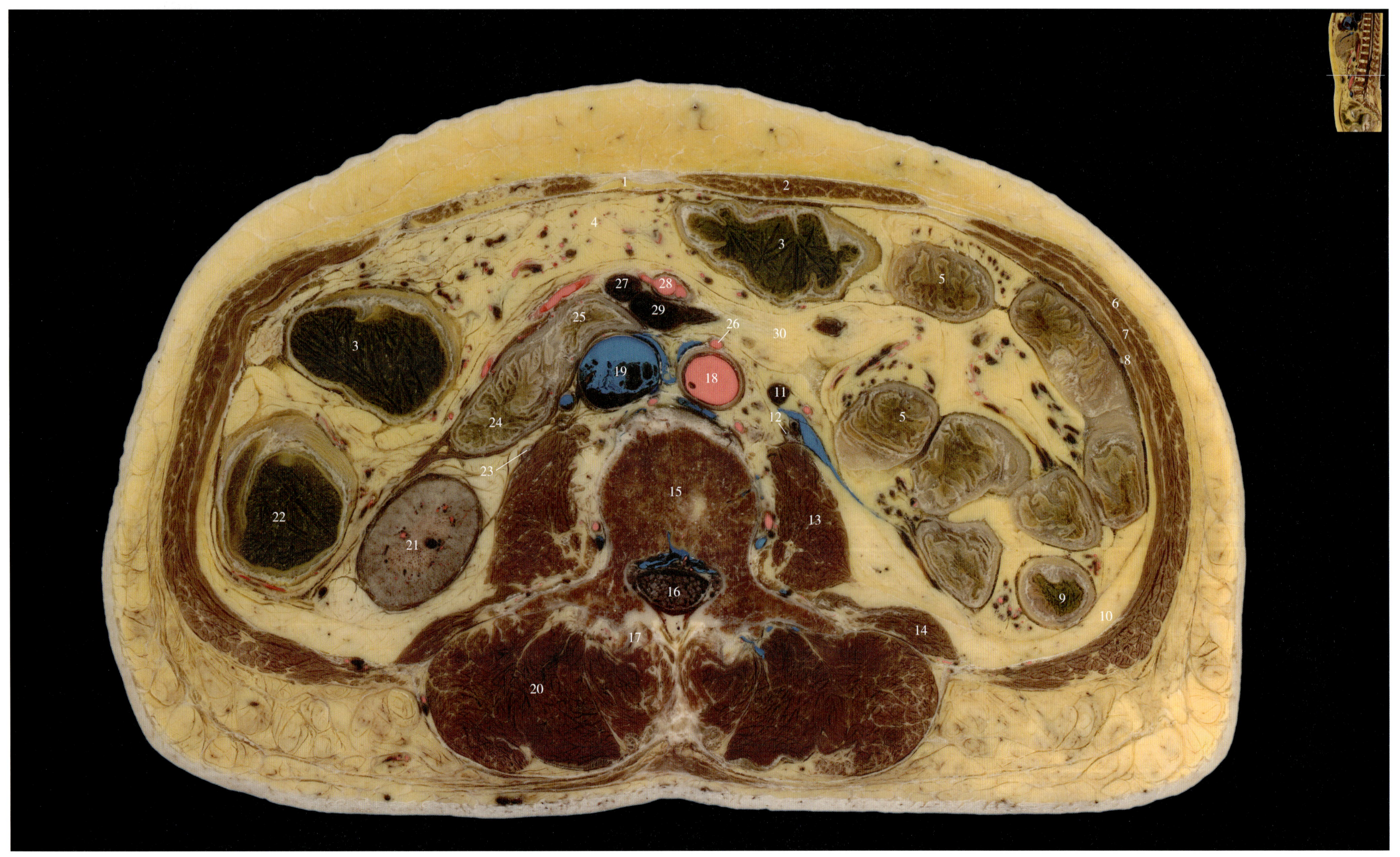

A. 断层标本图像

1. 肝圆韧带 ligamentum teres hepatis
2. 腹直肌 rectus abdominis
3. 横结肠 transverse colon
4. 大网膜 greater omentum
5. 空肠 jejunum
6. 腹外斜肌 obliquus externus abdominis
7. 腹内斜肌 obliquus internus abdominis
8. 腹横肌 transverses abdominis
9. 降结肠 descending colon
10. 腹膜外脂肪 extraperitoneal fat
11. 肠系膜下静脉 inferior mesenteric vein
12. 左输尿管 left ureter
13. 腰大肌 psoas major
14. 腰方肌 quadratus lumborum
15. 第 3 腰椎椎体 body of 3rd lumbar vertebra
16. 马尾 cauda equina
17. 关节突关节 zygapophysial joint
18. 腹主动脉 abdominal aorta
19. 下腔静脉 inferior vena cava
20. 竖脊肌 erector spinae
21. 右肾 right kidney
22. 升结肠 ascending colon
23. 右输尿管 right ureter
24. 十二指肠降部 descending part of duodenum
25. 十二指肠水平部 horizontal part of duodenum
26. 肠系膜下动脉 inferior mesenteric artery
27. 肠系膜上静脉 superior mesenteric vein
28. 肠系膜上动脉 superior mesenteric artery
29. 空肠静脉 jejunal vein
30. 肠系膜 mesentery

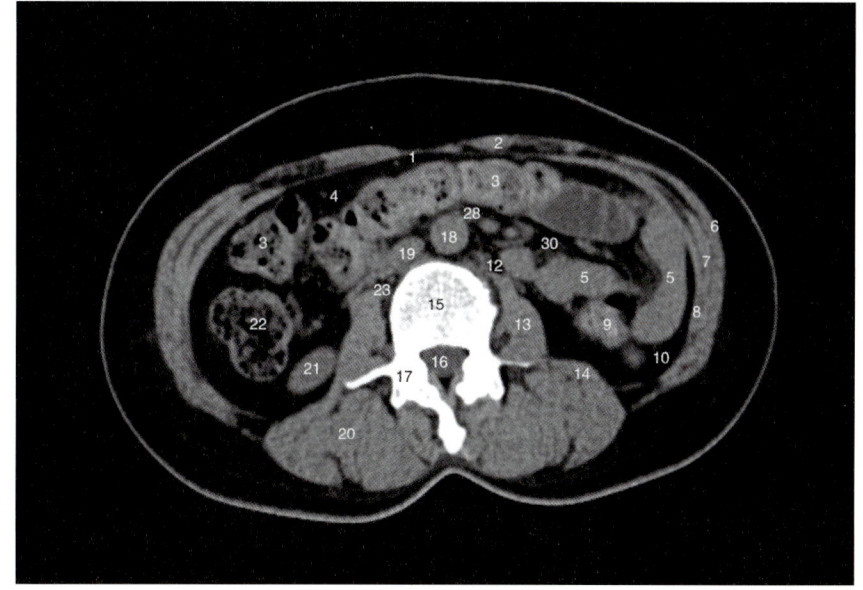

B. CT 平扫图像

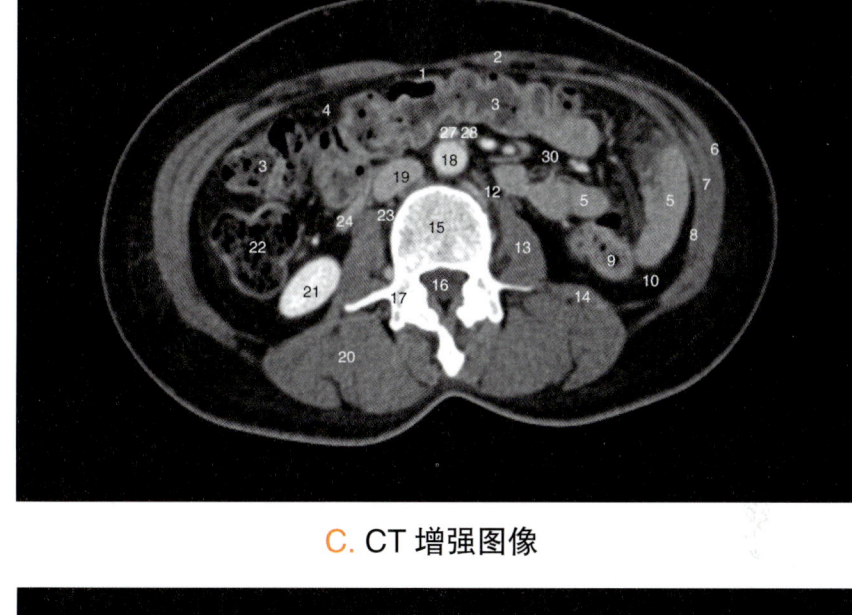

C. CT 增强图像

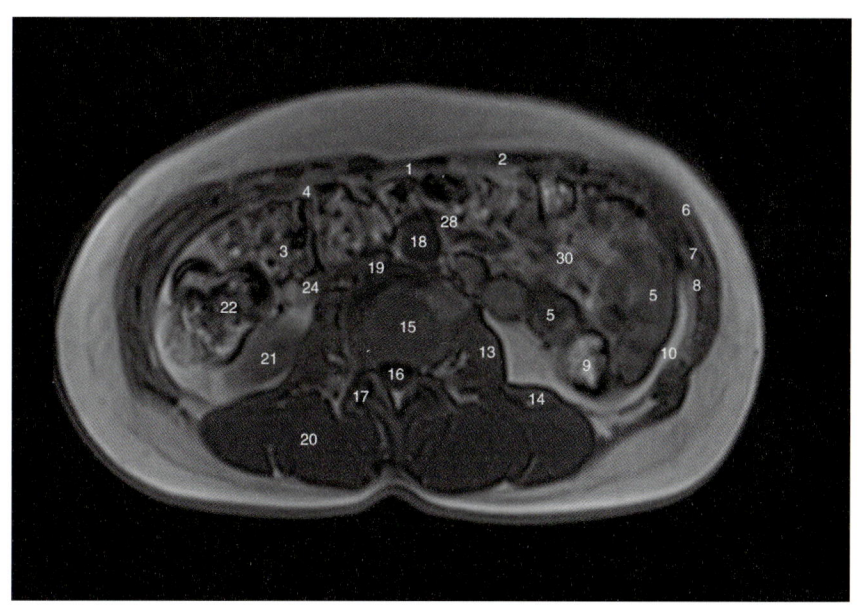

D. MR T1WI

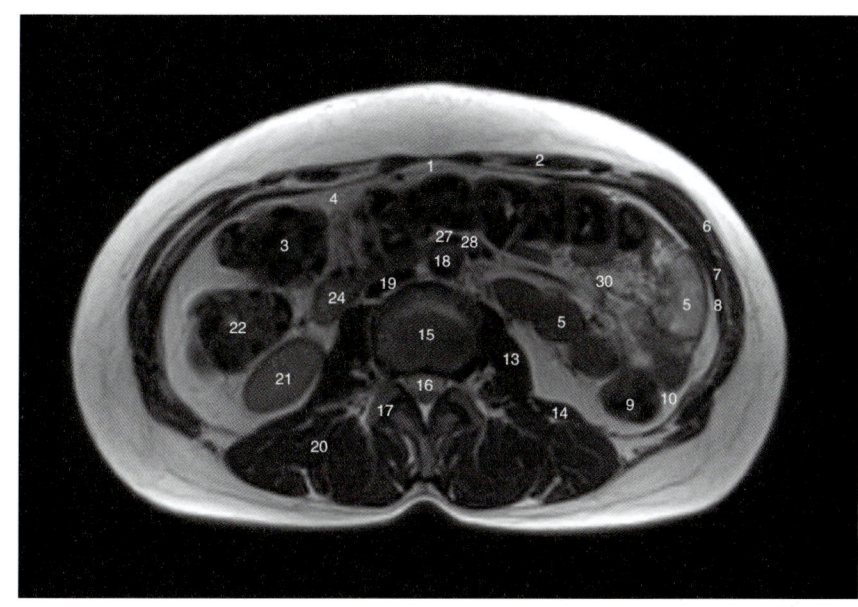

E. MR T2WI

关键结构：肠系膜上静脉，空肠静脉，腹主动脉。

此断面经第 3 腰椎椎体。

腹部中份由右向左可见十二指肠降部、十二指肠水平部、下腔静脉、肠系膜上静脉、肠系膜上动脉、腹主动脉和肠系膜下动脉等结构。空肠静脉向右前方注入十二指肠水平部前方的肠系膜上静脉是本断面的重要特征。肠系膜上静脉是中腹部的重要血管，其走行于小肠系膜内，于左侧和同名动脉伴行，收集十二指肠至结肠左曲以上肠管、部分胃和胰腺的静脉血，在幽门平面与脾静脉在胰颈后方汇合形成门静脉。肠系膜上静脉既是胰颈、钩突和左肾静脉的识别标志，又有助于辨识肠系膜根的起始段，还在中肠扭转不良的诊断中具有重要意义[7]。肠系膜上静脉的长度存在个体差异，短者仅有 2.2 cm，长者可达 17.0 cm，管径为 1.50 cm ± 0.34 cm[37]。最近的 CT、MRI 研究显示肠系膜上静脉多位于肠系膜上动脉的右前方，二者之间距离不超过 5 mm，静脉管径均大于或等于动脉，如发现静脉管径小于动脉并伴有静脉前移 >5 mm，即认为异常，需进一步查明病因。肠系膜上静脉血栓是最常见的肠系膜上静脉病变，原发性的血液高凝状态和肿瘤栓子是最常见的致病因素。影像学上表现为肠壁增厚、水肿，肠壁异常强化，肠管扩张，血管内充盈缺损、管腔扩张，肠系膜脂肪水肿，伴有腹水。

腹部连续横断层 89（FH.10150）

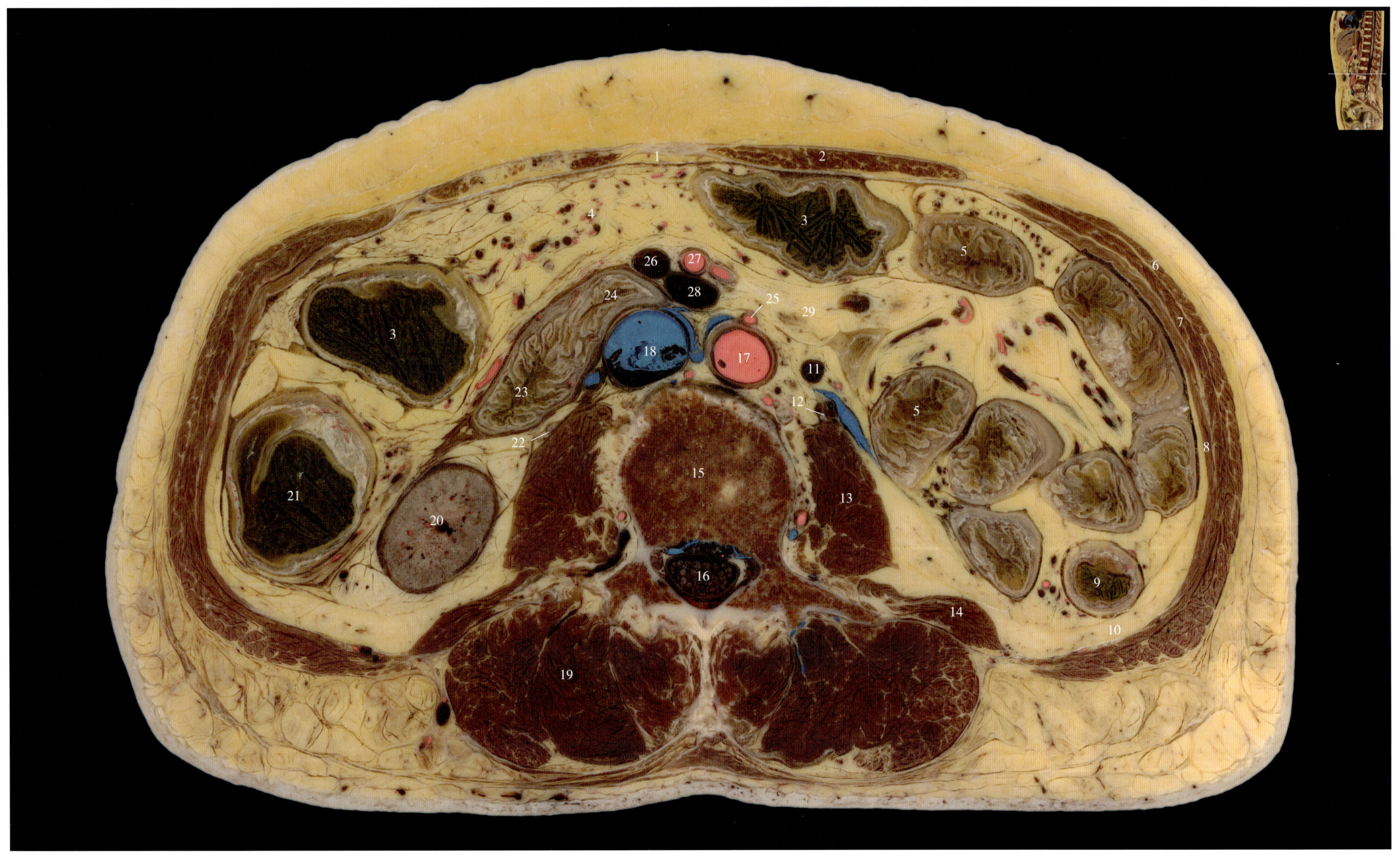

A. 断层标本图像

1. 肝圆韧带 ligamentum teres hepatis
2. 腹直肌 rectus abdominis
3. 横结肠 transverse colon
4. 大网膜 greater omentum
5. 空肠 jejunum
6. 腹外斜肌 obliquus externus abdominis
7. 腹内斜肌 obliquus internus abdominis
8. 腹横肌 transverses abdominis
9. 降结肠 descending colon
10. 腹膜外脂肪 extraperitoneal fat
11. 肠系膜下静脉 inferior mesenteric vein
12. 左输尿管 left ureter
13. 腰大肌 psoas major
14. 腰方肌 quadratus lumborum
15. 第3腰椎椎体 body of 3rd lumbar vertebra
16. 马尾 cauda equina
17. 腹主动脉 abdominal aorta
18. 下腔静脉 inferior vena cava
19. 竖脊肌 erector spinae
20. 右肾 right kidney
21. 升结肠 ascending colon
22. 右输尿管 right ureter
23. 十二指肠降部 descending part of duodenum
24. 十二指肠水平部 horizontal part of duodenum
25. 肠系膜下动脉 inferior mesenteric artery
26. 肠系膜上静脉 superior mesenteric vein
27. 肠系膜上动脉 superior mesenteric artery
28. 空肠静脉 jejunal vein
29. 肠系膜 mesentery

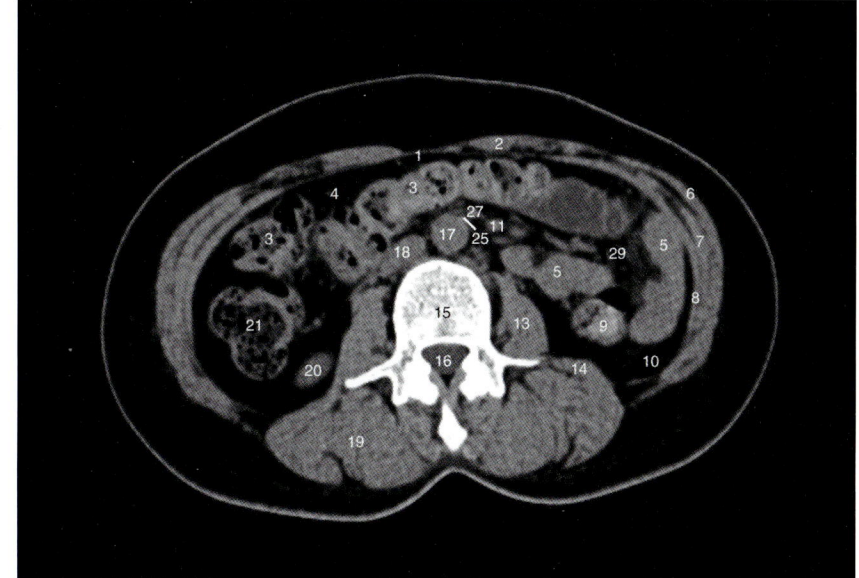

B. CT 平扫图像

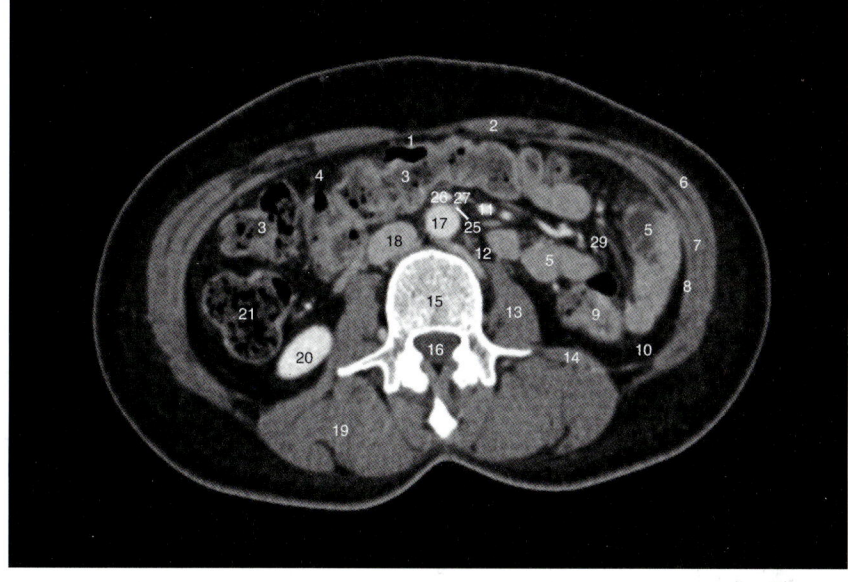

C. CT 增强图像

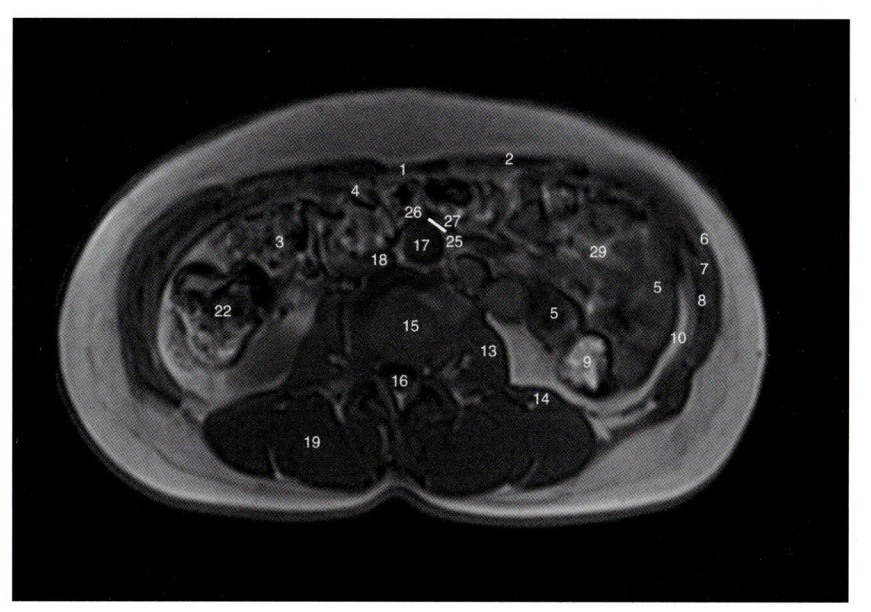

D. MR T1WI

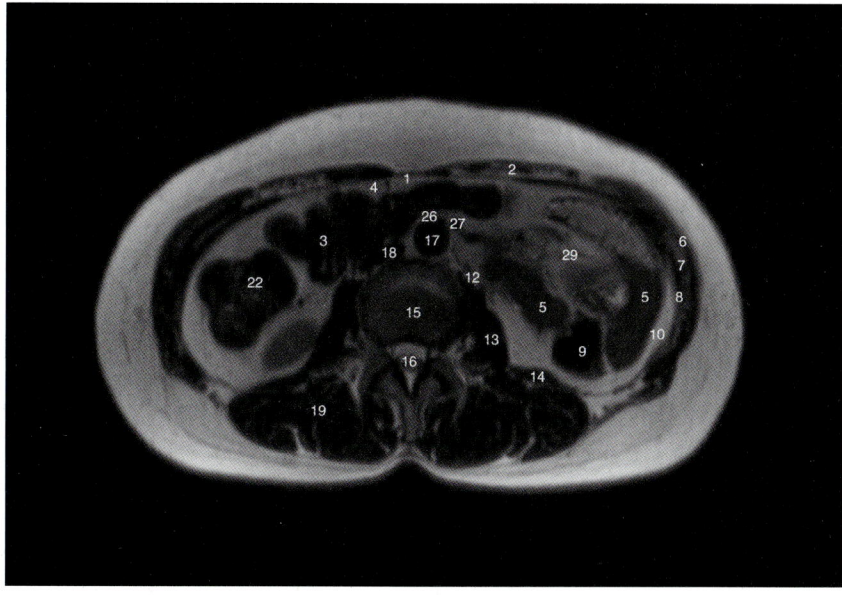

E. MR T2WI

关键结构：肠系膜下动脉，肠系膜下静脉，肠系膜。

此断面经过第3腰椎椎体。

腹主动脉于脊柱的左前方继续下行，下腔静脉位于其右侧。在腹主动脉的左前方和左后方，可见肠系膜下动脉和肠系膜下静脉，二者相隔一段距离。肠系膜下动脉一般在第3腰椎的高度发自腹主动脉的前壁，外径平均约4 mm，行向左下方，发出左结肠动脉、乙状结肠动脉和直肠上动脉分布于结肠左曲到直肠上部的结构，其小分支向上与肠系膜上动脉的细小分支吻合，向下与直肠下动脉的分支吻合。肠系膜上、下动脉的各结肠支间相互吻合，形成一条完整的动脉弓，称边缘动脉，若肠系膜上动脉或肠系膜下动脉慢性阻塞时，边缘动脉可以扩张，形成侧支循环。在横结肠右侧和降结肠上部之间的区域内，除了边缘动脉外，尚可存在由中结肠动脉和左结肠动脉主干或一级分支吻合成的 Riolan 弓，是肠系膜上、下动脉直接交通动脉。肠系膜下静脉是肝门静脉的重要属支，收纳同名动脉供应区域的静脉血，上行至胰颈后方注入脾静脉或肠系膜上静脉，有时亦与此两条静脉共同汇合形成肝门静脉。当患者行肠系膜动脉 CTA 检查时，肠系膜下动脉的最大密度投影的重建通常在矢状位图像上进行，可见其主干几乎紧贴腹主动脉向下延伸。此外，临床上在行结肠手术分离、切除肠脂垂时，不可牵拉，以免损伤结肠动脉长支，影响肠壁反应。

腹部连续横断层 90（FH.10130）

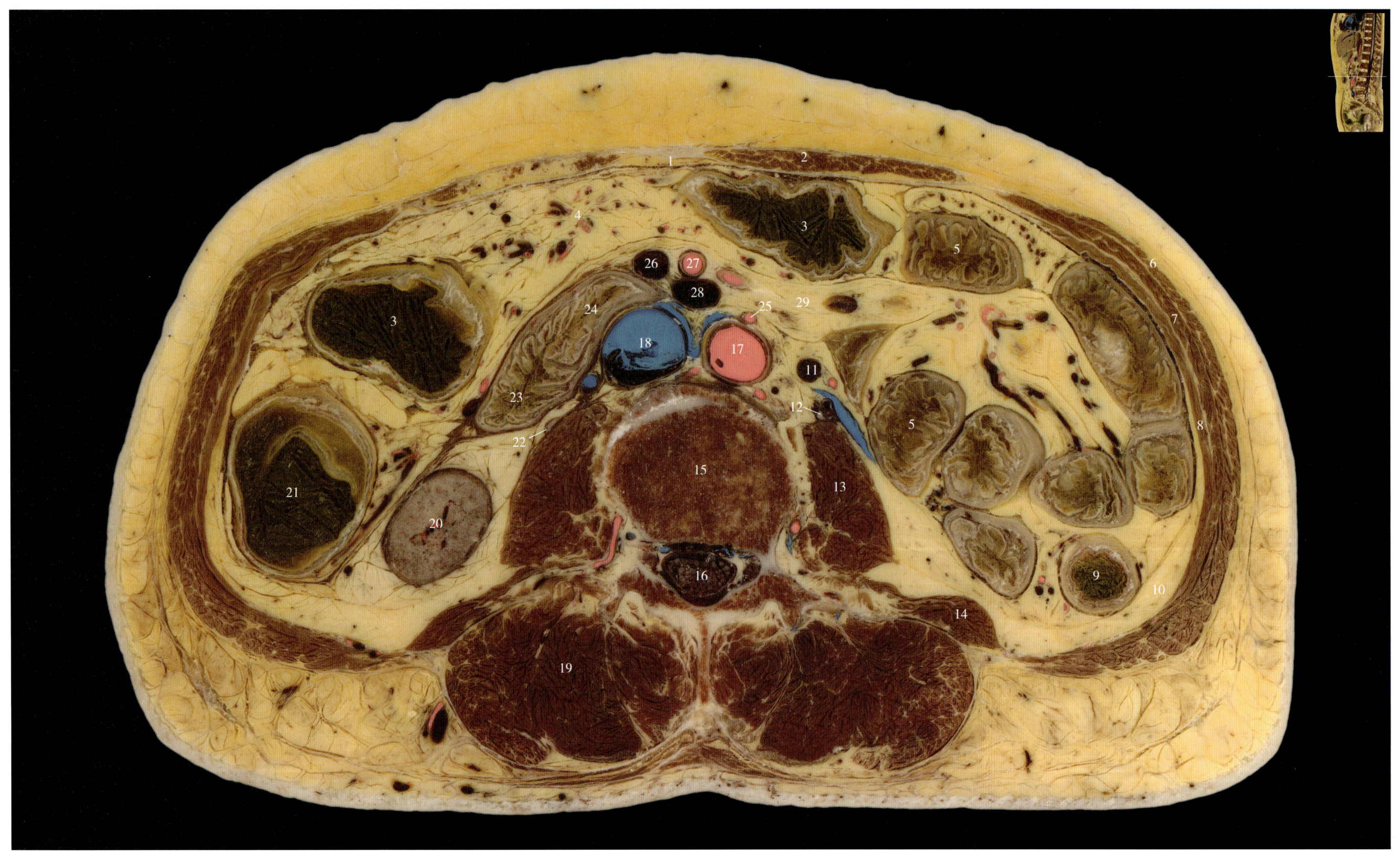

A. 断层标本图像

1. 肝圆韧带 ligamentum teres hepatis
2. 腹直肌 rectus abdominis
3. 横结肠 transverse colon
4. 大网膜 greater omentum
5. 空肠 jejunum
6. 腹外斜肌 obliquus externus abdominis
7. 腹内斜肌 obliquus internus abdominis
8. 腹横肌 transverses abdominis
9. 降结肠 descending colon
10. 腹膜外脂肪 extraperitoneal fat
11. 肠系膜下静脉 inferior mesenteric vein
12. 左输尿管 left ureter
13. 腰大肌 psoas major
14. 腰方肌 quadratus lumborum
15. 第 3 腰椎椎体 body of 3rd lumbar vertebra
16. 马尾 cauda equina
17. 腹主动脉 abdominal aorta
18. 下腔静脉 inferior vena cava
19. 竖脊肌 erector spinae
20. 右肾 right kidney
21. 升结肠 ascending colon
22. 右输尿管 right ureter
23. 十二指肠降部 descending part of duodenum
24. 十二指肠水平部 horizontal part of duodenum
25. 肠系膜下动脉 inferior mesenteric artery
26. 肠系膜上静脉 superior mesenteric vein
27. 肠系膜上动脉 superior mesenteric artery
28. 空肠静脉 jejunal vein
29. 肠系膜 mesentery

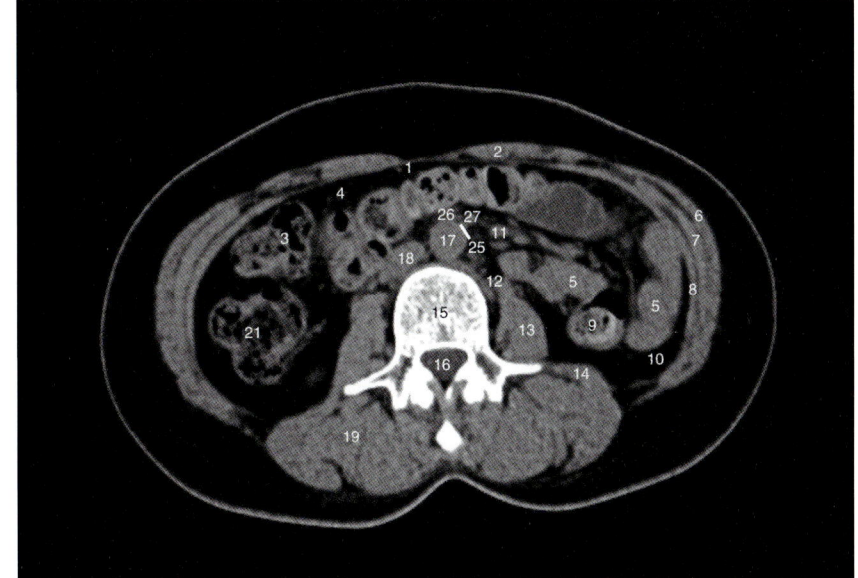
B. CT 平扫图像

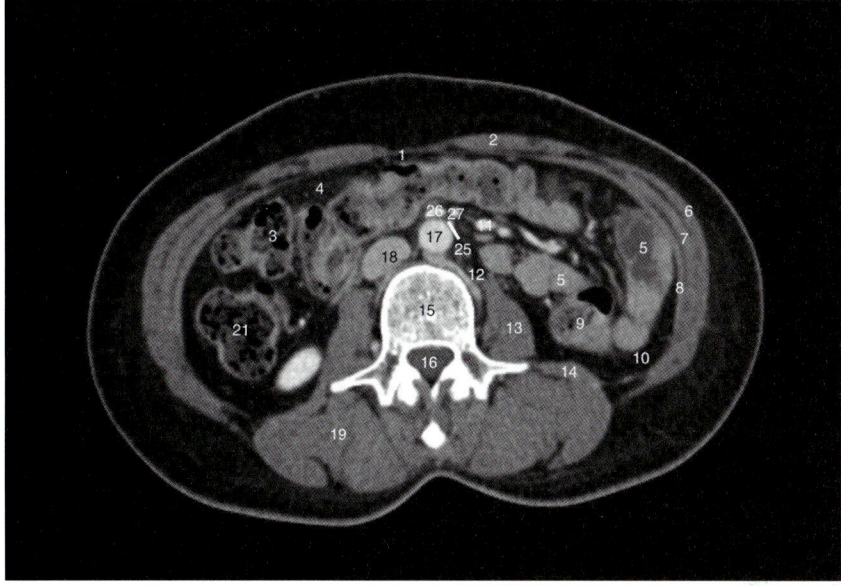
C. CT 增强图像

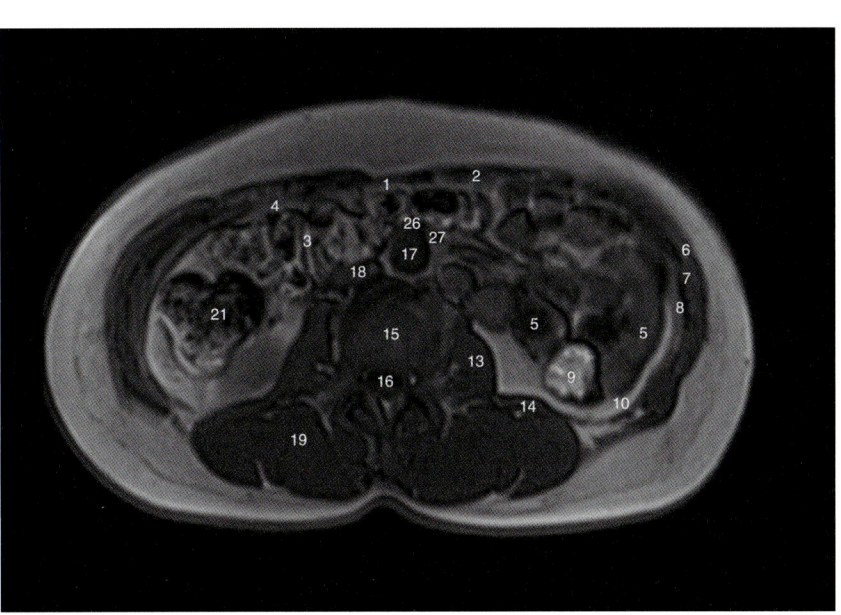
D. MR T1WI

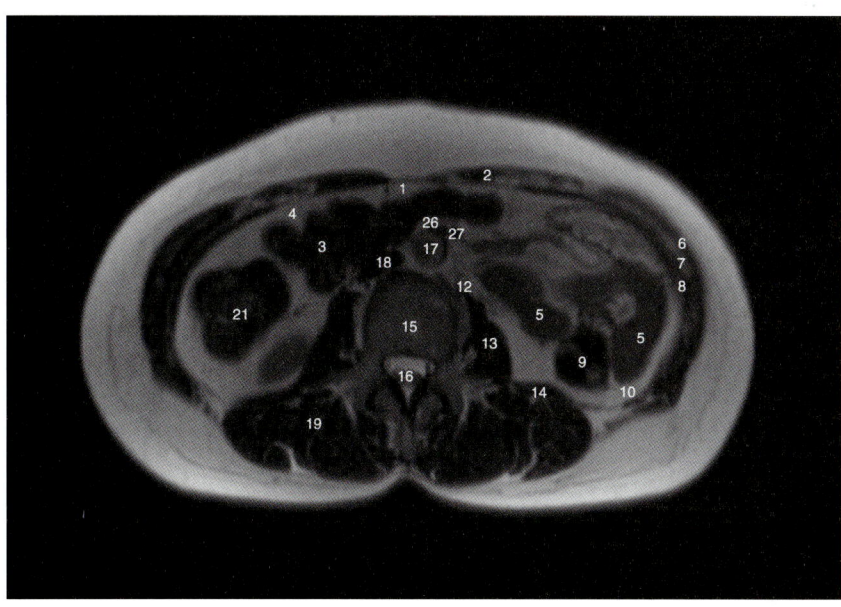
E. MR T2WI

关键结构：左、右输尿管，腰大肌。

此断面经过第 3 腰椎椎体。

脊柱两侧为粗壮的腰大肌，左输尿管位于左侧腰大肌的前方，肠系膜下静脉的后方，右输尿管在右腰大肌前外侧、十二指肠降部后方下行。输尿管是位于腹膜外位的肌性管道，平第 2 腰椎上缘，起自肾盂末端，终于膀胱，长 20~30 cm，管径为 0.5~1.0 cm[91]。输尿管全长可分为腹部、盆部及壁内部 3 段。输尿管腹部经腰大肌前面下行至其中点附近，与卵巢血管（女性）或睾丸血管（男性）交叉，左侧输尿管越过左髂总动脉末端前方，右侧输尿管越过右髂外动脉起始部入盆腔。输尿管盆部经盆腔侧壁、髂内血管、腰骶干和骶髂关节前方下行，跨过闭孔神经血管束达坐骨棘水平。男性输尿管在输精管后方与之交叉，女性输尿管经子宫颈外侧 2.5 cm，从子宫动脉后下方绕过。输尿管壁内部为长约 1.5 cm 斜行的管道，在膀胱空虚时，膀胱三角内的两输尿管口间距约 2.5 cm。输尿管全程有 3 处狭窄：①上狭窄位于肾盂输尿管移行处；②中狭窄位于小骨盆上口，输尿管跨过髂血管处；③下狭窄位于输尿管壁内部。急性输尿管结石是最常见的急腹症之一，结石多停留在输尿管 3 个生理狭窄部位，患者可出现绞痛。输尿管结石常为数毫米大小，长圆形，长轴与输尿管的纵轴平行，影像学上呈高密度（CT 平扫）或高回声（B 超）显影，其周围可见软组织密度环，代表受累肿胀的输尿管壁；结石嵌顿于输尿管内，亦可引起肾盂积水[92]。

腹部连续横断层 91（FH.10110）

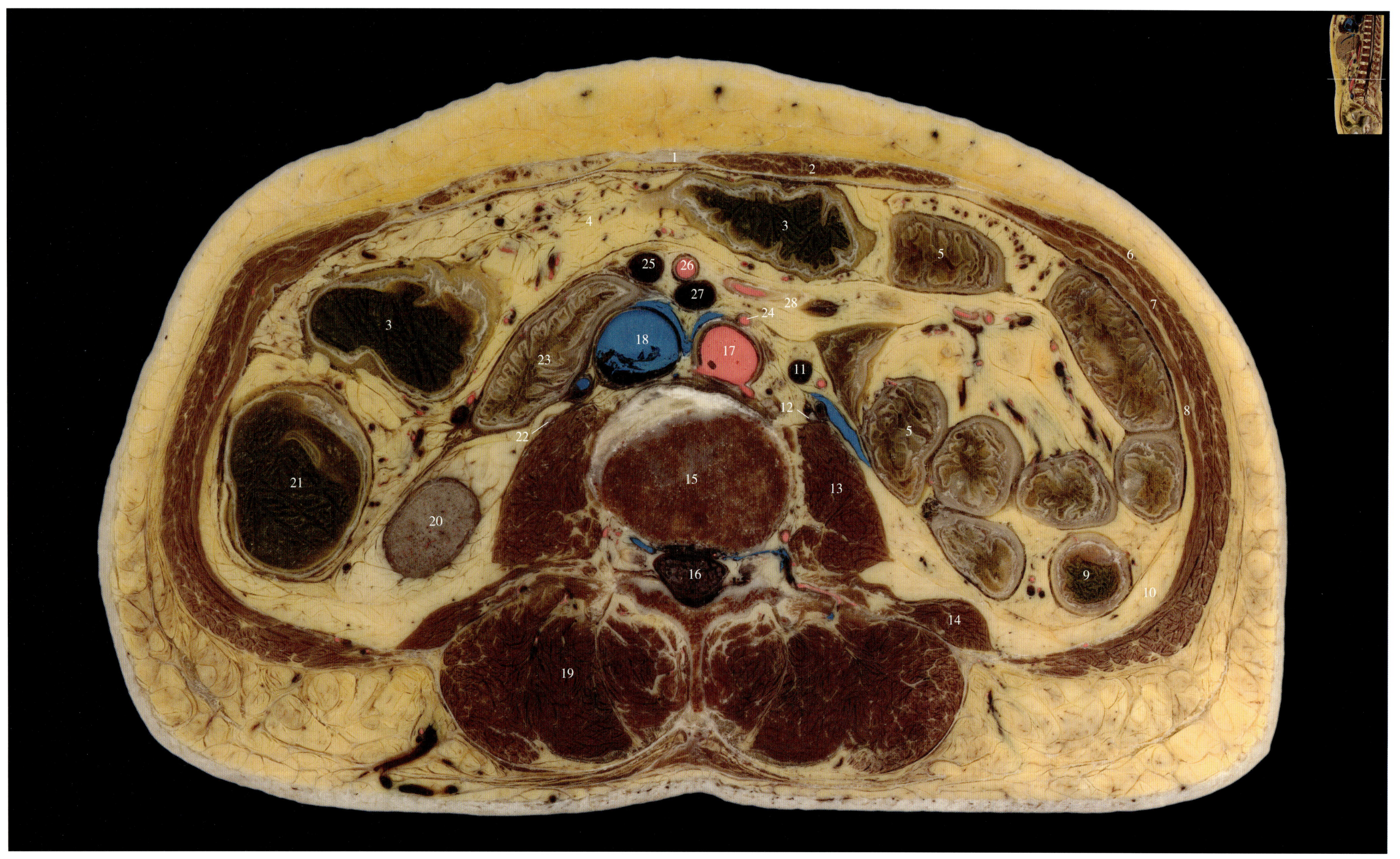

A. 断层标本图像

1. 肝圆韧带 ligamentum teres hepatis
2. 腹直肌 rectus abdominis
3. 横结肠 transverse colon
4. 大网膜 greater omentum
5. 空肠 jejunum
6. 腹外斜肌 obliquus externus abdominis
7. 腹内斜肌 obliquus internus abdominis
8. 腹横肌 transverses abdominis
9. 降结肠 descending colon
10. 腹膜外脂肪 extraperitoneal fat
11. 肠系膜下静脉 inferior mesenteric vein
12. 左输尿管 left ureter
13. 腰大肌 psoas major
14. 腰方肌 quadratus lumborum
15. 第 3 腰椎椎体 body of 3rd lumbar vertebra
16. 马尾 cauda equina
17. 腹主动脉 abdominal aorta
18. 下腔静脉 inferior vena cava
19. 竖脊肌 erector spinae
20. 右肾 right kidney
21. 升结肠 ascending colon
22. 右输尿管 right ureter
23. 十二指肠水平部 horizontal part of duodenum
24. 肠系膜下动脉 inferior mesenteric artery
25. 肠系膜上静脉 superior mesenteric vein
26. 肠系膜上动脉 superior mesenteric artery
27. 空肠静脉 jejunal vein
28. 肠系膜 mesentery

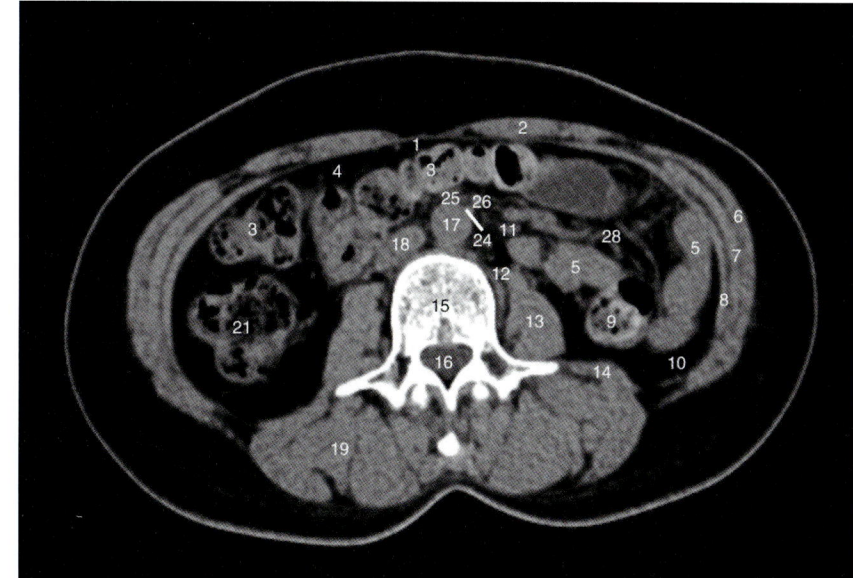

B. CT 平扫图像

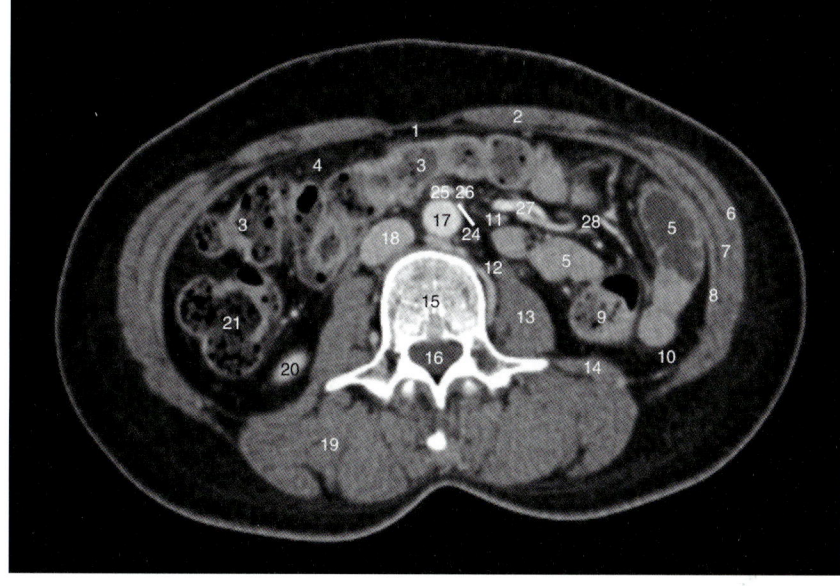

C. CT 增强图像

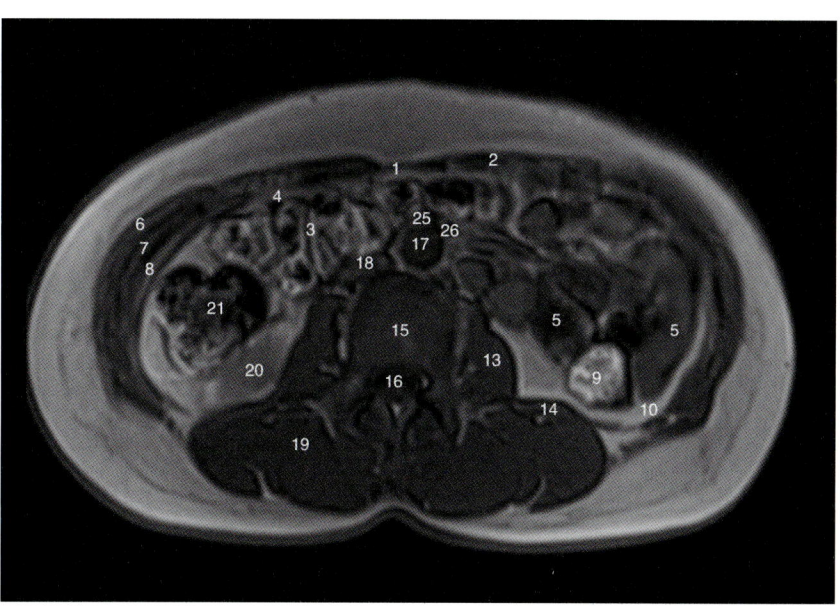

D. MR T1WI

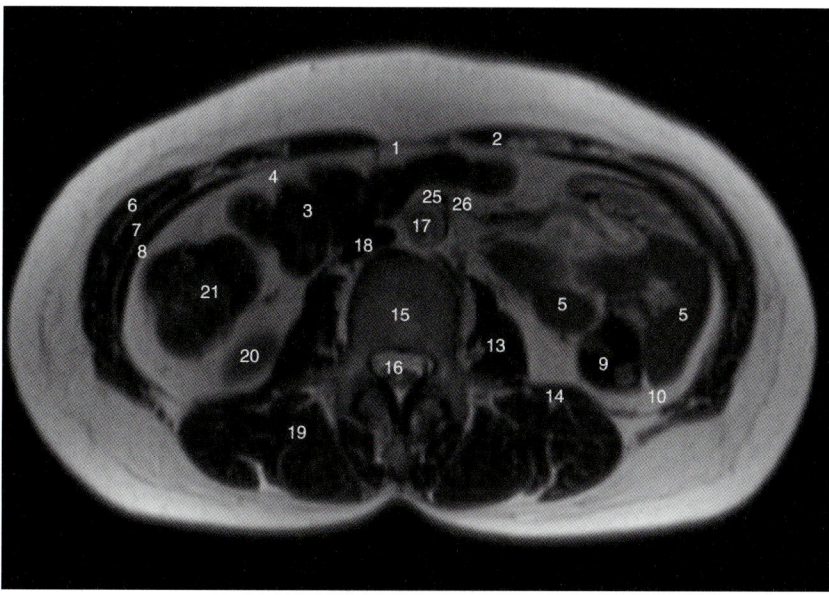

E. MR T2WI

关键结构：腹前外侧壁，腹直肌鞘。

此断面经过第 3 腰椎椎体和 L3-4 椎间盘。

腹腔的前外侧壁由前外侧肌群构成，腹直肌位于腹前壁中线两侧，腹外斜肌、腹内斜肌和腹横肌由外向内依次排列。3 块扁肌的腱膜构成的腹直肌鞘清晰可见，分前后 2 层包绕腹直肌。腹直肌有 3~4 条横行的腱划将肌腹分成多个，腱划与腹直肌鞘前层紧密结合。腹直肌鞘的上 2/3，前层由腹外斜肌腱膜和腹内斜肌腱膜的前层构成，后层由腹内斜肌腱膜的后层与腹横肌腱膜构成。鞘下 1/3 部，3 块扁肌的腱膜构成前层，后层阙如。腹前外侧肌群的功能是保护腹腔脏器，维持腹内压。在 B 超图像上，腹壁结构如腹直肌鞘、腹股沟管深环等均易显示，CT 可显示腹壁上的肌群和皮下脂肪组织，二者对区分一些腹壁的疾病有重要临床价值，如疝、血肿、肿瘤等。其中，韧带样瘤是腹前外侧壁常见的病变，主要为肌肉内结缔组织及其被覆的筋膜或腱膜的单克隆纤维细胞性肿瘤。CT 主要表现为无包膜，单发或多发的肿块；单发者多见，大小不一，直径可达 1.5 cm 或更大。在平扫图像上呈等或稍低密度，密度较均匀，边界较光整，坏死少见，增强后呈轻 - 中度强化。较大损害可发生黏液样变性或囊性变[93]。

腹部连续横断层 92（FH.10090）

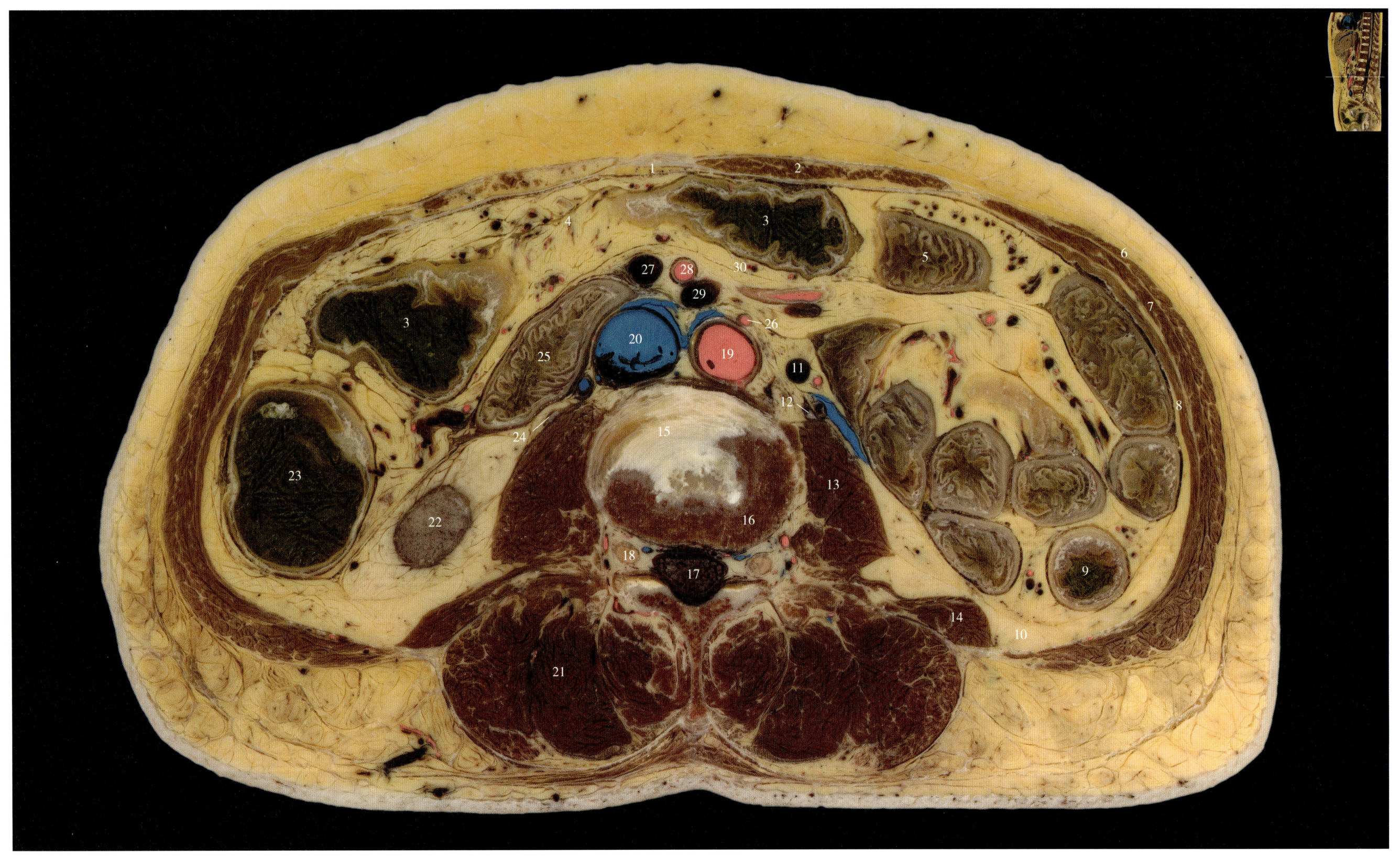

A. 断层标本图像

1. 肝圆韧带 ligamentum teres hepatis
2. 腹直肌 rectus abdominis
3. 横结肠 transverse colon
4. 大网膜 greater omentum
5. 空肠 jejunum
6. 腹外斜肌 obliquus externus abdominis
7. 腹内斜肌 obliquus internus abdominis
8. 腹横肌 transverses abdominis
9. 降结肠 descending colon
10. 腹膜外脂肪 extraperitoneal fat
11. 肠系膜下静脉 inferior mesenteric vein
12. 左输尿管 left ureter
13. 腰大肌 psoas major
14. 腰方肌 quadratus lumborum
15. L3-4 椎间盘 L3-4 intervertebral disc
16. 第 3 腰椎椎体 body of 3rd lumbar vertebra
17. 马尾 cauda equina
18. 第 3 腰神经 3rd lumbar nerve
19. 腹主动脉 abdominal aorta
20. 下腔静脉 inferior vena cava
21. 竖脊肌 erector spinae
22. 右肾 right kidney
23. 升结肠 ascending colon
24. 右输尿管 right ureter
25. 十二指肠水平部 horizontal part of duodenum
26. 肠系膜下动脉 inferior mesenteric artery
27. 肠系膜上静脉 superior mesenteric vein
28. 肠系膜上动脉 superior mesenteric artery
29. 空肠静脉 jejunal vein
30. 肠系膜 mesentery

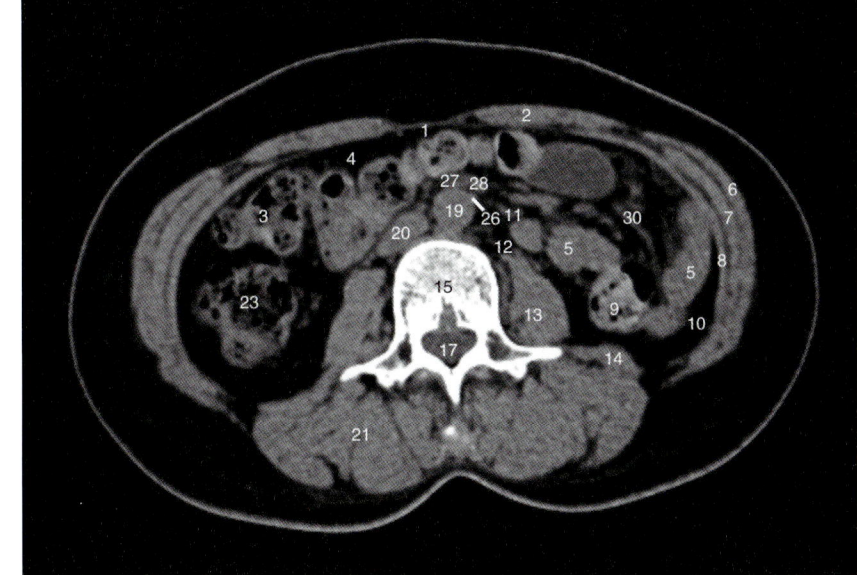

B. CT 平扫图像

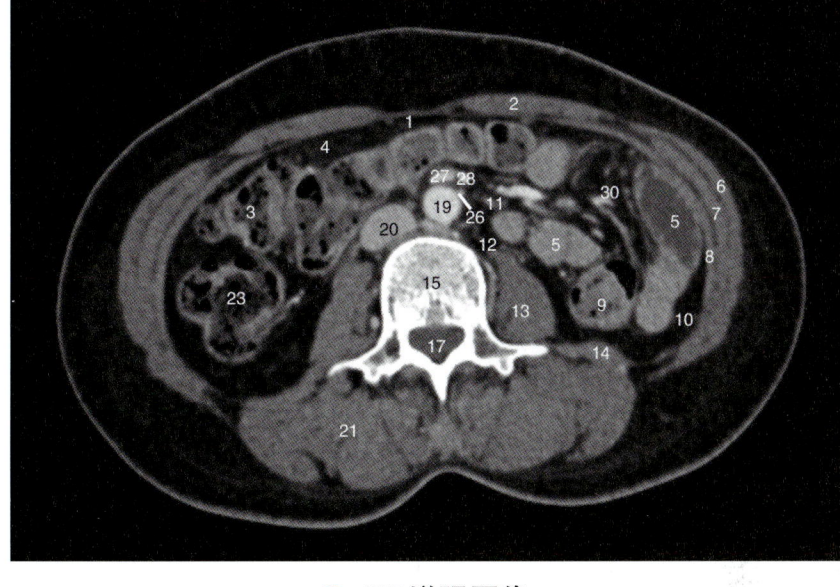

C. CT 增强图像

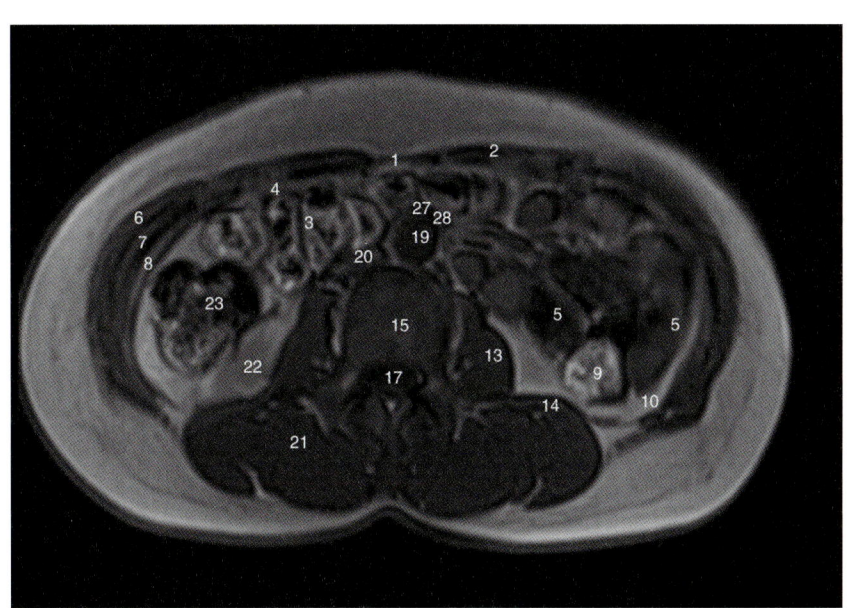

D. MR T1WI

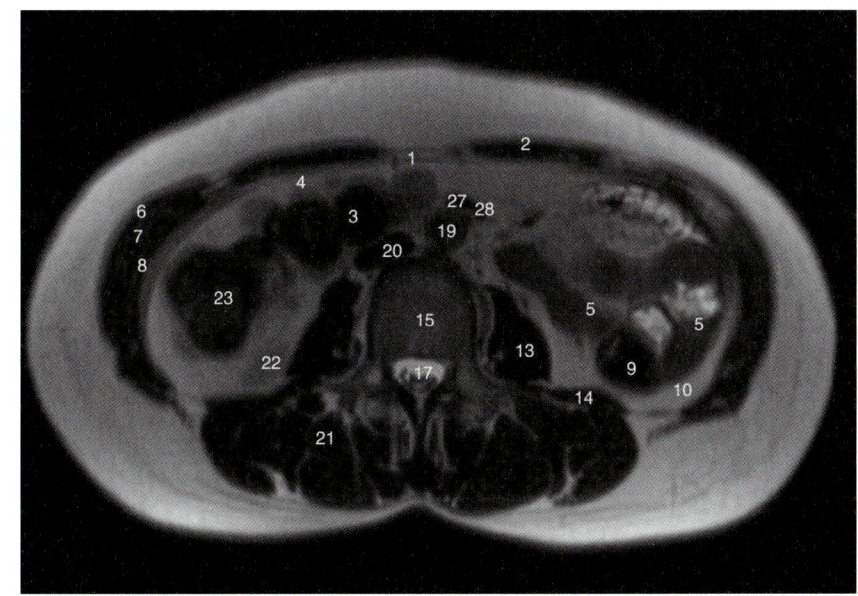

E. MR T2WI

关键结构：下腔静脉，L3-4 椎间盘。

此断面经过第 3 腰椎椎体和 L3-4 椎间盘。

脊柱前方，下腔静脉断面呈圆形，腹主动脉沿其左侧下行。腹腔内结构配布大致同上一断层。下腔静脉由左、右髂总静脉在第 4 或第 5 腰椎的右前方汇合而成，沿腹主动脉右侧和脊柱右前方上行，经肝的腔静脉沟，穿膈的腔静脉孔进入胸腔，最后注入右心房，全长为 20.70~30.70 cm。左、右髂总静脉汇合处的外径为 2.00~3.20 cm，角度在 71.50°~80.50°[37]。下腔静脉常见变异和畸形，畸形发生率高达 1.5%~4.4%，由于畸形的下腔静脉容易在断层影像上误诊，故应引起重视。常见下腔静脉畸形有：①双下腔静脉，发生率 2.2%~2.8%；②左下腔静脉，发生率 0.2%~0.45%；③奇静脉通连，发生率 0.3%；④下腔静脉后输尿管，发生率 0.1%[7]。腹部静脉和双下肢静脉的血栓容易通过下腔静脉进入肺动脉，引起肺动脉栓塞。腔静脉过滤器是一种预防肺动脉栓塞的介入放射学手段，用非外科插管技术在下腔静脉置入滤器，不仅明显降低肺动脉栓塞发病率，而且创伤小。下腔静脉 CT 造影能有效地观察下腔静脉与腔静脉滤器的解剖位置关系，腔静脉滤器在 CT 上呈现明显高密度影，多数呈伞状，尖端朝向近心端，容易辨认[93]。

腹部连续横断层 93（FH.10070）

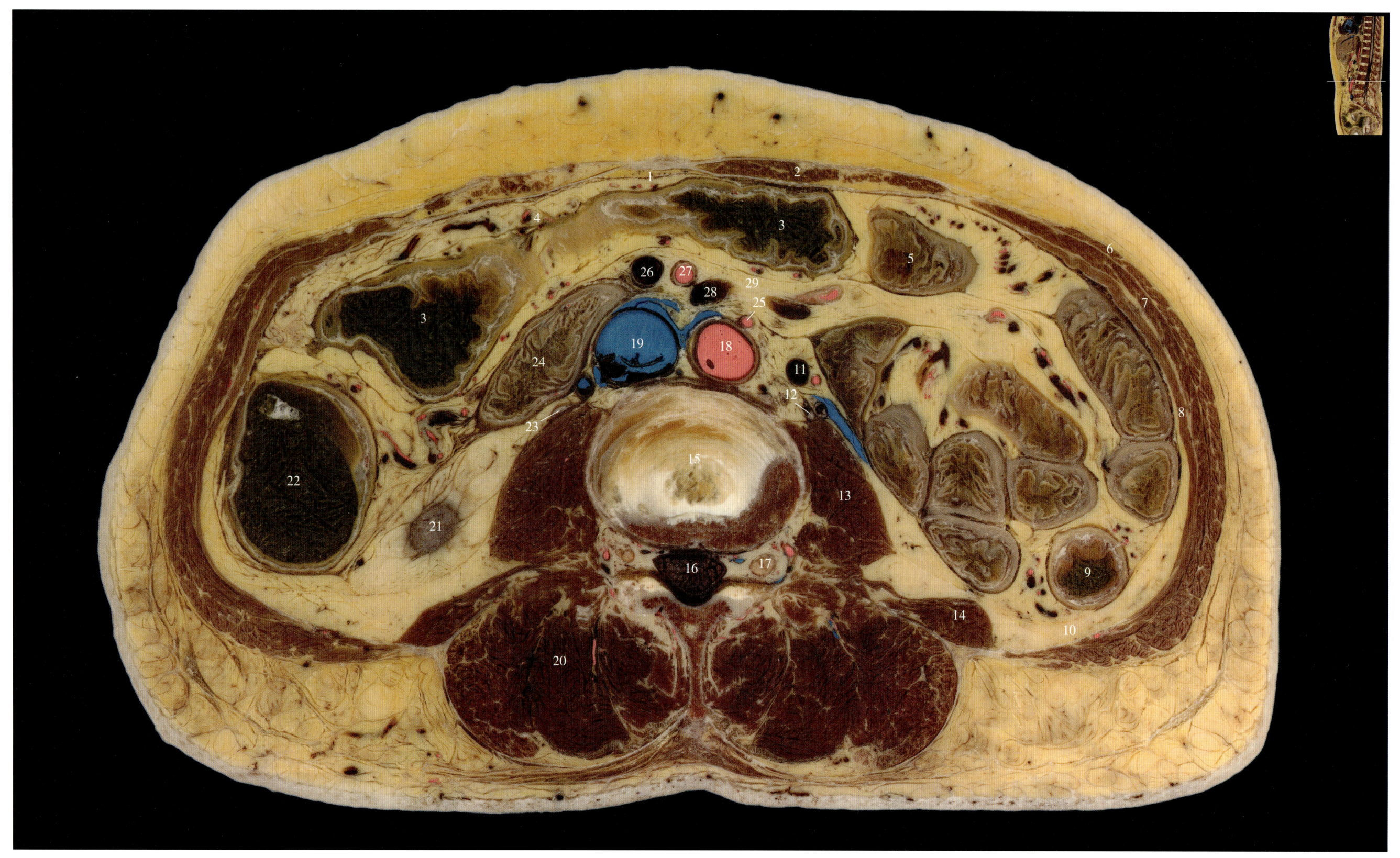

A. 断层标本图像

1. 肝圆韧带 ligamentum teres hepatis
2. 腹直肌 rectus abdominis
3. 横结肠 transverse colon
4. 大网膜 greater omentum
5. 空肠 jejunum
6. 腹外斜肌 obliquus externus abdominis
7. 腹内斜肌 obliquus internus abdominis
8. 腹横肌 transverses abdominis
9. 降结肠 descending colon
10. 腹膜外脂肪 extraperitoneal fat
11. 肠系膜下静脉 inferior mesenteric vein
12. 左输尿管 left ureter
13. 腰大肌 psoas major
14. 腰方肌 quadratus lumborum
15. L3-4 椎间盘 L3-4 intervertebral disc
16. 马尾 cauda equina
17. 第 3 腰神经 3rd lumbar nerve
18. 腹主动脉 abdominal aorta
19. 下腔静脉 inferior vena cava
20. 竖脊肌 erector spinae
21. 右肾 right kidney
22. 升结肠 ascending colon
23. 右输尿管 right ureter
24. 十二指肠水平部 horizontal part of duodenum
25. 肠系膜下动脉 inferior mesenteric artery
26. 肠系膜上静脉 superior mesenteric vein
27. 肠系膜上动脉 superior mesenteric artery
28. 空肠静脉 jejunal vein
29. 肠系膜 mesentery
30. 第 3 腰椎椎体 body of 3rd lumbar vertebra

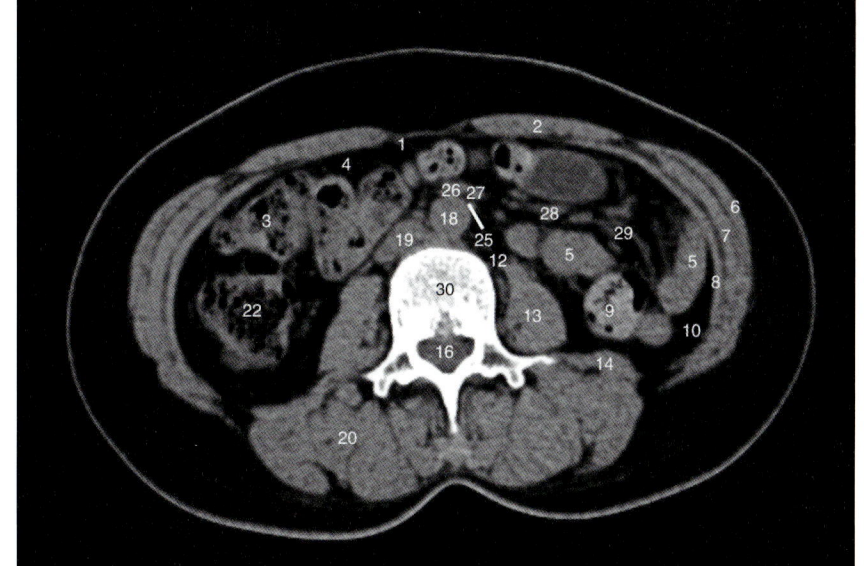

B. CT 平扫图像

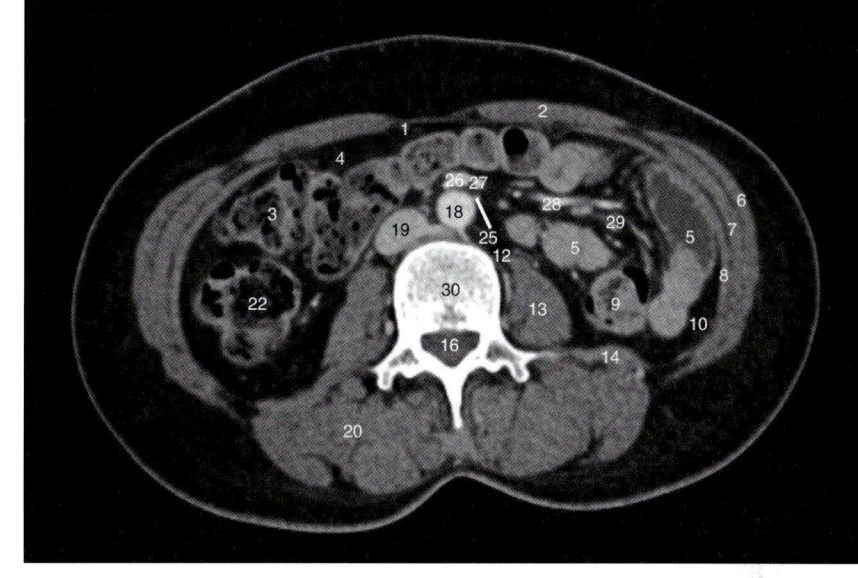

C. CT 增强图像

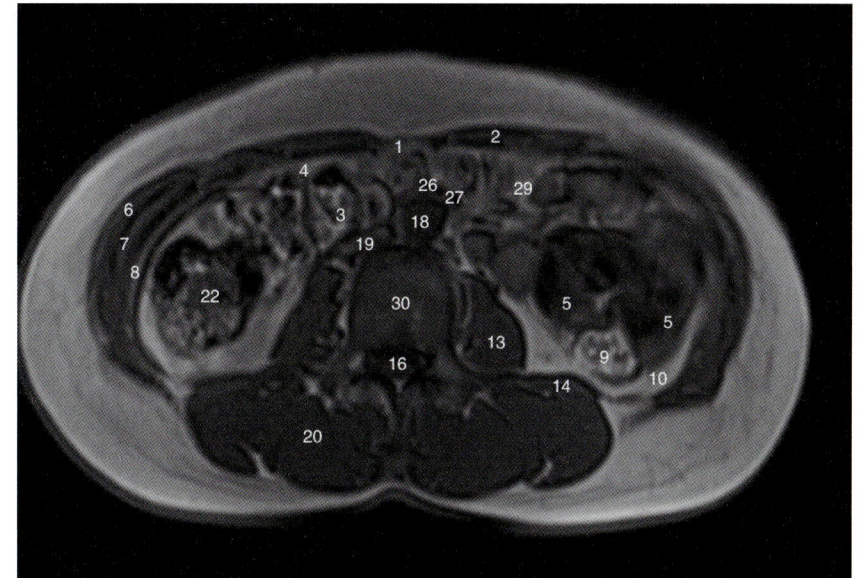

D. MR T1WI

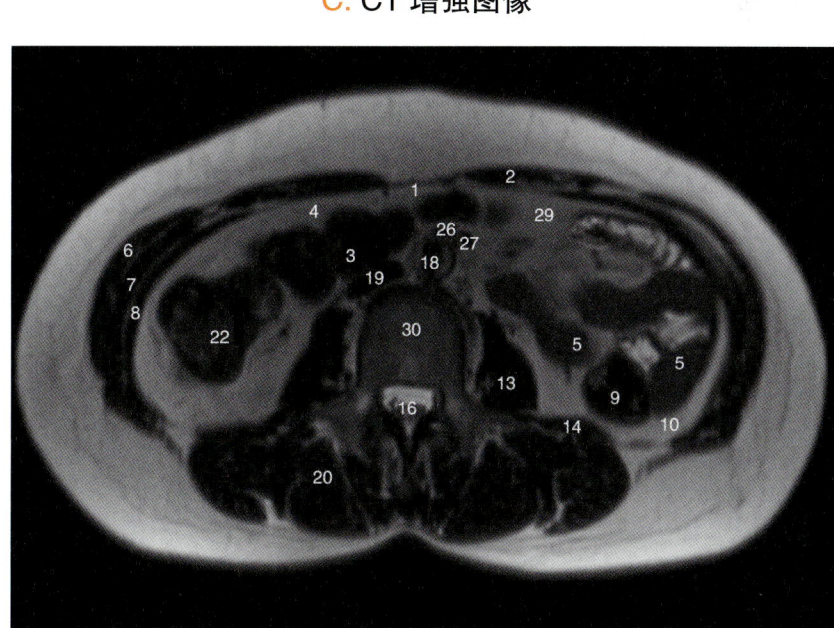

E. MR T2WI

关键结构：马尾，第 3 腰神经，肠系膜上动、静脉。

　　此断面经过第 3 腰椎椎体和 L3-4 椎间盘。

　　腹腔内的结构主要为肠管、系膜及血管。脊柱后方为三角形的椎管，椎管内容纳马尾，其两侧为第 3 腰神经。马尾由腰、骶、尾部的脊神经根在脊髓圆锥下方围绕终丝聚集形成，成人因第 1 腰椎以下已无脊髓，故临床上进行脊髓蛛网膜下隙穿刺抽取脑脊液或麻醉时，常选择第 3、4 腰椎棘突间进针，以免损伤脊髓。虽然副神经节瘤在马尾区少见，但马尾神经副神经节瘤与该区发生的室管膜瘤及神经鞘瘤在鉴别上存在一定困难，这可能会对治疗方案的制订及术后预期产生误导。鉴别诊断的首选检查为 MRI，一般在 T1WI 呈低至等信号，T2WI 呈中至高信号，有时 T2WI 信号可不均匀。迂曲血管及沉积于肿瘤边缘的含铁血黄素有助于鉴别副神经节瘤。迂曲血管位于肿瘤上方的椎管内，迂曲的血管流空信号影可见于肿瘤周围，迂曲血管在增强扫描时可见异常强化[94]。第 3 腰神经从腰神经通道穿出，主要分布于腰丛的股外侧皮神经、股神经、闭孔神经等。腰神经通道可分为神经根管和椎间管两段，此通道任何部分的病变均可刺激或压迫神经根，引起腰腿疼。神经根管有几处狭窄：①盘黄间隙，位于椎间盘与黄韧带之间；②上关节突旁沟；③侧隐窝；④椎弓根下沟，位于椎弓根内下缘与椎间盘之间，在椎间盘后方膨出时更为明显。腰神经根呈圆形或椭圆形，直径为 2~3 mm，两侧对称，在 CT 图像上可清楚显示，如一侧神经根后移则是椎间盘突出的重要征象[7]。

腹部连续横断层 94（FH.10050）

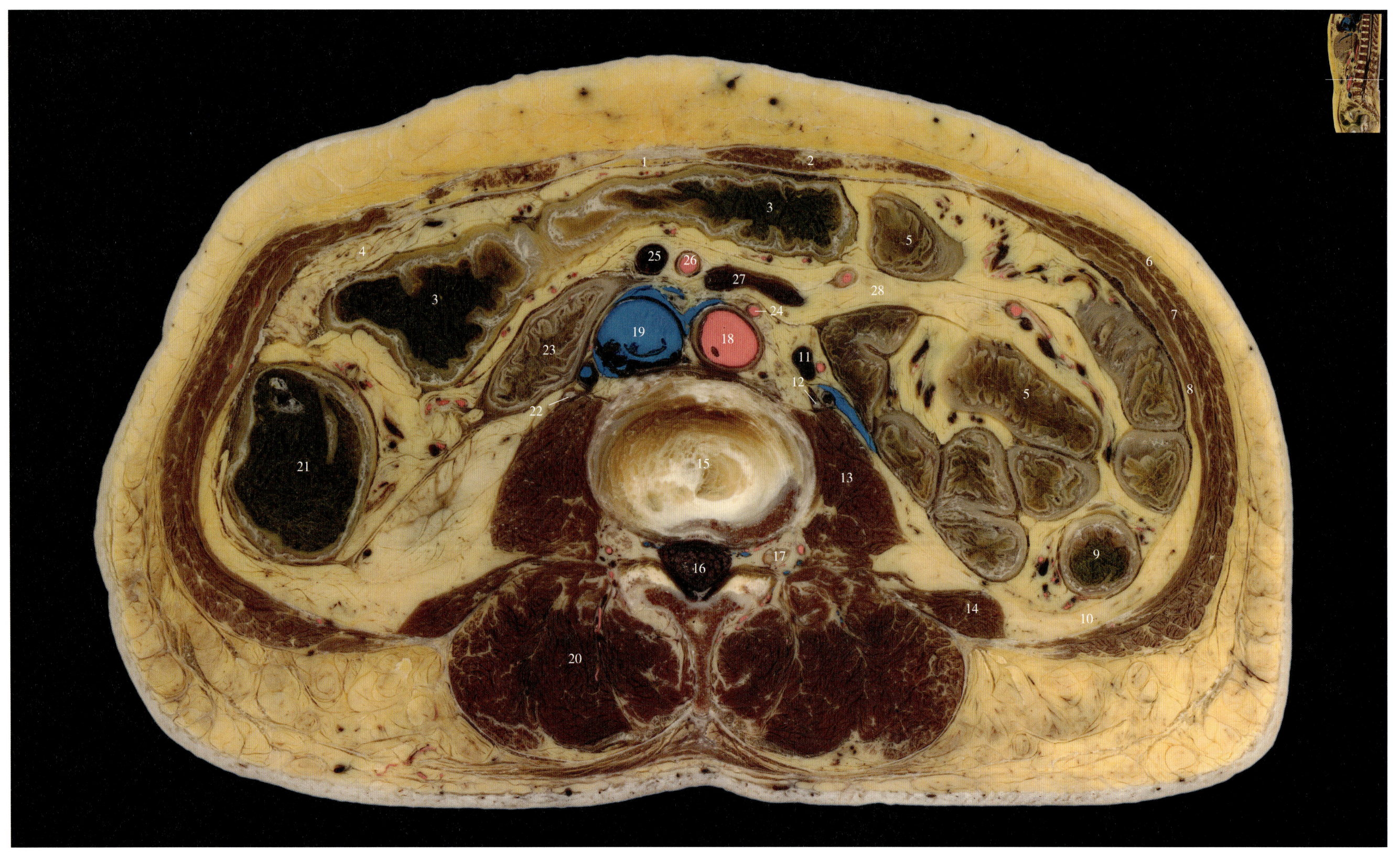

A. 断层标本图像

1. 肝圆韧带 ligamentum teres hepatis
2. 腹直肌 rectus abdominis
3. 横结肠 transverse colon
4. 大网膜 greater omentum
5. 空肠 jejunum
6. 腹外斜肌 obliquus externus abdominis
7. 腹内斜肌 obliquus internus abdominis
8. 腹横肌 transverses abdominis
9. 降结肠 descending colon
10. 腹膜外脂肪 extraperitoneal fat
11. 肠系膜下静脉 inferior mesenteric vein
12. 左输尿管 left ureter
13. 腰大肌 psoas major
14. 腰方肌 quadratus lumborum
15. L3-4 椎间盘 L3-4 intervertebral disc
16. 马尾 cauda equina
17. 第 3 腰神经 3rd lumbar nerve
18. 腹主动脉 abdominal aorta
19. 下腔静脉 inferior vena cava
20. 竖脊肌 erector spinae
21. 升结肠 ascending colon
22. 右输尿管 right ureter
23. 十二指肠水平部 horizontal part of duodenum
24. 肠系膜下动脉 inferior mesenteric artery
25. 肠系膜上静脉 superior mesenteric vein
26. 肠系膜上动脉 superior mesenteric artery
27. 空肠静脉 jejunal vein
28. 肠系膜 mesentery
29. 第 3 腰椎椎体 body of 3rd lumbar vertebra

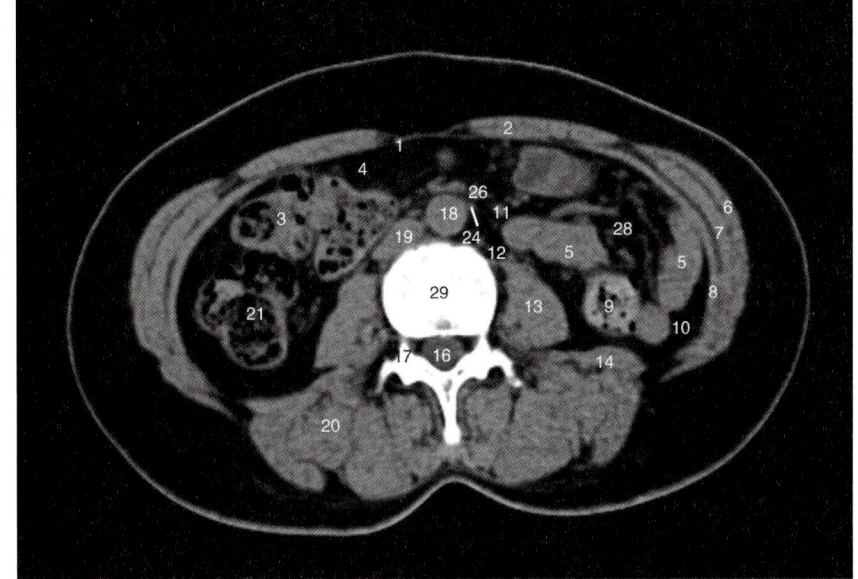

B. CT 平扫图像

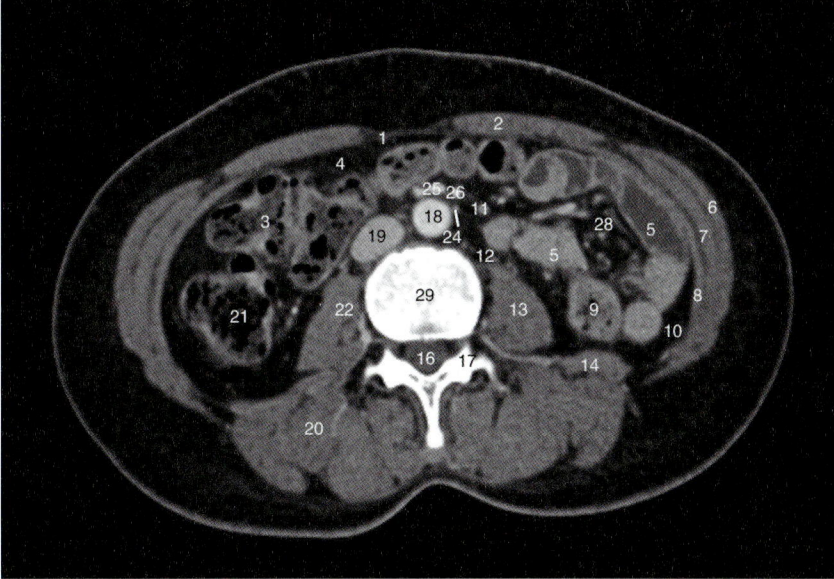

C. CT 增强图像

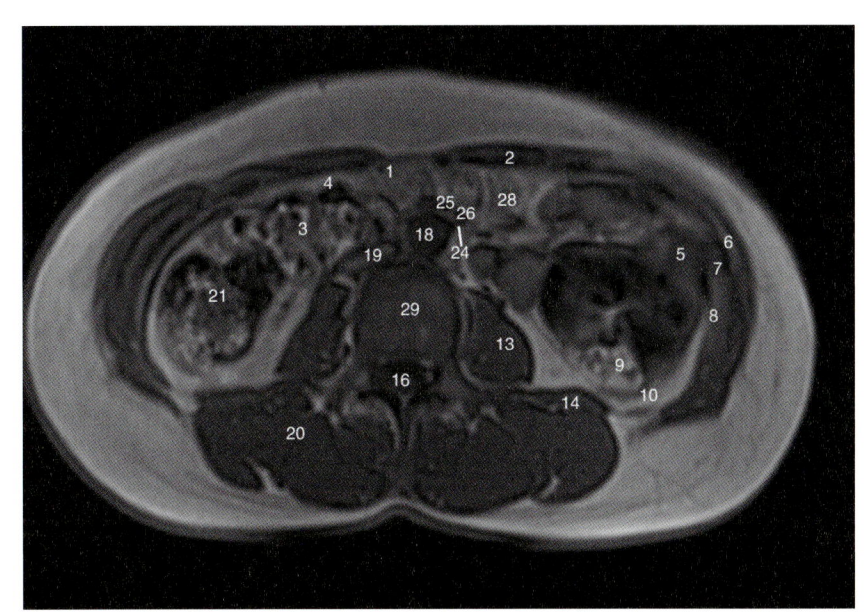

D. MR T1WI

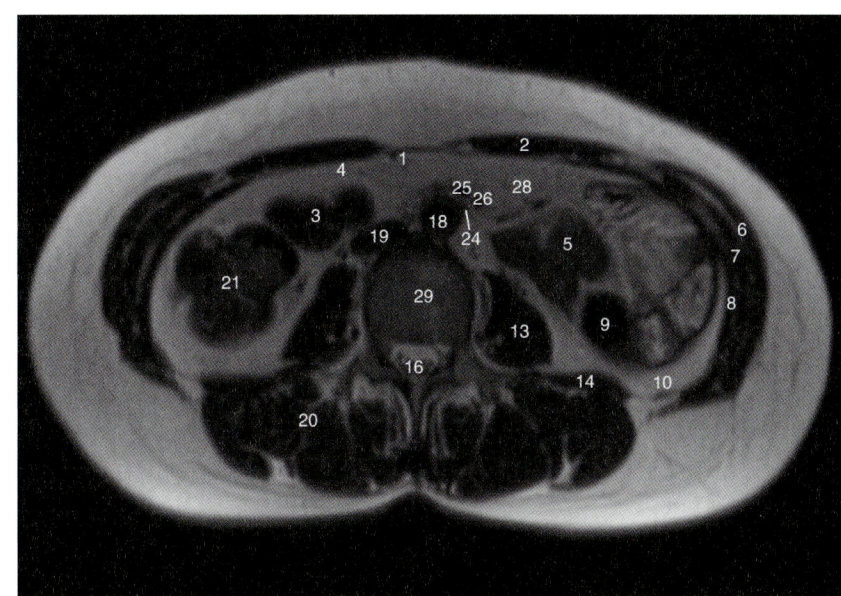

E. MR T2WI

关键结构：L3-4 椎间盘，腰大肌，腰方肌。

此断面经过 L3-4 椎间盘。

脊柱两侧为粗壮的腰大肌，其后外侧为腰方肌，腹腔内结构分布同上，右肾消失。腰椎间盘的大小和形态与相邻椎体基本相似，髓核位于中央偏后，周围为纤维环。在 CT 和 MR 图像上，腰椎间盘呈肾形或椭圆形，直径为 30~50 mm。腰椎间盘可向椎体的上、下面膨出，因此，在经腰椎体上、下面的横断层内，可见在椎体后部出现两个圆形的椎间盘断面，称为"猫头鹰眼征"。脊柱腰段运动幅度大，在急转、过度劳损或暴力撞击时，常引起纤维环破裂，导致髓核突入椎管或椎间孔，压迫神经出现腰椎间盘脱出症，脱出常发生在纤维环后外侧薄弱处，以 L4-5 椎间盘和 L5-S1 椎间盘最为常见。腰大肌起自腰椎体两侧面及横突，向下与髂肌组成髂腰肌。腰方肌位于腹后壁脊柱两侧后方，起自髂嵴后部，向上止于第 12 肋和第 1~4 腰椎横突。脊柱椎体是结核的常见发病部位，当发生腰椎椎体结核时，病变会累及腰大肌，结核杆菌会聚集于腰大肌旁，形成脓肿，称为"冷脓肿"，当脓肿增大，张力增高时，常自行破溃并沿较薄弱的组织间隙蔓延形成窦道。在 CT 上表现为脓肿向皮肤延伸的不连续的、形态不规则、内壁不光整的含气腔隙，开口部皮肤凹陷或呈火山口状改变[95]。

腹部连续横断层 95（FH.10030）

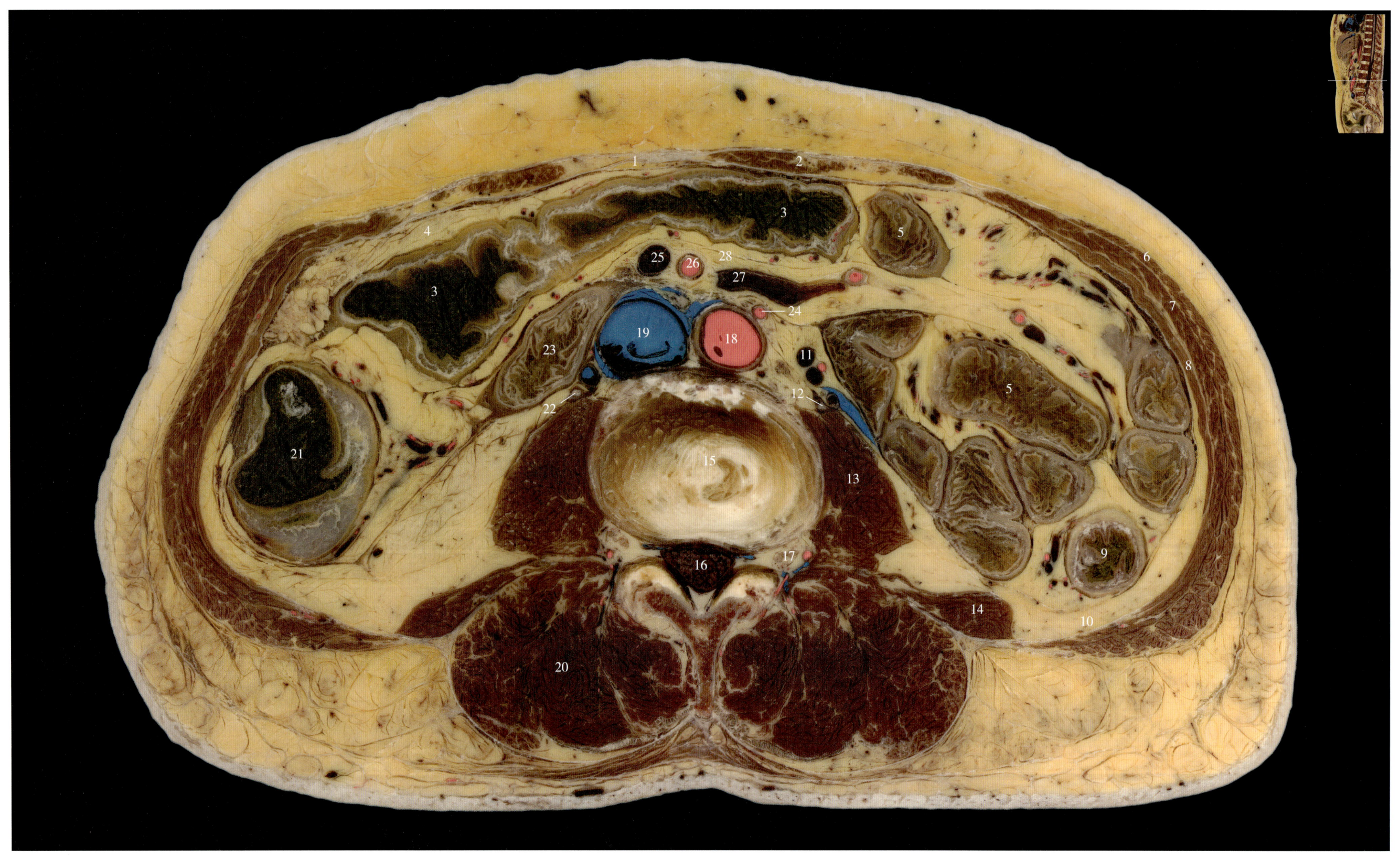

A. 断层标本图像

1. 肝圆韧带 ligamentum teres hepatis
2. 腹直肌 rectus abdominis
3. 横结肠 transverse colon
4. 大网膜 greater omentum
5. 空肠 jejunum
6. 腹外斜肌 obliquus externus abdominis
7. 腹内斜肌 obliquus internus abdominis
8. 腹横肌 transverses abdominis
9. 降结肠 descending colon
10. 腹膜外脂肪 extraperitoneal fat
11. 肠系膜下静脉 inferior mesenteric vein
12. 左输尿管 left ureter
13. 腰大肌 psoas major
14. 腰方肌 quadratus lumborum
15. L3-4 椎间盘 L3-4 intervertebral disc
16. 马尾 cauda equina
17. 第 3 腰神经 3rd lumbar nerve
18. 腹主动脉 abdominal aorta
19. 下腔静脉 inferior vena cava
20. 竖脊肌 erector spinae
21. 升结肠 ascending colon
22. 右输尿管 right ureter
23. 十二指肠水平部 horizontal part of duodenum
24. 肠系膜下动脉 inferior mesenteric artery
25. 肠系膜上静脉 superior mesenteric vein
26. 肠系膜上动脉 superior mesenteric artery
27. 空肠静脉 jejunal vein
28. 肠系膜 mesentery
29. 第 3 腰椎椎体 body of 3rd lumbar vertebra

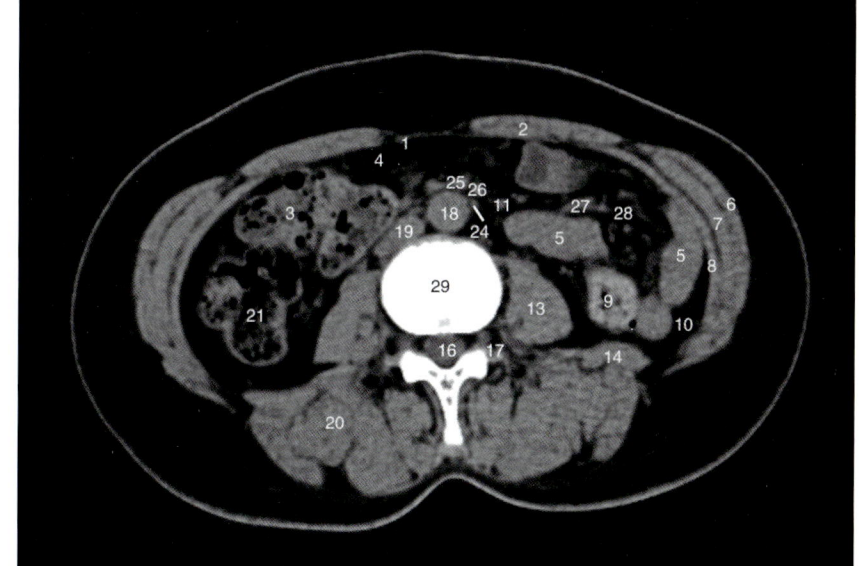

B. CT 平扫图像

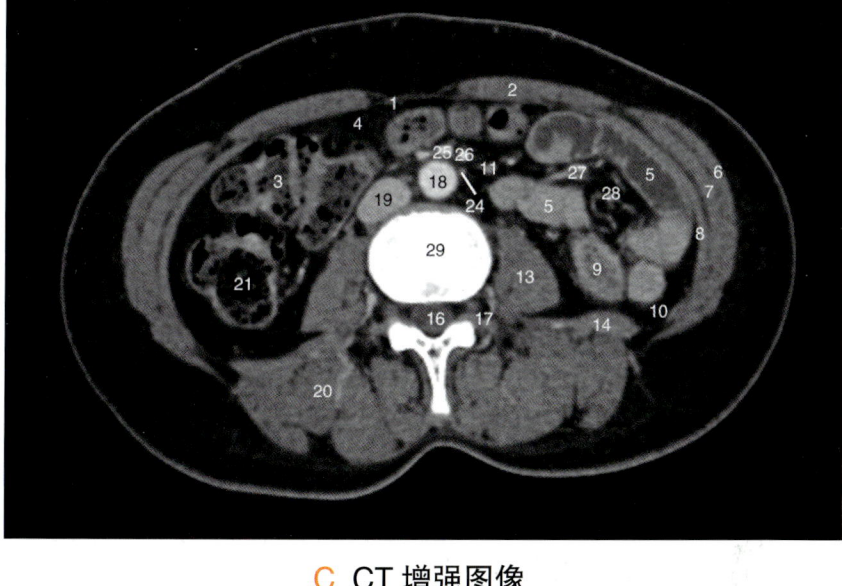

C. CT 增强图像

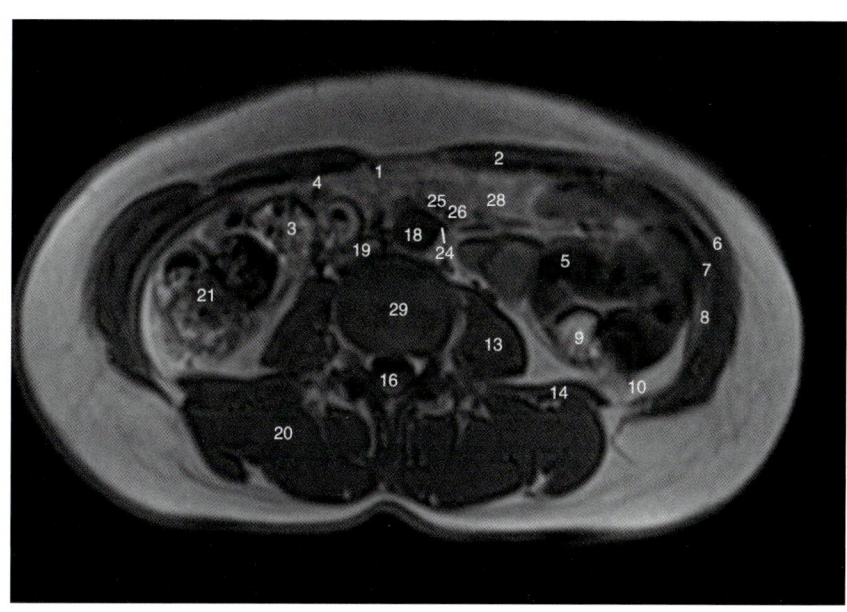

D. MR T1WI

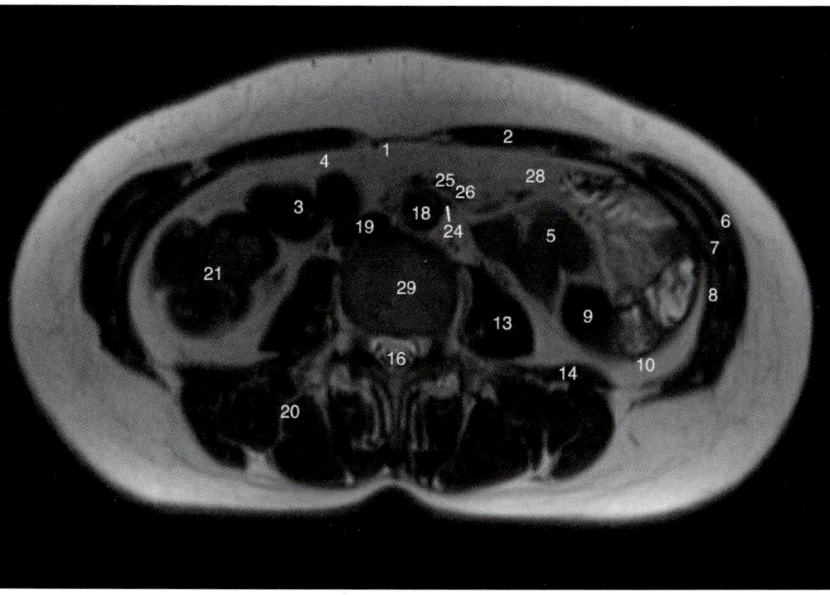

E. MR T2WI

关键结构：升结肠，降结肠，左、右结肠旁沟。

此断面经过 L3-4 椎间盘。

下腔静脉和腹主动脉位于脊柱前方，肠系膜下动脉逐渐远离腹主动脉，向左前方走行。腹腔内左右两侧可见升结肠和降结肠的断面。升结肠长约 18 cm，下连盲肠，沿腰方肌上升，至肝右叶下方，折转向左前方形成结肠右曲，移行为横结肠。升结肠右侧与腹壁之间为右结肠旁沟，此沟上通右肝下间隙，下达髂窝及盆腔。因此，右肝周脓肿可沿此沟流入右髂窝，甚至盆腔，右髂窝的炎症如阑尾化脓可向上蔓延至膈下。降结肠长约 20 cm，自结肠左曲向下，在腰方肌左侧下行，至左髂嵴高度，移行于乙状结肠。降结肠左侧与腹壁之间可见左结肠旁沟，此沟上方受阻于左膈结肠韧带，故其积液只能向下流入盆腔。升结肠和降结肠以系膜固定于腹后壁，位置较固定。克罗恩病是右半结肠的常见疾病，溃疡呈裂隙状、纵行刀切样，可直达浆膜，是形成肠瘘的病理基础。CT 及 MRI 表现为多发节段性、跳跃性病变，管壁明显增厚，可达 10 mm 以上，肠腔不对称狭窄，但不易发生肠梗阻。若浆膜层及黏膜层明显强化，黏膜下层水肿增宽，横断面可呈"靶征"，提示病变处于活动期；若管壁不强化或轻度强化，无分层，提示病变处于静止期或慢性期[96]。

腹部连续横断层 96（FH.10010）

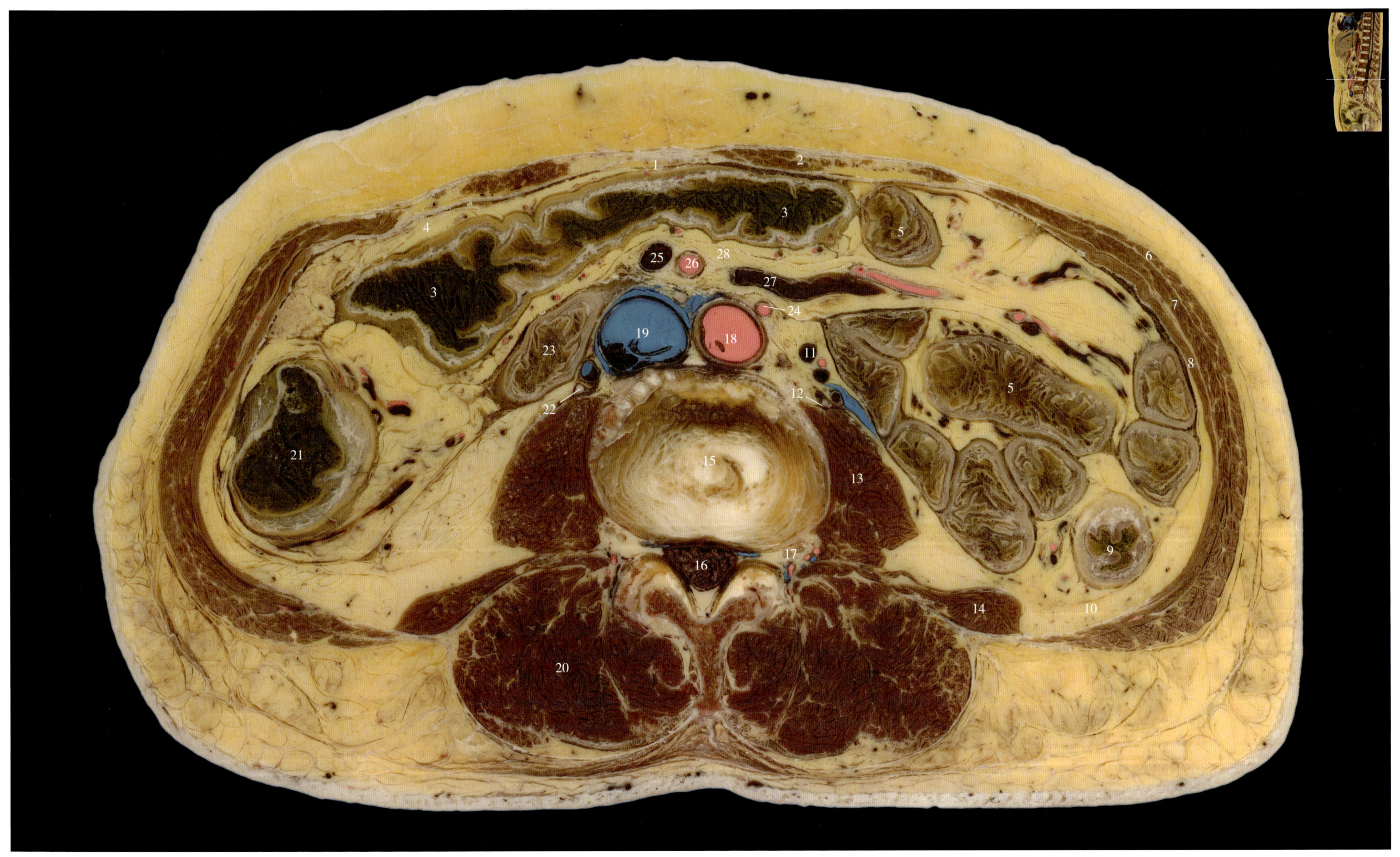

A. 断层标本图像

1. 肝圆韧带 ligamentum teres hepatis
2. 腹直肌 rectus abdominis
3. 横结肠 transverse colon
4. 大网膜 greater omentum
5. 空肠 jejunum
6. 腹外斜肌 obliquus externus abdominis
7. 腹内斜肌 obliquus internus abdominis
8. 腹横肌 transverses abdominis
9. 降结肠 descending colon
10. 腹膜外脂肪 extraperitoneal fat
11. 肠系膜下静脉 inferior mesenteric vein
12. 左输尿管 left ureter
13. 腰大肌 psoas major
14. 腰方肌 quadratus lumborum
15. L3-4 椎间盘 L3-4 intervertebral disc
16. 马尾 cauda equina
17. 第 3 腰神经 3rd lumbar nerve
18. 腹主动脉 abdominal aorta
19. 下腔静脉 inferior vena cava
20. 竖脊肌 erector spinae
21. 升结肠 ascending colon
22. 右输尿管 right ureter
23. 十二指肠水平部 horizontal part of duodenum
24. 肠系膜下动脉 inferior mesenteric artery
25. 肠系膜上静脉 superior mesenteric vein
26. 肠系膜上动脉 superior mesenteric artery
27. 空肠静脉 jejunal vein
28. 肠系膜 mesentery

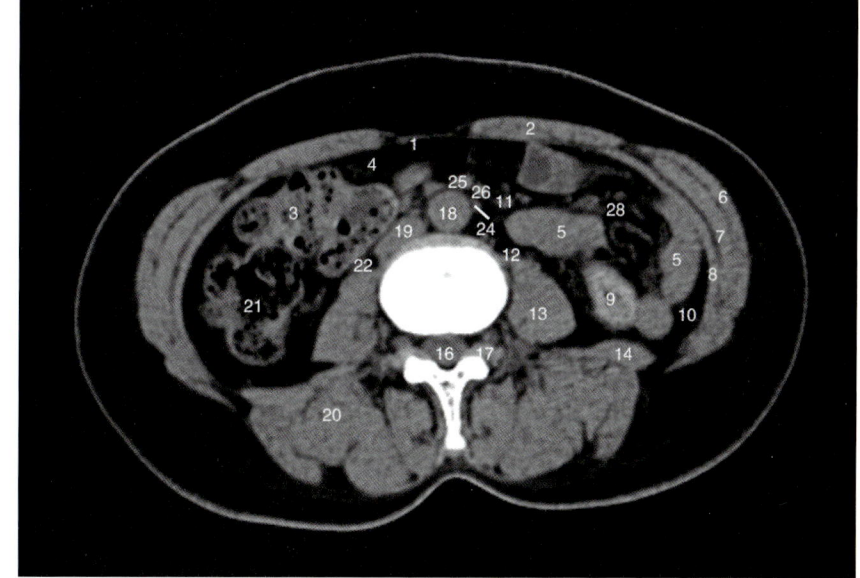

B. CT 平扫图像

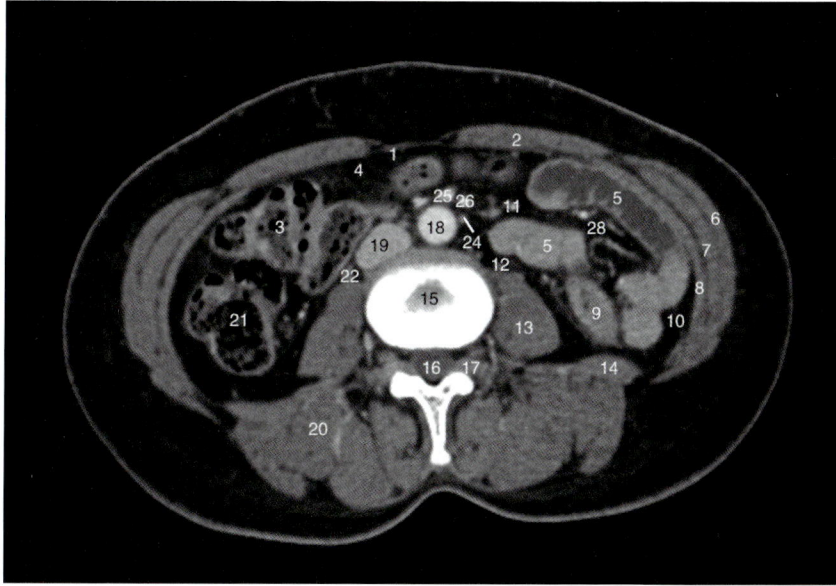

C. CT 增强图像

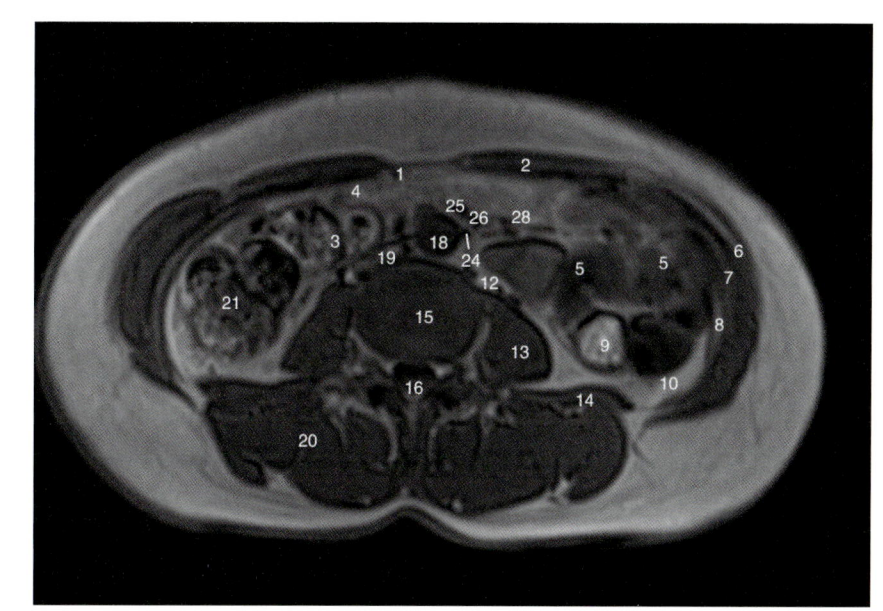

D. MR T1WI

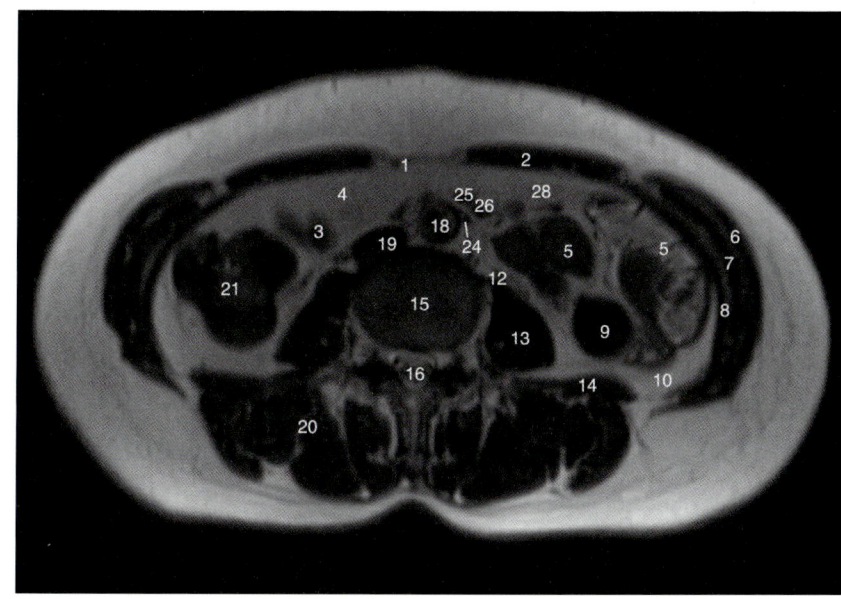

E. MR T2WI

关键结构：竖脊肌，空肠，十二指肠水平部。

此断面经过 L3-4 椎间盘。

肠道和肠系膜及内部血管占据腹腔的大部分区域，下腔静脉和腹主动脉均接近其分叉处。肠道可大致分为两层排列，前层为横结肠、十二指肠水平部和空肠，后层为升结肠、空肠和降结肠。脊柱两侧为腰大肌，后方为粗大的竖脊肌。竖脊肌位于棘突两侧、斜方肌和背阔肌的深面，是背肌中最长最大者，起自骶骨背面、髂嵴后部和腰椎棘突，肌纤维向外上分为 3 组，沿途分别止于椎骨、肋骨及颞骨乳突，又称骶棘肌。作用为一侧收缩使脊柱同向侧屈，两侧同时收缩时使脊柱后伸并仰头。许多腰痛、背痛，甚至头痛头晕可由竖脊肌劳损引起，竖脊肌的形态和病变在 CT 和 MRI 上容易辨认。此外，超声引导下竖脊肌平面阻滞被逐步应用在胸部、腹部、髋关节、妇科和脊柱手术及其术后镇痛。即在高频超声线阵探头引导下，通过神经阻滞穿刺针将局麻药物注射到竖脊肌与横突之间的筋膜内，局麻药物在此筋膜内扩散，可以使注药点附近的脊神经被阻滞[97]。

腹部连续横断层 97（FH.9990）

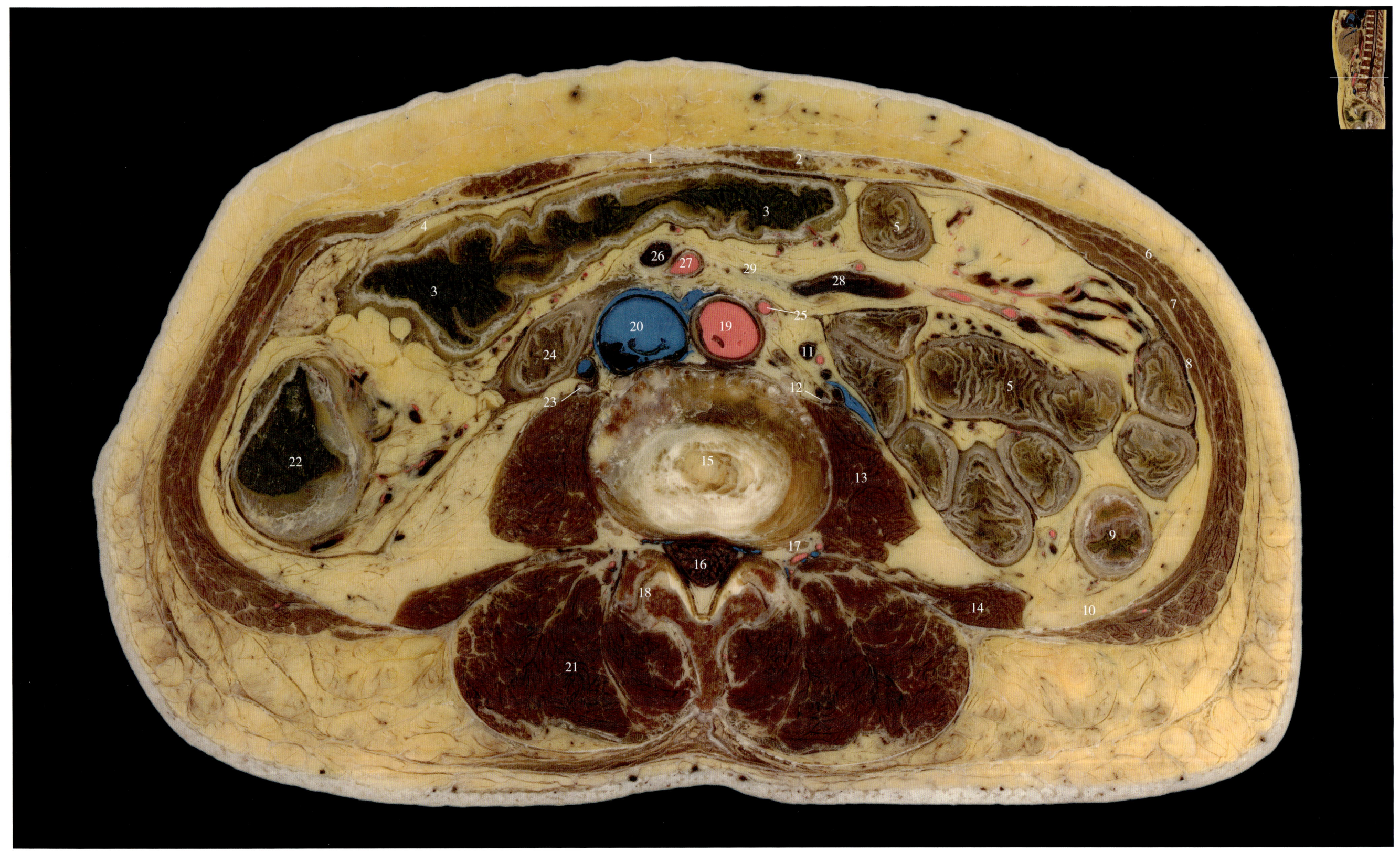

A. 断层标本图像

1. 肝圆韧带 ligamentum teres hepatis
2. 腹直肌 rectus abdominis
3. 横结肠 transverse colon
4. 大网膜 greater omentum
5. 空肠 jejunum
6. 腹外斜肌 obliquus externus abdominis
7. 腹内斜肌 obliquus internus abdominis
8. 腹横肌 transverses abdominis
9. 降结肠 descending colon
10. 腹膜外脂肪 extraperitoneal fat
11. 肠系膜下静脉 inferior mesenteric vein
12. 左输尿管 left ureter
13. 腰大肌 psoas major
14. 腰方肌 quadratus lumborum
15. L3-4 椎间盘 L3-4 intervertebral disc
16. 马尾 cauda equina
17. 第 3 腰神经 3rd lumbar nerve
18. 关节突关节 zygapophysial joint
19. 腹主动脉 abdominal aorta
20. 下腔静脉 inferior vena cava
21. 竖脊肌 erector spinae
22. 升结肠 ascending colon
23. 右输尿管 right ureter
24. 十二指肠水平部 horizontal part of duodenum
25. 肠系膜下动脉 inferior mesenteric artery
26. 肠系膜上静脉 superior mesenteric vein
27. 肠系膜上动脉 superior mesenteric artery
28. 空肠静脉 jejunal vein
29. 肠系膜 mesentery

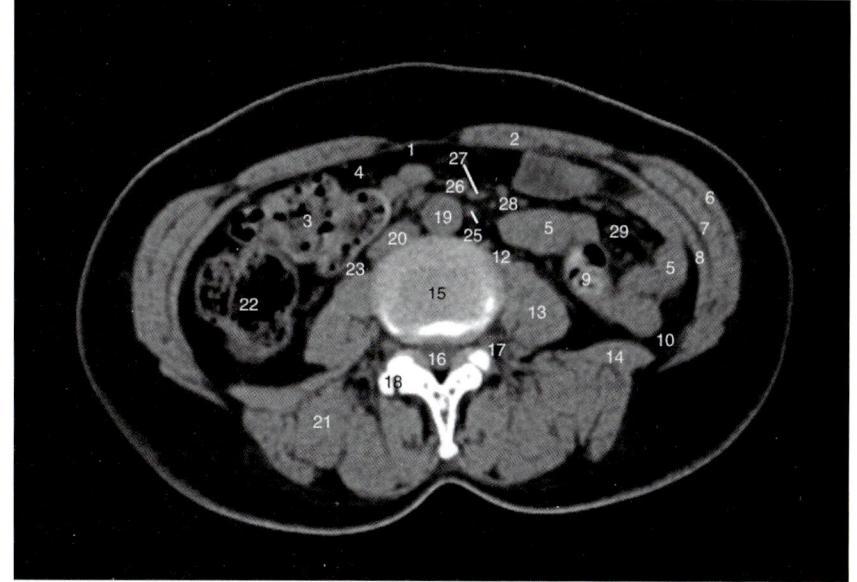

B. CT 平扫图像

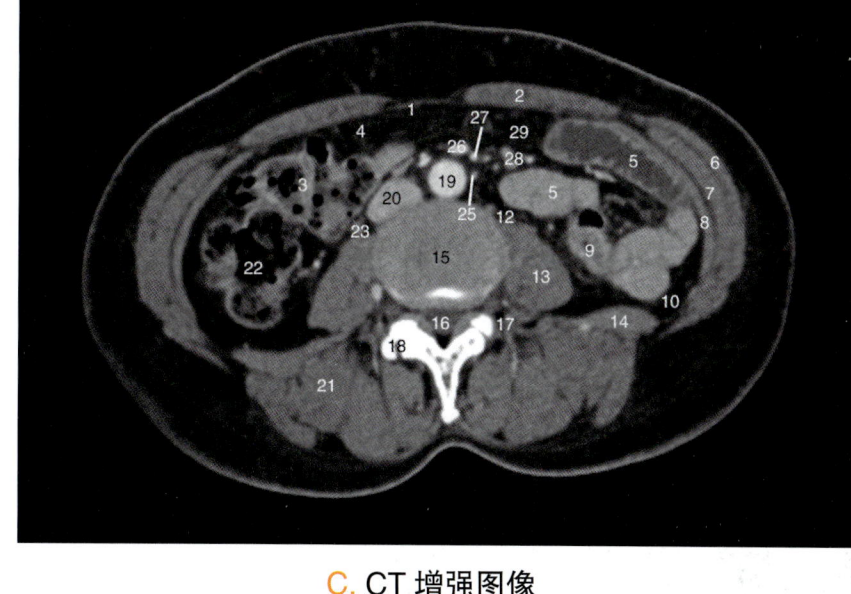

C. CT 增强图像

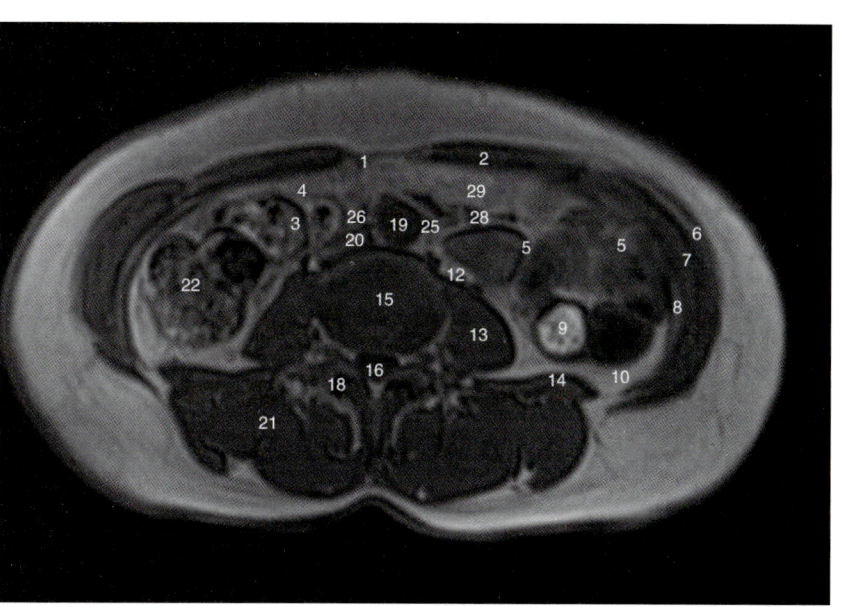

D. MR T1WI

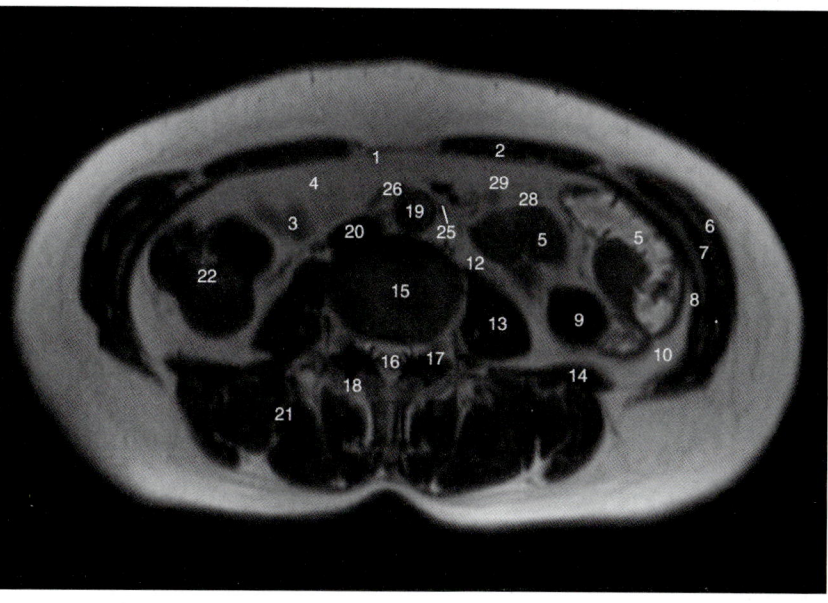

E. MR T2WI

关键结构：横结肠，横结肠肠系膜，升结肠。

此断面经过 L3-4 椎间盘。

肠管占据腹腔的大部分区域，其配布特点如下：升结肠和十二指肠水平部位于右腹部；横结肠横卧腹腔前方，已有中部下垂部分，外覆大网膜；空肠和降结肠居右腹部。横结肠长约 50 cm，自结肠右曲（又称肝曲）行向左前下方，形成略向下垂的弓形弯曲，至左季肋区脾脏面下份折转成结肠左曲（又称脾曲），向下续于降结肠[98]。横结肠为腹膜内位器官，由横结肠系膜连于腹后壁，活动性较大，前中间部分可下垂至脐或低于脐平面，但是脾曲与肝区位置相对固定，并且脾曲较肝曲位置高，在影像图上观察时需注意此特点。横结肠系膜根部起自结肠右曲，向左跨右肾中部、十二指肠降部、胰前缘至左肾中部，止于结肠左曲，其附着线在腹前壁的体表投影约与脐上线一致。该系膜内含有中结肠血管，左、右结肠血管的分支，淋巴管、淋巴结和神经丛等。溃疡性结肠炎是常见的慢性非特异性炎症性疾病，病变局限于大肠黏膜及黏膜下层，病程漫长，反复发作。CT 及 MRI 上表现为连续性病变，管壁增厚一般小于 10 mm，肠腔可略窄，较对称。管壁分层强化，横断面呈"靶征"，可见肠壁积气、肠系膜血管末端分支增多、纤维脂肪增多[99]。

腹部连续横断层 98（FH.9970）

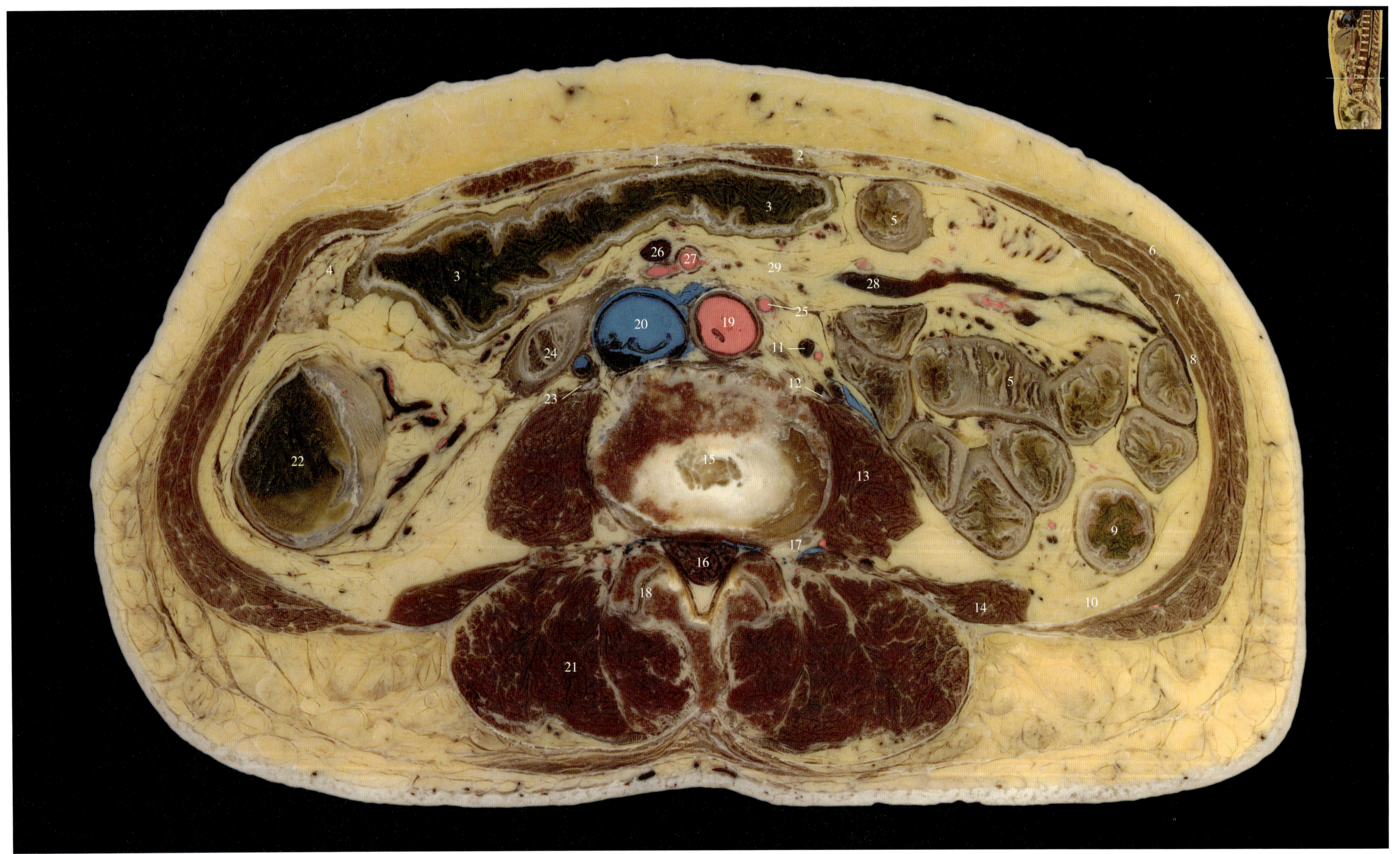

A. 断层标本图像

1. 肝圆韧带 ligamentum teres hepatis
2. 腹直肌 rectus abdominis
3. 横结肠 transverse colon
4. 大网膜 greater omentum
5. 空肠 jejunum
6. 腹外斜肌 obliquus externus abdominis
7. 腹内斜肌 obliquus internus abdominis
8. 腹横肌 transverses abdominis
9. 降结肠 descending colon
10. 腹膜外脂肪 extraperitoneal fat
11. 肠系膜下静脉 inferior mesenteric vein
12. 左输尿管 left ureter
13. 腰大肌 psoas major
14. 腰方肌 quadratus lumborum
15. L3-4 椎间盘 L3-4 intervertebral disc
16. 马尾 cauda equina
17. 第 3 腰神经 3rd lumbar nerve
18. 关节突关节 zygapophysial joint
19. 腹主动脉 abdominal aorta
20. 下腔静脉 inferior vena cava
21. 竖脊肌 erector spinae
22. 升结肠 ascending colon
23. 右输尿管 right ureter
24. 十二指肠水平部 horizontal part of duodenum
25. 肠系膜下动脉 inferior mesenteric artery
26. 肠系膜上静脉 superior mesenteric vein
27. 肠系膜上动脉 superior mesenteric artery
28. 空肠静脉 jejunal vein
29. 肠系膜 mesentery

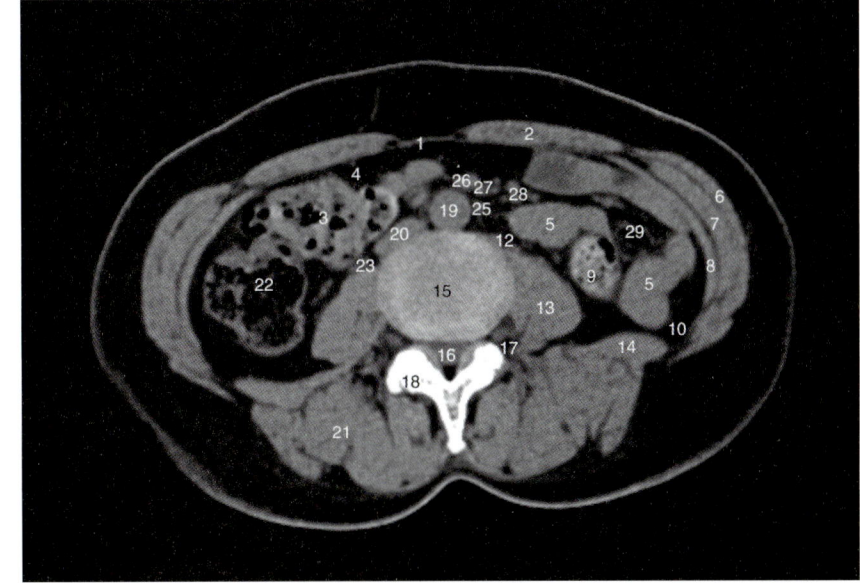

B. CT 平扫图像

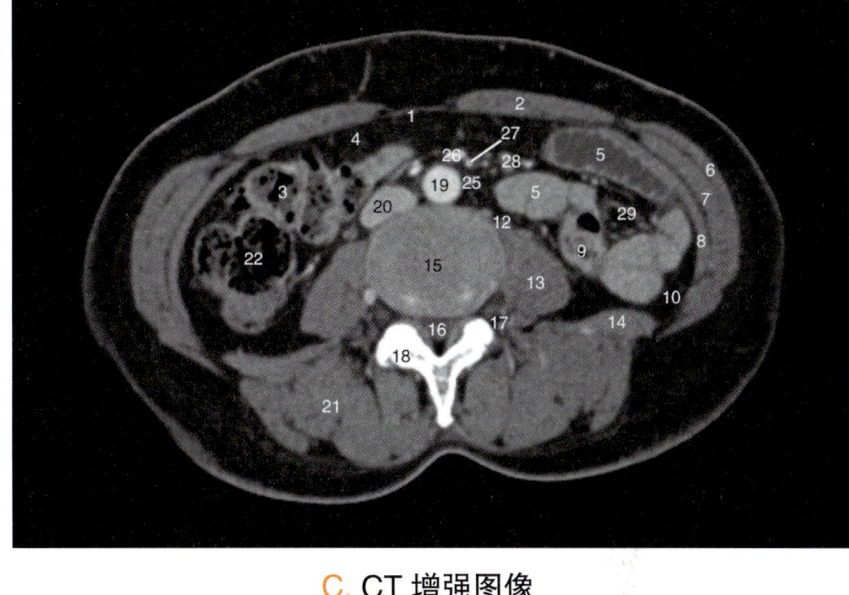

C. CT 增强图像

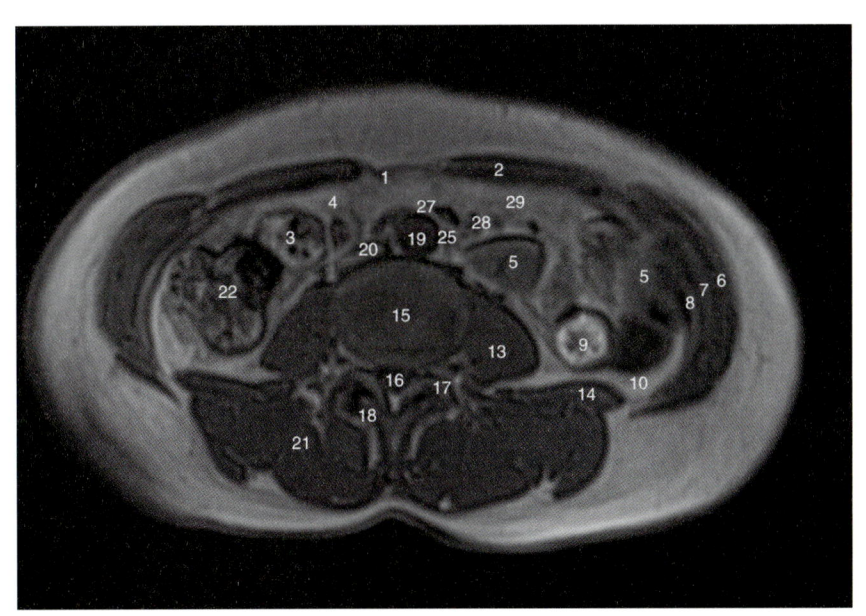

D. MR T1WI

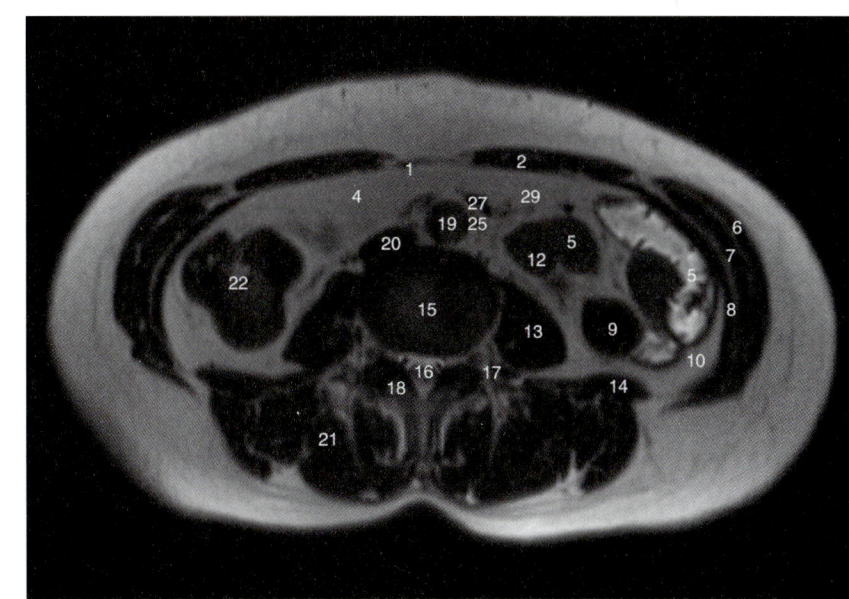

E. MR T2WI

关键结构：大网膜，降结肠，横结肠。

此断面经过 L3-4 椎间盘和第 4 腰椎椎体。

腹腔内，横结肠中间部和空肠位于前方，升结肠、十二指肠水平部、空肠和降结肠在后方由右向左依次排列，大网膜覆盖于肠道前方。大网膜连接于胃大弯与横结肠之间，呈围裙状下垂，由 4 层腹膜折叠而成，前 2 层由胃前、后壁浆膜延续而成，向下伸至脐平面或稍下方，然后向后反折，并向上附着于横结肠，形成前后 2 层。成年人大网膜前两层和后两层通常愈着，遂使前 2 层上部直接由胃大弯连至横结肠，形成胃结肠韧带。大网膜含脂肪及吞噬细胞，具有重要的防御功能，小儿大网膜较短，当下腹部器官发生炎症尤其是穿孔时，易形成弥漫性腹膜炎。特发性大网膜节段性梗死是临床上少见的急腹症，主要表现为大网膜的急性血液循环障碍，急性腹痛是患者就医的首要症状，患者为突发性右下腹疼痛，有反跳痛，个别情况下可触及包块。典型 CT 表现为单个较大不同密度的网膜肿块，增强扫描一般不见强化，常位于右下腹，腹直肌深部和横结肠前方。尽管网膜梗死与急性肠脂垂炎相似，但它缺乏急性肠脂垂炎的高密度环，还缺乏其中心的病变，且网膜梗死的危险性一般较急性肠脂垂炎更大[100]。

腹部连续横断层99（FH.9950）

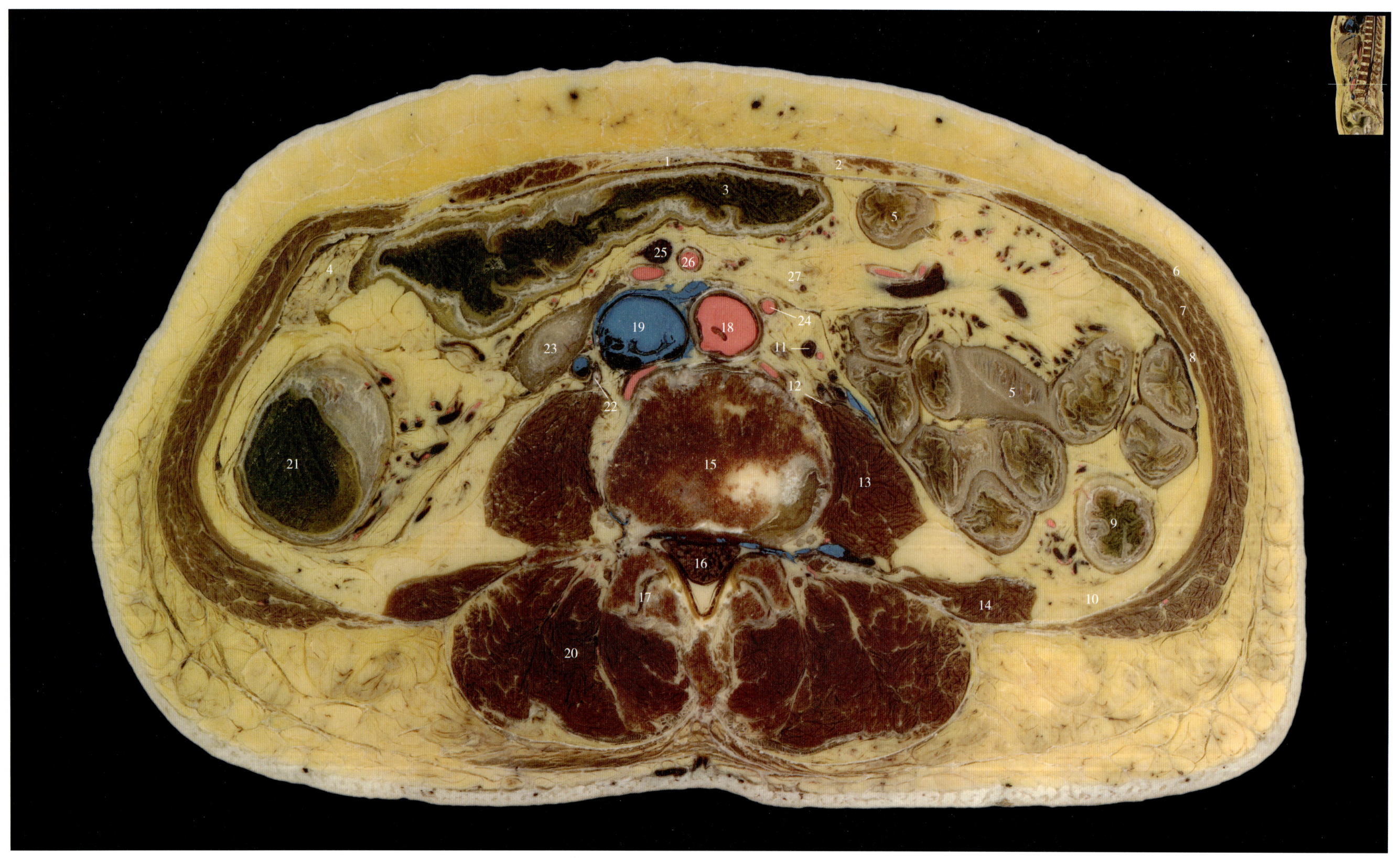

A. 断层标本图像

1. 肝圆韧带 ligamentum teres hepatis
2. 腹直肌 rectus abdominis
3. 横结肠 transverse colon
4. 大网膜 greater omentum
5. 空肠 jejunum
6. 腹外斜肌 obliquus externus abdominis
7. 腹内斜肌 obliquus internus abdominis
8. 腹横肌 transverses abdominis
9. 降结肠 descending colon
10. 腹膜外脂肪 extraperitoneal fat
11. 肠系膜下静脉 inferior mesenteric vein
12. 左输尿管 left ureter
13. 腰大肌 psoas major
14. 腰方肌 quadratus lumborum
15. 第4腰椎椎体 body of 4th lumbar vertebra
16. 马尾 cauda equina
17. 关节突关节 zygapophysial joint
18. 腹主动脉 abdominal aorta
19. 下腔静脉 inferior vena cava
20. 竖脊肌 erector spinae
21. 升结肠 ascending colon
22. 右输尿管 right ureter
23. 十二指肠水平部 horizontal part of duodenum
24. 肠系膜下动脉 inferior mesenteric artery
25. 肠系膜上静脉 superior mesenteric vein
26. 肠系膜上动脉 superior mesenteric artery
27. 肠系膜 mesentery
28. L3-4椎间盘 L3-4 intervertebral disc

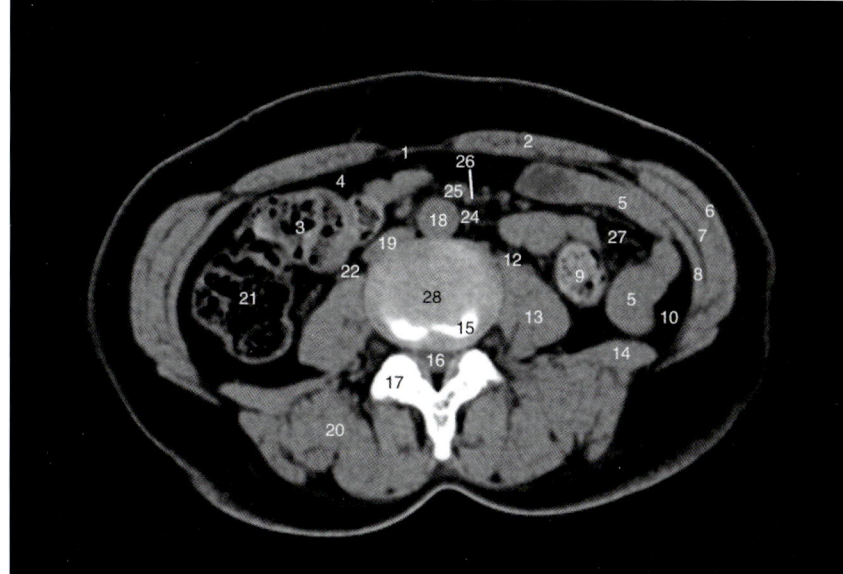

B. CT 平扫图像

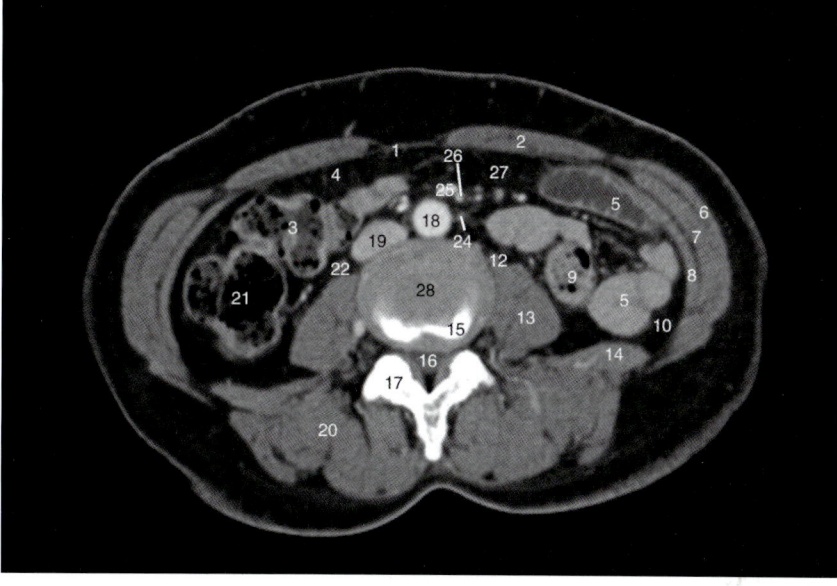

C. CT 增强图像

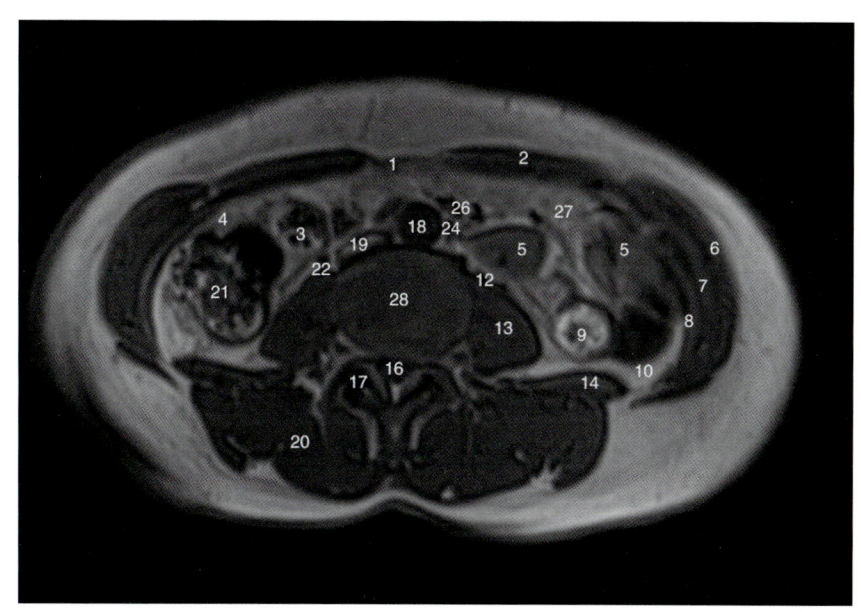

D. MR T1WI

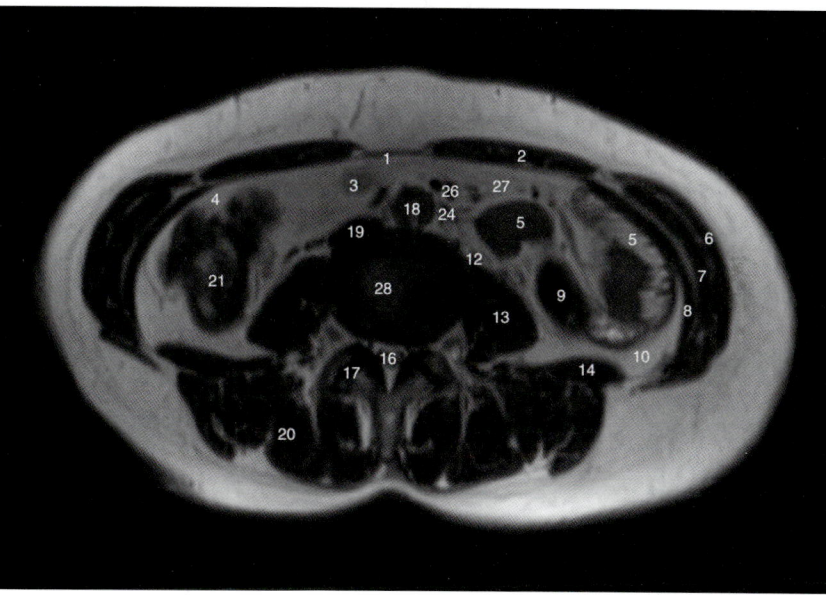

E. MR T2WI

关键结构：第4腰椎，关节突关节，输尿管。

此断面经过第4腰椎椎体。

第4腰椎椎体位于断面中央，两侧腰大肌的前方可见左、右输尿管。肠系膜动、静脉，肠道结构的配布与之前的断面相似，十二指肠水平部逐渐消失。椎体横断面呈肾形，前面凸，后面略凹，后方为三角形的椎孔，内容马尾，椎体静脉向后汇入椎体后静脉。在椎弓根与椎弓板结合处可见关节突关节，其由相邻椎骨的上、下关节突的关节面构成。在CT和MR图像上均能清晰地显示关节腔间隙，正常宽度为2~4 mm。关节囊后外侧壁较薄，前内侧壁被黄韧带加强而明显增厚。腰椎不稳使关节突关节所产生的异常应力和异常活动增多，反复发生易导致关节突关节退变，患者常表现为腰痛及腰部活动受限。腰椎关节突关节退行性病变在影像学上可呈炎性增生性改变，可见小关节肥大及骨赘形成，甚至小关节骨质融合；同时关节软骨硬化，MR T2WI信号可增高（提示炎性水肿或炎性反应），进而引起关节间隙狭窄[101]。

腹部连续横断层 100（FH.9930）

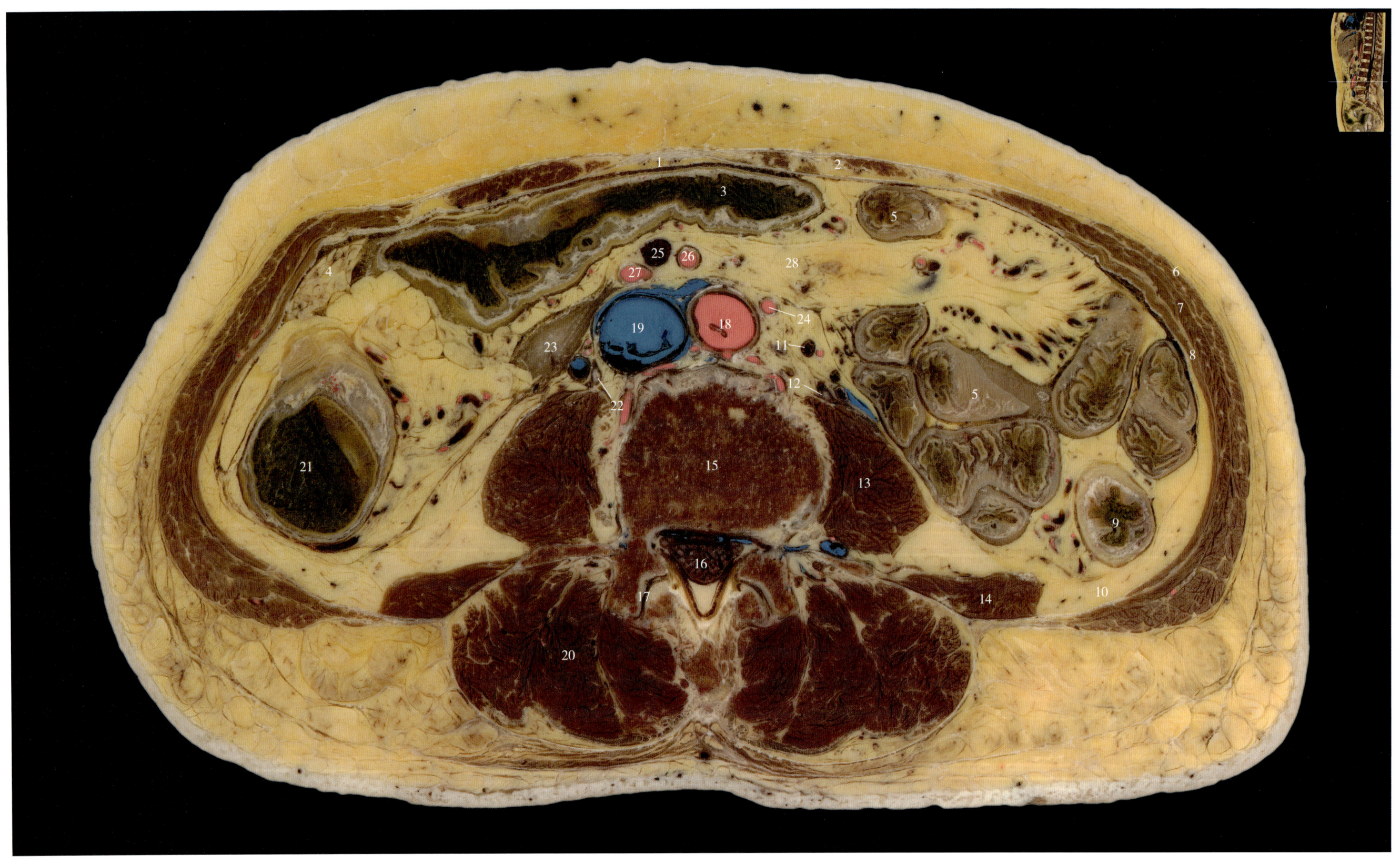

A. 断层标本图像

1. 肝圆韧带 ligamentum teres hepatis
2. 腹直肌 rectus abdominis
3. 横结肠 transverse colon
4. 大网膜 greater omentum
5. 空肠 jejunum
6. 腹外斜肌 obliquus externus abdominis
7. 腹内斜肌 obliquus internus abdominis
8. 腹横肌 transverses abdominis
9. 降结肠 descending colon
10. 腹膜外脂肪 extraperitoneal fat
11. 肠系膜下静脉 inferior mesenteric vein
12. 左输尿管 left ureter
13. 腰大肌 psoas major
14. 腰方肌 quadratus lumborum
15. 第 4 腰椎椎体 body of 4th lumbar vertebra
16. 马尾 cauda equina
17. 关节突关节 zygapophysial joint
18. 腹主动脉 abdominal aorta
19. 下腔静脉 inferior vena cava
20. 竖脊肌 erector spinae
21. 升结肠 ascending colon
22. 右输尿管 right ureter
23. 十二指肠水平部 horizontal part of duodenum
24. 肠系膜下动脉 inferior mesenteric artery
25. 肠系膜上静脉 superior mesenteric vein
26. 肠系膜上动脉 superior mesenteric artery
27. 结肠动脉 colic artery
28. 肠系膜 mesentery

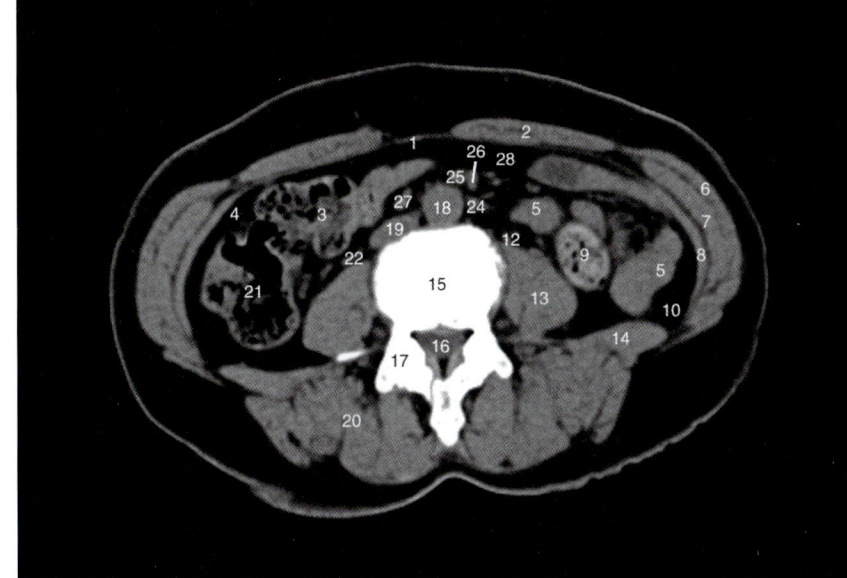

B. CT 平扫图像

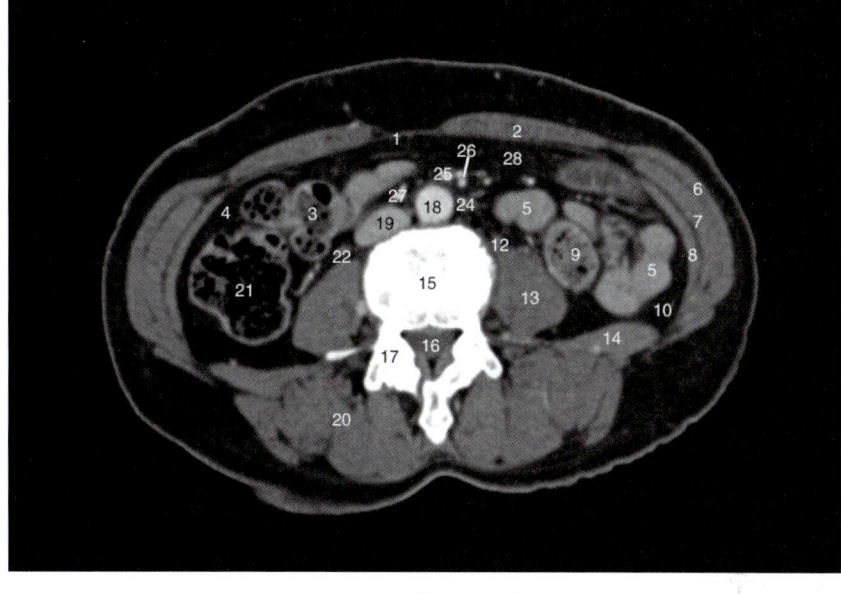

C. CT 增强图像

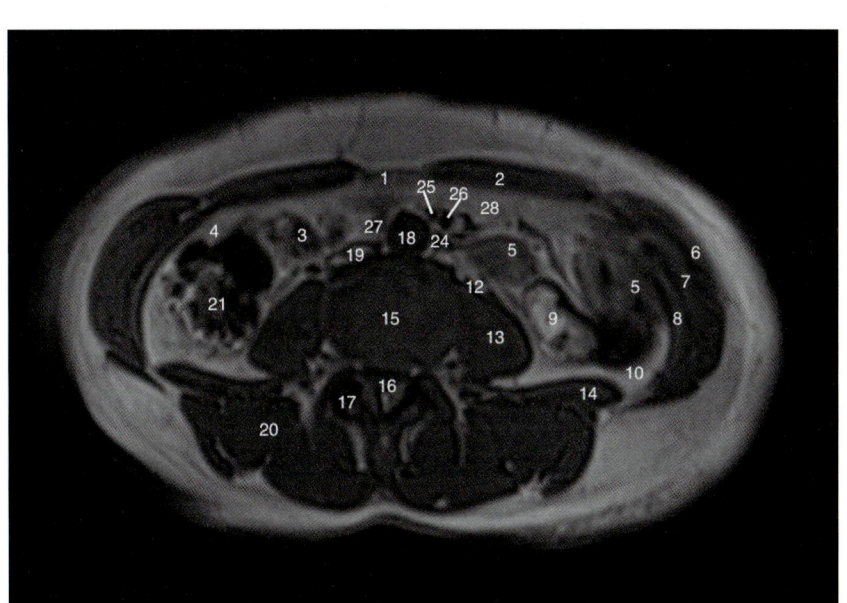

D. MR T1WI

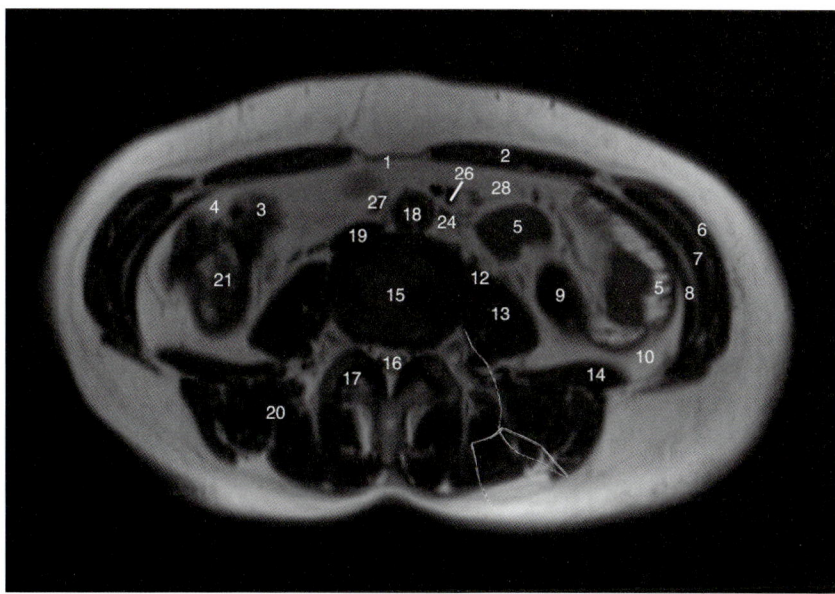

E. MR T2WI

关键结构：肝圆韧带，腹直肌。

此断面经过第 4 腰椎椎体。

腹直肌位于腹前壁正中线两侧，居腹直肌鞘内，其中间稍后方可见肝圆韧带贴于腹前壁中线偏右位置，腹腔内结构位置变化不大。肝圆韧带由胎儿时期的脐静脉闭锁而成，经肝镰状韧带的游离缘内行至脐，肝圆韧带保留了血管壁的结构特征，分为内膜、中膜和外膜 3 层。肝圆韧带的长度为 19.28 cm，可分为肝内段和肝外段，1 岁以内为 10.40 cm[37]。由于镰状韧带偏中线右侧，脐以上腹壁正中切口需向下延长时，应偏向中线左侧，以避免损伤肝圆韧带及伴其内走行的附脐静脉。在肝门静脉高压时 MRI 可发现肝圆韧带内有血流入脐。在 B 超图像上，开放的肝圆韧带呈现高回声中出现圆形的暗区现象，直径 3~7 mm，状若牛眼，故称"牛眼征"。另外，肝圆韧带在肝圆韧带 – 下腔静脉分流术、脐静脉 – 大隐静脉转流术、侧脑室 – 门静脉分流术等临床应用中发挥重要作用[102]。腹直肌上宽下窄，起自耻骨联合和耻骨嵴，肌束向上止于胸骨剑突和第 5~7 肋软骨的前面。肌的全长被 3~4 条横行腱划分成多个肌腹，腱划与腹直肌鞘的前层紧密结合，而后面不愈合。腹直肌鞘由腹外斜肌、腹内斜肌和腹横肌的腱膜构成，其上 2/3，前层由腹外斜肌腱膜和腹内斜肌腱膜的前层构成，后层由腹内斜肌腱膜的后层与腹横肌腱膜构成。鞘下 1/3 部，3 块扁肌的腱膜构成前层，后层阙如。两侧腹直肌收缩使脊柱前屈，一侧收缩，使脊柱侧屈；上方固定时，两侧收缩使骨盆后倾。腹直肌与腹外斜肌、腹内斜肌和腹横肌共同构成腹腔的前外侧壁。

腹部连续横断层 101（FH.9910）

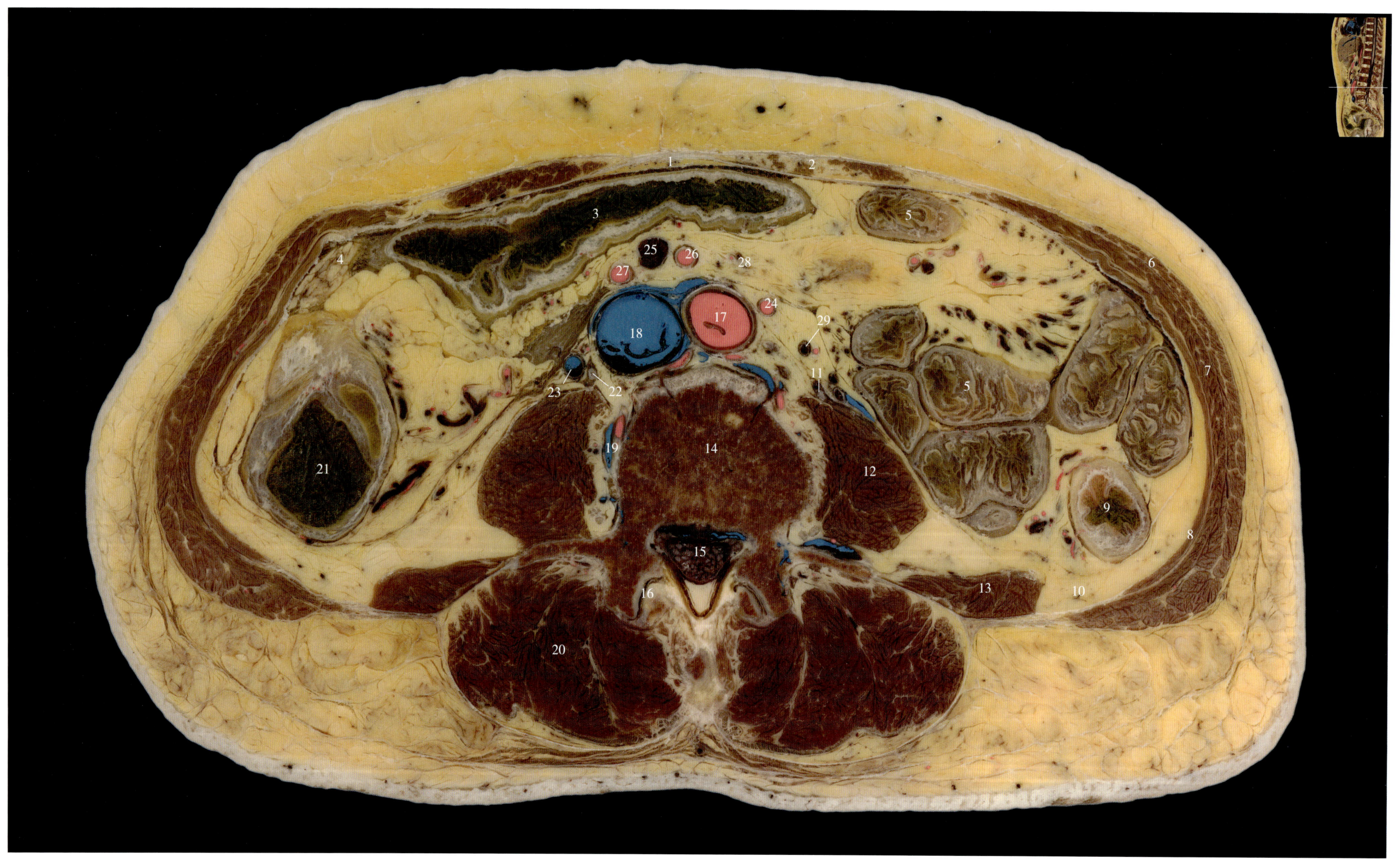

A. 断层标本图像

1. 肝圆韧带 ligamentum teres hepatis
2. 腹直肌 rectus abdominis
3. 横结肠 transverse colon
4. 大网膜 greater omentum
5. 空肠 jejunum
6. 腹外斜肌 obliquus externus abdominis
7. 腹内斜肌 obliquus internus abdominis
8. 腹横肌 transverses abdominis
9. 降结肠 descending colon
10. 腹膜外脂肪 extraperitoneal fat
11. 左输尿管 left ureter
12. 腰大肌 psoas major
13. 腰方肌 quadratus lumborum
14. 第4腰椎椎体 body of 4th lumbar vertebra
15. 马尾 cauda equina
16. 关节突关节 zygapophysial joint
17. 腹主动脉 abdominal aorta
18. 下腔静脉 inferior vena cava
19. 腰动、静脉 lumbar artery and vein
20. 竖脊肌 erector spinae
21. 升结肠 ascending colon
22. 右输尿管 right ureter
23. 右卵巢静脉 right ovarian vein
24. 肠系膜下动脉 inferior mesenteric artery
25. 肠系膜上静脉 superior mesenteric vein
26. 肠系膜上动脉 superior mesenteric artery
27. 结肠动脉 colic artery
28. 肠系膜 mesentery
29. 肠系膜下静脉 inferior mesenteric vein

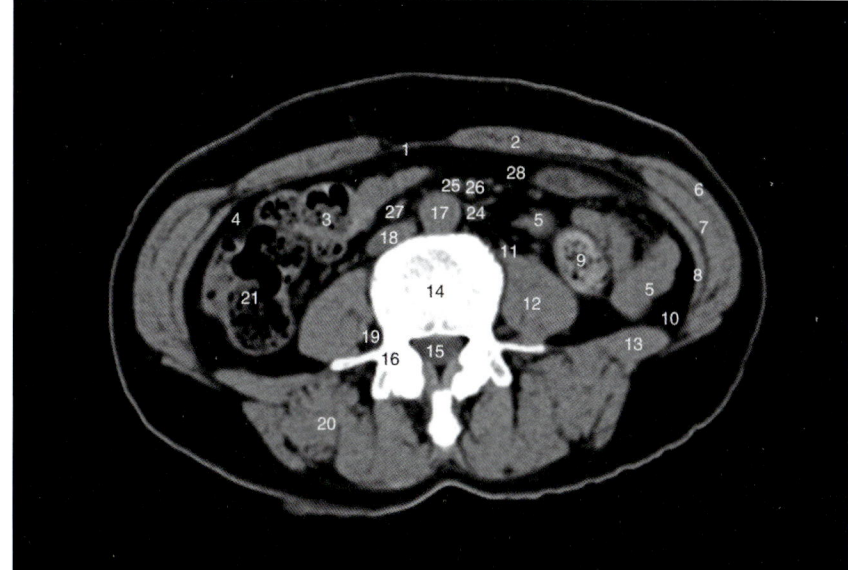

B. CT 平扫图像

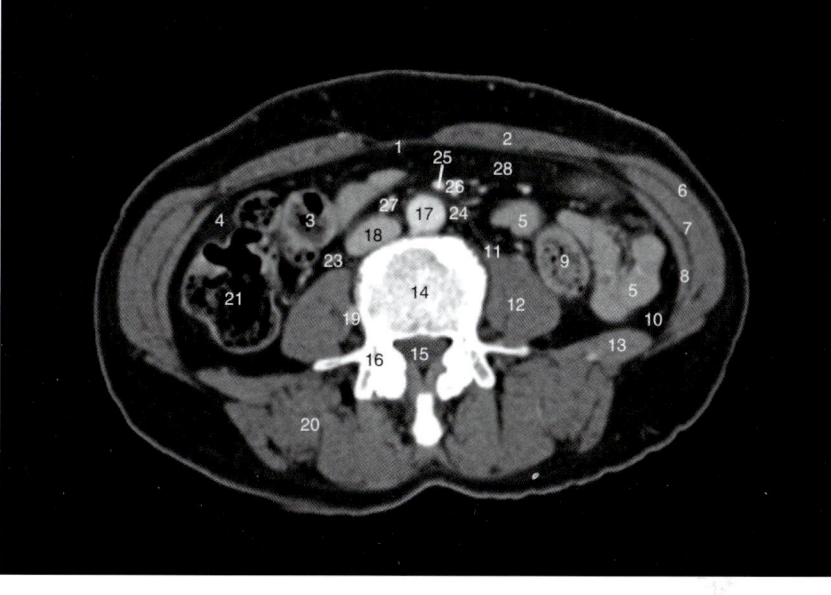

C. CT 增强图像

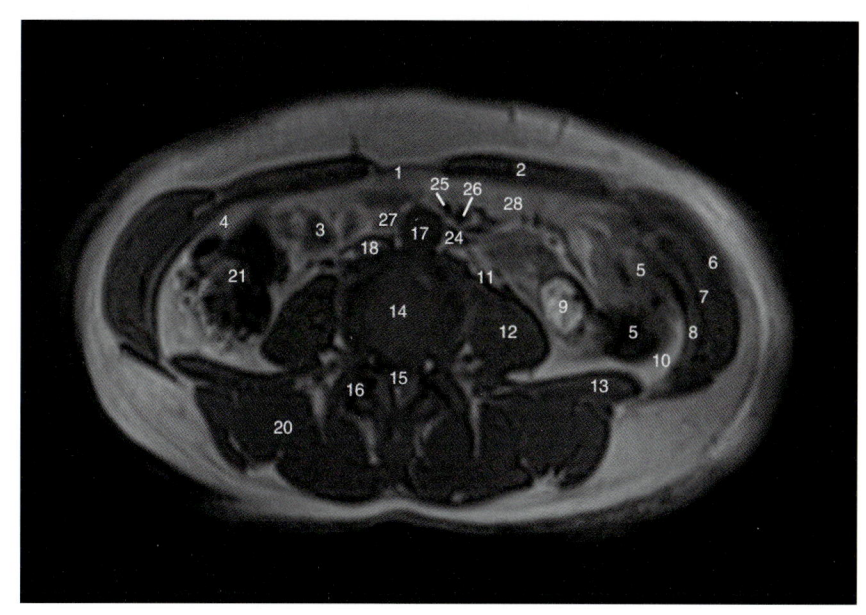

D. MR T1WI

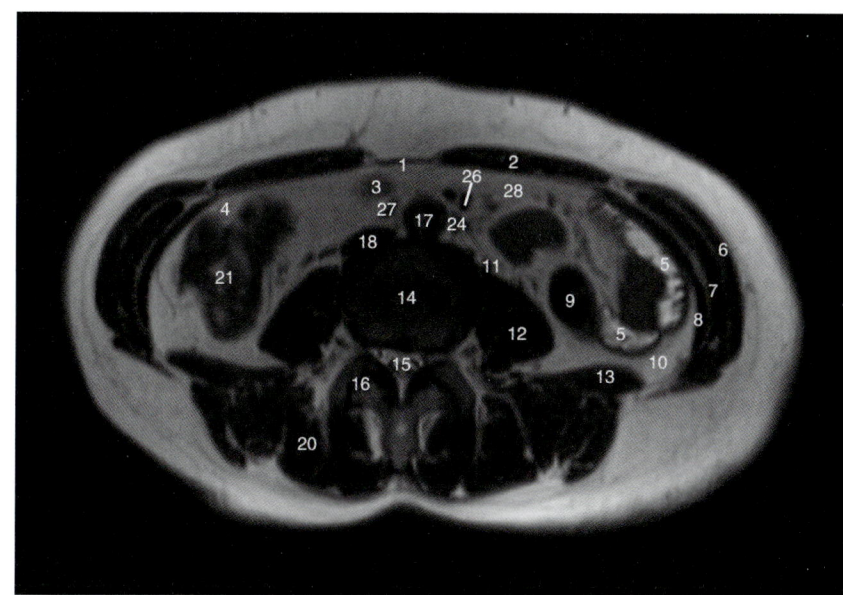

E. MR T2WI

关键结构：结肠动脉，肠系膜上静脉，肠系膜上动脉。

此断面经过第4腰椎椎体。

下腔静脉与腹主动脉沿脊柱前方走行，其前方由右向左依次可见结肠动脉、肠系膜上静脉和肠系膜上动脉，十二指肠消失，腹腔内其他肠管位置不变。结肠动脉分为右结肠动脉、中结肠动脉及左结肠动脉，此结肠动脉应为中结肠动脉。中结肠动脉在胰下缘的附近起于肠系膜上动脉，向前并稍偏右侧进入横结肠系膜，达横结肠系膜缘分为左、右两支，分别与左、右结肠动脉的分支吻合，沿途分支营养横结肠。节段性动脉中层溶解症是一种相对罕见的非动脉粥样硬化性或炎性动脉血管病变，易引起中年人自发性的腹腔出血，病理特征为动脉中层的平滑肌层溶解。结肠动脉是其好发部位之一，而经结肠动脉栓塞是治疗节段性动脉中层溶解症的重要手段。CTA 是诊断节段性动脉中层溶解症的有效方法，主要表现为结肠或腹腔内出血，多发的腹部内脏动脉改变，包括梭形动脉瘤、血管管腔狭窄、夹层和梗阻等[103]。

腹部连续横断层 102（FH.9890）

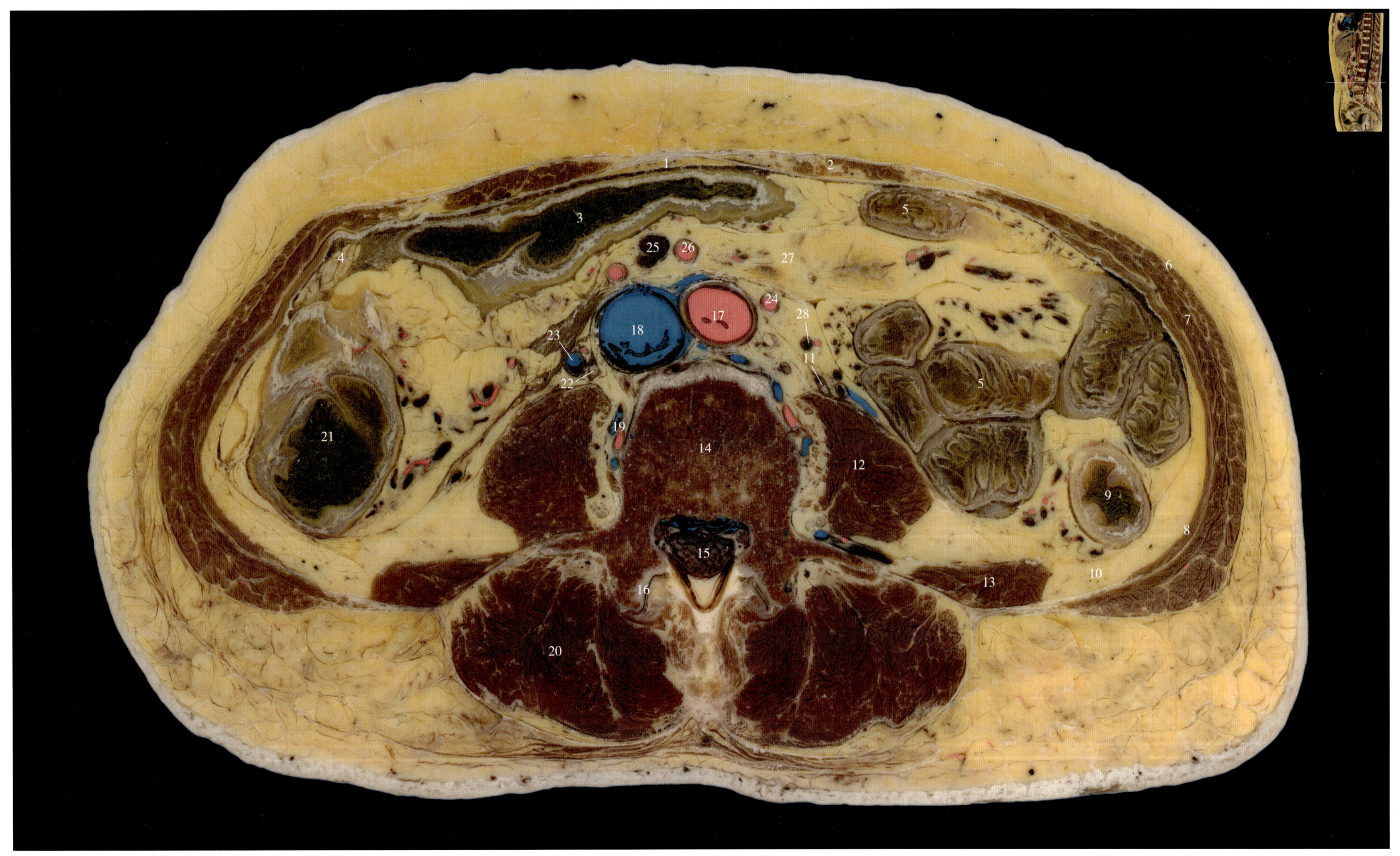

A. 断层标本图像

1. 肝圆韧带 ligamentum teres hepatis
2. 腹直肌 rectus abdominis
3. 横结肠 transverse colon
4. 大网膜 greater omentum
5. 空肠 jejunum
6. 腹外斜肌 obliquus externus abdominis
7. 腹内斜肌 obliquus internus abdominis
8. 腹横肌 transverses abdominis
9. 降结肠 descending colon
10. 腹膜外脂肪 extraperitoneal fat
11. 左输尿管 left ureter
12. 腰大肌 psoas major
13. 腰方肌 quadratus lumborum
14. 第4腰椎椎体 body of 4th lumbar vertebra
15. 马尾 cauda equina
16. 关节突关节 zygapophysial joint
17. 腹主动脉 abdominal aorta
18. 下腔静脉 inferior vena cava
19. 腰动、静脉 lumbar artery and vein
20. 竖脊肌 erector spinae
21. 升结肠 ascending colon
22. 右输尿管 right ureter
23. 右卵巢静脉 right ovarian vein
24. 肠系膜下动脉 inferior mesenteric artery
25. 肠系膜上静脉 superior mesenteric vein
26. 肠系膜上动脉 superior mesenteric artery
27. 肠系膜 mesentery
28. 肠系膜下静脉 inferior mesenteric vein

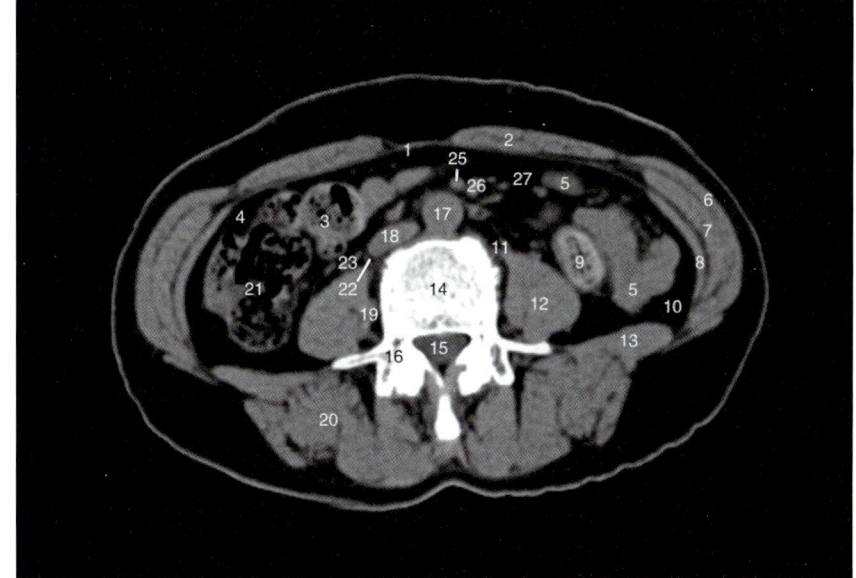

B. CT 平扫图像

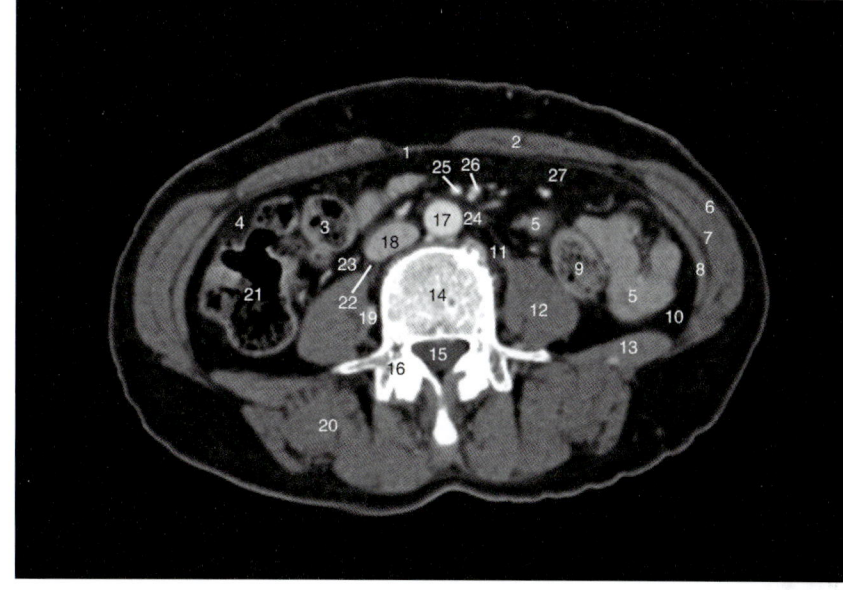

C. CT 增强图像

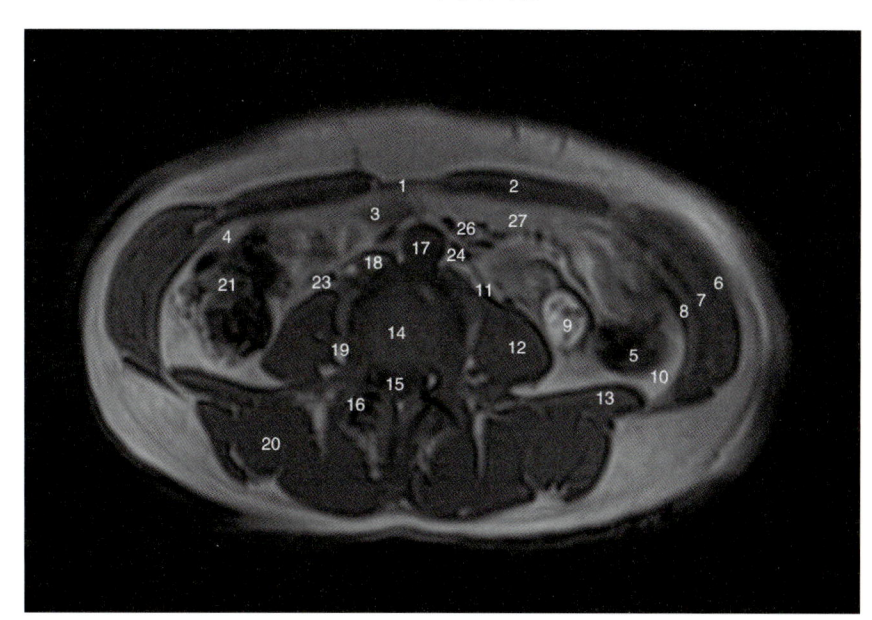

D. MR T1WI

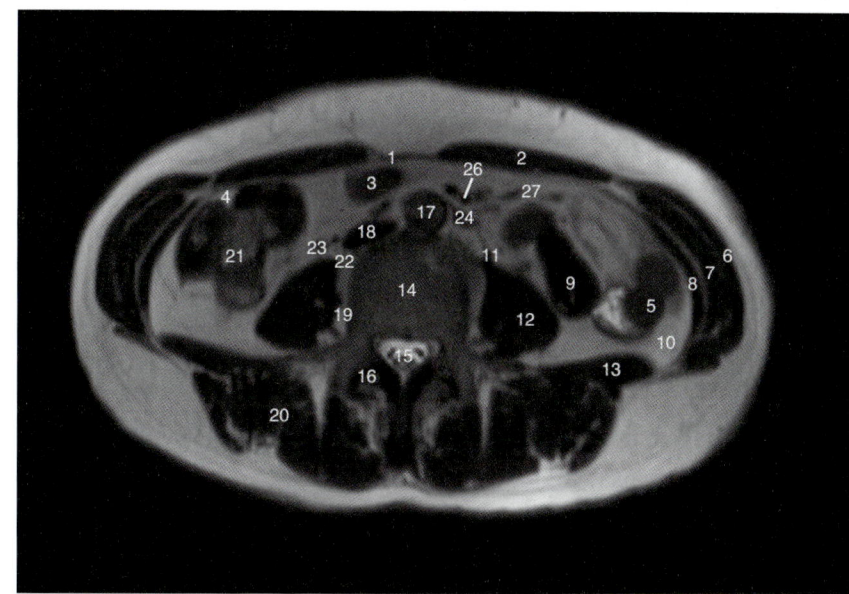

E. MR T2WI

关键结构：右卵巢静脉，右输尿管。

此断面经过第4腰椎椎体。

下腔静脉位于脊柱前方，与腹主动脉伴行。在其右后方和腰大肌前方的区域可见右卵巢静脉和右输尿管的断面，在右卵巢静脉的左前方可见与之伴行的右卵巢动脉。右卵巢动脉起自腹主动脉前壁，沿腰大肌前面斜向外下，在第4腰椎下缘处与输尿管交叉，经腹股沟管环入腹股沟管，在小骨盆上缘处，进入卵巢悬韧带，再向下进入子宫阔韧带，分支分布于卵巢和输卵管的外侧部，并于子宫阔韧带内与子宫动脉的分支相吻合。右卵巢静脉起自卵巢静脉丛，在卵巢悬韧带内合成卵巢静脉，向上以锐角注入下腔静脉。卵巢静脉血栓性静脉炎是产褥期最常见的并发症之一，其典型表现为发热、腹痛，查体下腹部可有压痛，但一般无肌紧张及反跳痛。约80%的病例为右侧卵巢静脉血栓性静脉炎，且可以延伸到下腔静脉。卵巢静脉因血栓扩张，增强扫描可见对比剂充盈缺损及条状血栓，这种扩张亦可导致静脉壁强化和血管周围炎性改变[104]。

腹部连续横断层 103（FH.9870）

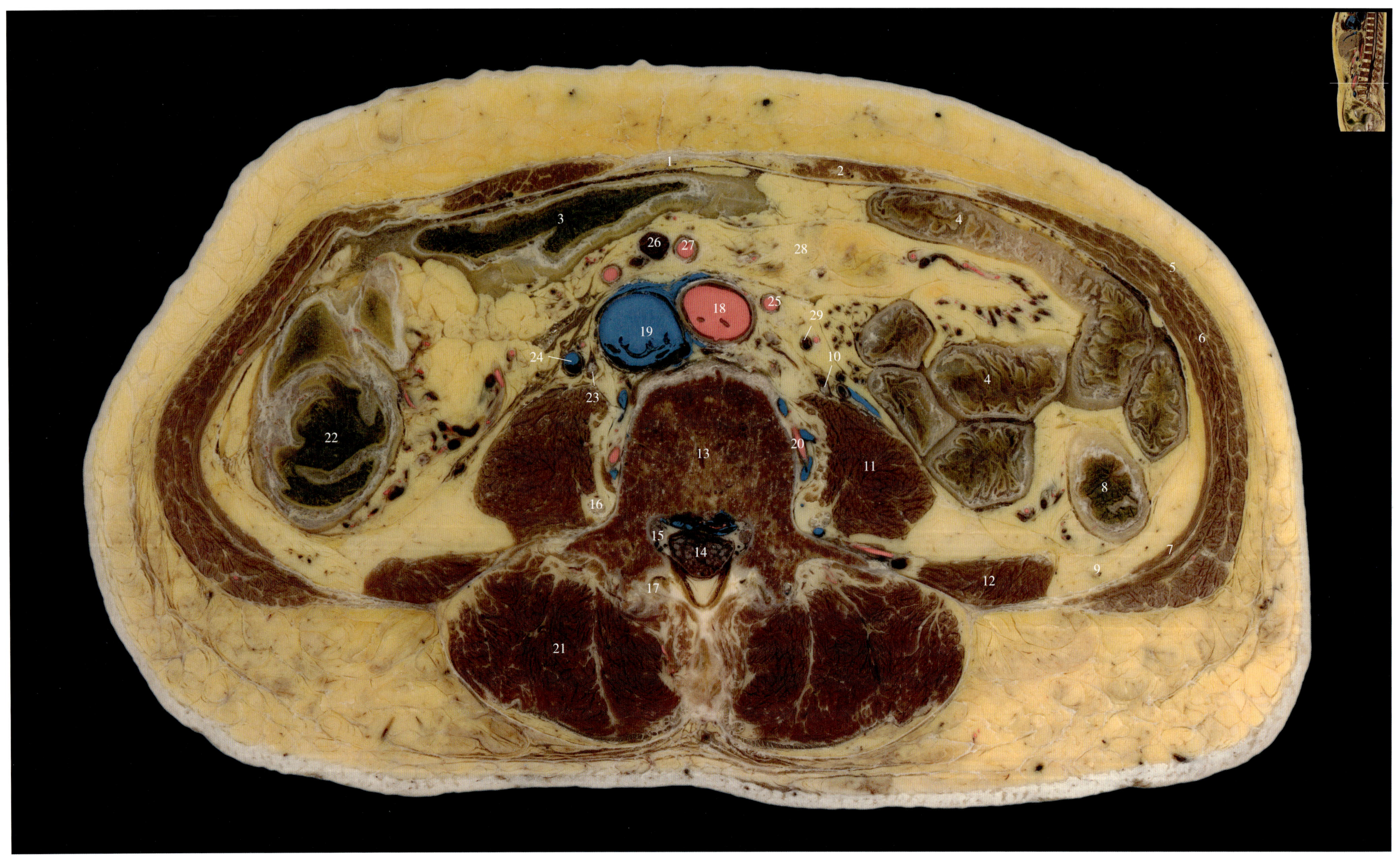

A. 断层标本图像

1. 肝圆韧带 ligamentum teres hepatis
2. 腹直肌 rectus abdominis
3. 横结肠 transverse colon
4. 空肠 jejunum
5. 腹外斜肌 obliquus externus abdominis
6. 腹内斜肌 obliquus internus abdominis
7. 腹横肌 transverses abdominis
8. 降结肠 descending colon
9. 腹膜外脂肪 extraperitoneal fat
10. 左输尿管 left ureter
11. 腰大肌 psoas major
12. 腰方肌 quadratus lumborum
13. 第 4 腰椎椎体 body of 4th lumbar vertebra
14. 马尾 cauda equina
15. 第 4 腰神经 4th lumbar nerve
16. 第 3 腰神经 3rd lumbar nerve
17. 关节突关节 zygapophysial joint
18. 腹主动脉 abdominal aorta
19. 下腔静脉 inferior vena cava
20. 腰动、静脉 lumbar artery and vein
21. 竖脊肌 erector spinae
22. 升结肠 ascending colon
23. 右输尿管 right ureter
24. 右卵巢静脉 right ovarian vein
25. 肠系膜下动脉 inferior mesenteric artery
26. 肠系膜上静脉 superior mesenteric vein
27. 肠系膜上动脉 superior mesenteric artery
28. 肠系膜 mesentery
29. 肠系膜下静脉 inferior mesenteric vein

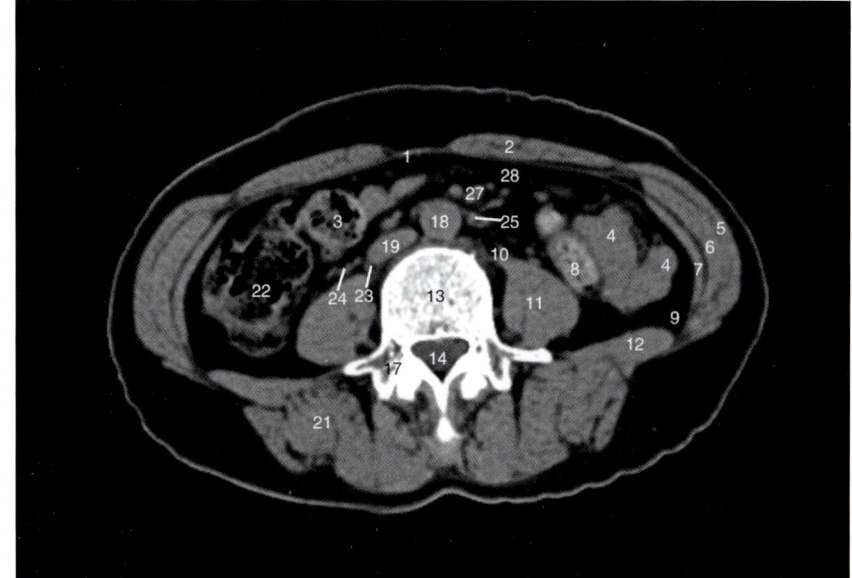

B. CT 平扫图像

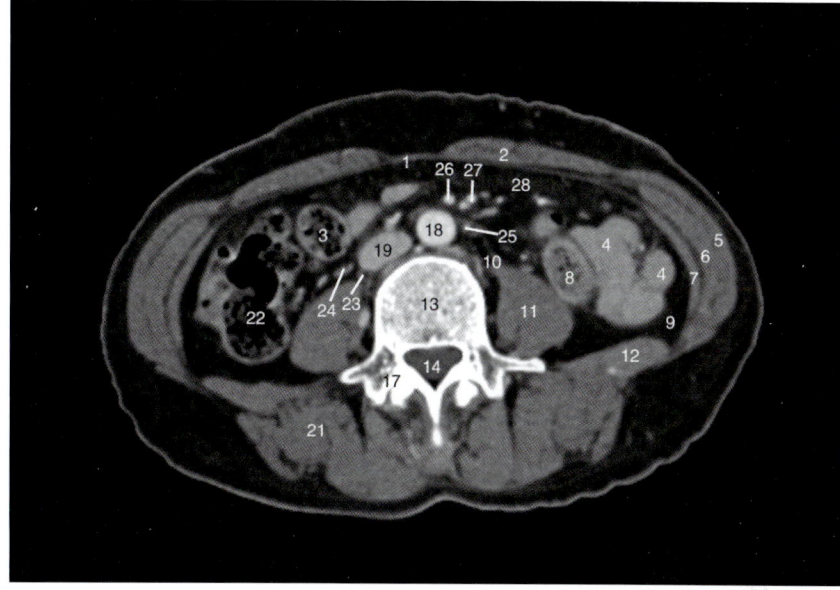

C. CT 增强图像

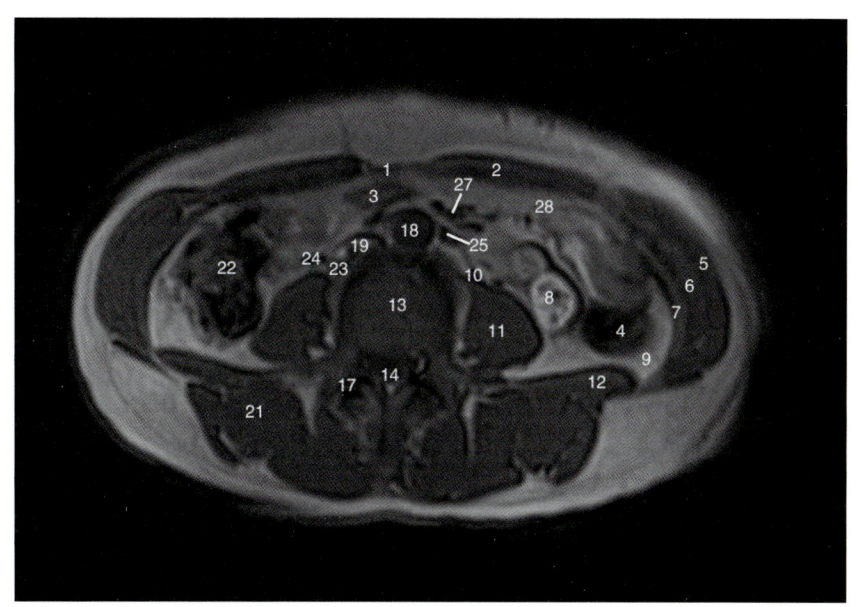

D. MR T1WI

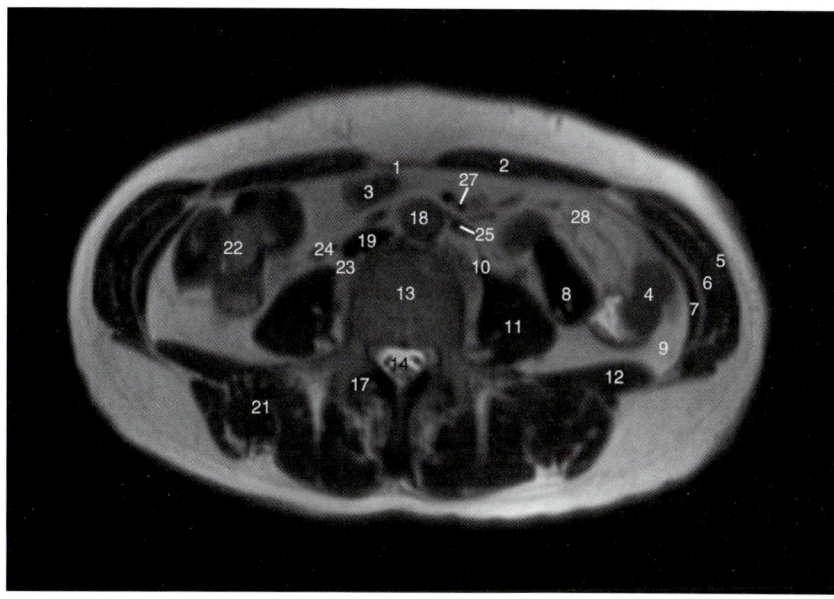

E. MR T2WI

关键结构：腰动、静脉，腰大肌。

此断面经过第 4 腰椎椎体。

左、右腰动、静脉位于椎体与两侧腰大肌之间。在椎体与腰大肌之间靠后的部位有第 3 腰神经从上方椎间孔穿出向下走行，与其他腰神经组成腰丛，椎管内可见马尾与第 4 腰神经。腰动脉共 4 对，从腹主动脉后壁的两侧发出，横越腰椎体前面及侧面，与腰静脉伴行，在腰大肌内侧缘处分出背侧支和腹侧支。背侧支分布到背部的肌、皮肤及脊柱，腹侧支分布至腹壁，并与腹前外侧壁其他动脉吻合。由于腰动脉紧贴腰椎体横行，当行腰椎结核病灶清除术时，主要结扎有关动脉，防止出血。腰静脉与椎内静脉丛相通，收集腰部组织的静脉血，汇入下腔静脉。腰静脉间的纵行交通支为腰升静脉，是上、下腔静脉系间联系通道。经皮椎间孔镜术在治疗腰椎间盘突出症时有着良好的疗效，虽然经皮椎间孔镜术引起的大出血比较少见，但是一旦发生大出血，处理往往比较困难。腰动脉是重要的栓塞入路，有研究表明腰动脉栓塞治疗经皮椎间孔镜术引起的大出血安全有效[105]。

腹部连续横断层 104（FH.9850）

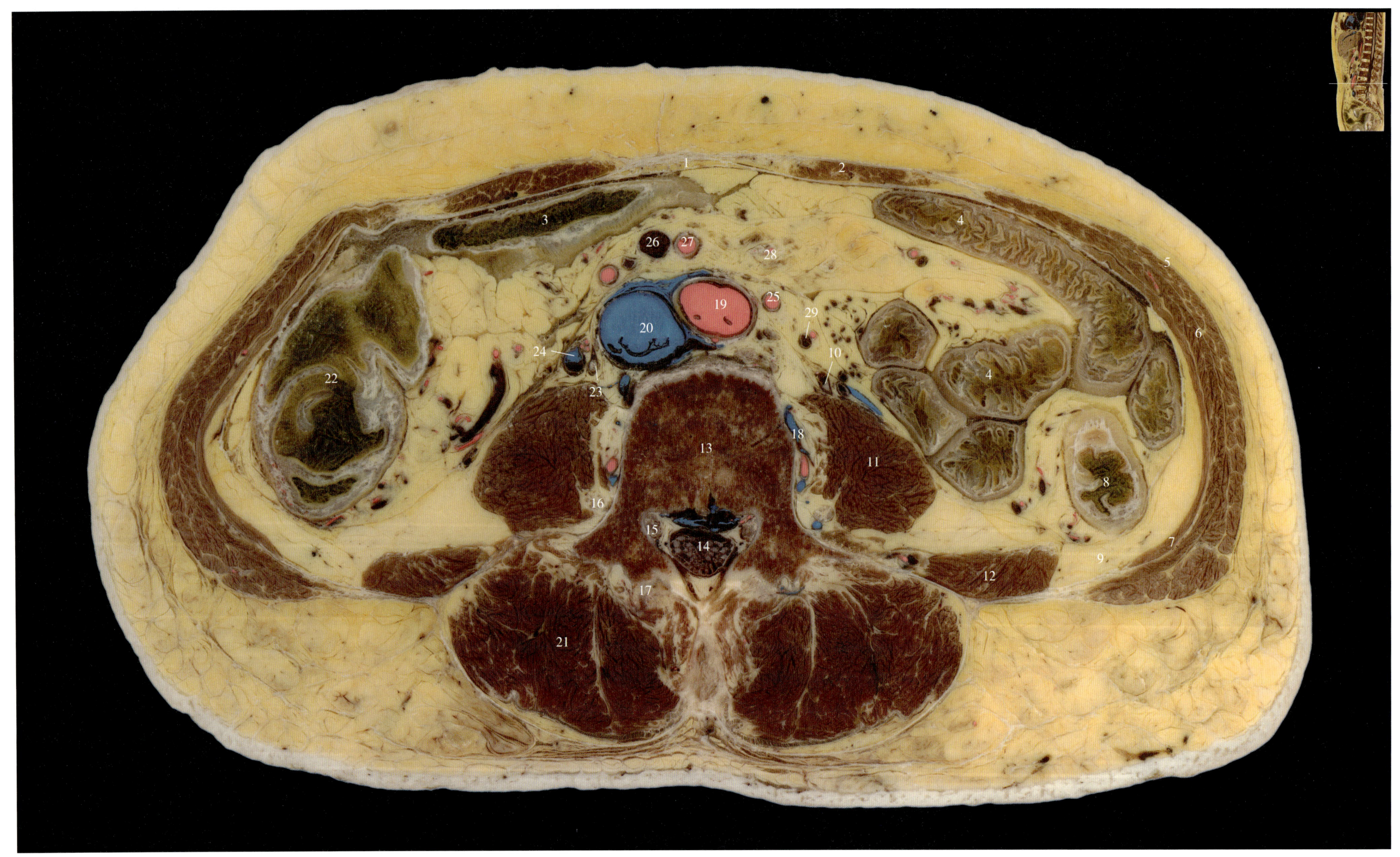

A. 断层标本图像

1. 肝圆韧带 ligamentum teres hepatis
2. 腹直肌 rectus abdominis
3. 横结肠 transverse colon
4. 空肠 jejunum
5. 腹外斜肌 obliquus externus abdominis
6. 腹内斜肌 obliquus internus abdominis
7. 腹横肌 transverses abdominis
8. 降结肠 descending colon
9. 腹膜外脂肪 extraperitoneal fat
10. 左输尿管 left ureter
11. 腰大肌 psoas major
12. 腰方肌 quadratus lumborum
13. 第4腰椎椎体 body of 4th lumbar vertebra
14. 马尾 cauda equina
15. 第4腰神经 4th lumbar nerve
16. 第3腰神经 3rd lumbar nerve
17. 关节突关节 zygapophysial joint
18. 腰动、静脉 lumbar artery and vein
19. 腹主动脉 abdominal aorta
20. 下腔静脉 inferior vena cava
21. 竖脊肌 erector spinae
22. 升结肠 ascending colon
23. 右输尿管 right ureter
24. 右卵巢静脉 right ovarian vein
25. 肠系膜下动脉 inferior mesenteric artery
26. 肠系膜上静脉 superior mesenteric vein
27. 肠系膜上动脉 superior mesenteric artery
28. 肠系膜 mesentery
29. 肠系膜下静脉 inferior mesenteric vein

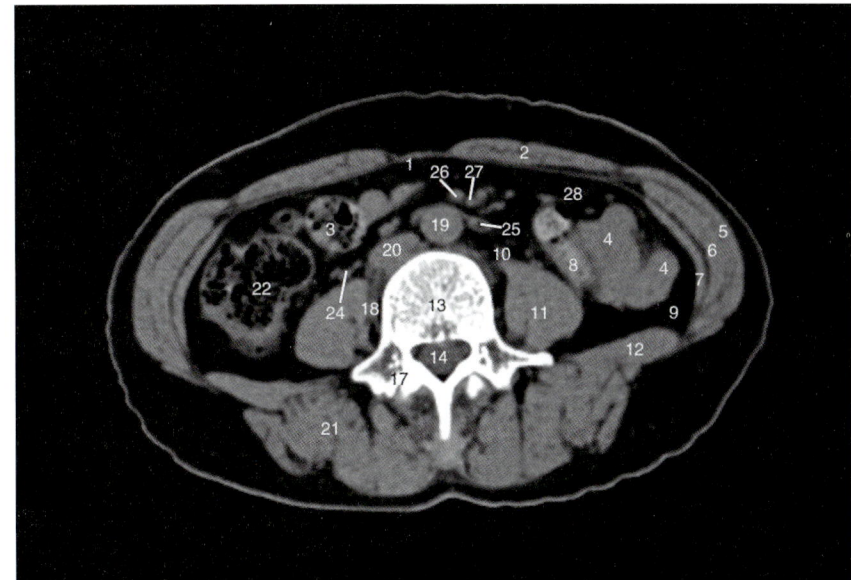

B. CT 平扫图像

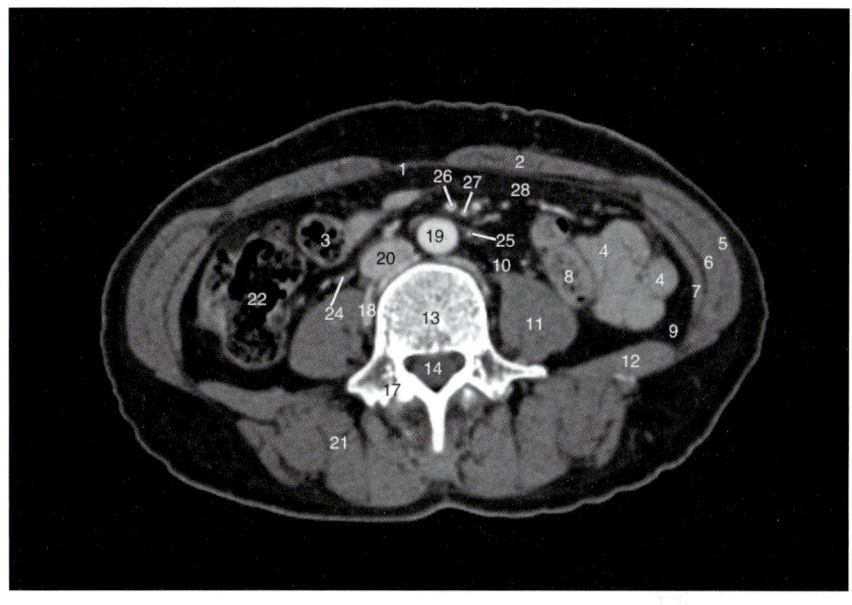

C. CT 增强图像

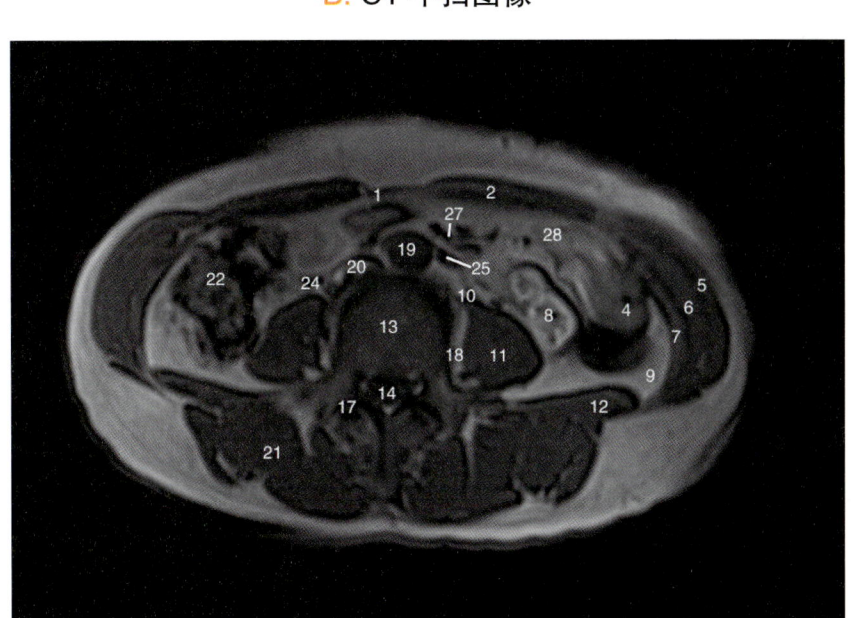

D. MR T1WI

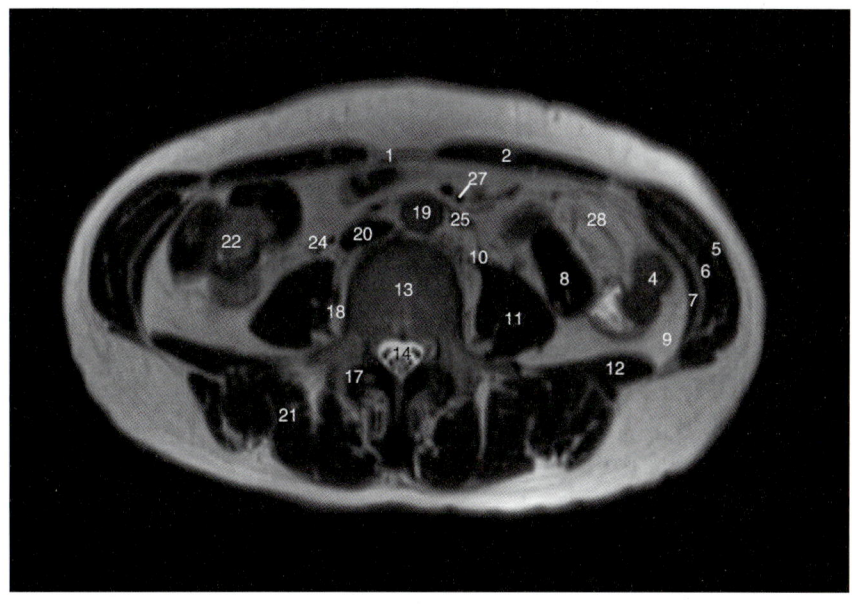

E. MR T2WI

关键结构：第 4 腰神经，马尾，腰动、静脉。

此断面经过第4腰椎椎体下缘。

椎体位于断面中央，其前方为下腔静脉和腹主动脉，两侧为腰大肌及腰动、静脉，后方为三角形的椎管，内容马尾，第4腰神经从椎管内穿出。腹腔内的肠管结构分布同上一断层，横结肠的断面逐渐变小。第4腰神经前支的一部分与第12胸神经前支的一部分、第1~3腰神经前支组成腰丛，而前支的剩余部分和第5腰神经前支合成腰骶干，向下加入骶丛。马尾位于椎体后方的椎孔内，由腰、骶、尾部的脊神经根在脊髓圆锥下方围绕终丝聚集形成，脊髓蛛网膜下隙穿刺抽取脑脊液或麻醉时，常选择第3、4腰椎棘突间进针，以免损伤脊髓。终丝脂肪变是临床较常见的一种终丝退变表现，当终丝发生脂肪变性，受外力牵拉或过度屈伸时脊髓受到损伤的可能性增加，可引起脊髓栓系综合征，出现下肢感觉功能运动障碍，甚至大小便功能障碍。MRI表现为椎管内点状或条状异常信号，T1WI表现椎管内呈点状或条状高信号；T2WI终丝脂肪沉积和脑脊液均表现为高信号；T2WI-FS序列椎管内显示为条状低信号。横断位CT扫描呈现小类圆形脂肪低密度灶。当终丝脂肪沉积呈瘤状表现时，称为终丝脂肪瘤[106]。

腹部连续横断层 105（FH.9830）

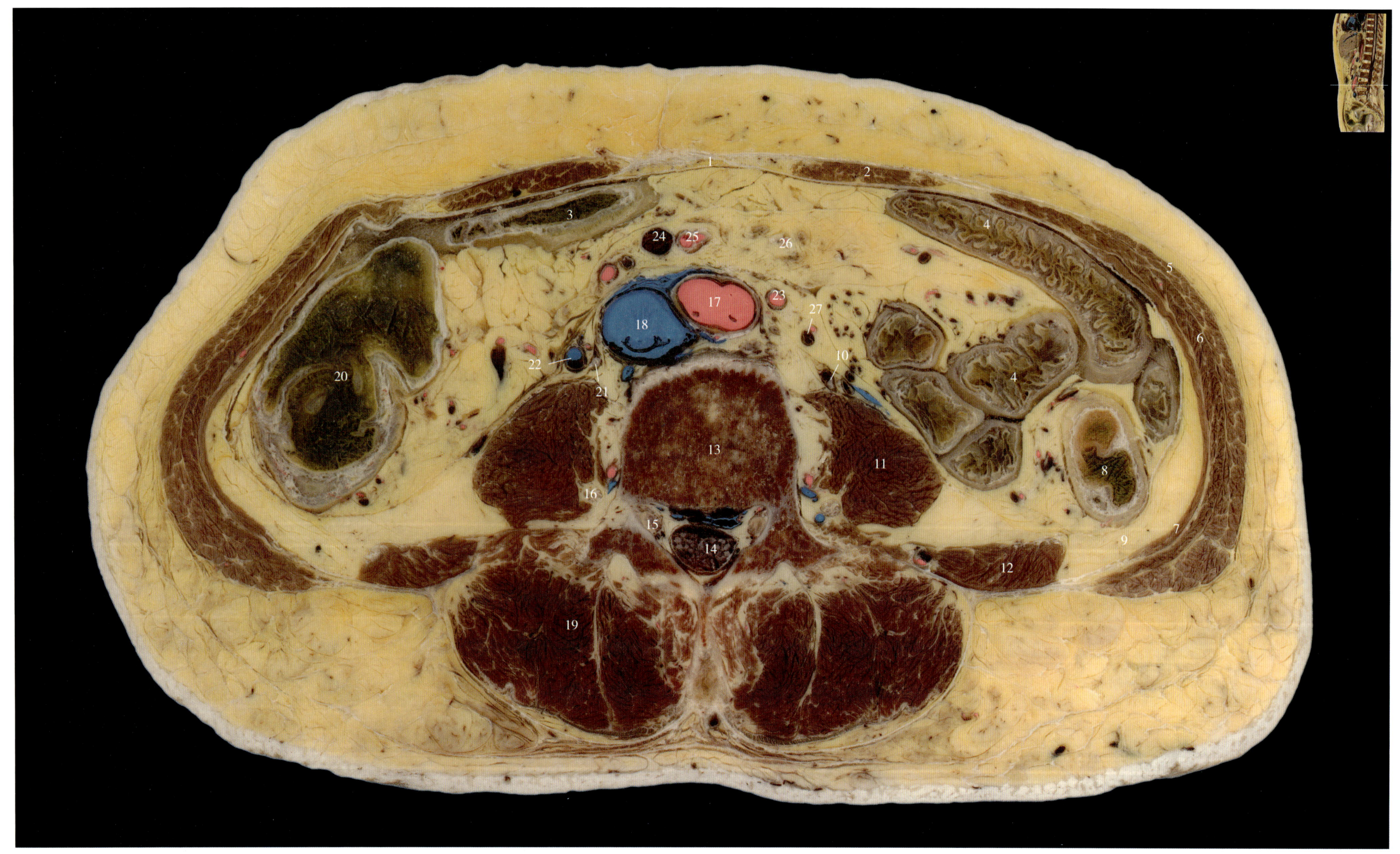

A. 断层标本图像

1. 肝圆韧带 ligamentum teres hepatis
2. 腹直肌 rectus abdominis
3. 横结肠 transverse colon
4. 空肠 jejunum
5. 腹外斜肌 obliquus externus abdominis
6. 腹内斜肌 obliquus internus abdominis
7. 腹横肌 transverses abdominis
8. 降结肠 descending colon
9. 腹膜外脂肪 extraperitoneal fat
10. 左输尿管 left ureter
11. 腰大肌 psoas major
12. 腰方肌 quadratus lumborum
13. 第 4 腰椎椎体 body of 4th lumbar vertebra
14. 马尾 cauda equina
15. 第 4 腰神经 4th lumbar nerve
16. 第 3 腰神经 3rd lumbar nerve
17. 腹主动脉 abdominal aorta
18. 下腔静脉 inferior vena cava
19. 竖脊肌 erector spinae
20. 升结肠 ascending colon
21. 右输尿管 right ureter
22. 右卵巢静脉 right ovarian vein
23. 肠系膜下动脉 inferior mesenteric artery
24. 肠系膜上静脉 superior mesenteric vein
25. 肠系膜上动脉 superior mesenteric artery
26. 肠系膜 mesentery
27. 肠系膜下静脉 inferior mesenteric vein

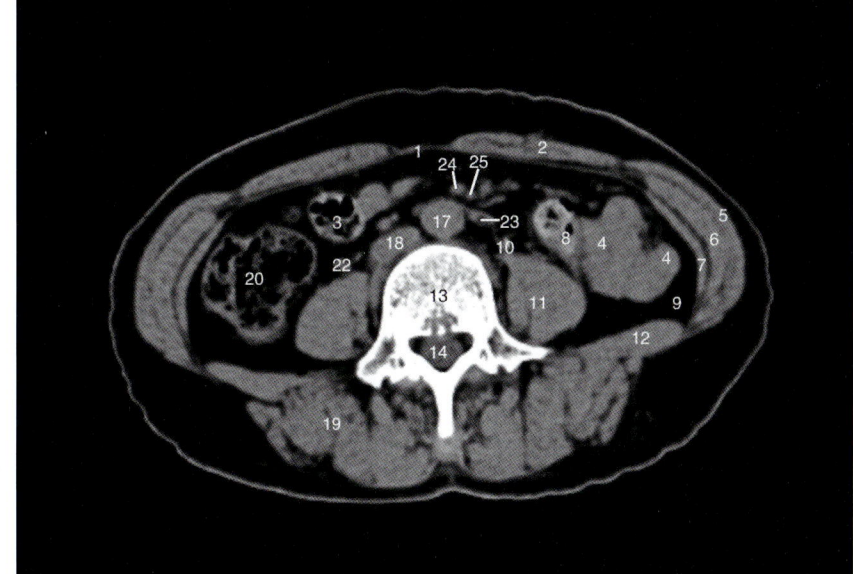

B. CT 平扫图像

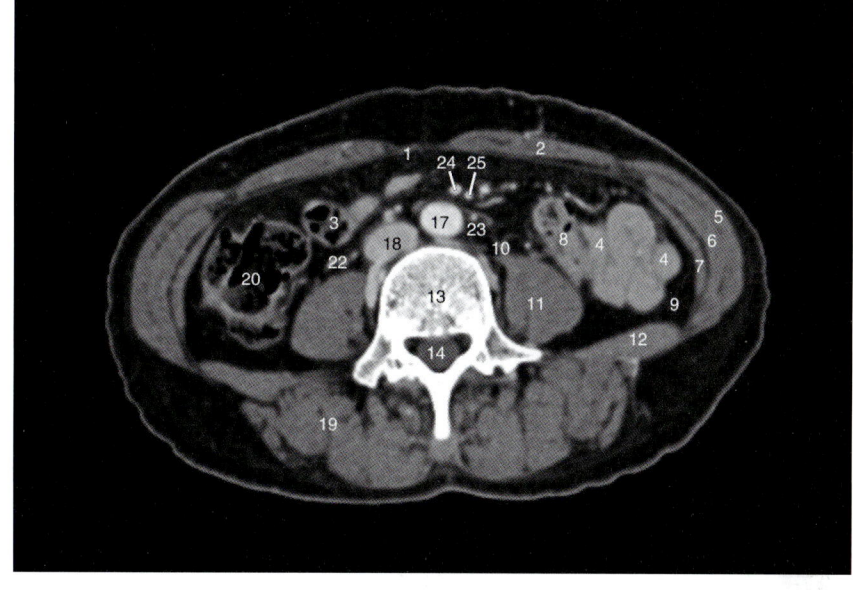

C. CT 增强图像

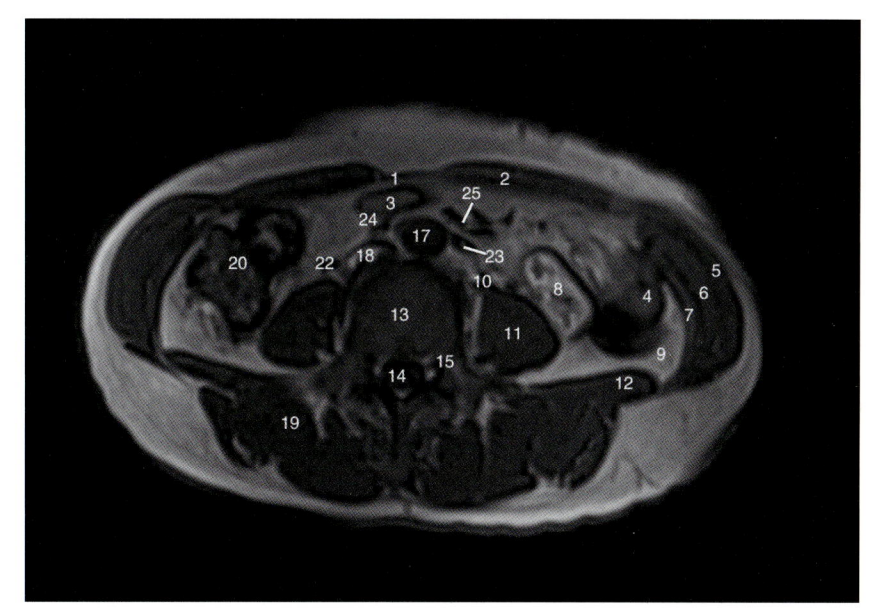

D. MR T1WI

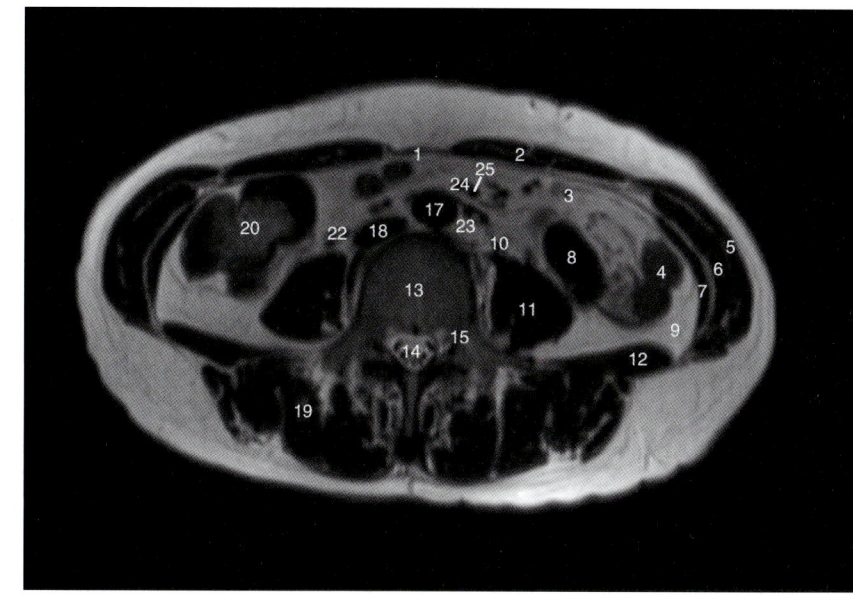

E. MR T2WI

关键结构：腹主动脉，下腔静脉，肠系膜。

此断面经过第 4 腰椎椎体下缘。

腹主动脉位于脊柱前方，其右侧有下腔静脉伴行，二者前方和两侧有肠系膜及位于肠系膜内的血管及其分支，肠道结构分布同上。在此平面上，可见腹主动脉从圆形变成前后稍扁的椭圆形管腔，表示其即将分成左、右髂总动脉。腹主动脉是腹部的动脉主干，于主动脉裂孔处由胸主动脉移行而来，沿脊柱腰段的左前方下降，至第 4 腰椎椎体下缘或第 5 腰椎前方分为左、右髂总动脉。成人全长为 145.23 cm ± 14.15 cm，上端直径为 18.31 mm ± 3.92 mm，中段为 15.85 mm ± 3.02 mm，下端为 16.42 mm ± 2.94 mm[37]。腹主动脉分支有壁支与脏支，壁支小，主要有膈下动脉、腰动脉与骶正中动脉；脏支粗大，主要有肾上腺动脉、肾动脉、睾丸动脉、腹腔干、肠系膜上动脉与肠系膜下动脉等。腹主动脉的形态和周围结构在 CT 和 MRI 上都能清晰辨认。腹主动脉瘤和腹主动脉夹层是威胁患者生命安全的严重病变。当腹主动脉瘤样扩张的直径超过正常腹主动脉直径的 1.5 倍或直径超过 3 cm 时，可以诊断为腹主动脉瘤。当发生主动脉夹层时，CTA 可以看到真腔、假腔及撕裂的内膜片，通常真腔小、假腔大，真腔强化程度弱于假腔。CTA 也是腹主动脉瘤及主动脉夹层支架置入术后最常用的随访观察手段[107,108]。

腹部连续横断层 106 (FH.9810)

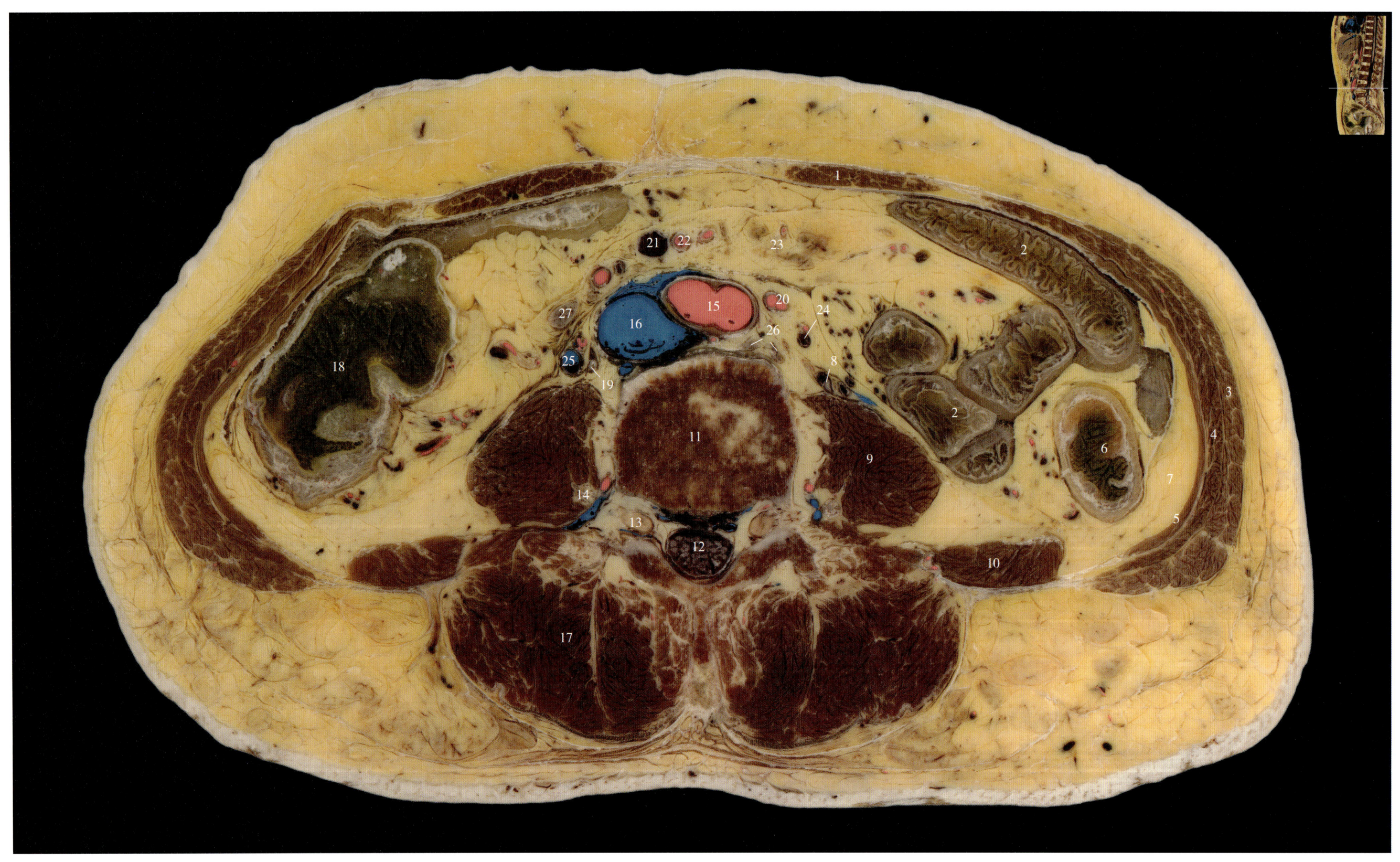

A. 断层标本图像

1. 腹直肌 rectus abdominis
2. 空肠 jejunum
3. 腹外斜肌 obliquus externus abdominis
4. 腹内斜肌 obliquus internus abdominis
5. 腹横肌 transverses abdominis
6. 降结肠 descending colon
7. 腹膜外脂肪 extraperitoneal fat
8. 左输尿管 left ureter
9. 腰大肌 psoas major
10. 腰方肌 quadratus lumborum
11. 第4腰椎椎体 body of 4th lumbar vertebra
12. 马尾 cauda equina
13. 第4腰神经 4th lumbar nerve
14. 第3腰神经 3rd lumbar nerve
15. 腹主动脉 abdominal aorta
16. 下腔静脉 inferior vena cava
17. 竖脊肌 erector spinae
18. 升结肠 ascending colon
19. 右输尿管 right ureter
20. 肠系膜下动脉 inferior mesenteric artery
21. 肠系膜上静脉 superior mesenteric vein
22. 肠系膜上动脉 superior mesenteric artery
23. 肠系膜 mesentery
24. 肠系膜下静脉 inferior mesenteric vein
25. 右卵巢静脉 right ovarian vein
26. 腰淋巴结 lumbar lymph nodes
27. 淋巴结 lymph node

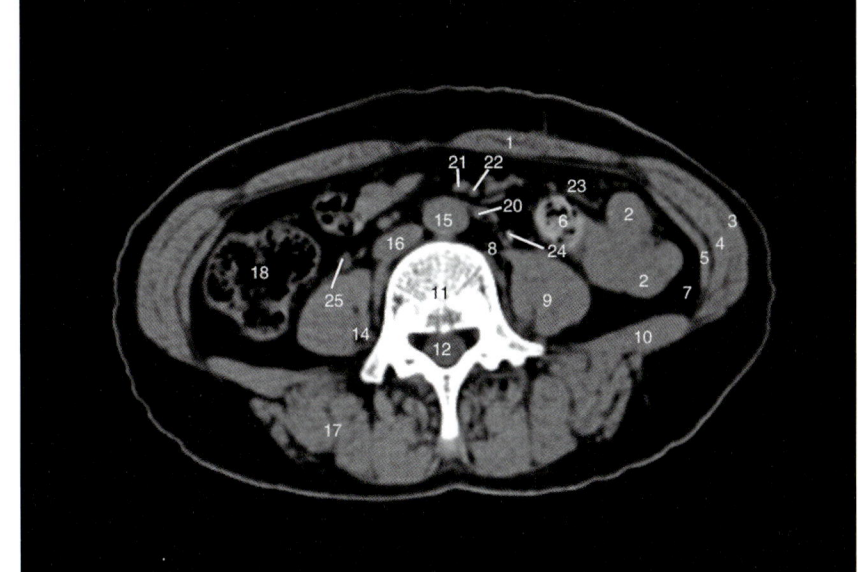

B. CT 平扫图像

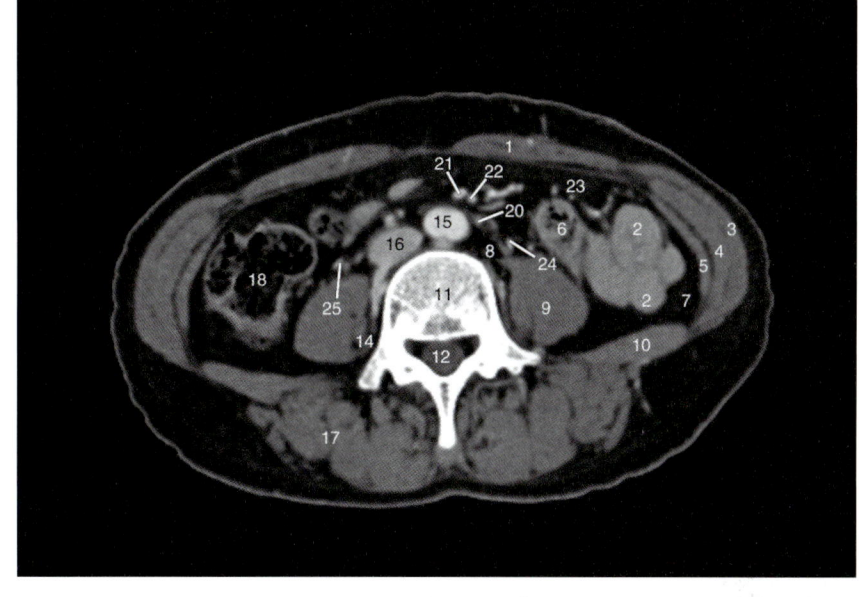

C. CT 增强图像

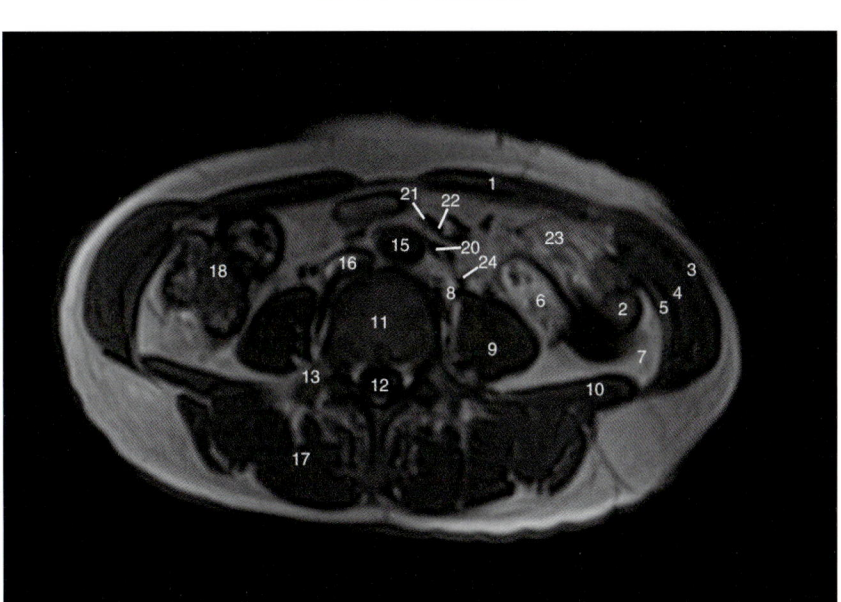

D. MR T1WI

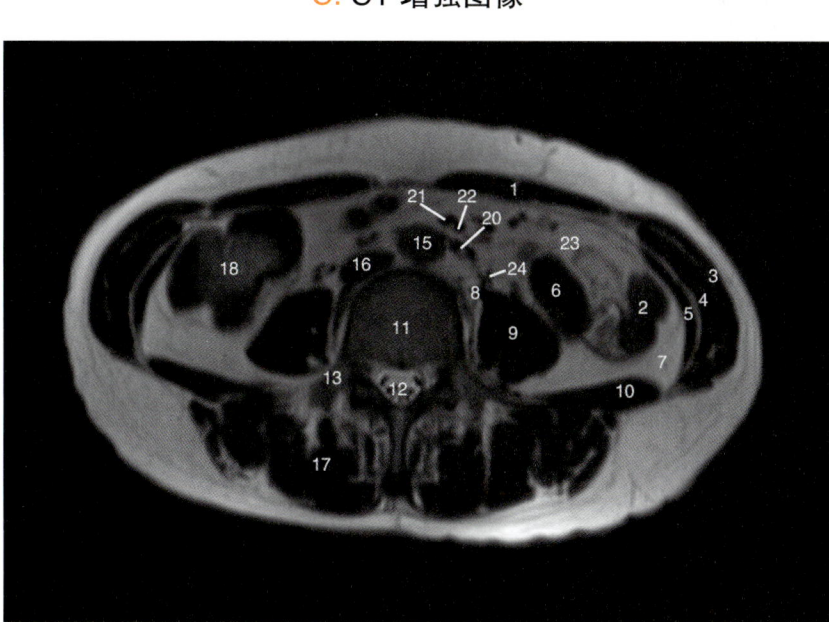

E. MR T2WI

关键结构：淋巴结，左、右髂总动脉，腰淋巴结。

此断面经过第4腰椎椎体下缘。

脊柱前方为腹主动脉和下腔静脉，腹主动脉逐渐分成左、右髂总动脉，下腔静脉也有两侧髂总静脉汇合的趋势。腹主动脉和脊柱间可见数个腰淋巴结，下腔静脉右侧亦有淋巴结存在。横结肠逐渐消失，肠管结构主要为升结肠、降结肠和空肠。腰淋巴结通常有30~50个，可分为左、中、右3群，沿腹主动脉和下腔静脉周围配布，主要收纳腹后壁深淋巴管、髂总淋巴结的输出管及腹腔内成对脏器的淋巴管，输出管组成左、右腰干，参与乳糜池的构成。CT 可显示腰淋巴结，表现为大血管旁点状软组织密度影，直径一般不超过10 mm。腹腔器官的淋巴结主要沿腹腔干、肠系膜上动脉、肠系膜下动脉及其分支排列，输出管分别注入腹腔淋巴结、肠系膜上淋巴结和肠系膜下淋巴结，最后汇合成肠干。肠系膜淋巴结位于肠系膜内，总数约为300个，其配布的位置可分为3列：第1列沿肠壁排列，在肠系膜缘；第2列在肠系膜中份位于肠血管襻之间，第3列位于肠系膜根部[7]。CT 可显示第2、3列肠系膜淋巴结，如脂肪含量充足，CT 有时可显示出直径小至5 mm 的肠系膜淋巴结，并可沿肠系膜血管追踪至肝门静脉，以观察疾病的淋巴播散情况。腹腔恶性肿瘤会发生淋巴结的转移，表现为淋巴结的明显增大，增强扫描可见强化，但是 CT 和 MRI 并不能有效地鉴别淋巴结反应性增生引起的增大和恶性肿瘤引起的增大。PET-CT 通过评估肿大淋巴结的同位素摄取情况为鉴别诊断提供一定的价值，但是病理诊断仍然是金标准[109]。

腹部连续横断层 107（FH.9790）

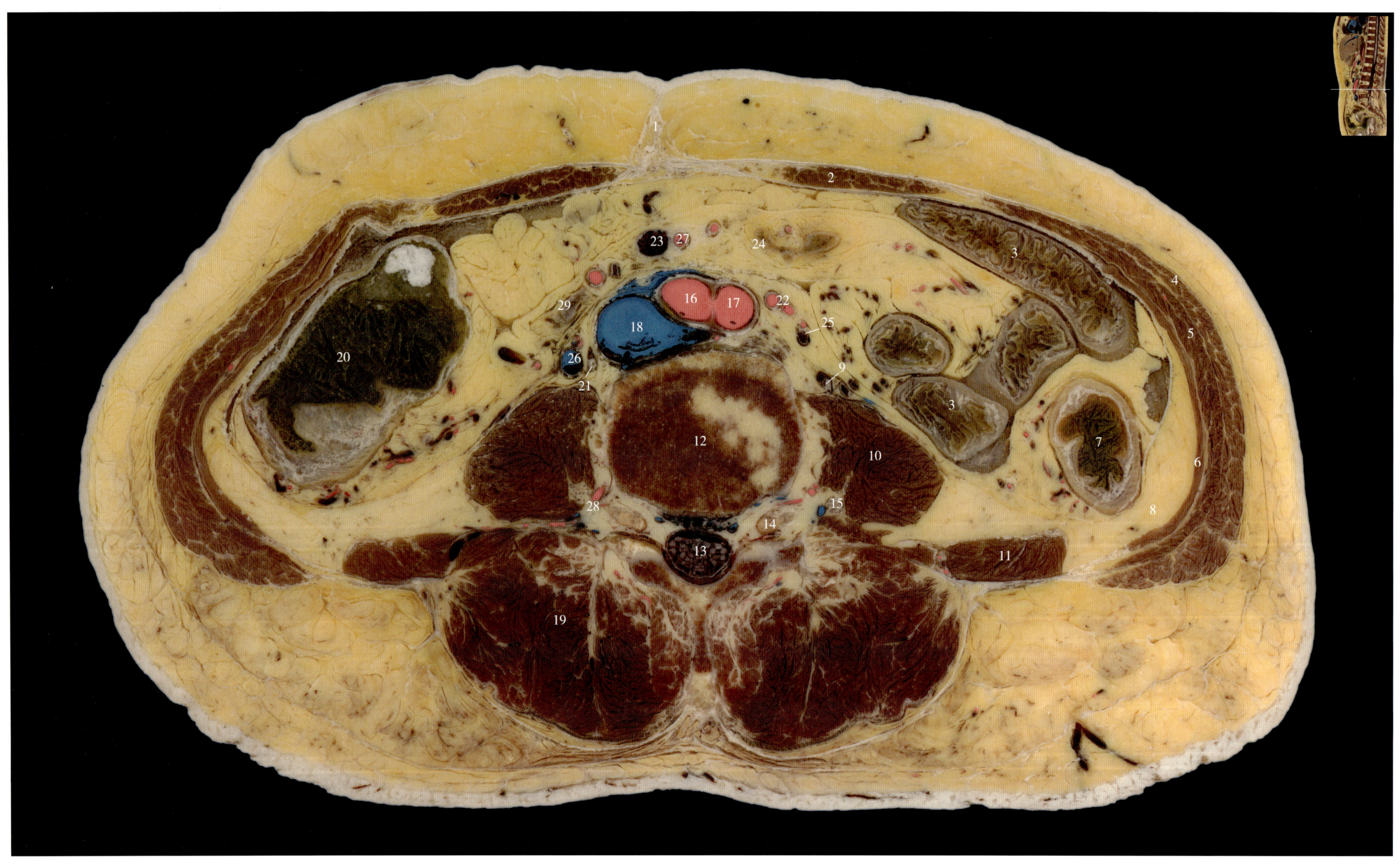

A. 断层标本图像

1. 脐 umbilicus
2. 腹直肌 rectus abdominis
3. 空肠 jejunum
4. 腹外斜肌 obliquus externus abdominis
5. 腹内斜肌 obliquus internus abdominis
6. 腹横肌 transverses abdominis
7. 降结肠 descending colon
8. 腹膜外脂肪 extraperitoneal fat
9. 左输尿管 left ureter
10. 腰大肌 psoas major
11. 腰方肌 quadratus lumborum
12. 第 4 腰椎椎体 body of 4th lumbar vertebra
13. 马尾 cauda equina
14. 第 4 腰神经 4th lumbar nerve
15. 第 3 腰神经 3rd lumbar nerve
16. 右髂总动脉 right common iliac artery
17. 左髂总动脉 left common iliac artery
18. 下腔静脉 inferior vena cava
19. 竖脊肌 erector spinae
20. 升结肠 ascending colon
21. 右输尿管 right ureter
22. 肠系膜下动脉 inferior mesenteric artery
23. 肠系膜上静脉 superior mesenteric vein
24. 肠系膜 mesentery
25. 肠系膜下静脉 inferior mesenteric vein
26. 右卵巢静脉 right ovarian vein
27. 肠系膜上动脉 superior mesenteric artery
28. 腰丛 lumbar plexus
29. 淋巴结 lymph node

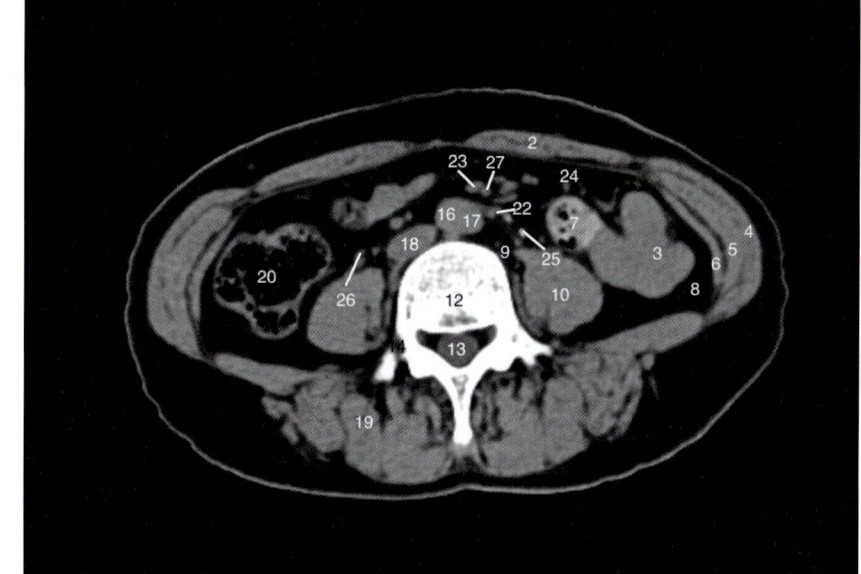

B. CT 平扫图像

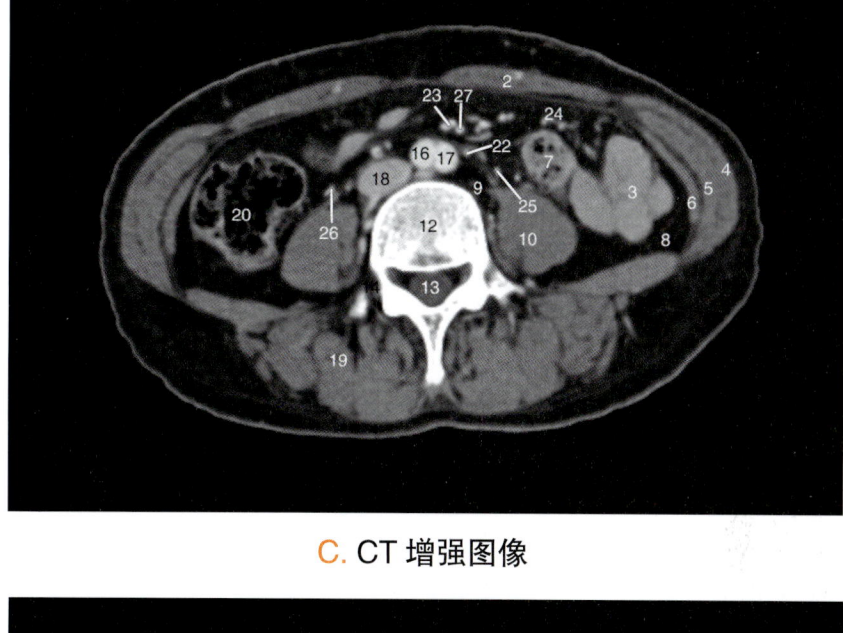

C. CT 增强图像

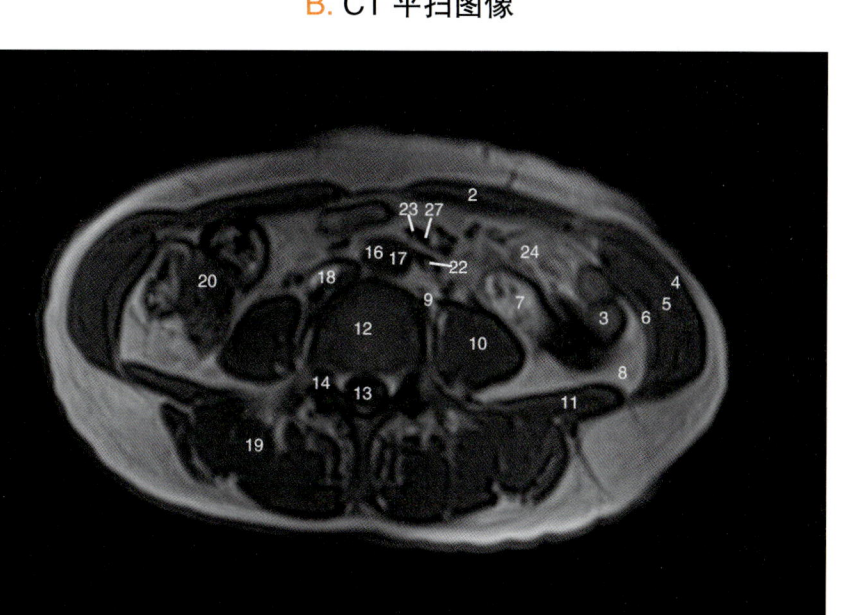

D. MR T1WI

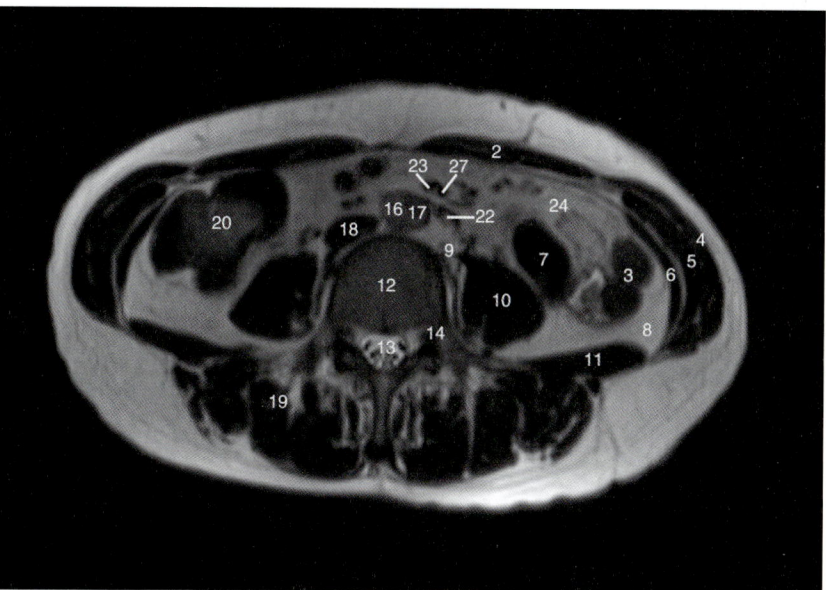

E. MR T2WI

关键结构：腰大肌，腰神经丛。

此断面经第 4 腰椎椎体下份。

腰大肌位于腰部横突和椎体之间的沟内，起自第 12 胸椎和 5 个腰椎横突前方，并以 5 个肌齿起自相邻的 2 个椎体和椎间盘，肌齿与腰椎椎体之间有腱弓可容腰动脉、腰静脉和腰交感干的小支通过。腰大肌跨骶髂关节前方，沿小骨盆入口向前下，在腹股沟韧带深面跨过髋关节前方，进入大腿，形成肌腱，与其外侧的髂肌合并，共同止于股骨小转子。腰大肌由腰大肌筋膜包绕，腰大肌筋膜在髂窝与髂筋膜愈合成髂腰肌筋膜。腰椎结核引起的冷性脓肿可沿筋膜深面向下蔓延，可以波及髂窝、骶髂关节或髋关节，由于腰大肌止于大腿根部的小转子，故冷性脓肿可出现在腹股沟韧带下方的股三角内。腰神经丛位于腰椎横突前方、腰方肌内侧，腰大肌深面和外侧。腰丛由第 1~3 腰神经前支和部分第 4 腰神经前支组成，尚有部分第 12 胸神经前支参加组成。上述各支均发出肌支配腰大肌和腰方肌，各支在参与腰丛组成以前，通过灰交通支接交感神经节后纤维，这些交感神经节后纤维随腰丛的分布到皮肤的汗腺和立毛肌。腰丛的分支分布到腹壁、盆壁和下肢[26]。腰神经丛损伤较常见，但是 X 线、CT、超声和核素成像并不能全面显示神经的形态、病变和毗邻关系。MRI 是最常用的评估腰神经丛损伤的无创成像手段，背景信号抑制扩散加权体部成像序列（DWIBS）和三维压脂 T2WI 是磁共振周围神经成像常用的手段，影像学表现为神经丛肿胀，信号明显增高[110]。

腹部连续横断层 108（FH.9770）

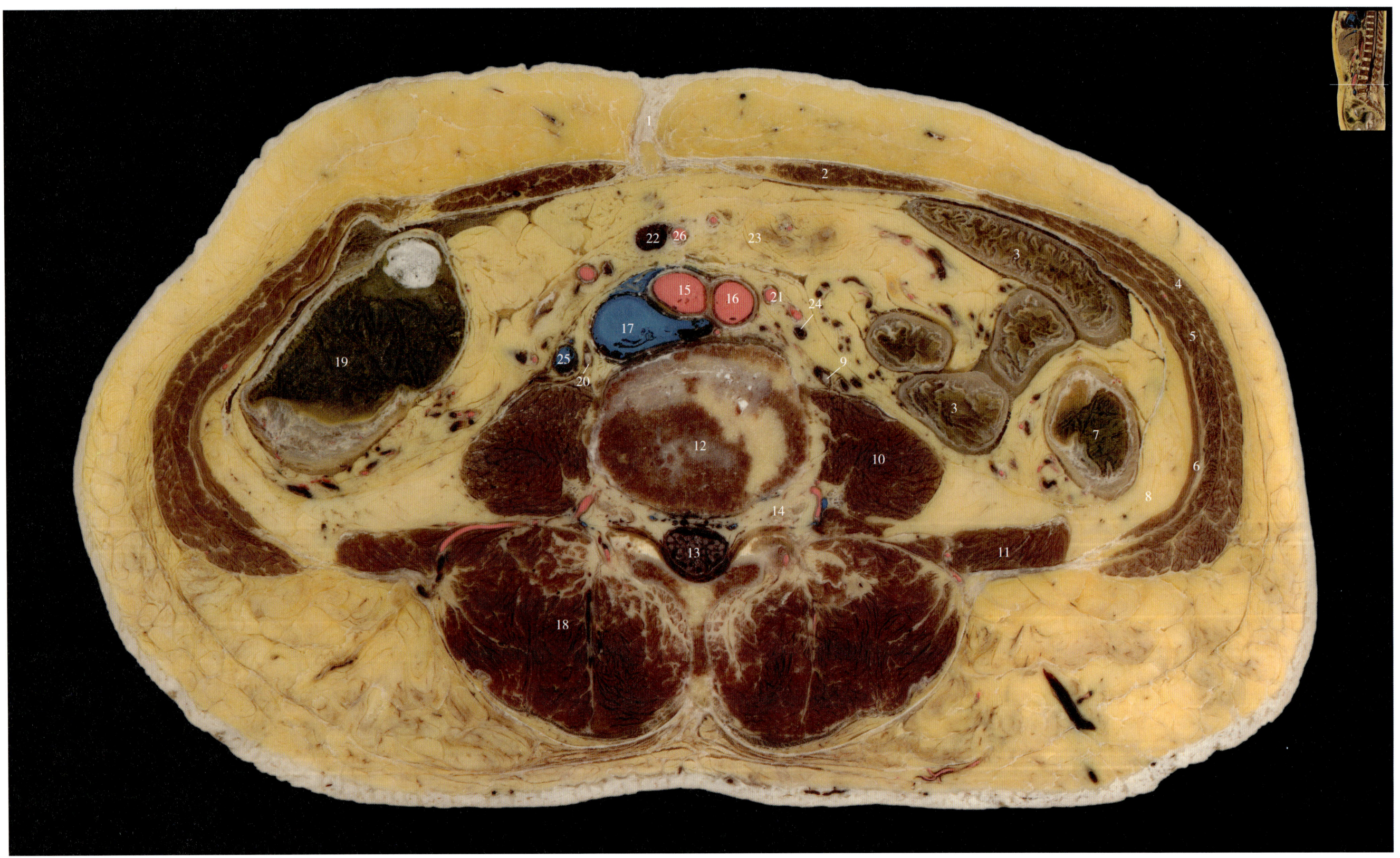

A. 断层标本图像

1. 脐 umbilicus
2. 腹直肌 rectus abdominis
3. 空肠 jejunum
4. 腹外斜肌 obliquus externus abdominis
5. 腹内斜肌 obliquus internus abdominis
6. 腹横肌 transverses abdominis
7. 降结肠 descending colon
8. 腹膜外脂肪 extraperitoneal fat
9. 左输尿管 left ureter
10. 腰大肌 psoas major
11. 腰方肌 quadratus lumborum
12. 第 4 腰椎椎体 body of 4th lumbar vertebra
13. 马尾 cauda equina
14. 第 4 腰神经 4th lumbar nerve
15. 右髂总动脉 right common iliac artery
16. 左髂总动脉 left common iliac artery
17. 下腔静脉 inferior vena cava
18. 竖脊肌 erector spinae
19. 升结肠 ascending colon
20. 右输尿管 right ureter
21. 肠系膜下动脉 inferior mesenteric artery
22. 肠系膜上静脉 superior mesenteric vein
23. 肠系膜 mesentery
24. 肠系膜下静脉 inferior mesenteric vein
25. 右卵巢静脉 right ovarian vein
26. 肠系膜上动脉 superior mesenteric artery

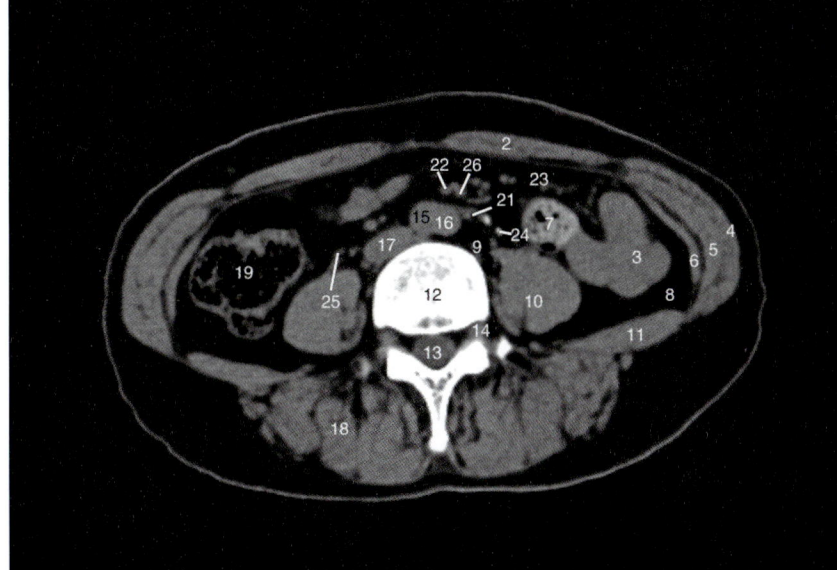

B. CT 平扫图像

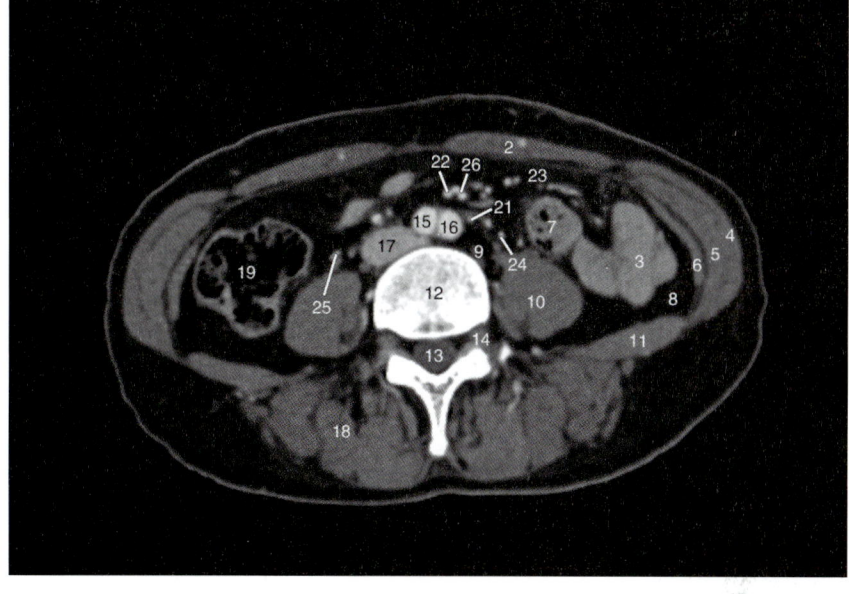

C. CT 增强图像

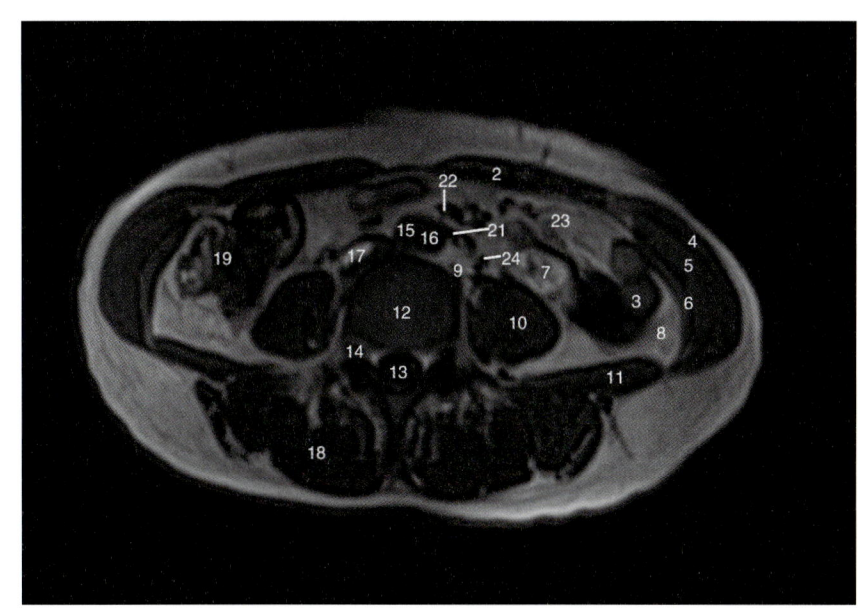

D. MR T1WI

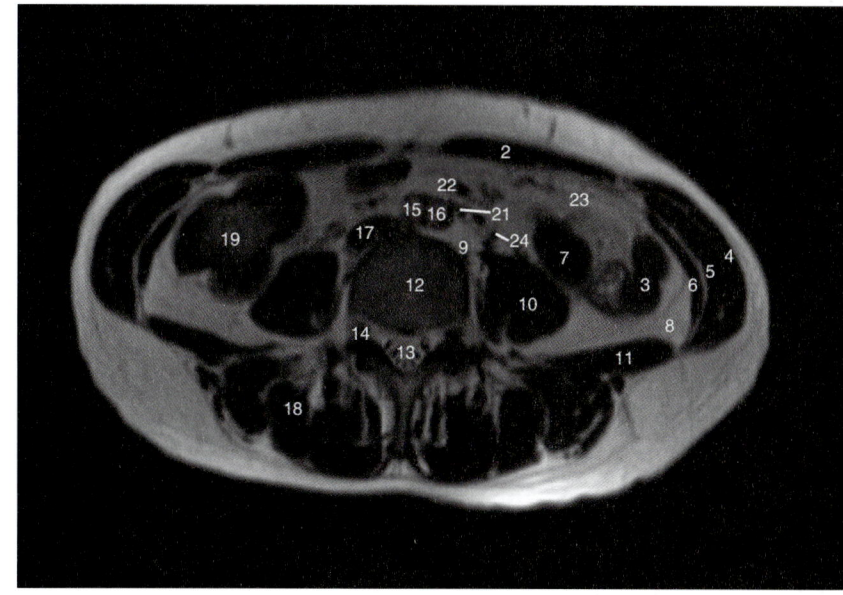

E. MR T2WI

关键结构：左、右髂总动脉，第 4 腰椎椎体。

此断面经第 4 腰椎椎体下份。

腹主动脉在第 3 腰椎椎体平面以下靠脊柱左前方下行，于第 3 腰椎至 L5~S1 椎间盘前方分为左、右髂总动脉。右髂总动脉沿下腔静脉前方及右髂总静脉前内侧下行，左髂总动脉走行于左髂总静脉的外侧，二者均在骶髂关节水平处分为髂内、髂外动脉，左髂总动脉长度大于右髂总动脉长度，壁厚度基本相同，约为 1 mm。此外还有 1 支骶正中动脉起自于腹主动脉末端背侧[111]。骶正中动脉栓塞在骶骨肿瘤术前栓塞治疗中具有重要意义：尽管骶骨肿瘤的发病率很低，但其发病隐匿，症状不明显，发现时瘤体往往巨大，且对放化疗敏感者不多；而且该部位肿瘤具有位置深、不易暴露、局部血液循环丰富等特点，常因术中出血凶猛致手术视野不清。造成肿瘤切除不完全，易复发。因此对于骶骨肿瘤，术前栓塞除常规髂内动脉栓塞外，应考虑到有骶正中动脉等多支供血的特点，尽量栓塞彻底以减少术中出血[112]。

腹部连续横断层 109（FH.9750）

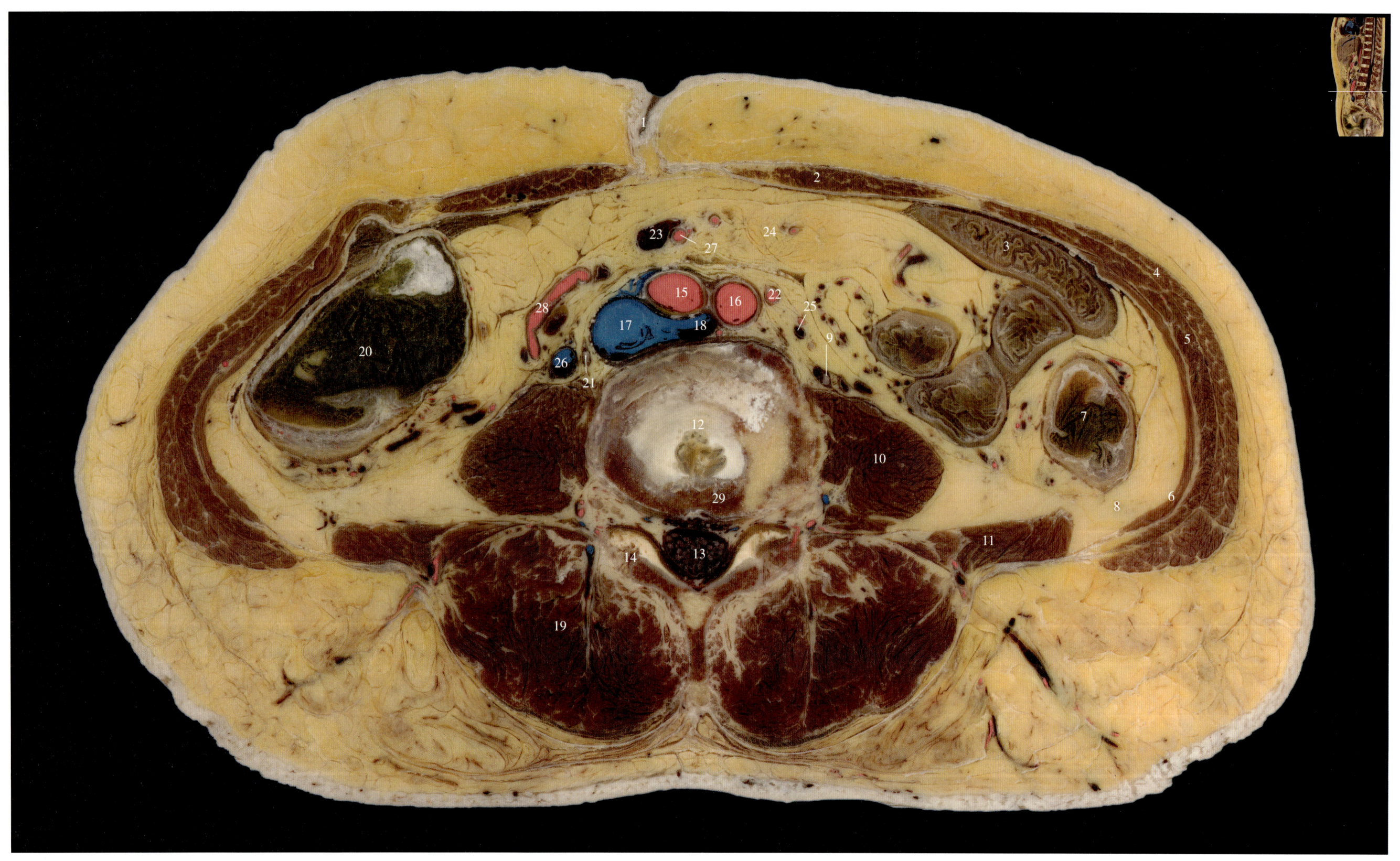

A. 断层标本图像

1. 脐 umbilicus
2. 腹直肌 rectus abdominis
3. 空肠 jejunum
4. 腹外斜肌 obliquus externus abdominis
5. 腹内斜肌 obliquus internus abdominis
6. 腹横肌 transverses abdominis
7. 降结肠 descending colon
8. 腹膜外脂肪 extraperitoneal fat
9. 左输尿管 left ureter
10. 腰大肌 psoas major
11. 腰方肌 quadratus lumborum
12. L4-5 椎间盘 L4-5 intervertebral disc
13. 马尾 cauda equina
14. 关节突关节 zygapophysial joint
15. 右髂总动脉 right common iliac artery
16. 左髂总动脉 left common iliac artery
17. 右髂总静脉 right common iliac vein
18. 左髂总静脉 left common iliac vein
19. 竖脊肌 erector spinae
20. 升结肠 ascending colon
21. 右输尿管 right ureter
22. 肠系膜下动脉 inferior mesenteric artery
23. 肠系膜上静脉 superior mesenteric vein
24. 肠系膜 mesentery
25. 肠系膜下静脉 inferior mesenteric vein
26. 右卵巢静脉 right ovarian vein
27. 肠系膜上动脉 superior mesenteric artery
28. 结肠动脉 colic artery
29. 第 4 腰椎椎体 body of 4th lumbar vertebra

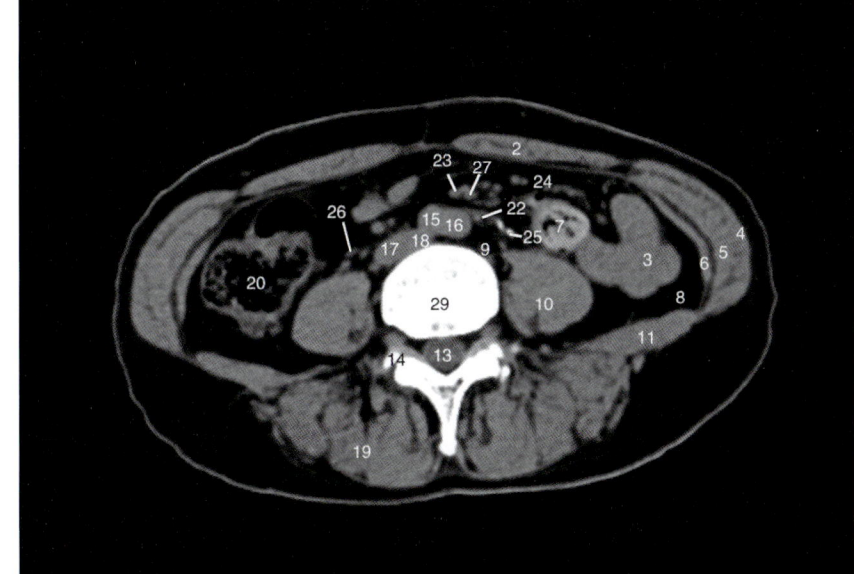

B. CT 平扫图像

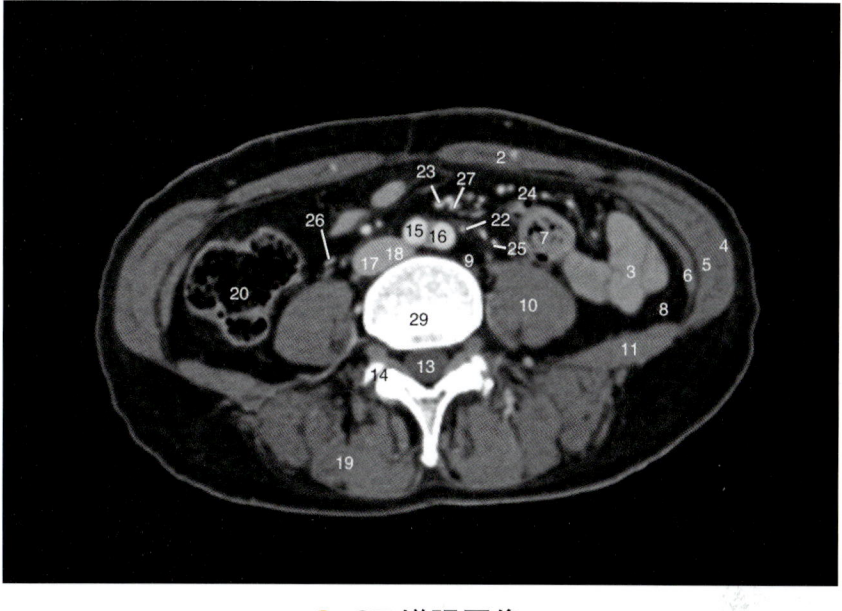

C. CT 增强图像

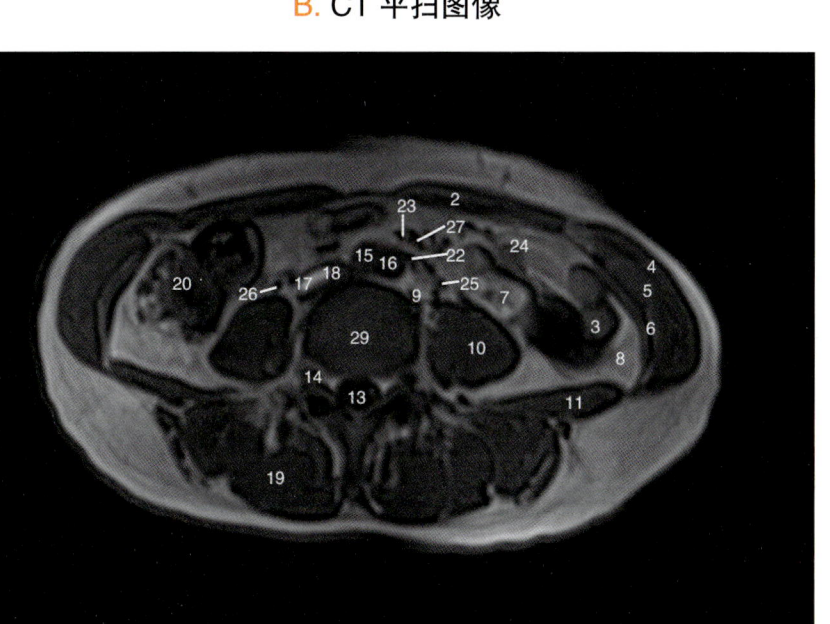

D. MR T1WI

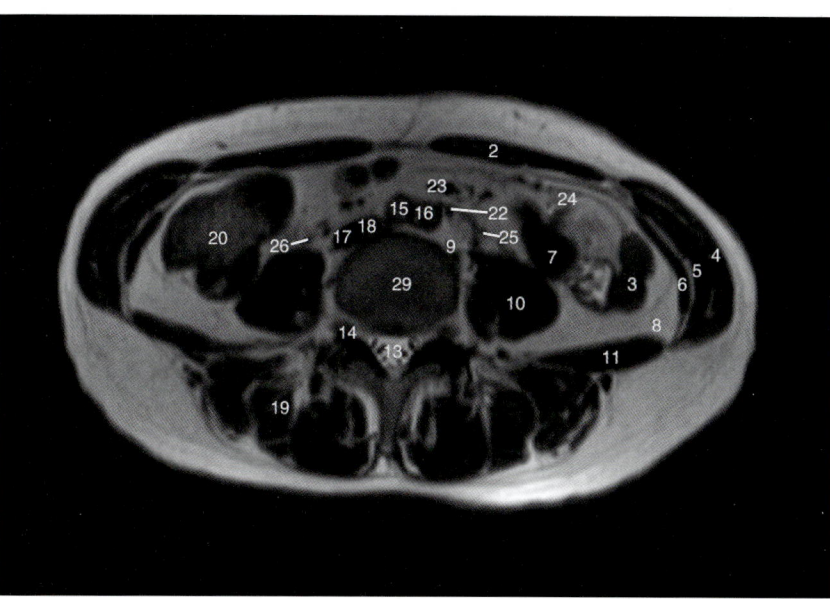

E. MR T2WI

关键结构：肠系膜，肠系膜窦。

此断面经 L4-5 椎间盘。

肠系膜是将空肠和回肠系于腹后壁的双层腹膜，整体形状如折扇。其附着于腹后壁的部分称肠系膜根，从第 2 腰椎椎体左侧起，斜向右下方，依次跨过十二指肠水平部、腹主动脉、下腔静脉、右侧输尿管和腰大肌，至右侧骶髂关节前方。肠系膜根长约为 15 cm，而小肠系膜缘长达 5~7 m，故小肠系膜形成许多皱褶。由肠系膜根至小肠系膜缘的距离以小肠系膜中部最长，可达 20 cm，而系膜上、下两端较短。小肠系膜内有肠系膜上动、静脉主干及其分支、淋巴管、淋巴结、神经和脂肪组织。右肠系膜窦是位于肠系膜根右侧与升结肠左侧壁腹膜之间的三角形间隙，上界是横结肠及其系膜右侧半，后界为腹后壁壁腹膜。右肠系膜窦下方有回肠末端相隔，周围相对封闭，故间隙内的炎性渗出物常积存于局部，不能向下直接扩散到盆腔。左肠系膜窦为位于肠系膜根左侧与升结肠右侧壁腹膜之间的斜方形间隙，上界是横结肠及其系膜左侧半，下界是乙状结肠及其系膜，后界为腹后壁壁腹膜。左肠系膜窦向下与腹膜腔盆部相通，窦内感染时易向下蔓延入盆腔[26]。在发生下消化道穿孔的情况时，肠系膜窦是常见的积气和积液部位。研究表明上消化道和下消化道穿孔时，肠系膜窦的积气积液存在明显统计学差异，故对诊断腹腔穿孔部位有一定的指导意义[113]。

腹部连续横断层 110（FH.9730）

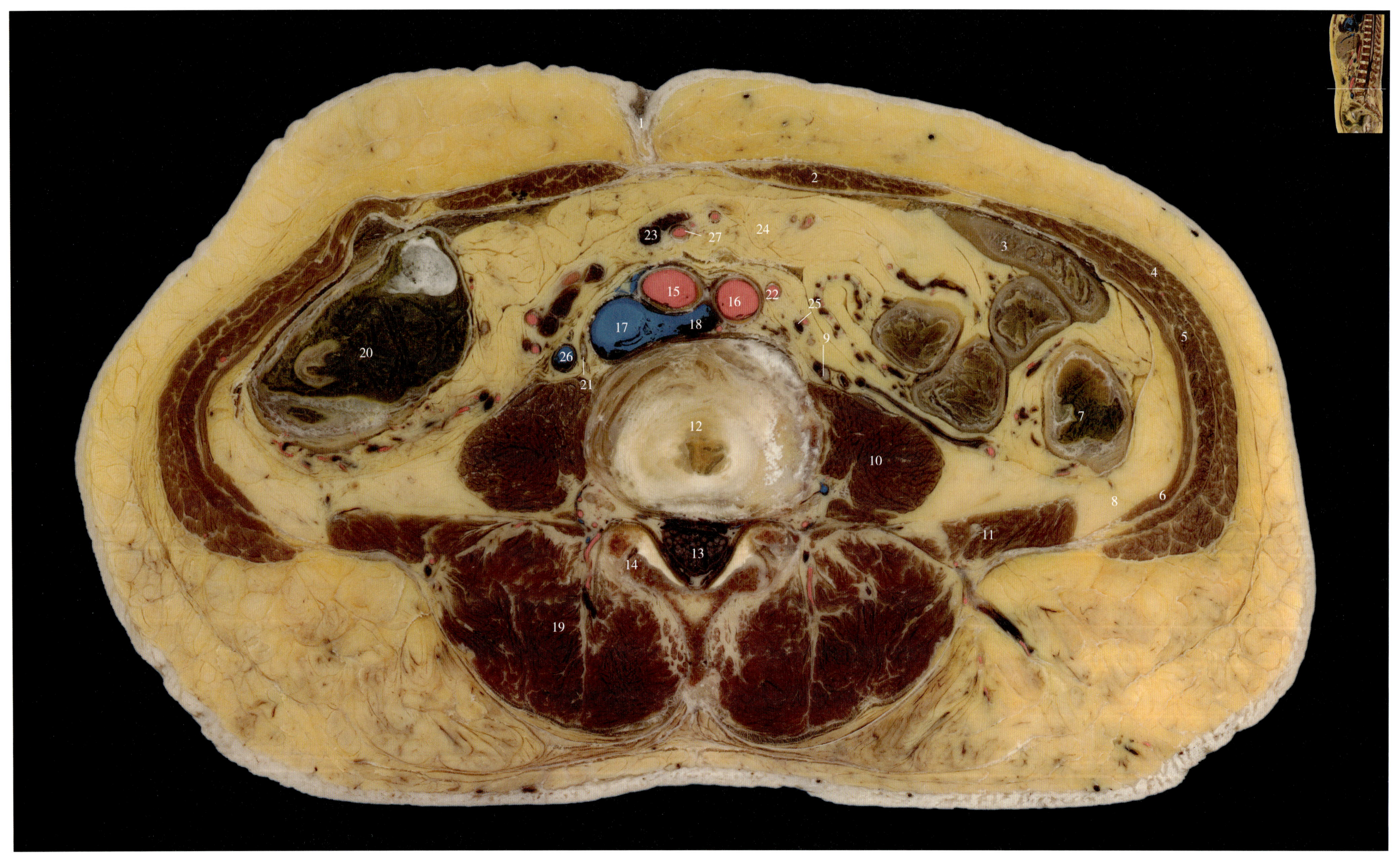

A. 断层标本图像

1. 脐 umbilicus
2. 腹直肌 rectus abdominis
3. 空肠 jejunum
4. 腹外斜肌 obliquus externus abdominis
5. 腹内斜肌 obliquus internus abdominis
6. 腹横肌 transverses abdominis
7. 降结肠 descending colon
8. 腹膜外脂肪 extraperitoneal fat
9. 左输尿管 left ureter
10. 腰大肌 psoas major
11. 腰方肌 quadratus lumborum
12. L4-5 椎间盘 L4-5 intervertebral disc
13. 马尾 cauda equina
14. 关节突关节 zygapophysial joint
15. 右髂总动脉 right common iliac artery
16. 左髂总动脉 left common iliac artery
17. 右髂总静脉 right common iliac vein
18. 左髂总静脉 left common iliac vein
19. 竖脊肌 erector spinae
20. 升结肠 ascending colon
21. 右输尿管 right ureter
22. 肠系膜下动脉 inferior mesenteric artery
23. 肠系膜上静脉 superior mesenteric vein
24. 肠系膜 mesentery
25. 肠系膜下静脉 inferior mesenteric vein
26. 右卵巢静脉 right ovarian vein
27. 肠系膜上动脉 superior mesenteric artery
28. 第 4 腰椎椎体 body of 4th lumbar vertebra

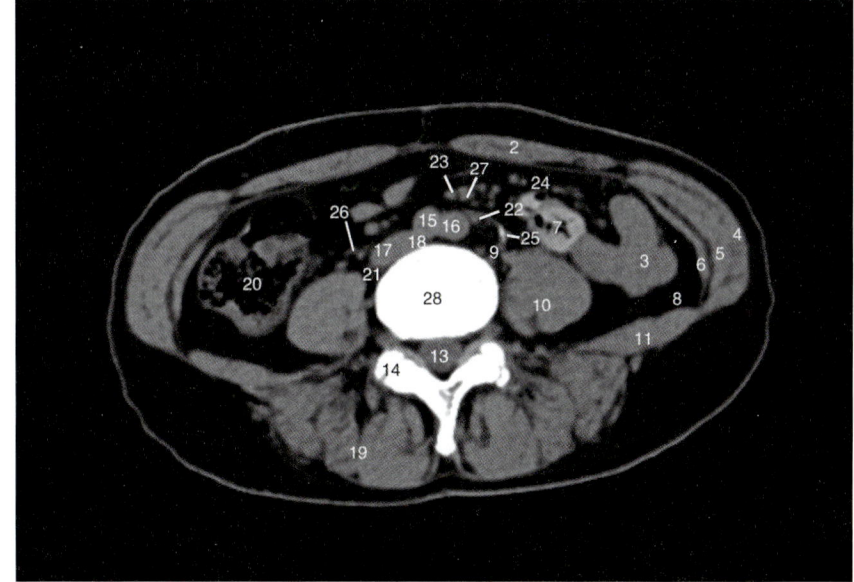

B. CT 平扫图像

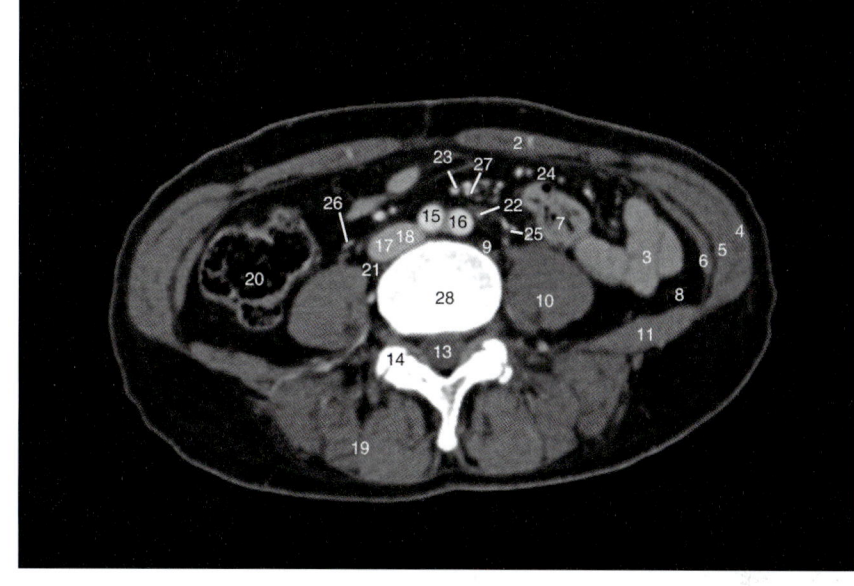

C. CT 增强图像

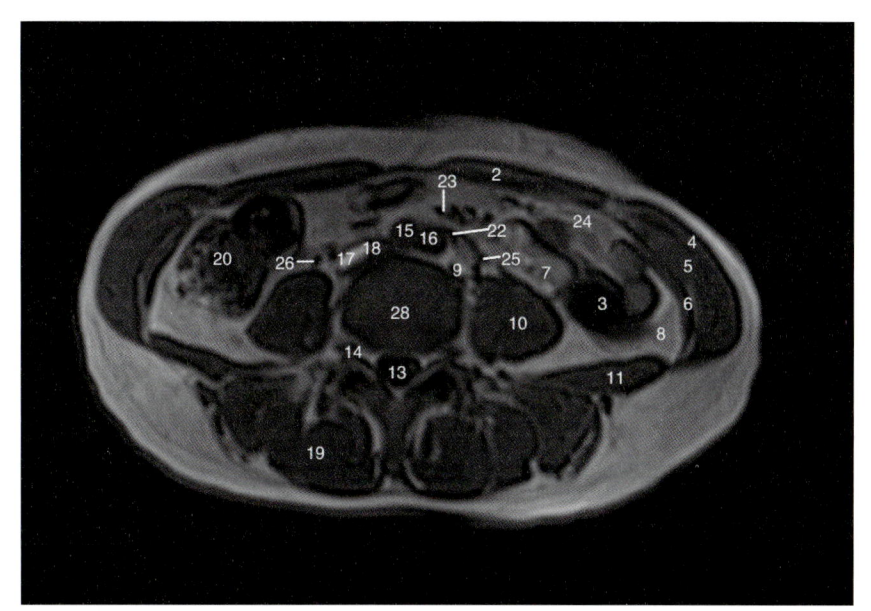

D. MR T1WI

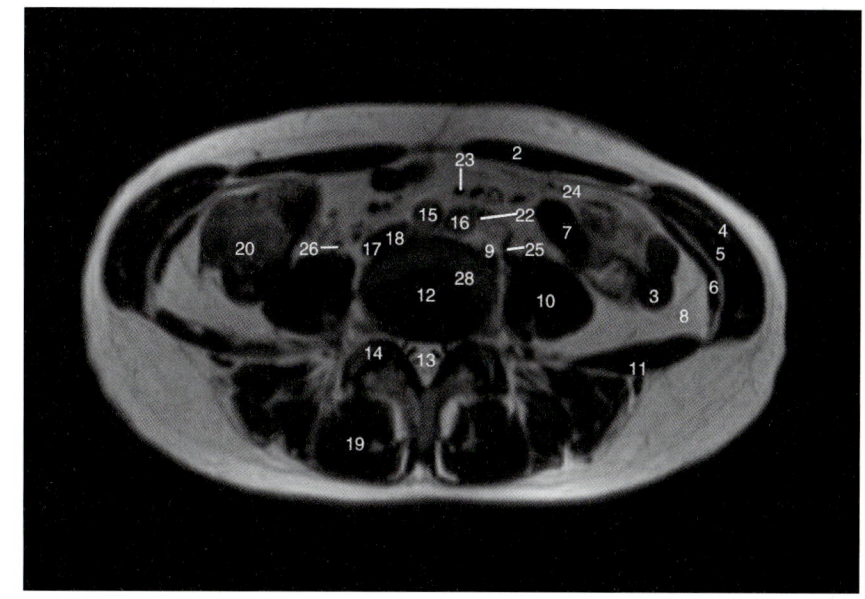

E. MR T2WI

关键结构：脐，L4-5 椎间盘，左、右髂总动脉。

此断面经 L4-5 椎间盘。

脐是一个纤维瘢痕，位于腹白线中点的稍下方，其表面覆盖着皮区。脐由皮肤、纤维层（肝圆韧带、脐正中韧带和两个脐内侧韧带融合的区域）、腹横筋膜、脐尿管及周围的筋膜和腹膜组成。在胎儿时期，脐部有脐血管、脐尿管、卵黄囊通过，出生几天后，卵黄囊闭锁，而血管和脐尿管的遗迹仍连于其深面。胎儿时期遗留下来的脐静脉形成肝圆韧带。闭锁的脐动脉形成脐内侧韧带，包裹在同名的腹膜皱襞内。部分闭锁的脐尿管遗迹以脐正中韧带的形式存在。先天性和获得性的脐疝很常见，大部分儿童脐疝可自然闭合，不需要手术修复。脐是腹腔镜探查腹膜腔最常见的位置[62]。

腰椎间盘突出症是因为腰椎间盘各部分（髓核、纤维环及软骨板），尤其是髓核，发生不同程度的退行性改变后，在外力因素的作用下，椎间盘的纤维环破裂，髓核组织从破裂之处突出（或脱出）于后方或椎管内，导致相邻脊神经根遭受刺激或压迫，从而产生腰腿部疼痛等临床症状。腰椎间盘突出症以 L4-5 椎间盘发病率最高。MRI 表现为腰椎间盘 T2WI 信号减低，腰椎间盘向后突出，严重者可见髓核脱出、压迫硬膜囊、椎管有效矢状径变窄、腰髓及马尾神经受压等。

腹部连续横断层 111（FH.9710）

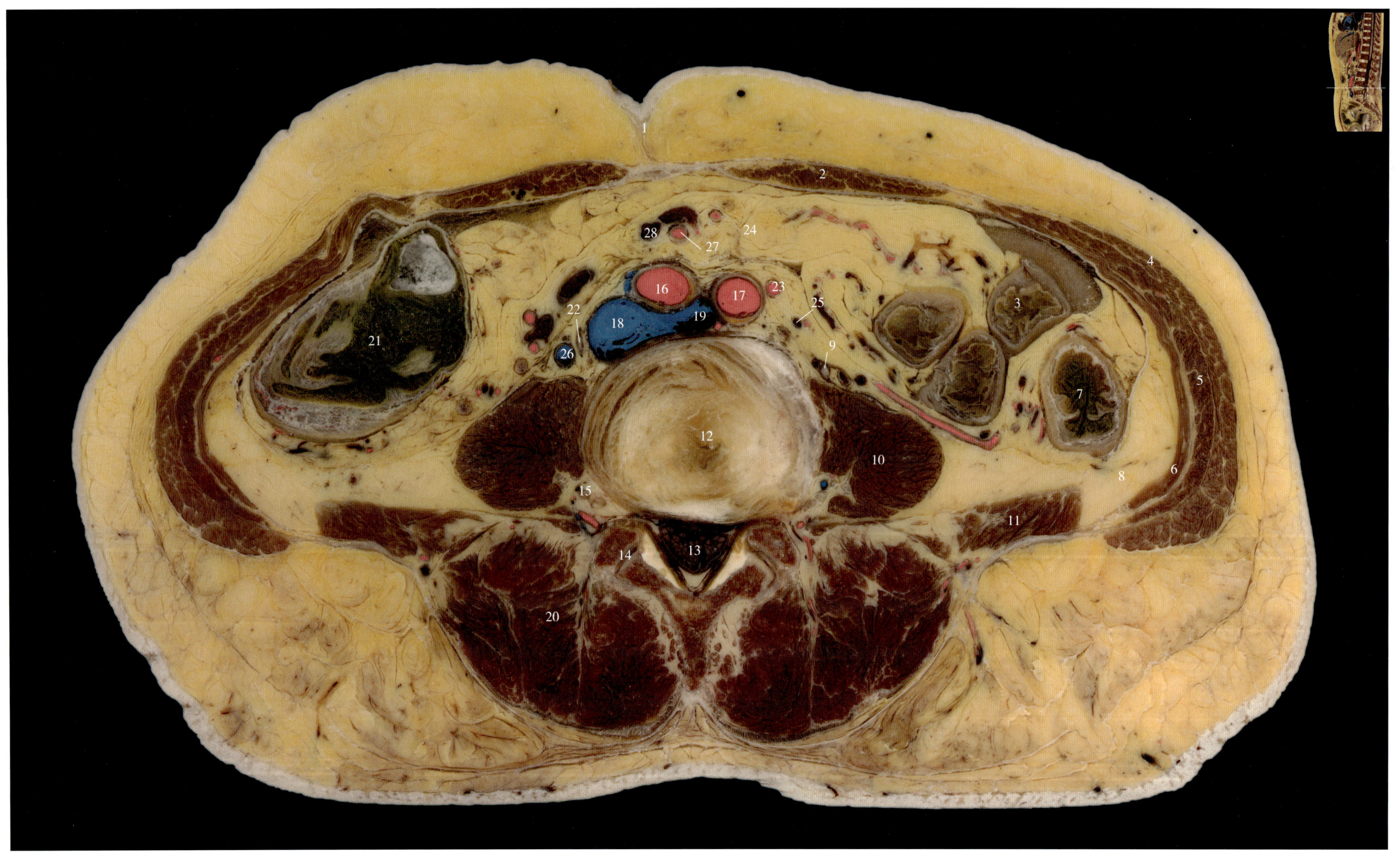

A. 断层标本图像

1. 脐 umbilicus
2. 腹直肌 rectus abdominis
3. 空肠 jejunum
4. 腹外斜肌 obliquus externus abdominis
5. 腹内斜肌 obliquus internus abdominis
6. 腹横肌 transverses abdominis
7. 乙状结肠 sigmoid colon
8. 腹膜外脂肪 extraperitoneal fat
9. 左输尿管 left ureter
10. 腰大肌 psoas major
11. 腰方肌 quadratus lumborum
12. L4-5 椎间盘 L4-5 intervertebral disc
13. 马尾 cauda equina
14. 关节突关节 zygapophysial joint
15. 第 4 腰神经 4th lumbar nerve
16. 右髂总动脉 right common iliac artery
17. 左髂总动脉 left common iliac artery
18. 右髂总静脉 right common iliac vein
19. 左髂总静脉 left common iliac vein
20. 竖脊肌 erector spinae
21. 升结肠 ascending colon
22. 右输尿管 right ureter
23. 肠系膜下动脉 inferior mesenteric artery
24. 肠系膜 mesentery
25. 肠系膜下静脉 inferior mesenteric vein
26. 右卵巢静脉 right ovarian vein
27. 肠系膜上动脉 superior mesenteric artery
28. 肠系膜上静脉 superior mesenteric vein

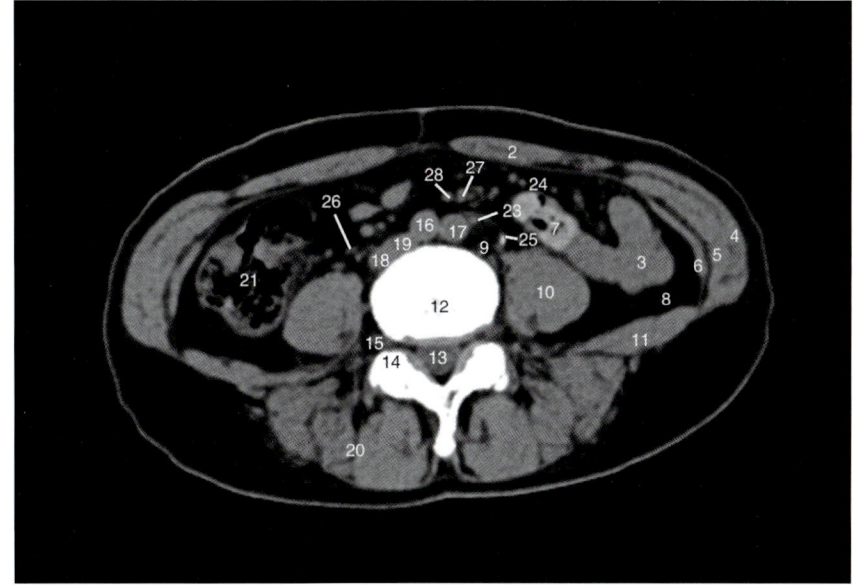

B. CT 平扫图像

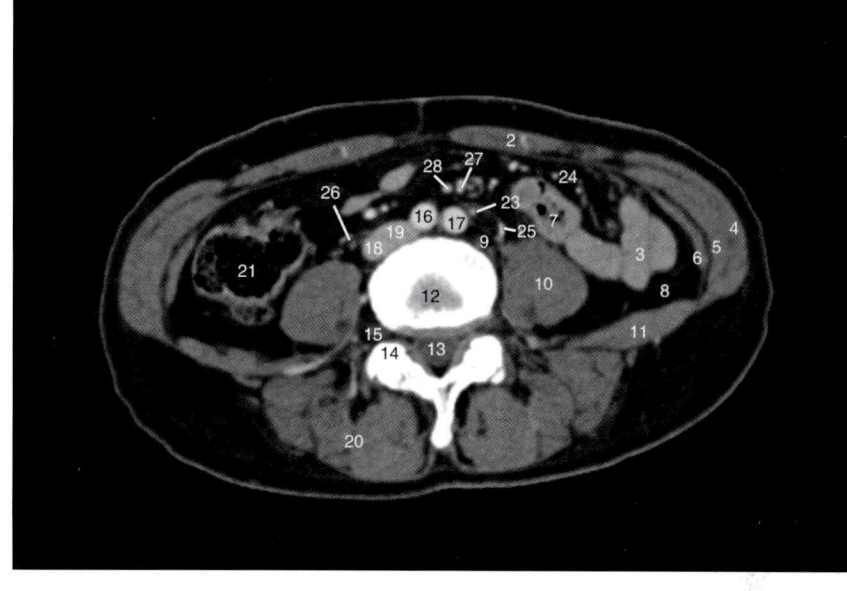

C. CT 增强图像

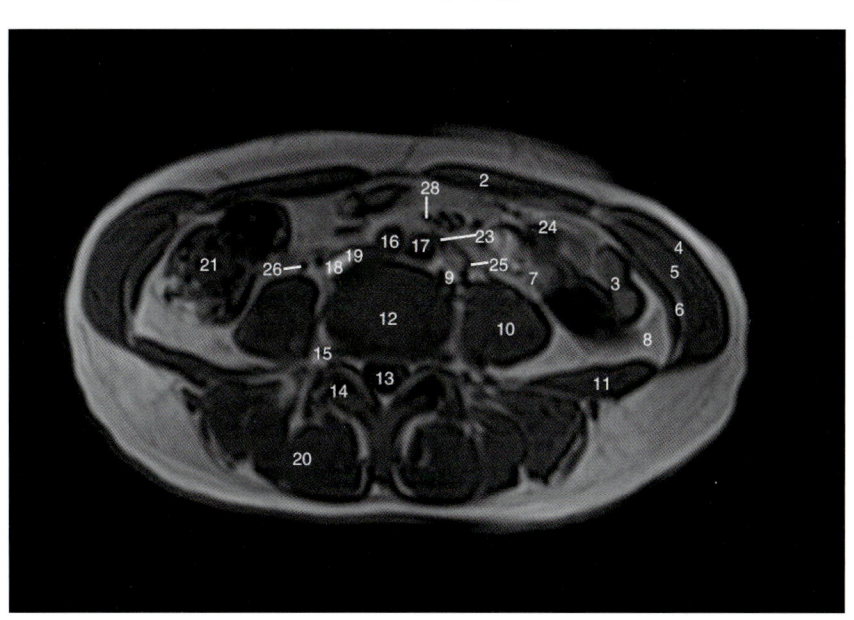

D. MR T1WI

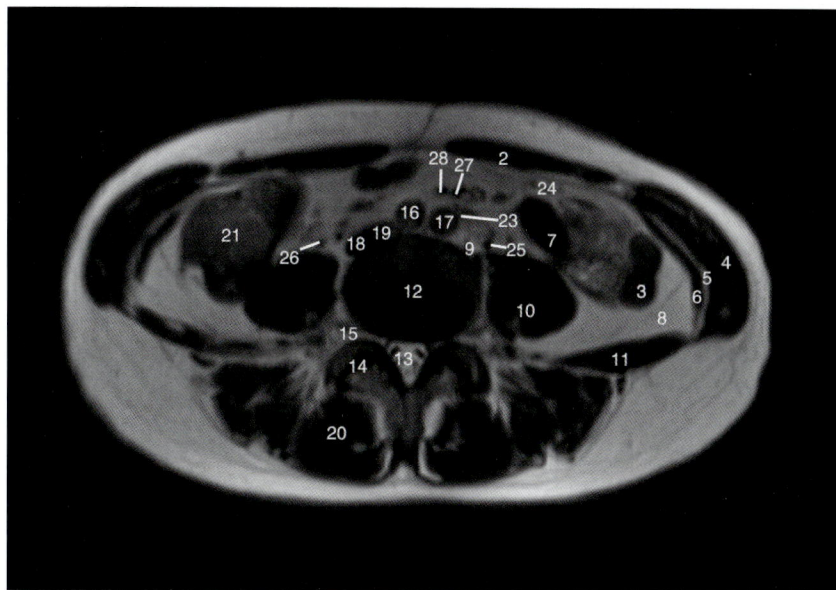

E. MR T2WI

关键结构：左、右髂总静脉。

此断面经 L4-5 椎间盘。

髂总静脉由髂外静脉和髂内静脉在骶髂关节前方组成，左髂总静脉起初与同名动脉相伴行并位于其内侧，后向正中线上升至右髂总动脉的后方，与右髂总静脉相结合；右髂总静脉起初在同名动脉的后方，垂直上行，至第 5 腰椎椎体的右前方，右髂总动脉的外侧，与左髂总静脉汇合成下腔静脉。

由于左髂总静脉被右髂总动脉越过而明显受压所产生的堵塞症状，有人称之为左髂总静脉压迫综合征。髂总静脉压迫不仅造成静脉回流障碍和下肢静脉高压，也是下肢静脉瓣膜功能不全和浅静脉曲张的原因之一，同时是继发髂-股静脉血栓的重要潜在因素。研究发现受压处静脉腔内常有异常结构存在，可促使静脉血栓形成并引起管腔狭窄和堵塞。髂总静脉还接收骶腰静脉和骶正中静脉（左髂总静脉）[26]。下肢顺行和/或股静脉插管造影是髂总静脉受压综合征诊断的金标准。血管彩超和 CTA 可显示髂静脉的管腔及其内部血流，并了解其与右侧髂总动脉、腰骶椎之间的关系，有利于诊断髂静脉压迫综合征[114]。

腹部连续横断层 112 (FH.9690)

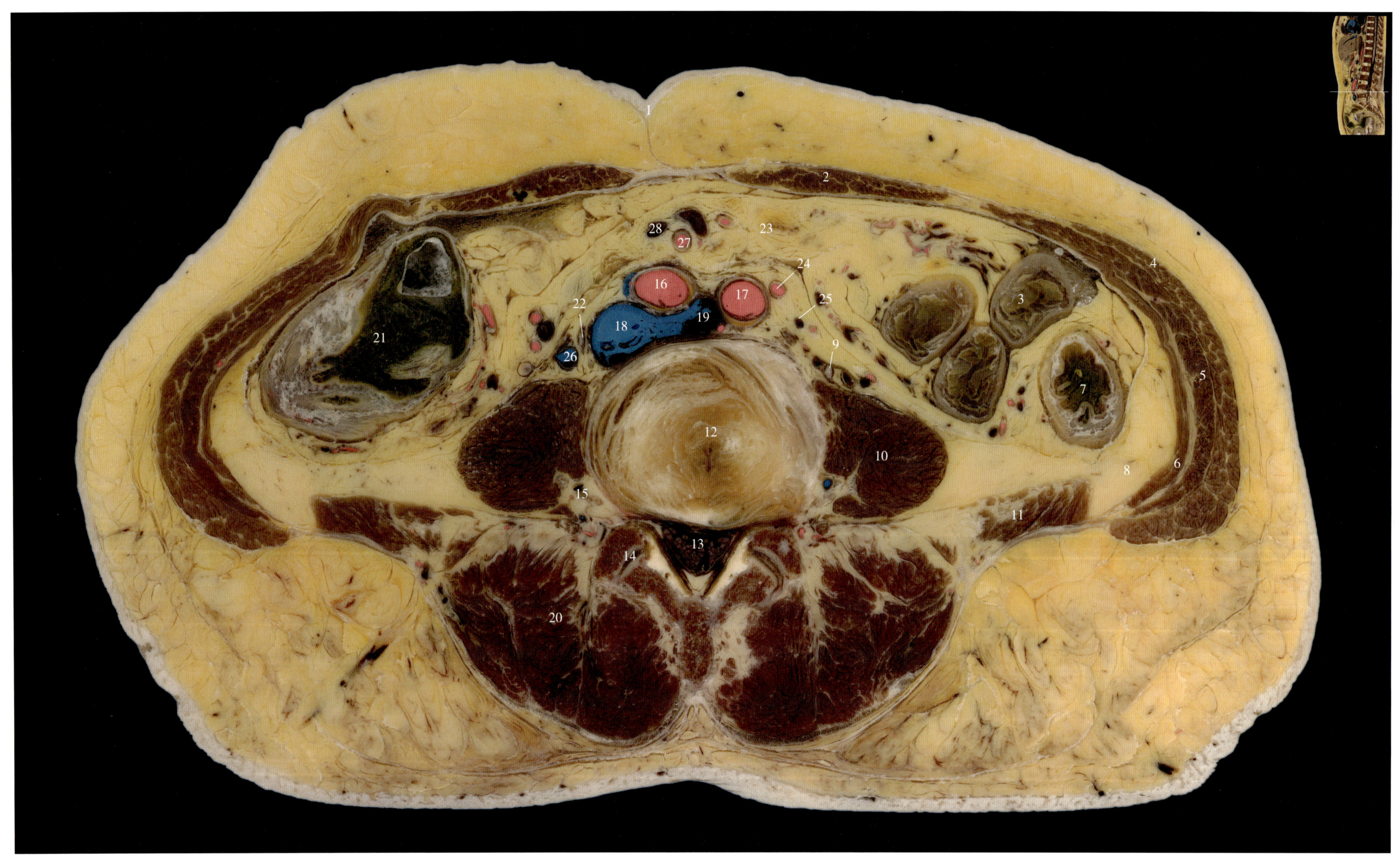

A. 断层标本图像

1. 脐 umbilicus
2. 腹直肌 rectus abdominis
3. 空肠 jejunum
4. 腹外斜肌 obliquus externus abdominis
5. 腹内斜肌 obliquus internus abdominis
6. 腹横肌 transverses abdominis
7. 乙状结肠 sigmoid colon
8. 腹膜外脂肪 extraperitoneal fat
9. 左输尿管 left ureter
10. 腰大肌 psoas major
11. 腰方肌 quadratus lumborum
12. L4-5 椎间盘 L4-5 intervertebral disc
13. 马尾 cauda equina
14. 关节突关节 zygapophysial joint
15. 第 4 腰神经 4th lumbar nerve
16. 右髂总动脉 right common iliac artery
17. 左髂总动脉 left common iliac artery
18. 右髂总静脉 right common iliac vein
19. 左髂总静脉 left common iliac vein
20. 竖脊肌 erector spinae
21. 升结肠 ascending colon
22. 右输尿管 right ureter
23. 肠系膜 mesentery
24. 肠系膜下动脉 inferior mesenteric artery
25. 肠系膜下静脉 inferior mesenteric vein
26. 右卵巢静脉 right ovarian vein
27. 肠系膜上动脉 superior mesenteric artery
28. 肠系膜上静脉 superior mesenteric vein

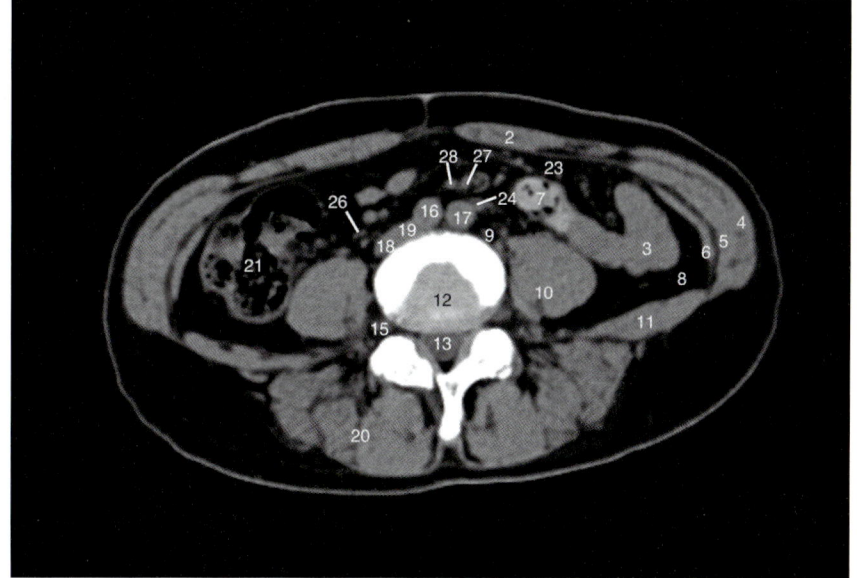

B. CT 平扫图像

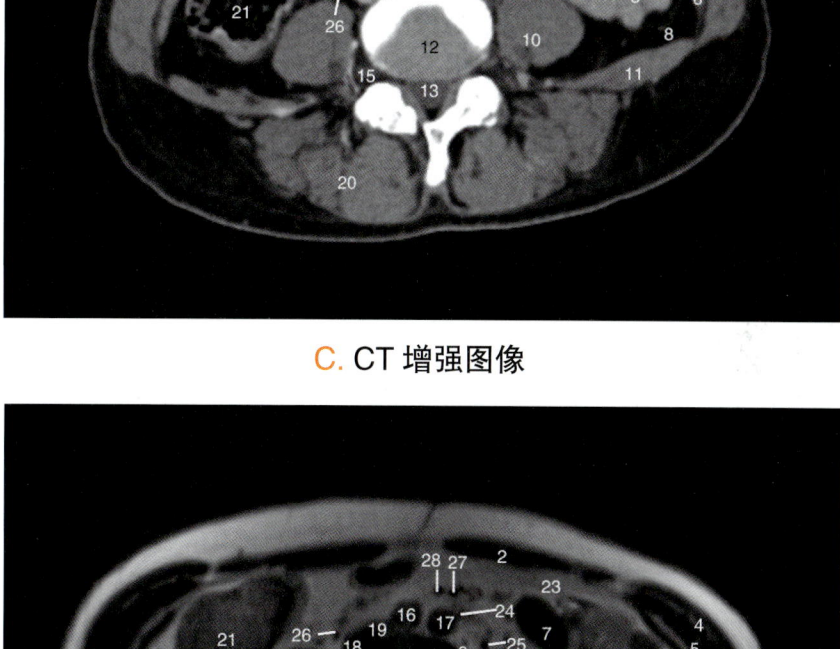

C. CT 增强图像

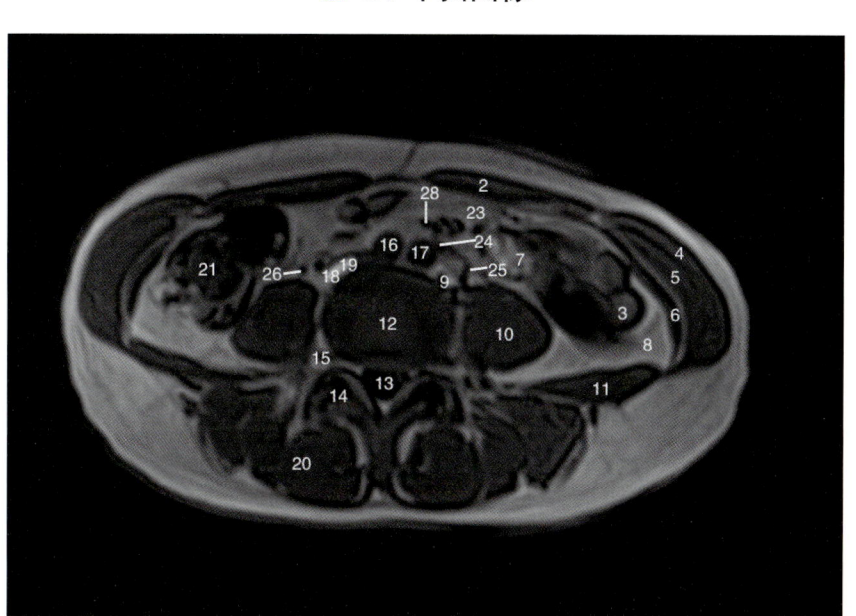

D. MR T1WI

E. MR T2WI

关键结构：升结肠，乙状结肠，结肠系膜。

此断面经 L4-5 椎间盘。

升结肠是盲肠的延续，沿腹腔右外侧区上行，至肝右叶下方转向左前下方移行为横结肠，所形成的弯曲称结肠右曲，又称肝曲。升结肠长 12~20 cm，较盲肠狭窄，一般为腹膜间位，其后面借疏松结缔组织与腹后壁相贴，因此，有时升结肠病变可累及腹膜后隙。少数人升结肠为腹膜内位，有系膜，活动度较大。升结肠的内侧为右肠系膜窦及回肠袢，外侧与腹壁间形成右结肠旁沟。此沟上通肝肾隐窝，下通右髂窝和盆腔，故膈下脓肿可经此沟流入右髂窝和盆腔，阑尾化脓时可向上蔓延至肝下。乙状结肠自左髂嵴起自降结肠至第 3 骶椎续于直肠，呈乙状弯曲，横过左侧髂腰肌、髂外血管、睾丸（卵巢）血管及输尿管前方降入盆腔。乙状结肠有较长的系膜，活动度较大，可入盆腔，也可移至右下腹遮盖回盲部，增加了阑尾切除术的难度。乙状结肠是结肠癌最常见的发病部位。患者早期多无症状，发现时多为晚期。肠道内对比剂充盈后，CT 可显示腔内软组织肿块影、不规则的管壁增厚和狭窄。肿瘤与周围脂肪界限不清，提示癌肿向腔外侵犯，增强扫描癌肿显示更清楚，尤其是对肠壁外浸润的评估。CT 仿真内镜（CTVE）可检出结肠内 0.5 cm 以上的隆起息肉，对腔内肿块或管腔狭窄的发现率极高，对显示狭窄后的情况有独到之处。癌肿在 T1WI 上信号低于结肠壁，T2WI 信号增高。此外，MRI 对癌肿侵犯深度及局部淋巴结转移的诊断价值更高。结肠癌术后复发时，T2WI 上信号高于手术瘢痕组织[115]。

腹部连续横断层 113（FH.9670）

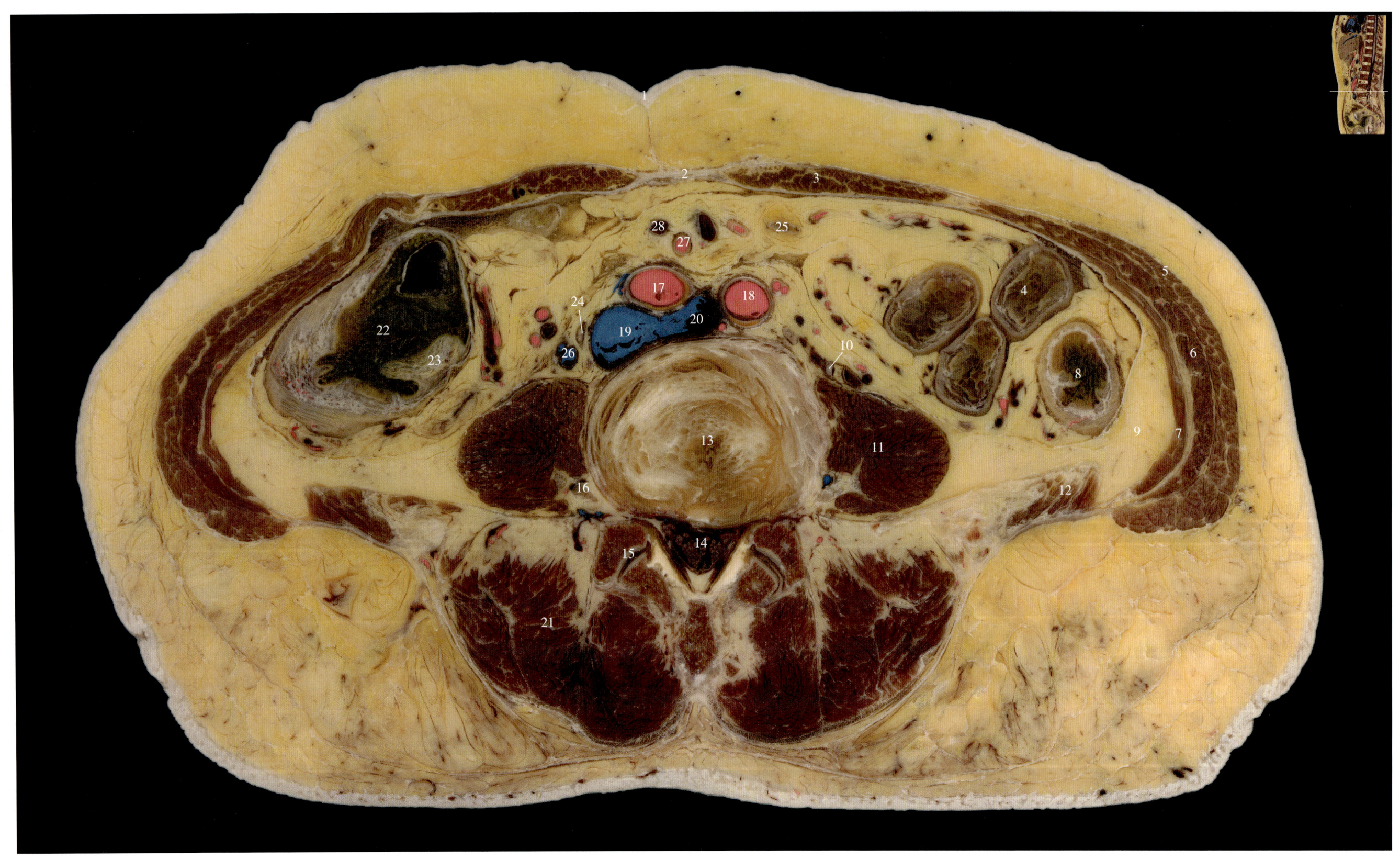

A. 断层标本图像

1. 脐 umbilicus
2. 白线 linea alba
3. 腹直肌 rectus abdominis
4. 空肠 jejunum
5. 腹外斜肌 obliquus externus abdominis
6. 腹内斜肌 obliquus internus abdominis
7. 腹横肌 transverses abdominis
8. 乙状结肠 sigmoid colon
9. 腹膜外脂肪 extraperitoneal fat
10. 左输尿管 left ureter
11. 腰大肌 psoas major
12. 腰方肌 quadratus lumborum
13. L4-5 椎间盘 L4-5 intervertebral disc
14. 马尾 cauda equina
15. 关节突关节 zygapophysial joint
16. 第 4 腰神经 4th lumbar nerve
17. 右髂总动脉 right common iliac artery
18. 左髂总动脉 left common iliac artery
19. 右髂总静脉 right common iliac vein
20. 左髂总静脉 left common iliac vein
21. 竖脊肌 erector spinae
22. 升结肠 ascending colon
23. 回盲瓣 ileocecal valve
24. 右输尿管 right ureter
25. 肠系膜 mesentery
26. 右卵巢静脉 right ovarian vein
27. 肠系膜上动脉 superior mesenteric artery
28. 肠系膜上静脉 superior mesenteric vein

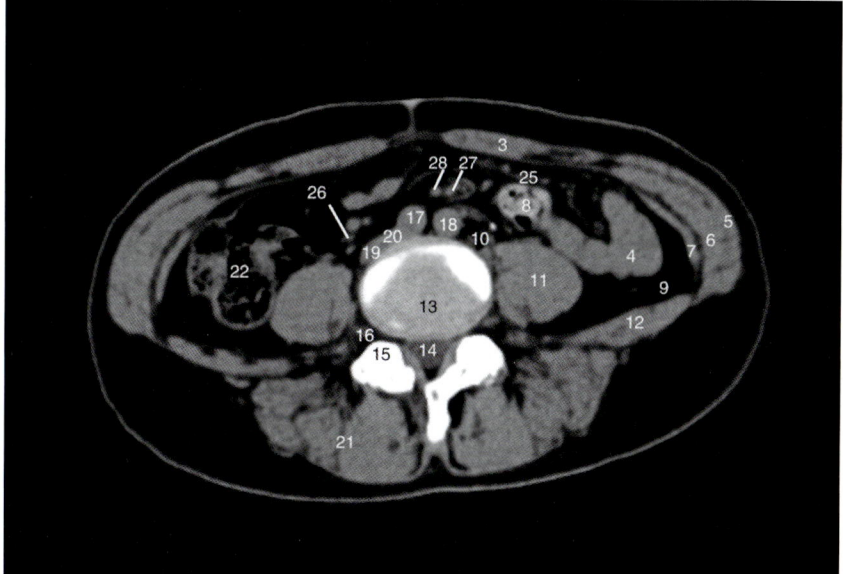

B. CT 平扫图像

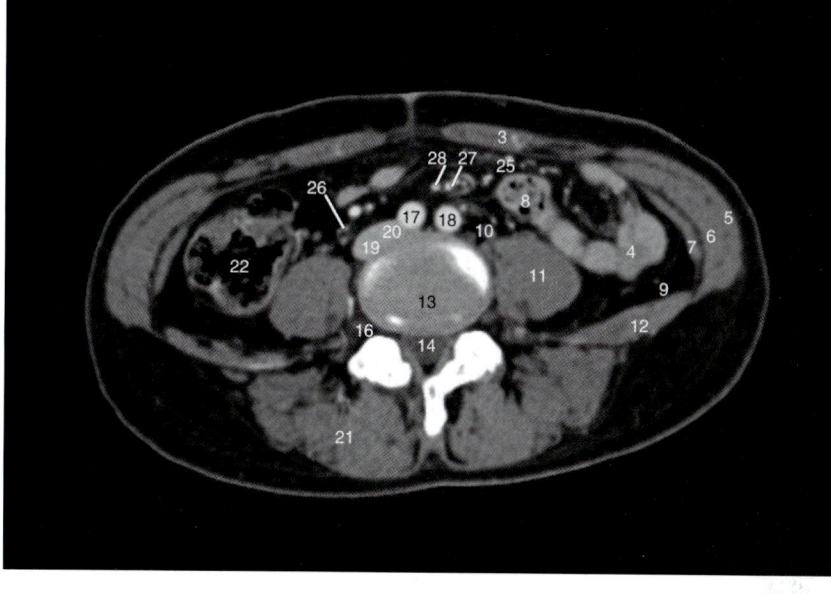

C. CT 增强图像

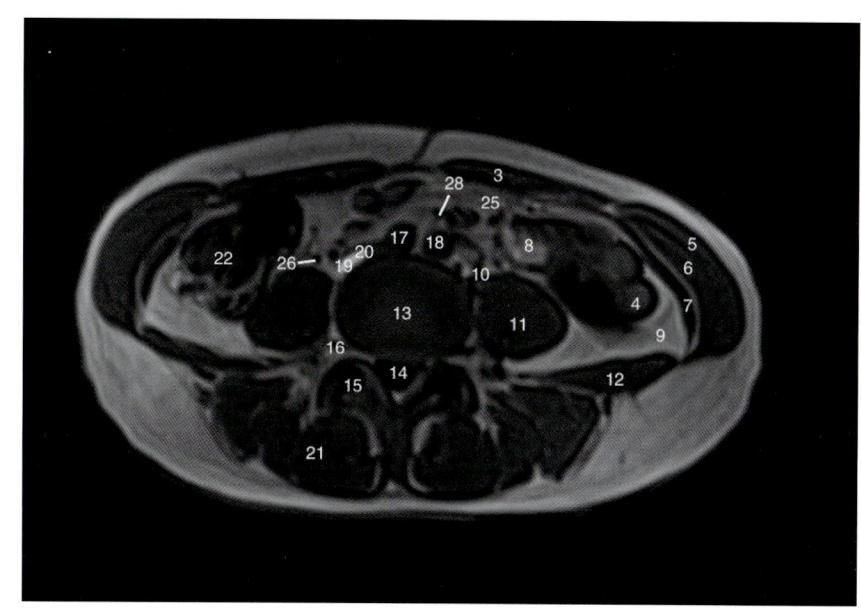

D. MR T1WI

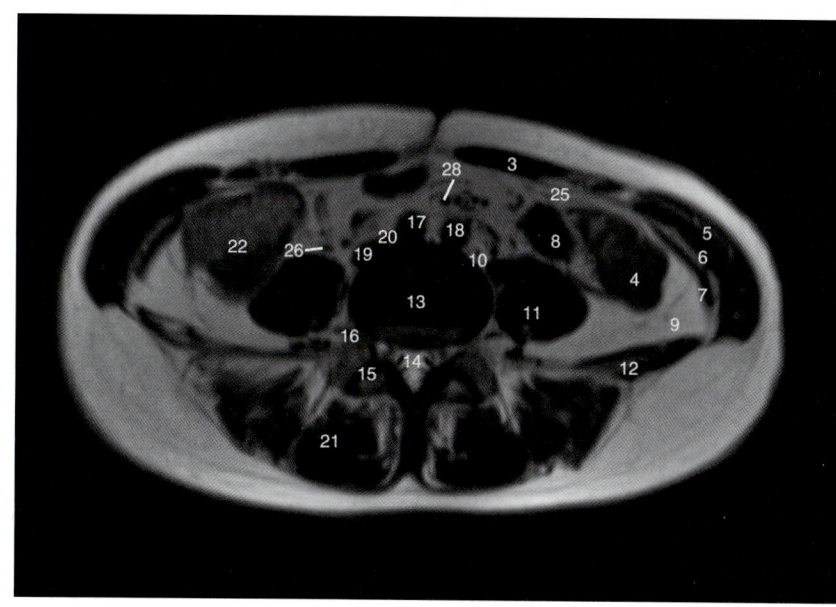

E. MR T2WI

关键结构：白线，腹直肌。

此断面经 L4-5 椎间盘。

白线亦称腹白线，由腹前外侧壁 3 层扁肌的腱膜在腹前正中线上互相交织而成，上宽下窄。脐以上白线宽 1~2 cm，较坚韧而血管较少，因此更明显。腹直肌为上宽下窄的带形多腹肌。肌纤维被 3~5 个腱划分隔。腱划与腹直肌鞘前层紧密相连、剥离困难，与腹直肌鞘后层不相连。手术时，切开腹直肌鞘前层后可向外侧牵拉腹直肌，暴露腹直肌鞘后层。但尽量不要向内侧牵拉，以防损伤胸神经前方三角形的小扁状肌—锥状肌[15]。在白线的中部有圆形的腱环，称脐环，其前面为皮肤，后面只有一层腹横筋膜，是腹壁的薄弱点之一，故易发生脐疝。在白线处（特别是脐以上），交错的腱膜纤维之间形成一些小孔或裂隙，如腹膜外组织甚至壁腹膜等由此突出，则形成白线疝。白线疝是发生在腹壁中线的腹外疝，绝大多数发生于脐与剑突之间（在二者中点的较多），故也称腹上疝。白线疝除肿块外多无显著症状，有时会误诊为腹壁脂肪瘤。实时超声显示疝囊内有肠管蠕动，CT 扫描显示腹壁肿物内有肠襻，内含造影剂或空气构形，也可以看到白线位置的缺损。手术是治愈白线疝的唯一有效方法。同时，由于腹白线处缺少血管、愈合差，故手术时不在此线上切口[116]。

腹部连续横断层 114（FH.9650）

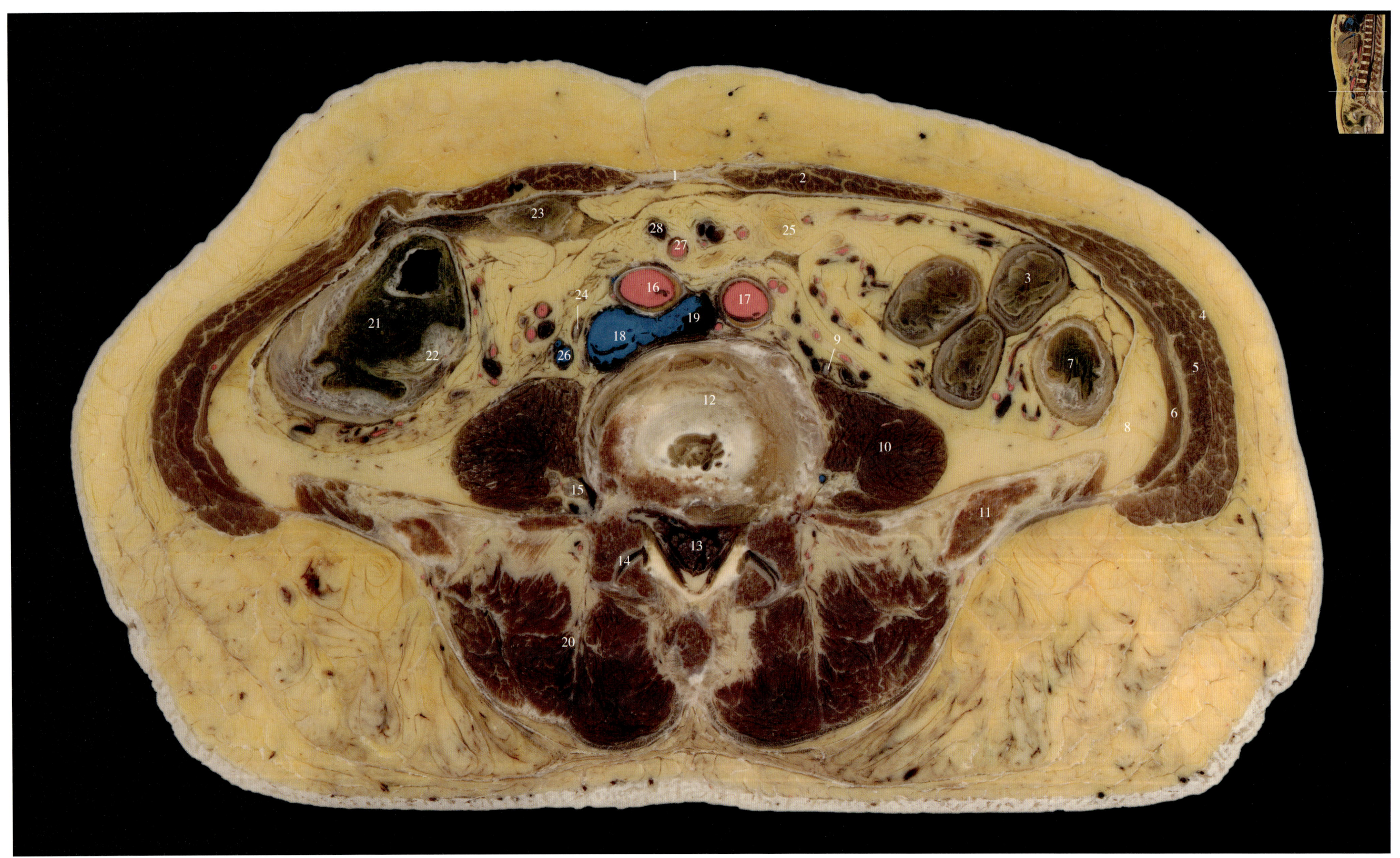

A. 断层标本图像

1. 白线 linea alba
2. 腹直肌 rectus abdominis
3. 空肠 jejunum
4. 腹外斜肌 obliquus externus abdominis
5. 腹内斜肌 obliquus internus abdominis
6. 腹横肌 transverses abdominis
7. 乙状结肠 sigmoid colon
8. 腹膜外脂肪 extraperitoneal fat
9. 左输尿管 left ureter
10. 腰大肌 psoas major
11. 髂嵴 iliac crest
12. L4-5 椎间盘 L4-5 intervertebral disc
13. 马尾 cauda equina
14. 关节突关节 zygapophysial joint
15. 第 4 腰神经 4th lumbar nerve
16. 右髂总动脉 right common iliac artery
17. 左髂总动脉 left common iliac artery
18. 右髂总静脉 right common iliac vein
19. 左髂总静脉 left common iliac vein
20. 竖脊肌 erector spinae
21. 升结肠 ascending colon
22. 回盲瓣 ileocecal valve
23. 回肠 ileum
24. 右输尿管 right ureter
25. 肠系膜 mesentery
26. 右卵巢静脉 right ovarian vein
27. 肠系膜上动脉 superior mesenteric artery
28. 肠系膜上静脉 superior mesenteric vein

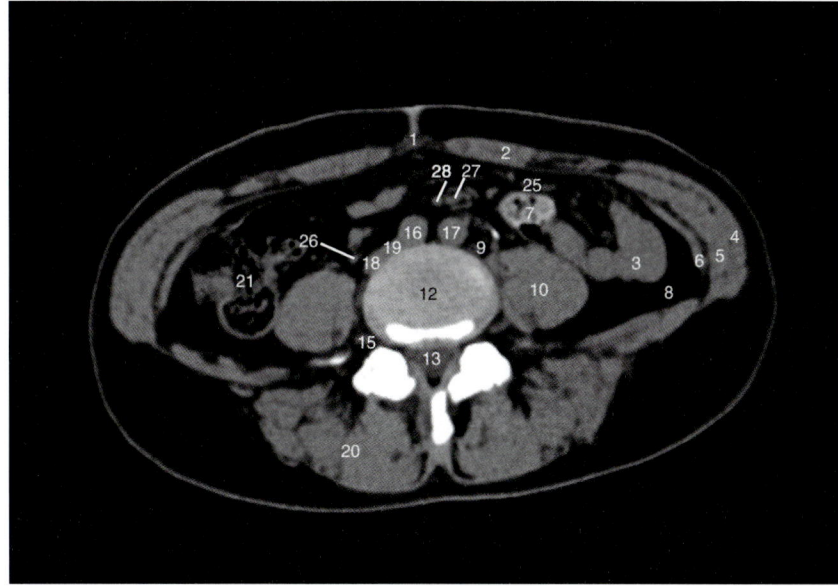

B. CT 平扫图像

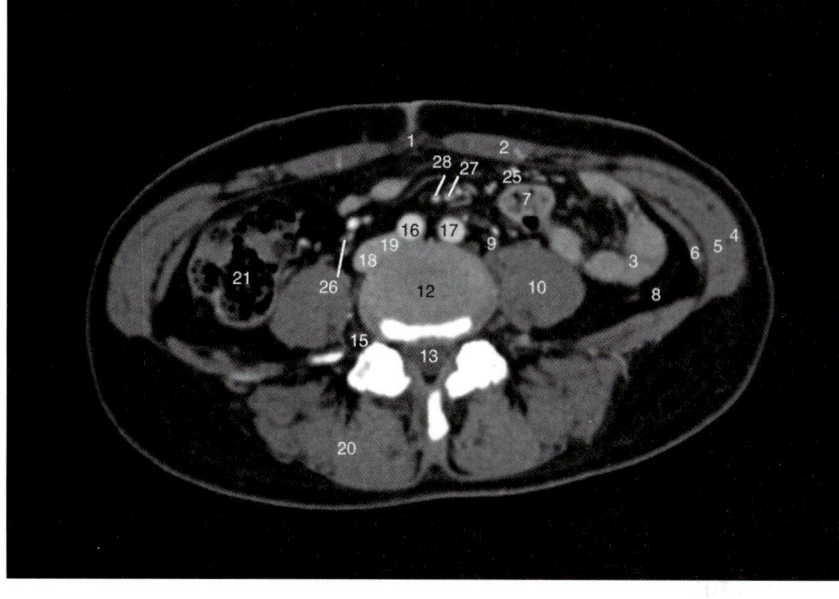

C. CT 增强图像

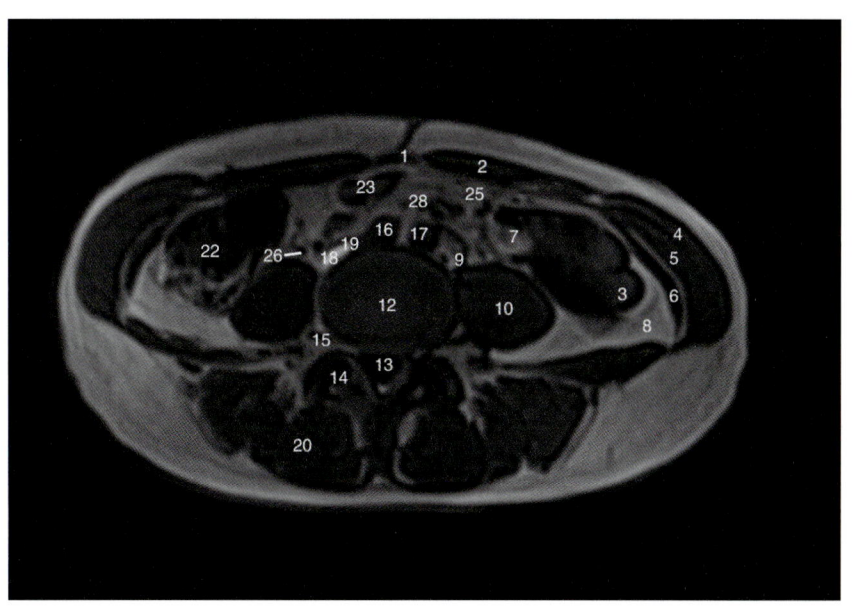

D. MR T1WI

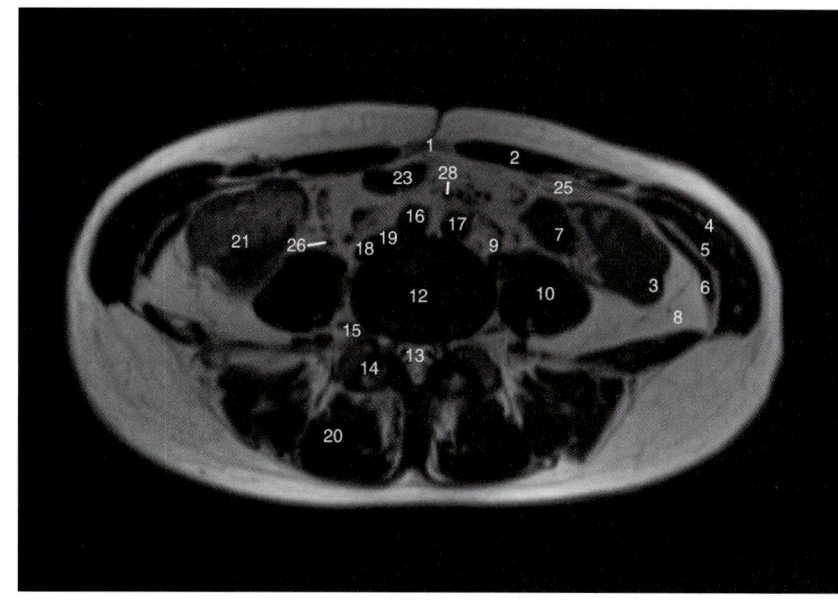

E. MR T2WI

关键结构：回盲瓣，升结肠，回肠。

此断面经 L4-5 椎间盘。

阑尾内口上方 2~3 cm，盲肠和升结肠移行处的左后内侧壁有回肠末端的开口，称回盲口，呈扁圆形的裂隙，口的上、下方各有一片唇状的结构，称回盲瓣。回盲瓣上、下唇分别向前后延伸为瓣系带，与半月襞相延续。回盲瓣是回肠末端肠壁突向盲肠壁而形成的结构，回肠的环肌参与其中。在盲肠排空的情况下，活体所见的回盲瓣大多形成乳头状，由内侧壁突向盲肠腔，系带不明显。回盲部具有括约肌的功能，不仅能防止盲肠的内容物逆流进入回肠，而且能阻止回肠的内容物过快地进入盲肠，有利于小肠进行消化吸收[26]。肠结核在回盲部发病率最高且常侵犯回盲瓣，这可能与肠内容物在该部停留时间较长和该部淋巴组织较丰富有关。病理上以溃疡型肠结核多见。CT 表现为病灶侵犯回盲肠肠壁全层，肠壁增厚甚至形成肿块，导致肠腔狭窄。增强扫描表现为增厚的肠壁明显强化，部分病变肠壁内外层呈高密度环形强化，中间层呈低密度形成"靶征"。肠系膜区淋巴结肿大最为常见，增强扫描时，肿大淋巴结表现为边缘环形强化，中间无强化的干酪样坏死[117]。

腹部连续横断层 115（FH.9630）

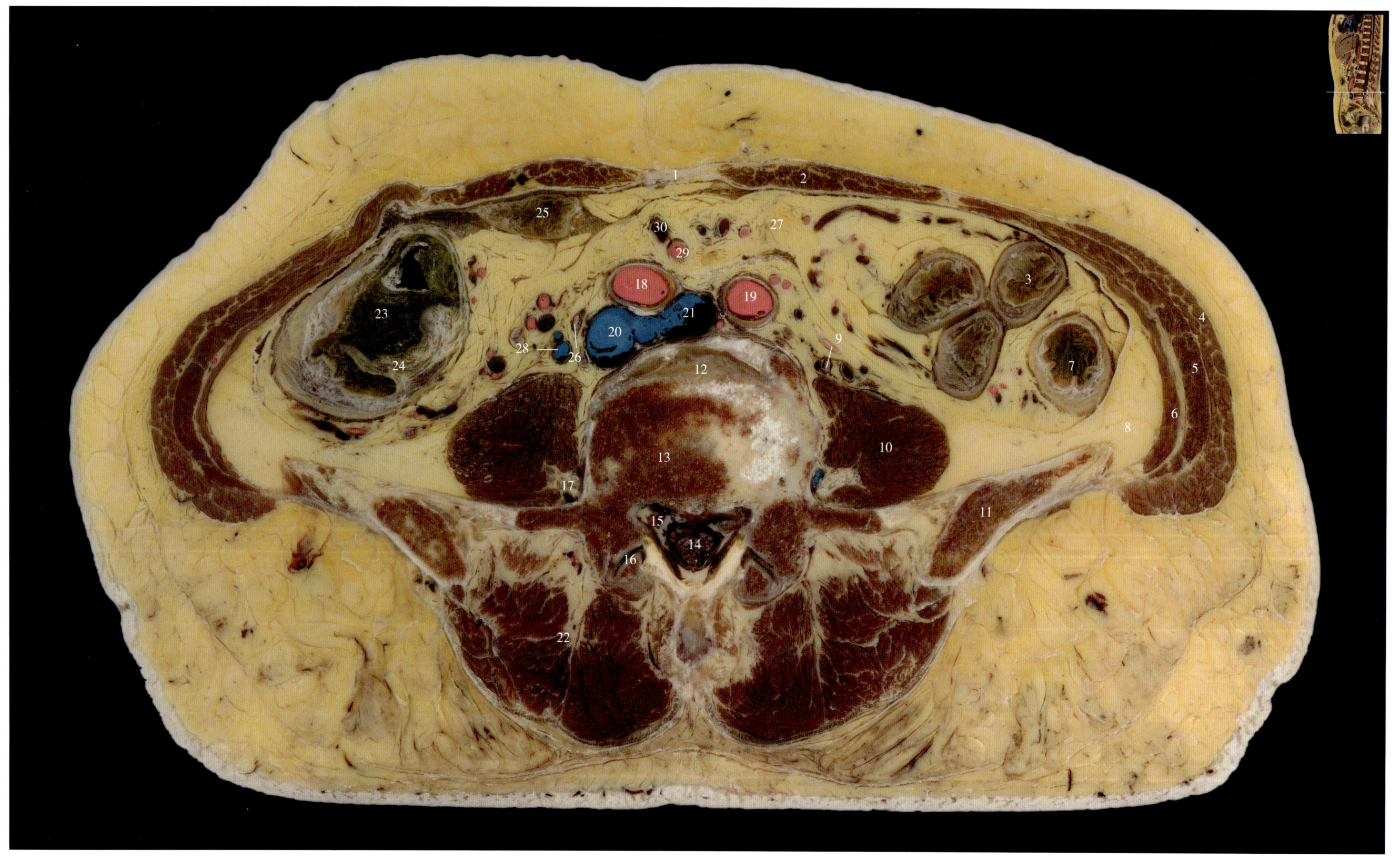

A. 断层标本图像

1. 白线 linea alba
2. 腹直肌 rectus abdominis
3. 空肠 jejunum
4. 腹外斜肌 obliquus externus abdominis
5. 腹内斜肌 obliquus internus abdominis
6. 腹横肌 transverses abdominis
7. 乙状结肠 sigmoid colon
8. 腹膜外脂肪 extraperitoneal fat
9. 左输尿管 left ureter
10. 腰大肌 psoas major
11. 髂嵴 iliac crest
12. L4-5 椎间盘 L4-5 intervertebral disc
13. 第 5 腰椎椎体 body of 5th lumbar vertebra
14. 马尾 cauda equina
15. 第 5 腰神经 5th lumbar nerve
16. 关节突关节 zygapophysial joint
17. 第 4 腰神经 4th lumbar nerve
18. 右髂总动脉 right common iliac artery
19. 左髂总动脉 left common iliac artery
20. 右髂总静脉 right common iliac vein
21. 左髂总静脉 left common iliac vein
22. 竖脊肌 erector spinae
23. 升结肠 ascending colon
24. 回盲瓣 ileocecal valve
25. 回肠 ileum
26. 右输尿管 right ureter
27. 肠系膜 mesentery
28. 右卵巢静脉 right ovarian vein
29. 肠系膜上动脉 superior mesenteric artery
30. 肠系膜上静脉 superior mesenteric vein

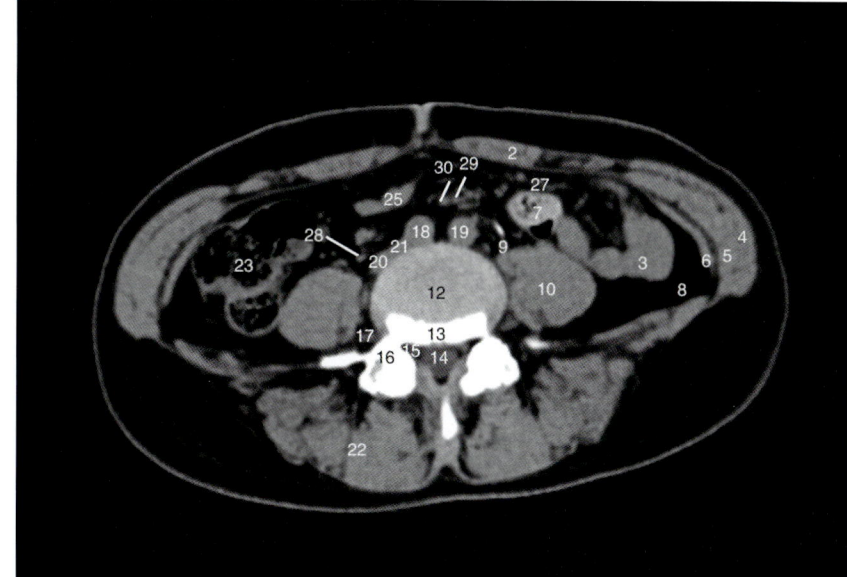

B. CT 平扫图像

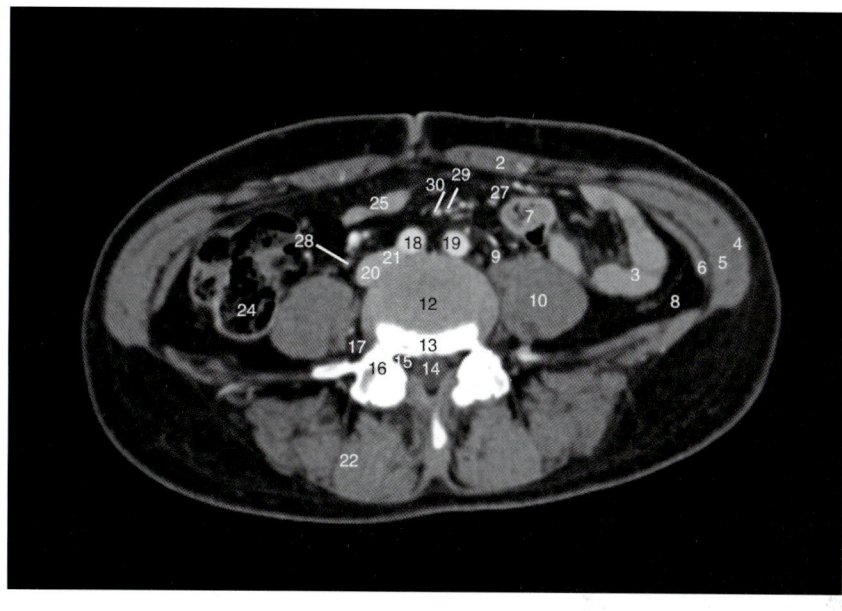

C. CT 增强图像

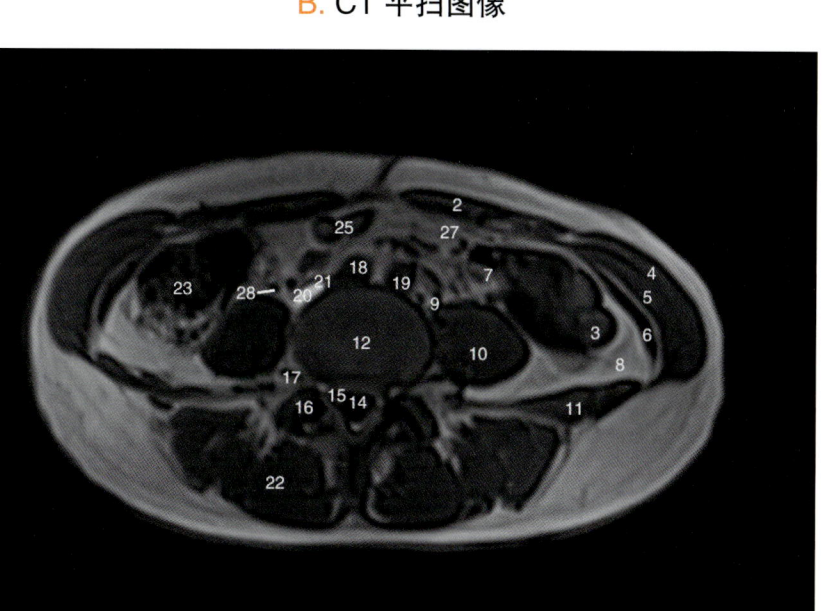

D. MR T1WI

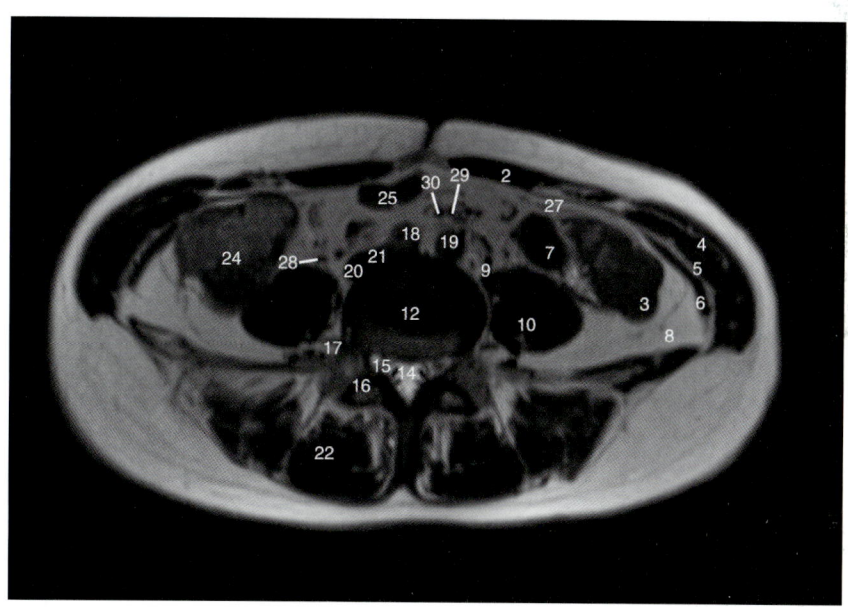

E. MR T2WI

关键结构：回肠，肠系膜上动脉，肠系膜上静脉。

此断面经第 5 腰椎椎体上份。

回肠位于结肠下区的右下部。人体直立时，回肠袢可垂入盆腔。管径一般约为 3.5 cm，肠壁较空肠略薄，血管较少而颜色稍白，血液供应较差，消化吸收功能减弱，黏膜环状皱襞少且低，黏膜内除有孤立淋巴滤泡外，还有集合淋巴滤泡，回肠系膜内血管弓级数较多，脂肪较丰富。回肠与空肠之间无明显的分界线。回肠的血液供应来自肠系膜上动脉。肠系膜上动脉发出供应空肠和回肠的血管为小肠动脉，其数目不定，少则 8 支，多达 24 支，一般为 13~18 支。其中供应空肠者称空肠动脉，供应回肠者称回肠动脉，二者行于肠系膜两层之间，皆分为两支，与相邻的小肠动脉分支吻合成动脉弓，由弓的突侧发出第 2 级分支，如此反复组成动脉弓，可达 3~5 级。原发性小肠淋巴瘤是原发于肠道黏膜固有层和黏膜下层淋巴组织的恶性肿瘤。大多数肠道淋巴瘤是全身性淋巴瘤的一种局部表现，小肠任何部位均可发生，但以淋巴组织丰富的回肠远端发生率最高，本病绝大多数属于 B 淋巴细胞来源。病变影像学表现：①分叶状软组织肿块，密度均匀，增强呈轻到中度强化；②肠壁阶段性及弥漫性增厚，肠腔扩张；③"夹心面包征"，肿大淋巴结包绕肠系膜血管及周围脂肪。其特征可以总结为长（病变范围长）、宽（病变段肠管扩张）、多（病变可累及多段肠管）、均（CT 扫描密度均匀）[118]。

腹部连续横断层 116（FH.9610）

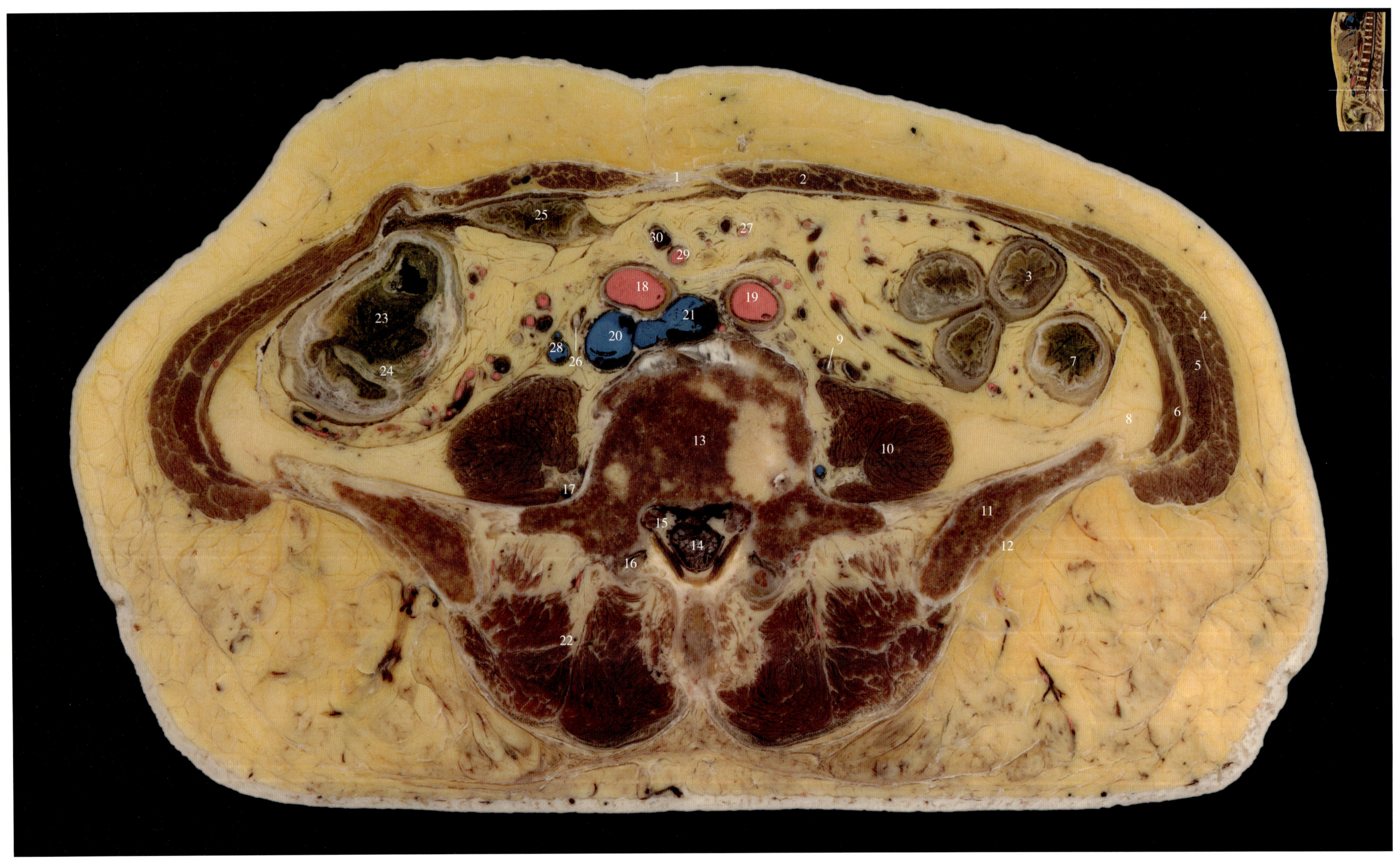

A. 断层标本图像

1. 白线 linea alba
2. 腹直肌 rectus abdominis
3. 空肠 jejunum
4. 腹外斜肌 obliquus externus abdominis
5. 腹内斜肌 obliquus internus abdominis
6. 腹横肌 transverses abdominis
7. 乙状结肠 sigmoid colon
8. 腹膜外脂肪 extraperitoneal fat
9. 左输尿管 left ureter
10. 腰大肌 psoas major
11. 髂嵴 iliac crest
12. 臀中肌 gluteus medius
13. 第5腰椎椎体 body of 5th lumbar vertebra
14. 马尾 cauda equina
15. 第5腰神经 5th lumbar nerve
16. 关节突关节 zygapophysial joint
17. 第4腰神经 4th lumbar nerve
18. 右髂总动脉 right common iliac artery
19. 左髂总动脉 left common iliac artery
20. 右髂总静脉 right common iliac vein
21. 左髂总静脉 left common iliac vein
22. 竖脊肌 erector spinae
23. 升结肠 ascending colon
24. 回盲瓣 ileocecal valve
25. 回肠 ileum
26. 右输尿管 right ureter
27. 肠系膜 mesentery
28. 右卵巢静脉 right ovarian vein
29. 肠系膜上动脉 superior mesenteric artery
30. 肠系膜上静脉 superior mesenteric vein

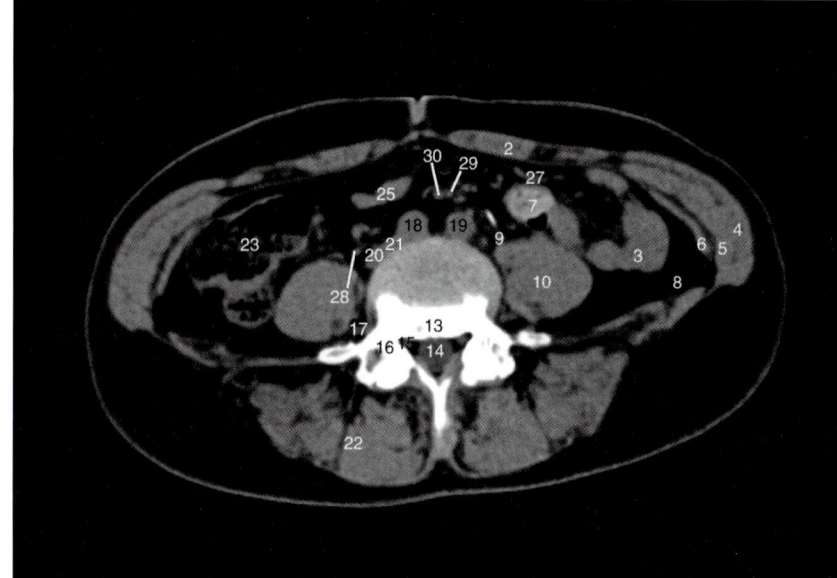

B. CT 平扫图像

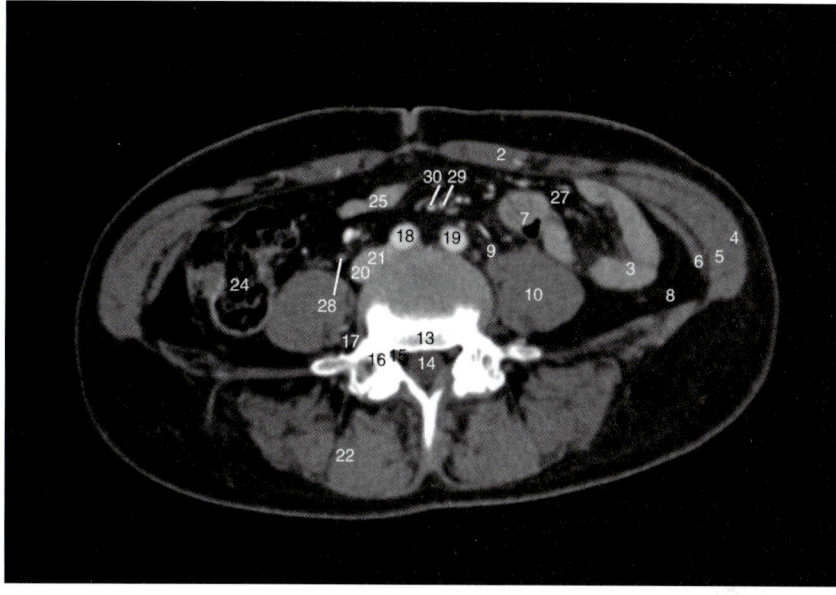

C. CT 增强图像

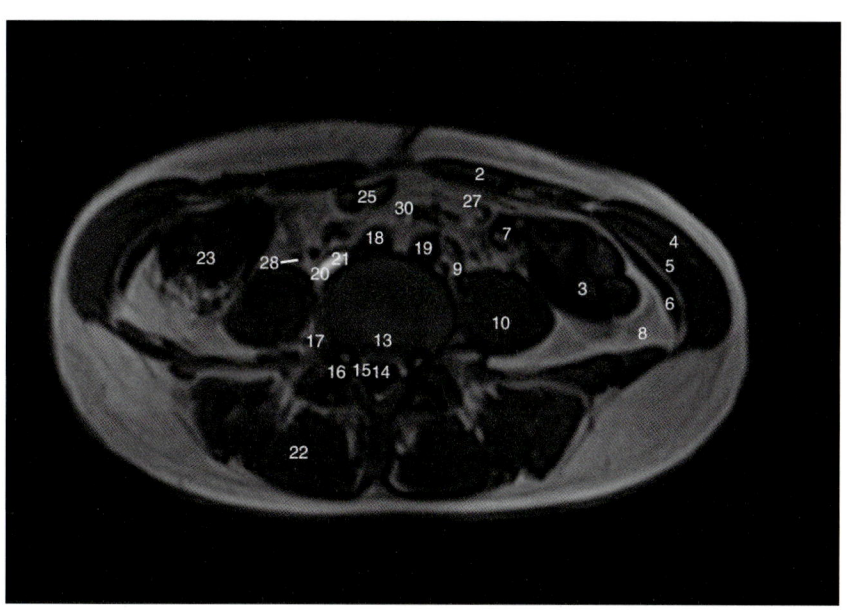

D. MR T1WI

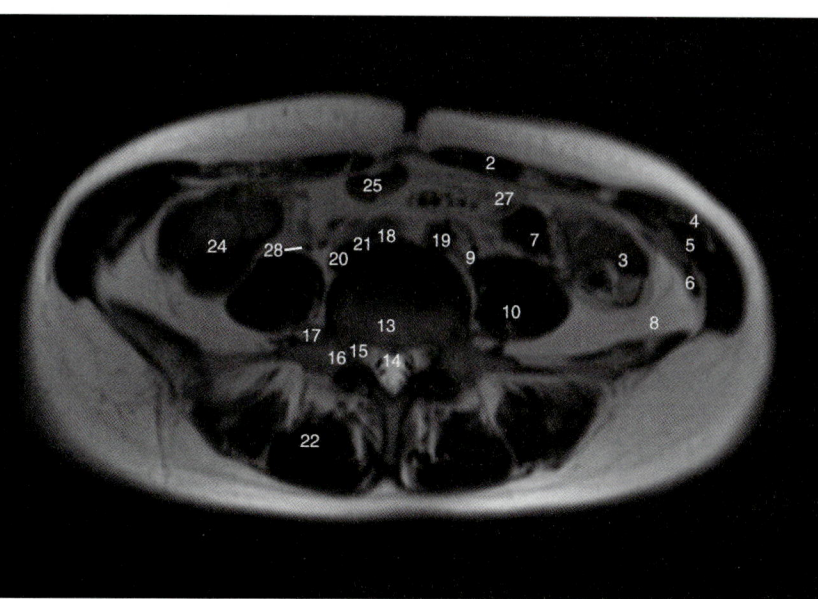

E. MR T2WI

关键结构：髂嵴，臀中肌，回盲瓣。

此断面经第5腰椎椎体上份。

髂骨翼的上缘肥厚并呈弓形向上凸弯，叫髂嵴，在皮下均可触及。两侧髂嵴最高点的连线约平齐第4腰椎棘突，是计数椎骨的标志。翼的前缘弯曲向下，达于髋骨和髂后下棘。髂后下棘下方有深陷的坐骨大切迹，两侧髂后上棘的连线约平第2骶椎。从髂前上棘向后上方5~7 cm处，髂嵴较厚且向外突出，为髂结节[26]。髂前上棘是临床上非常重要的一个解剖位点，许多器官和手术区的定位都是以髂前上棘作为解剖参考点。临床上骨髓穿刺也多采用髂穿的方式，即在髂前上棘稍外侧较平坦处作为骨髓穿刺针的入路点[119]。此外，可用髂前上棘作为标志来测量下肢的长度；也可根据与髂前上棘的关系来确定股动脉、股外侧皮神经、髂腹下神经和髂腹股沟神经的行程。

腹部连续横断层 117（FH.9590）

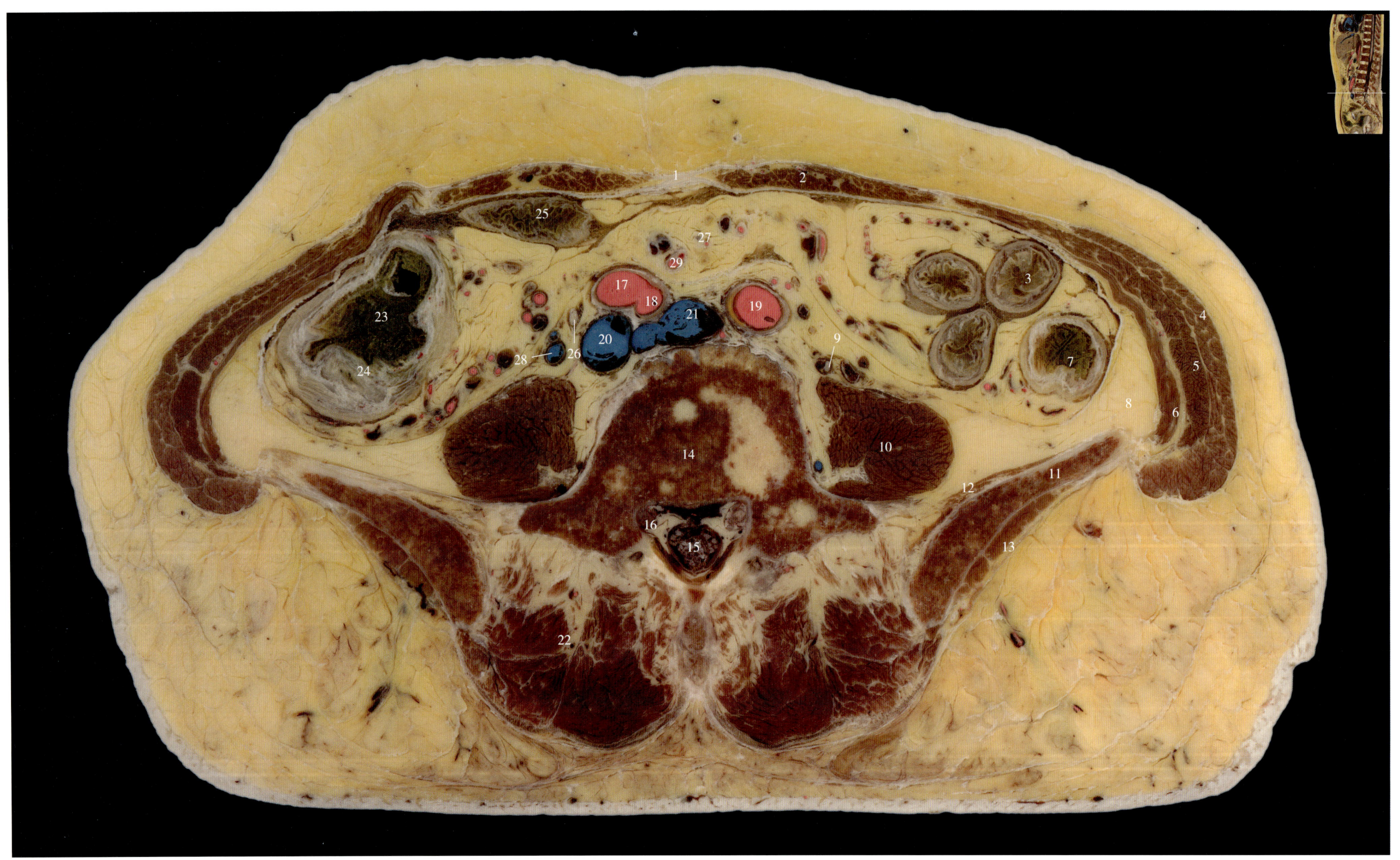

A. 断层标本图像

1. 白线 linea alba
2. 腹直肌 rectus abdominis
3. 空肠 jejunum
4. 腹外斜肌 obliquus externus abdominis
5. 腹内斜肌 obliquus internus abdominis
6. 腹横肌 transverses abdominis
7. 乙状结肠 sigmoid colon
8. 腹膜外脂肪 extraperitoneal fat
9. 左输尿管 left ureter
10. 腰大肌 psoas major
11. 髂骨翼 ala of ilium
12. 髂肌 iliacus
13. 臀中肌 gluteus medius
14. 第5腰椎椎体 body of 5th lumbar vertebra
15. 马尾 cauda equina
16. 第5腰神经 5th lumbar nerve
17. 右髂外动脉 right external iliac artery
18. 右髂内动脉 right internal iliac artery
19. 左髂总动脉 left common iliac artery
20. 右髂总静脉 right common iliac vein
21. 左髂总静脉 left common iliac vein
22. 竖脊肌 erector spinae
23. 升结肠 ascending colon
24. 回盲瓣 ileocecal valve
25. 回肠 ileum
26. 右输尿管 right ureter
27. 肠系膜 mesentery
28. 右卵巢静脉 right ovarian vein
29. 肠系膜上动脉 superior mesenteric artery
30. 右髂总动脉 right common iliac artery
31. 肠系膜上静脉 superior mesenteric vein

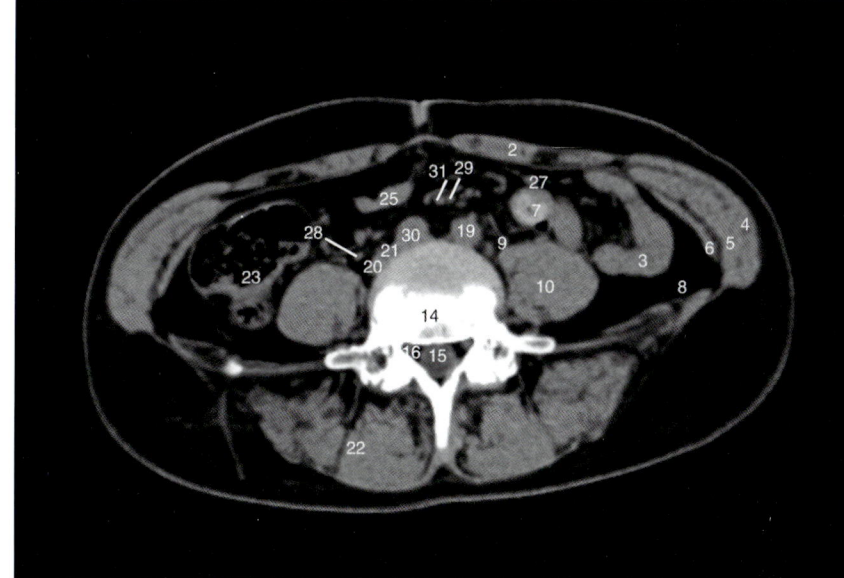

B. CT 平扫图像

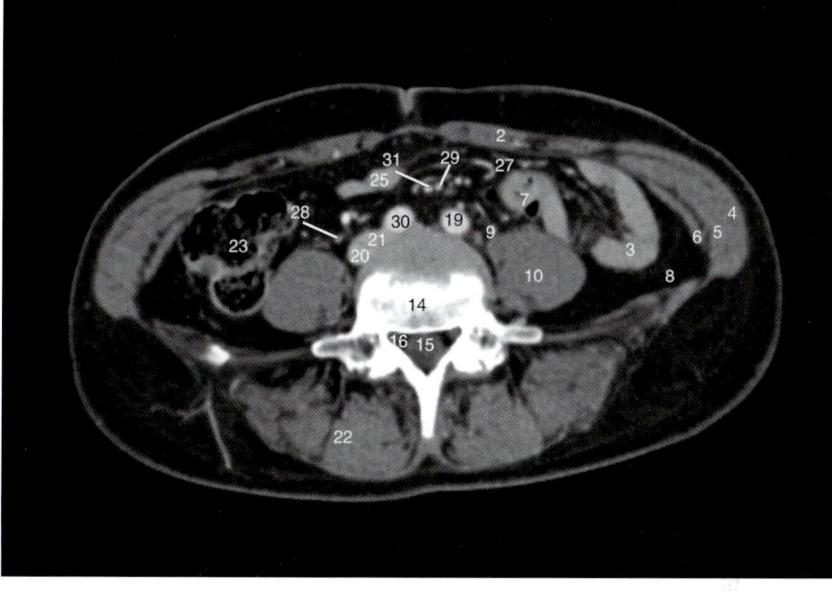

C. CT 增强图像

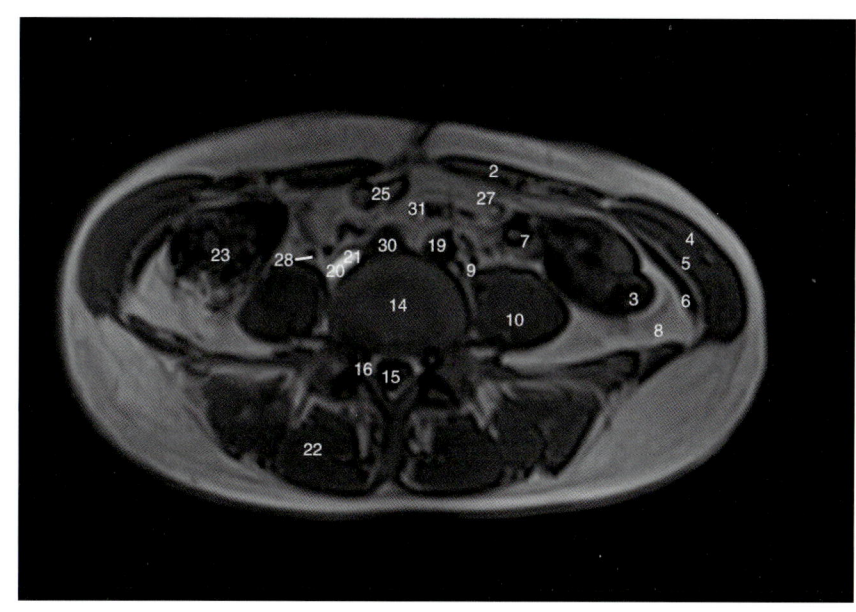

D. MR T1WI

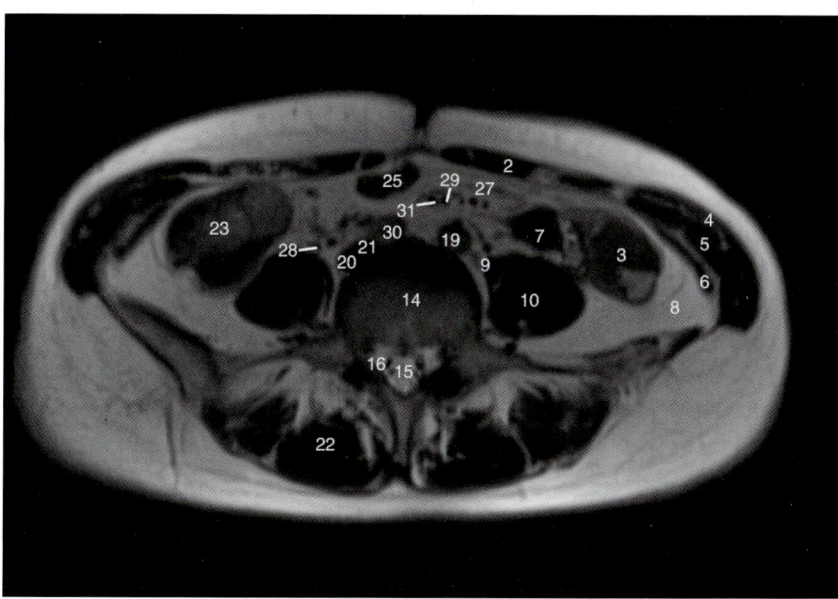

E. MR T2WI

关键结构：右髂外动脉，右髂内动脉，左髂总动脉。

此断面经过第5腰椎椎体上份。

椎体前方有左右髂总动、静脉走行，右髂总动脉将要分为右髂外动脉和右髂内动脉。椎体后方椎管内有马尾神经和第5腰神经走行，右侧腰大肌前方有右卵巢静脉经过。髂内动脉是一短干，自髂总动脉分出后，沿骨盆侧壁下行，分出脏、壁两支，分布于盆部及部分大腿。其中，壁支主要分支有髂腰动脉、骶外侧动脉、臀上动脉、臀下动脉和闭孔动脉等；脏支主要发出脐动脉、膀胱下动脉、直肠下动脉和子宫动脉等。髂外动脉经过股三角后移行为股动脉，沿途发出腹壁下动脉和旋髂深动脉。骨盆骨折，特别是粉碎性骨折时常引起髂内动脉壁支损伤，极易发生大出血，死亡率高达36.4%~54.0%。盆腔侧支循环丰富，栓塞两侧髂内动脉后，可在45~60分钟内形成侧支循环，因此，双侧髂内动脉栓塞既能有效止血又能维持盆腔脏器的血供，不会引起盆腔脏器的坏死，目前已成为骨盆骨折后合并动脉性出血止血的重要治疗手段之一[120]。

腹部连续横断层 118（FH.9570）

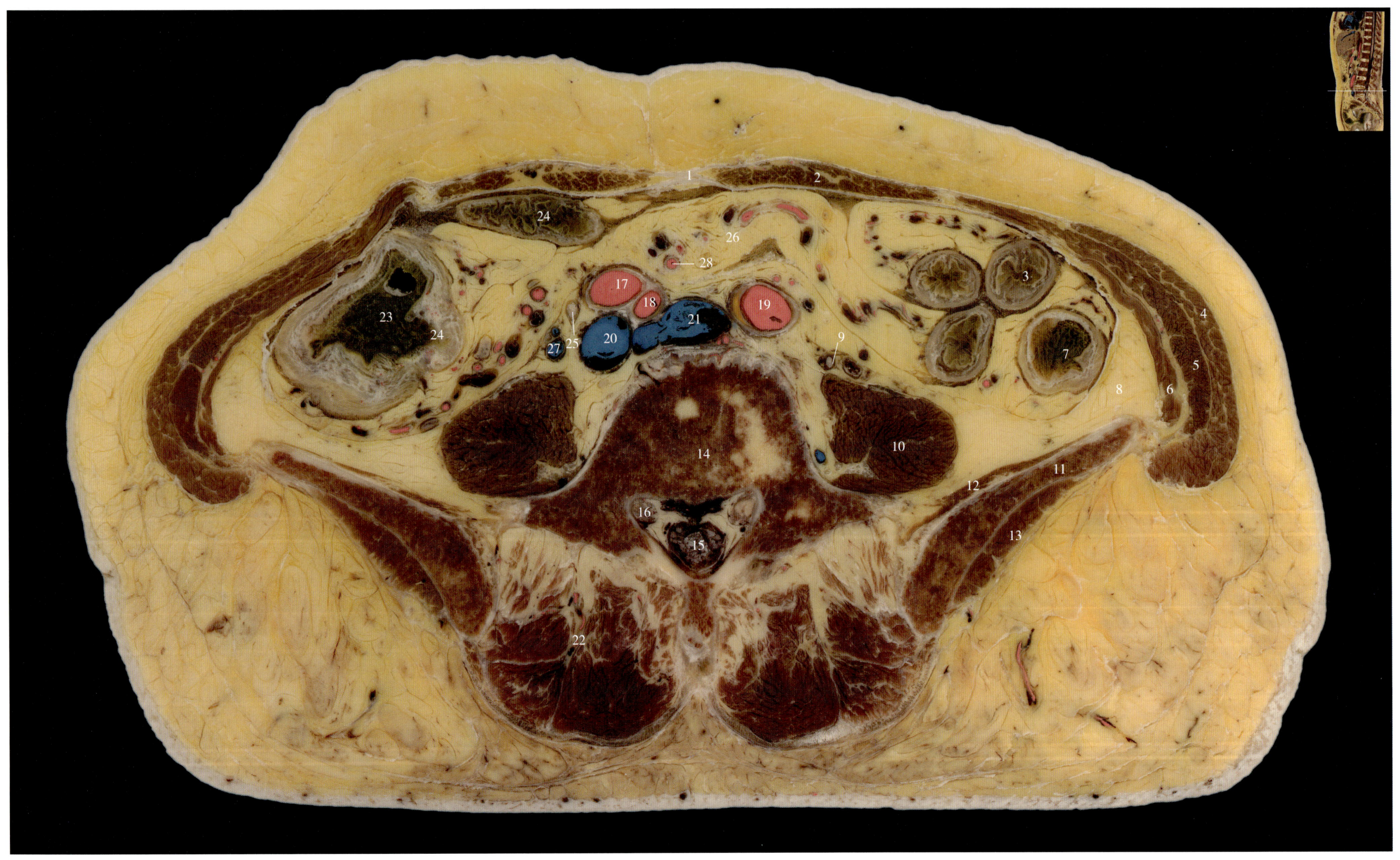

A. 断层标本图像

1. 白线 linea alba
2. 腹直肌 rectus abdominis
3. 空肠 jejunum
4. 腹外斜肌 obliquus externus abdominis
5. 腹内斜肌 obliquus internus abdominis
6. 腹横肌 transverses abdominis
7. 乙状结肠 sigmoid colon
8. 腹膜外脂肪 extraperitoneal fat
9. 左输尿管 left ureter
10. 腰大肌 psoas major
11. 髂骨翼 ala of ilium
12. 髂肌 iliacus
13. 臀中肌 gluteus medius
14. 第 5 腰椎椎体 body of 5th lumbar vertebra
15. 马尾 cauda equina
16. 第 5 腰神经 5th lumbar nerve
17. 右髂外动脉 right external iliac artery
18. 右髂内动脉 right internal iliac artery
19. 左髂总动脉 left common iliac artery
20. 右髂总静脉 right common iliac vein
21. 左髂总静脉 left common iliac vein
22. 竖脊肌 erector spinae
23. 盲肠 cecum
24. 回肠 ileum
25. 右输尿管 right ureter
26. 肠系膜 mesentery
27. 右卵巢静脉 right ovarian vein
28. 肠系膜上动脉 superior mesenteric artery
29. 右髂总动脉 right common iliac artery

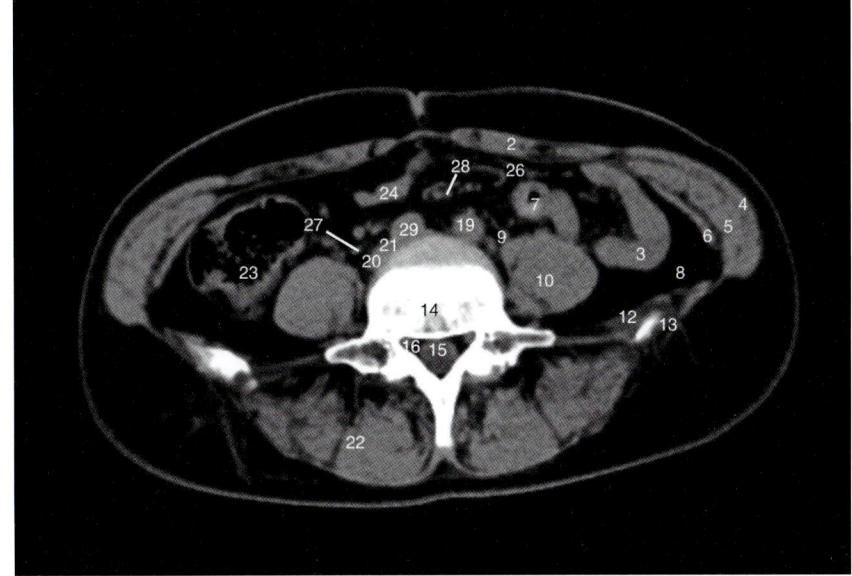

B. CT 平扫图像

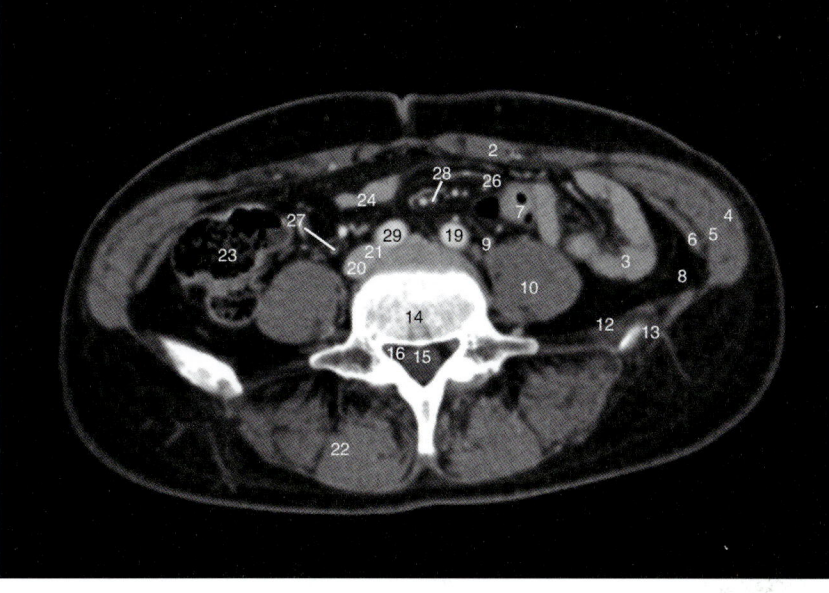

C. CT 增强图像

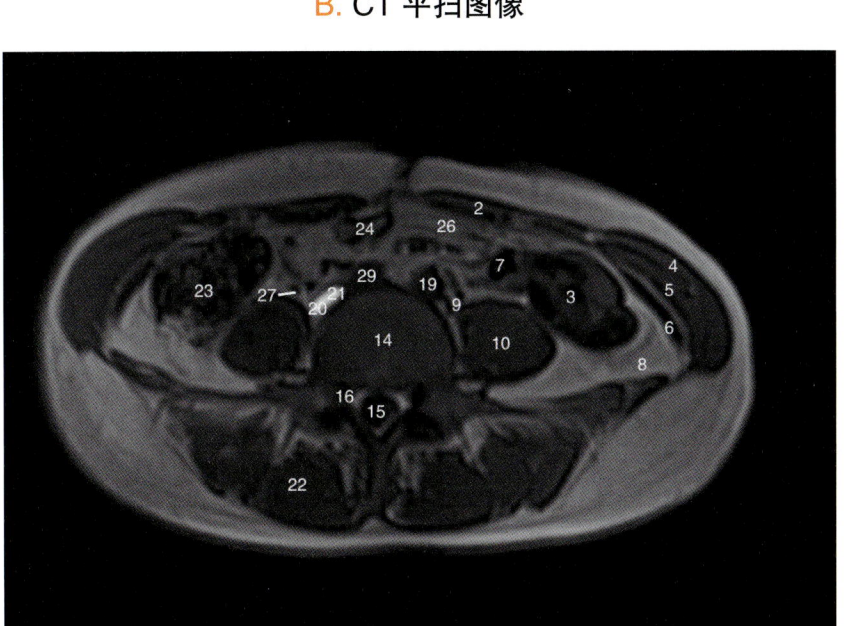

D. MR T1WI

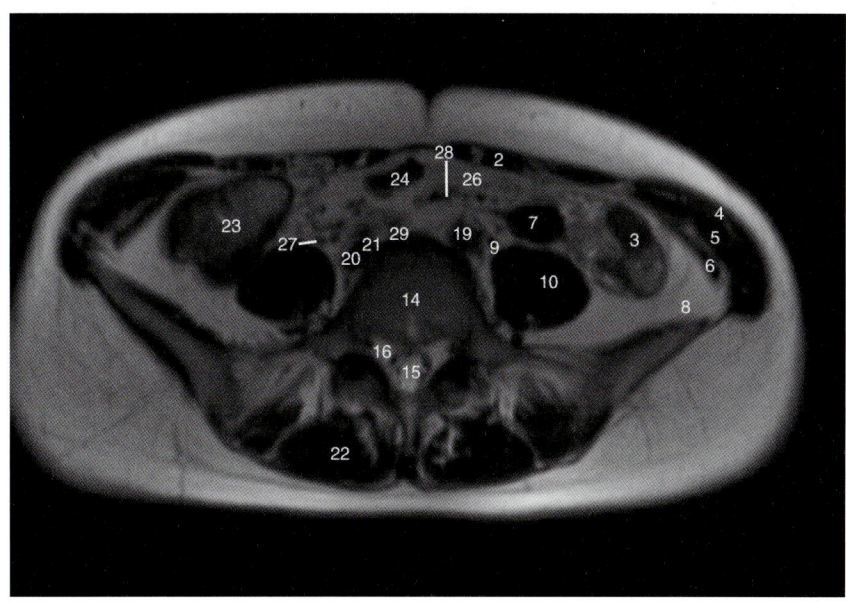

E. MR T2WI

关键结构：盲肠，回肠，右卵巢静脉。

此断面经过第 5 腰椎椎体上份。

消化系统管道、系膜、血管及神经的分布同上一断面。回肠占据小肠全长的远侧 3/5，多位于脐区、右腹股沟区和盆腔内，在右髂窝续于盲肠。盲肠是大肠的起始部，位于右髂窝内，呈盲囊状，左接回肠末端，上通升结肠，长 6~8 cm[37]。由于盲肠远端闭塞不通，故称之为盲肠。在盲肠远端伸出一小管，为阑尾，因其管腔细小，容易阻塞而发炎，形成阑尾炎。急性阑尾炎是最常见的急腹症之一，临床表现为腹痛、发热、腹肌紧张、麦氏点的压痛及反跳痛。典型的 CT 表现为阑尾增粗，壁水肿，阑尾周围渗出性改变及脂肪层模糊，多数患者可发现阑尾内的高密度粪石[121]。

腹部连续横断层 119（FH.9550）

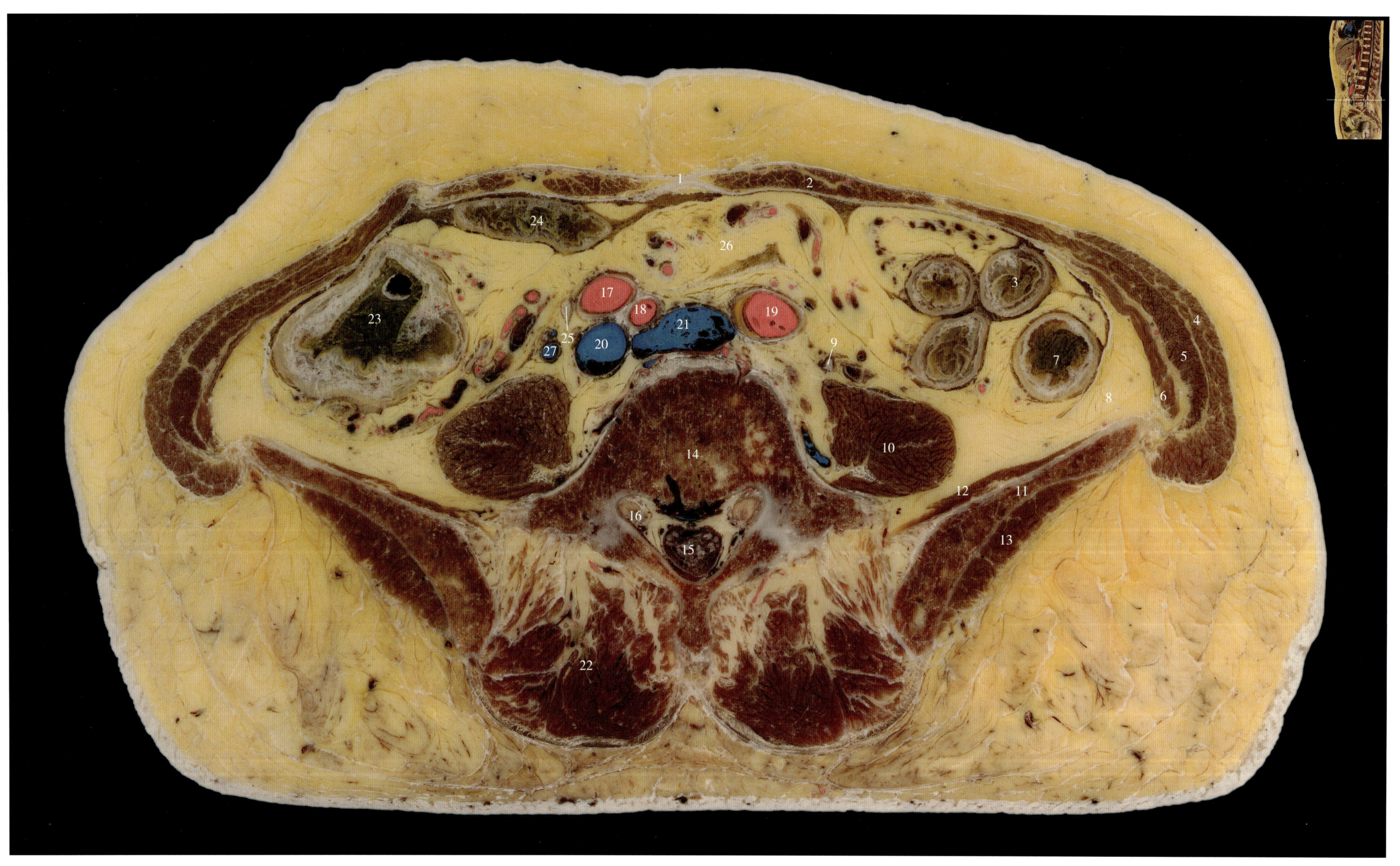

A. 断层标本图像

1. 白线 linea alba
2. 腹直肌 rectus abdominis
3. 空肠 jejunum
4. 腹外斜肌 obliquus externus abdominis
5. 腹内斜肌 obliquus internus abdominis
6. 腹横肌 transverses abdominis
7. 乙状结肠 sigmoid colon
8. 腹膜外脂肪 extraperitoneal fat
9. 左输尿管 left ureter
10. 腰大肌 psoas major
11. 髂骨翼 ala of ilium
12. 髂肌 iliacus
13. 臀中肌 gluteus medius
14. 第5腰椎椎体 body of 5th lumbar vertebra
15. 马尾 cauda equina
16. 第5腰神经 5th lumbar nerve
17. 右髂外动脉 right external iliac artery
18. 右髂内动脉 right internal iliac artery
19. 左髂总动脉 left common iliac artery
20. 右髂总静脉 right common iliac vein
21. 左髂总静脉 left common iliac vein
22. 竖脊肌 erector spinae
23. 盲肠 cecum
24. 回肠 ileum
25. 右输尿管 right ureter
26. 肠系膜 mesentery
27. 右卵巢静脉 right ovarian vein
28. 右髂总动脉 right common iliac artery

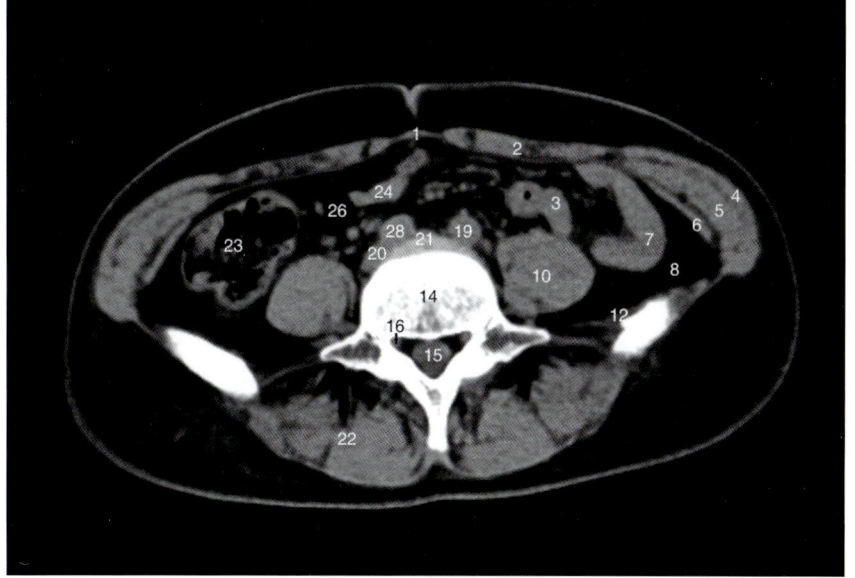

B. CT 平扫图像

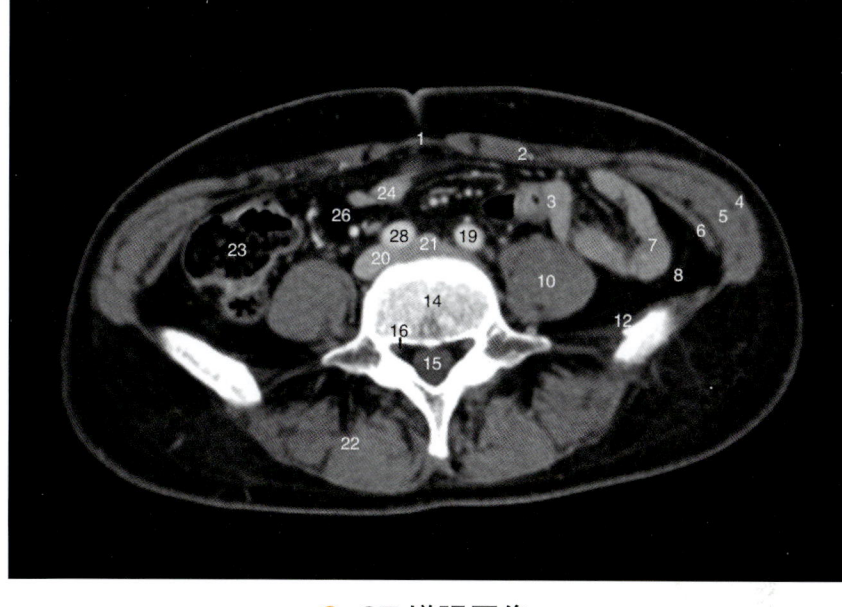

C. CT 增强图像

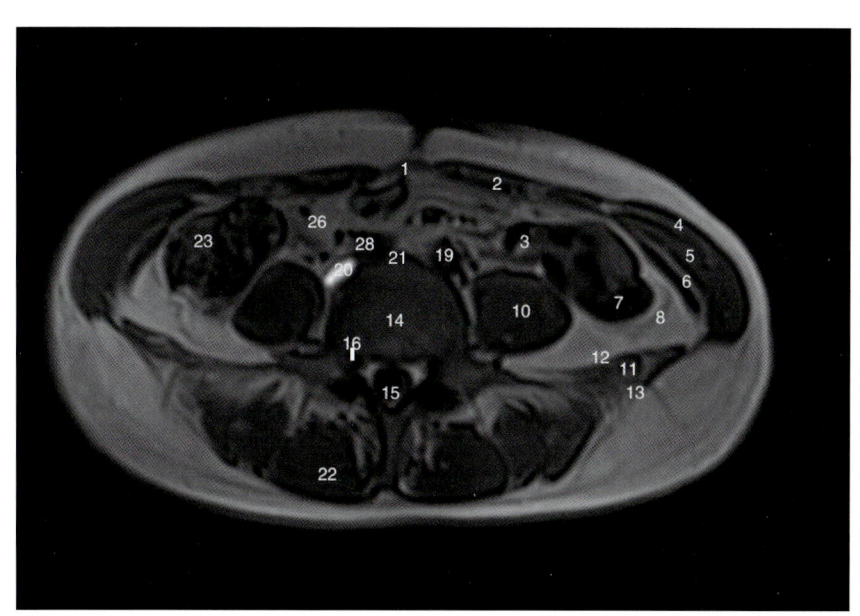

D. MR T1WI

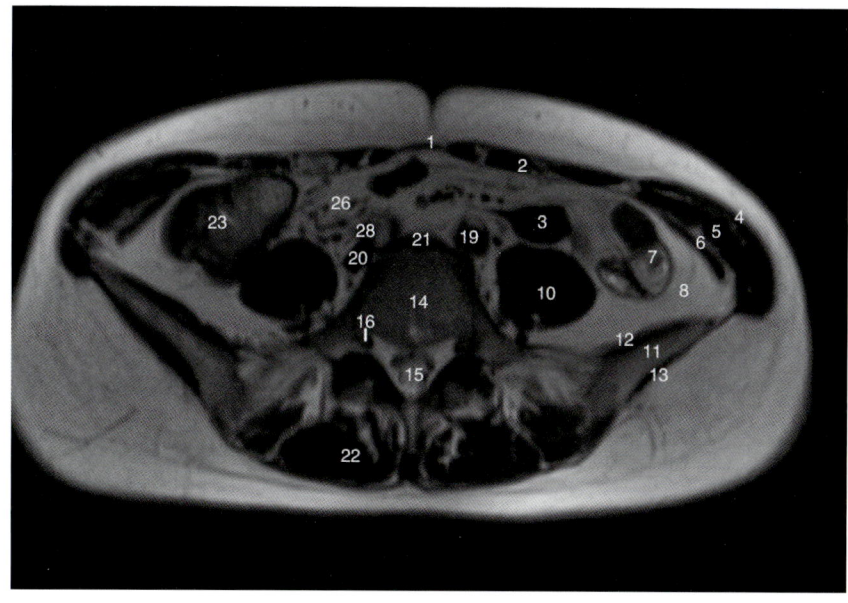

E. MR T2WI

关键结构：第5腰椎椎体，第5腰神经，输尿管。

此断面经过第5腰椎椎体。

右输尿管走行于回肠后方，肠系膜根部附着处的深面，右髂外动脉右侧。左输尿管居左腰大肌的前内侧、左髂总动脉外侧，其外为乙状结肠膜根的起始部[7]。第5腰椎是最后一块腰椎，与第4腰椎相接的椎间盘是腰椎间盘突出的好发部位，下接骶骨，与其形成腰骶角。各段相邻处的椎骨有时具有另一段的特征，称为移行椎。移行椎在腰椎处表现为腰椎骶化，如果在骶椎处就表现为骶椎腰化。腰椎骶化和骶椎腰化是产生腰背痛的原因之一。X线腰骶椎（包括骨盆）正位摄片，可确定腰椎骶化。CT腰骶椎矢状位重建也可观察到第5腰椎演变成骶椎样的形态，即第5腰椎与骶骨融合形成融合椎[122]。椎体后椎管内有马尾及第5腰神经走行。第5腰神经前支合成腰骶干向下加入骶丛。骶丛由腰骶干及全部骶神经和尾神经的前支组成，支配梨状肌、闭孔内肌等。

239

腹部连续横断层 120（FH.9530）

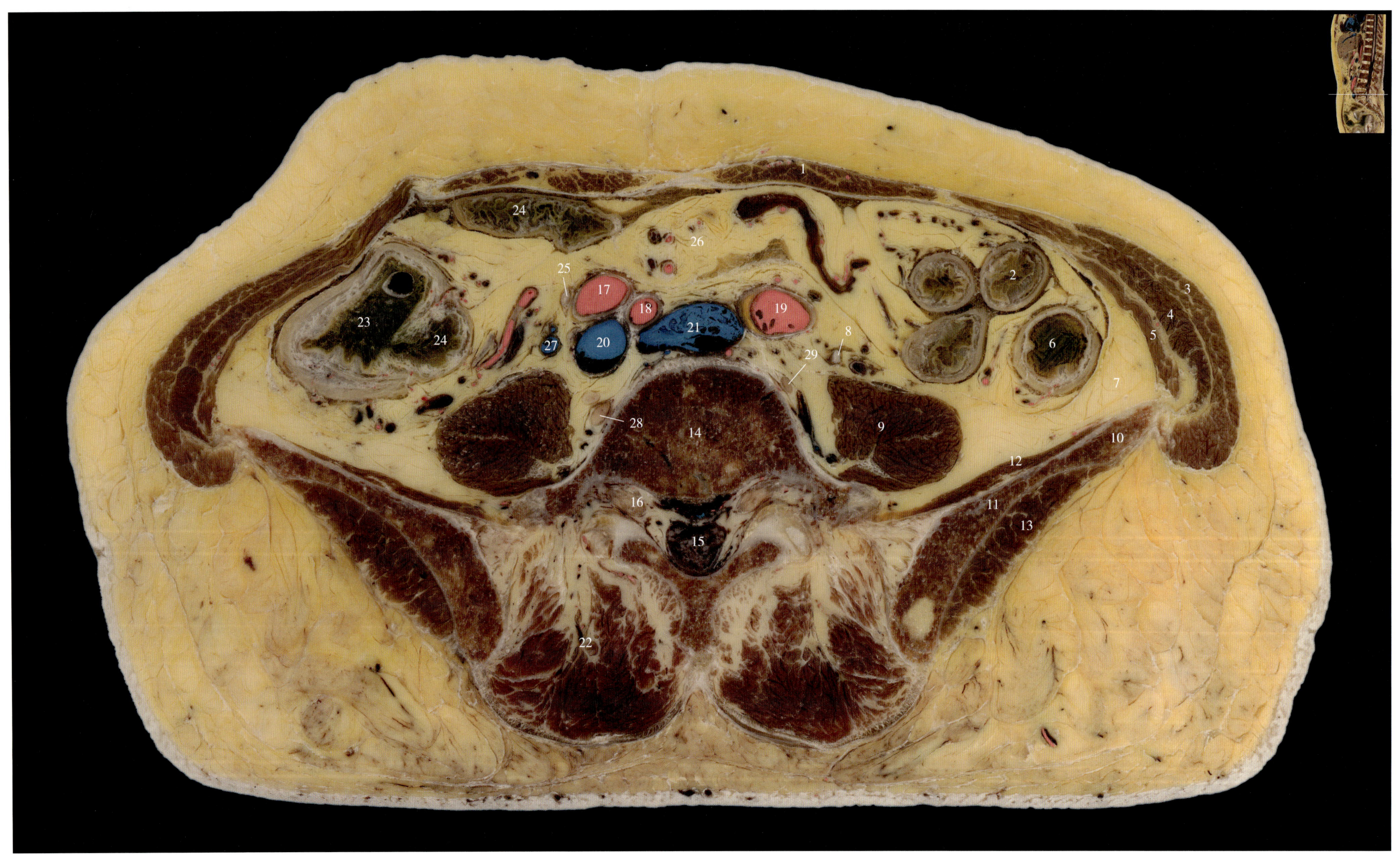

A. 断层标本图像

1. 腹直肌 rectus abdominis
2. 空肠 jejunum
3. 腹外斜肌 obliquus externus abdominis
4. 腹内斜肌 obliquus internus abdominis
5. 腹横肌 transverses abdominis
6. 乙状结肠 sigmoid colon
7. 腹膜外脂肪 extraperitoneal fat
8. 左输尿管 left ureter
9. 腰大肌 psoas major
10. 髂嵴 iliac crest
11. 髂骨翼 ala of ilium
12. 髂肌 iliacus
13. 臀中肌 gluteus medius
14. 第 5 腰椎椎体 body of 5th lumbar vertebra
15. 马尾 cauda equina
16. 第 5 腰神经 5th lumbar nerve
17. 右髂外动脉 right external iliac artery
18. 右髂内动脉 right internal iliac artery
19. 左髂总动脉 left common iliac artery
20. 右髂总静脉 right common iliac vein
21. 左髂总静脉 left common iliac vein
22. 竖脊肌 erector spinae
23. 盲肠 cecum
24. 回肠 ileum
25. 右输尿管 right ureter
26. 肠系膜 mesentery
27. 右卵巢静脉 right ovarian vein
28. 右交感干 right sympathetic trunk
29. 左交感干 left sympathetic trunk
30. 右髂总动脉 right common iliac artery

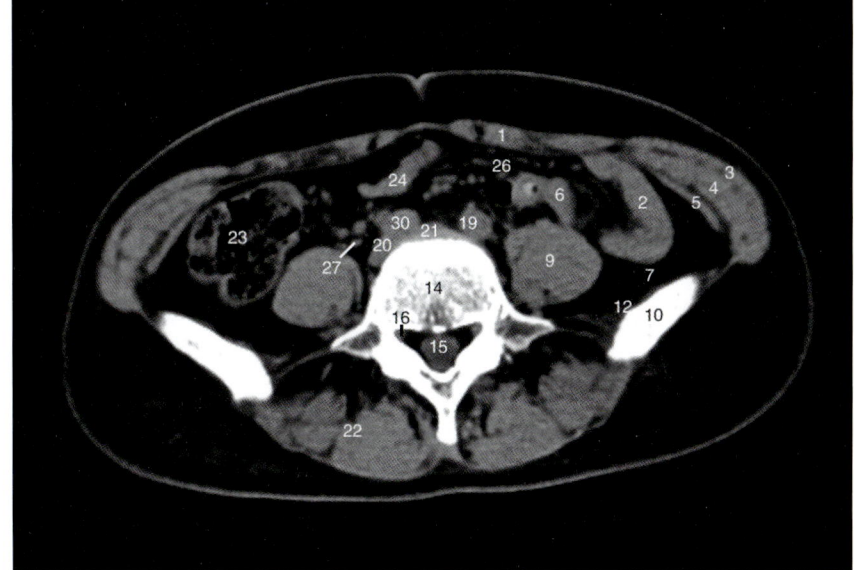

B. CT 平扫图像

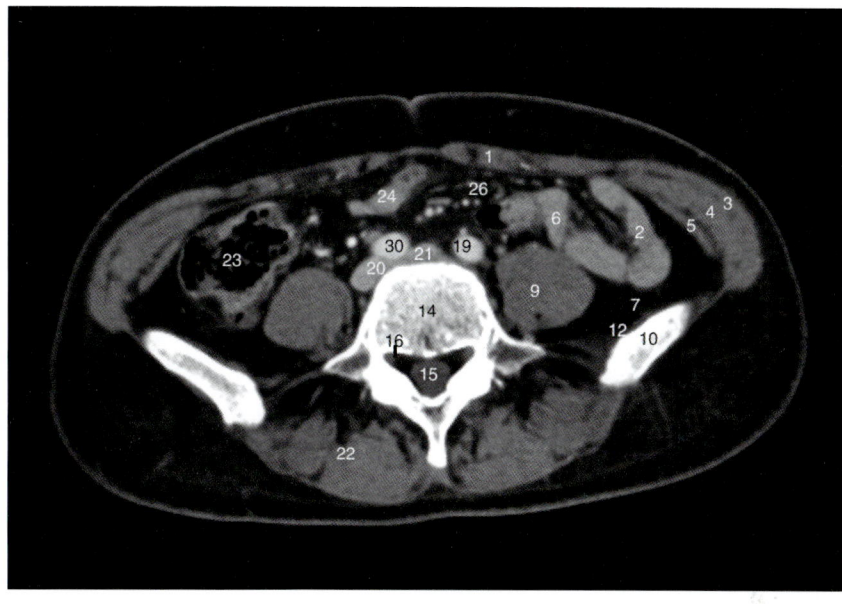

C. CT 增强图像

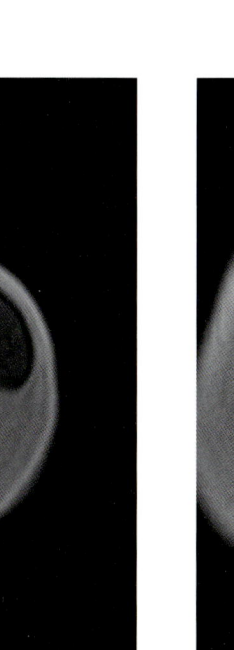

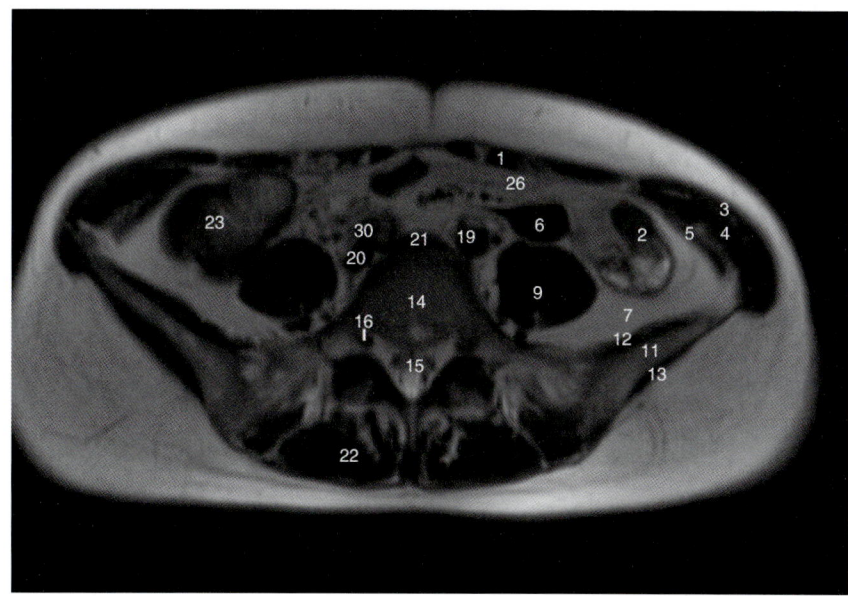

D. MR T1WI

E. MR T2WI

关键结构：交感干，右髂内动脉，右髂外动脉，左髂总动、静脉。

此断面经过第 5 腰椎椎体。

脊柱与右侧腰大肌之间可见右腰交感干，其前方为右髂总静脉和右髂内、外动脉。左侧腰大肌与脊柱的前方，可见左髂总动、静脉，二者与腰大肌之间可见左腰交感干。交感干是由一系列交感神经椎旁节借节间支连接构成，左右各一，位于脊椎两侧。交感干上起颅底，下至尾骨，两侧下端在尾骨前方合并。交感干借交通支与相应的脊神经相连。由于腰交感神经变异较大，局部解剖结构关系复杂，致使腰交感神经干/节切除手术难度系数大。有研究发现，中国人的腰交感神经节以 3~4 个节最多见[122]。腰交感干一般为一条连续的神经干，但有时亦可在某些地方分裂成 2 条或以上，文献报道腰交感干分裂的出现率为 36.4% ± 2.6%[37]。生殖股神经穿出点与腰交感干很近，特别是于腰大肌内侧缘处穿出者，在行腰交感神经切除时很容易损伤或误切该神经，导致手术失败或术后患者外阴部感觉迟钝，术中应格外小心[123]。

腹部连续横断层 121（FH.9510）

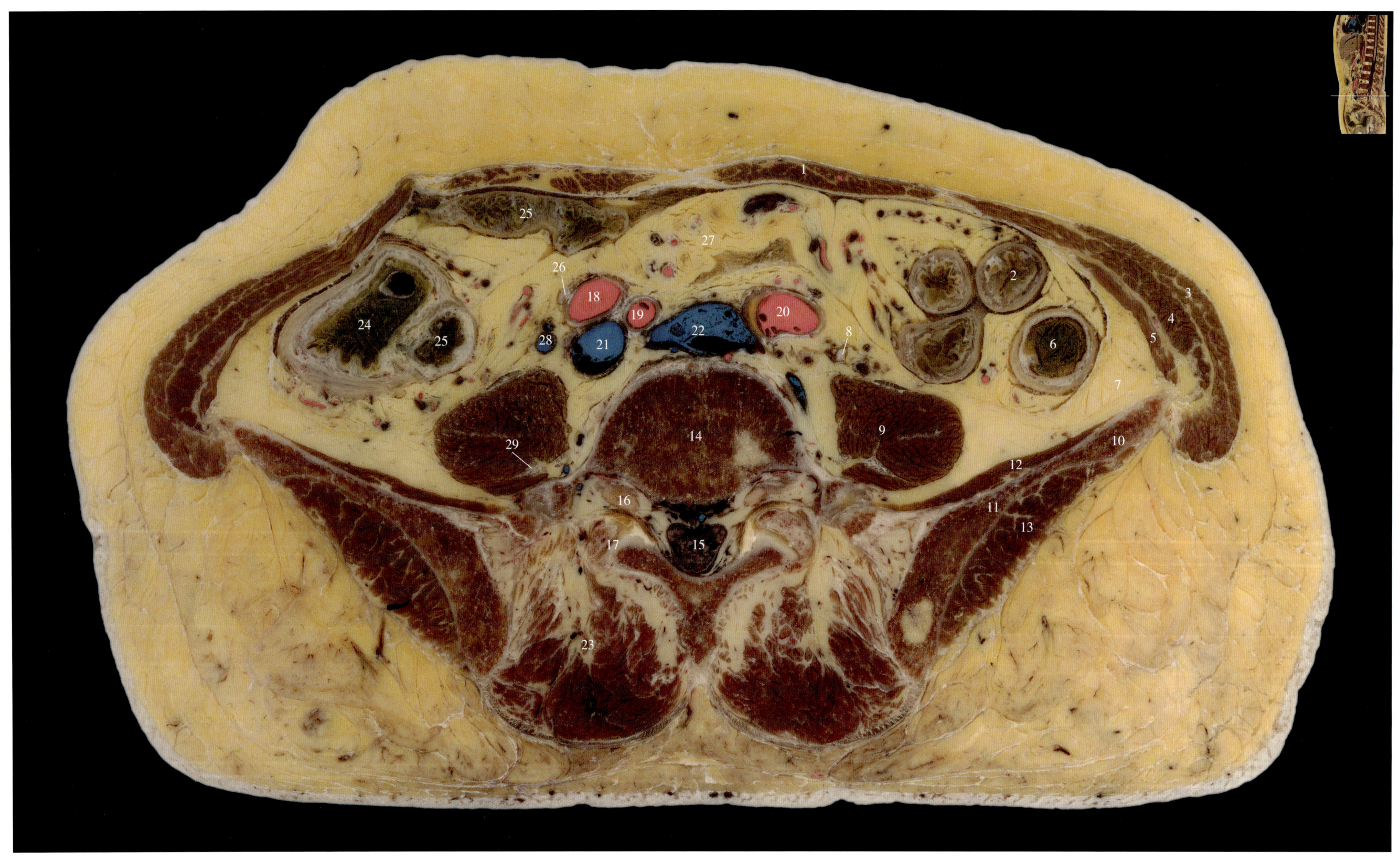

A. 断层标本图像

1. 腹直肌 rectus abdominis
2. 空肠 jejunum
3. 腹外斜肌 obliquus externus abdominis
4. 腹内斜肌 obliquus internus abdominis
5. 腹横肌 transverses abdominis
6. 乙状结肠 sigmoid colon
7. 腹膜外脂肪 extraperitoneal fat
8. 左输尿管 left ureter
9. 腰大肌 psoas major
10. 髂嵴 iliac crest
11. 髂骨翼 ala of ilium
12. 髂肌 iliacus
13. 臀中肌 gluteus medius
14. 第5腰椎椎体 body of 5th lumbar vertebra
15. 马尾 cauda equina
16. 第5腰神经 5th lumbar nerve
17. 关节突关节 zygapophysial joint
18. 右髂外动脉 right external iliac artery
19. 右髂内动脉 right internal iliac artery
20. 左髂总动脉 left common iliac artery
21. 右髂总静脉 right common iliac vein
22. 左髂总静脉 left common iliac vein
23. 竖脊肌 erector spinae
24. 盲肠 cecum
25. 回肠 ileum
26. 右输尿管 right ureter
27. 肠系膜 mesentery
28. 右卵巢静脉 right ovarian vein
29. 股神经 femoral nerve

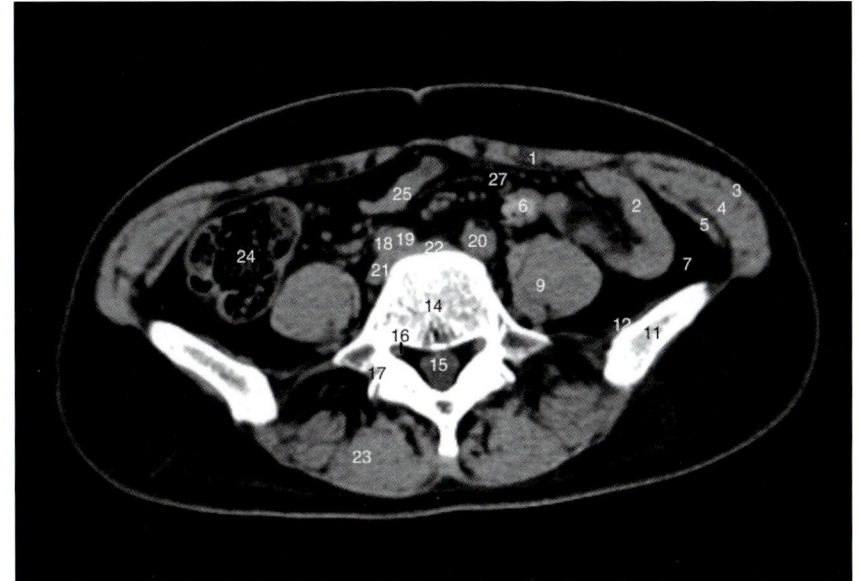
B. CT 平扫图像

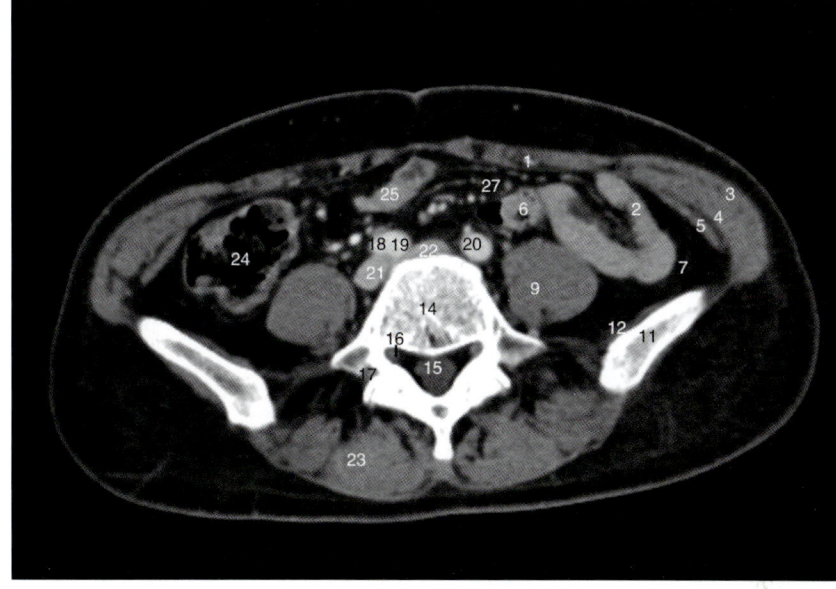
C. CT 增强图像

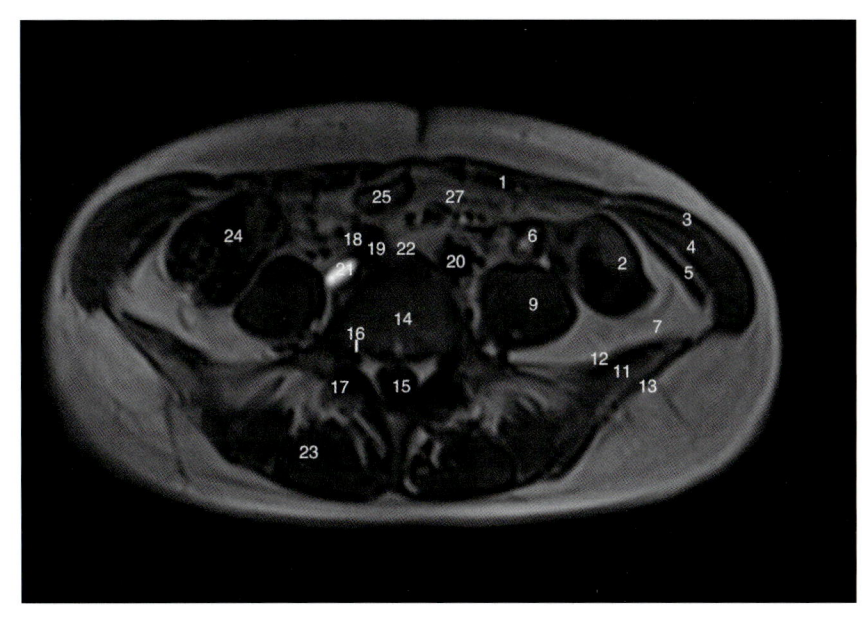
D. MR T1WI

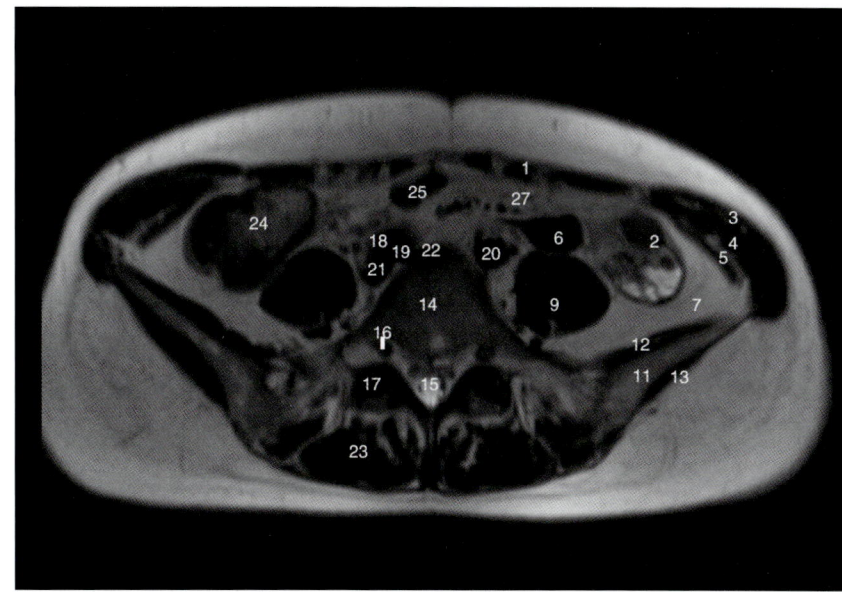
E. MR T2WI

关键结构：髂骨翼，髂肌，回盲部。

此断面经过第5腰椎椎体。

右髂窝内可见回盲部，左髂窝内为乙状结肠。于髂嵴平面以下，降结肠移行为乙状结肠。在断面的前份，可见右侧的回肠和左侧的空肠，大网膜覆盖于前方。髂骨翼是髂骨上部扁阔部分，其上缘为肥厚的弓形骨嵴，称为髂嵴。髂骨翼外侧面有臀中肌附着，内侧面有髂肌附着。髂骨翼内侧的浅凹为髂窝，髂肌起自髂窝，与腰大肌向下合并，经腹股沟韧带深面，止于股骨小转子。高处坠落或体育运动损伤引起髂肌撕裂、出血，使髂肌筋膜内张力增高，压迫股神经和股外侧皮神经可引起髂肌筋膜间隔综合征。组织内压测定可显示肌间隙内压力从正常的零骤升到 1.33~2.66 kPa（10~20 mmHg）甚至 3.99 kPa（30 mmHg）以上。筋膜间隙综合征的后果十分严重，可导致神经干及肌肉坏死，造成肢体畸形及神经麻痹，且后续修复困难。避免出现此种后果的唯一方法就是早期诊断、早期治疗[124]。

腹部连续横断层 122（FH.9490）

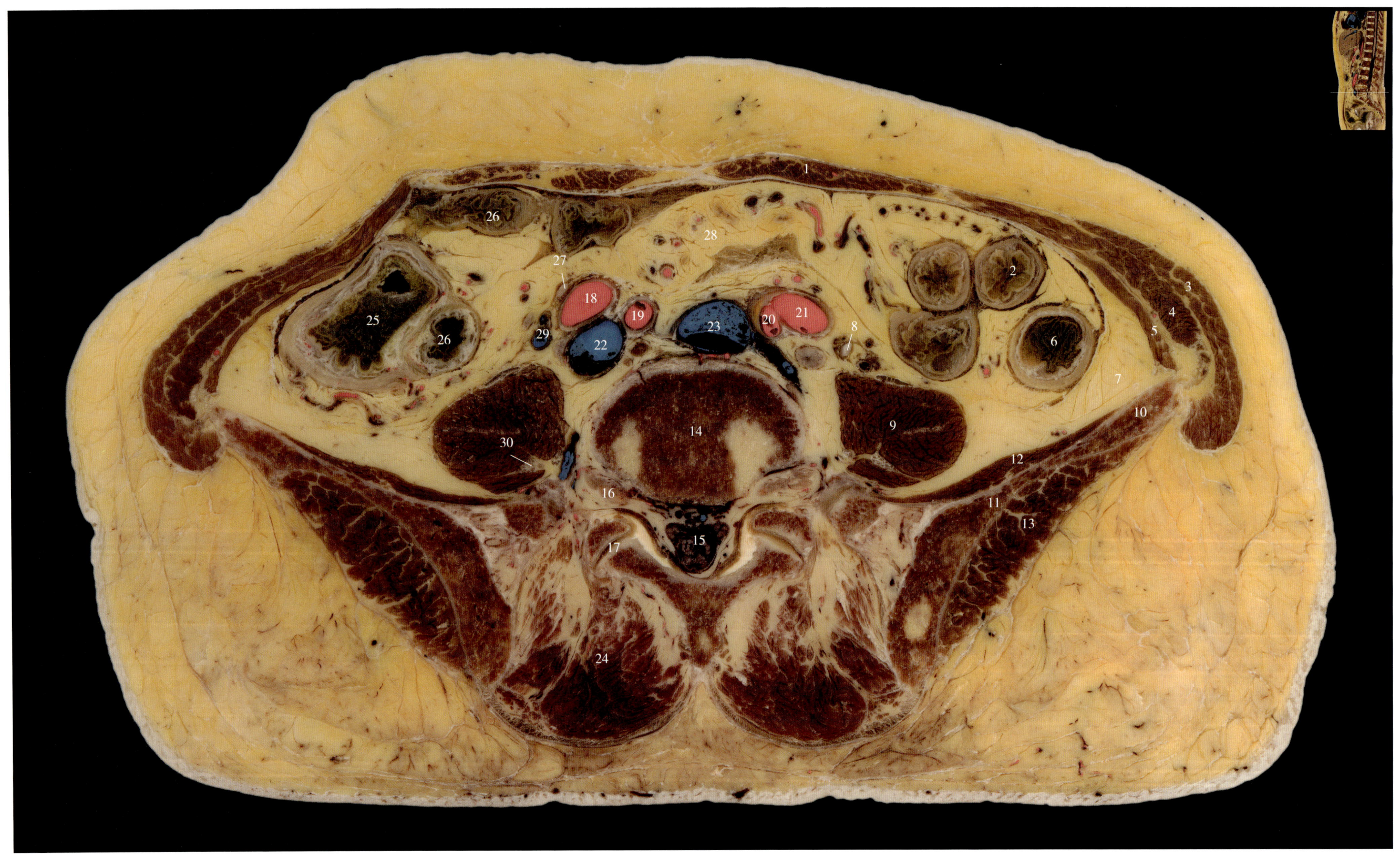

A. 断层标本图像

1. 腹直肌 rectus abdominis
2. 空肠 jejunum
3. 腹外斜肌 obliquus externus abdominis
4. 腹内斜肌 obliquus internus abdominis
5. 腹横肌 transverses abdominis
6. 乙状结肠 sigmoid colon
7. 腹膜外脂肪 extraperitoneal fat
8. 左输尿管 left ureter
9. 腰大肌 psoas major
10. 髂嵴 iliac crest
11. 髂骨翼 ala of ilium
12. 髂肌 iliacus
13. 臀中肌 gluteus medius
14. 第 5 腰椎椎体 body of 5th lumbar vertebra
15. 马尾 cauda equina
16. 第 5 腰神经 5th lumbar nerve
17. 关节突关节 zygapophysial joint
18. 右髂外动脉 right external iliac artery
19. 右髂内动脉 right internal iliac artery
20. 左髂内动脉 left internal iliac artery
21. 左髂外动脉 left external iliac artery
22. 右髂总静脉 right common iliac vein
23. 左髂总静脉 left common iliac vein
24. 竖脊肌 erector spinae
25. 盲肠 cecum
26. 回肠 ileum
27. 右输尿管 right ureter
28. 肠系膜 mesentery
29. 右卵巢静脉 right ovarian vein
30. 股神经 femoral nerve
31. 左髂总动脉 left common iliac artery

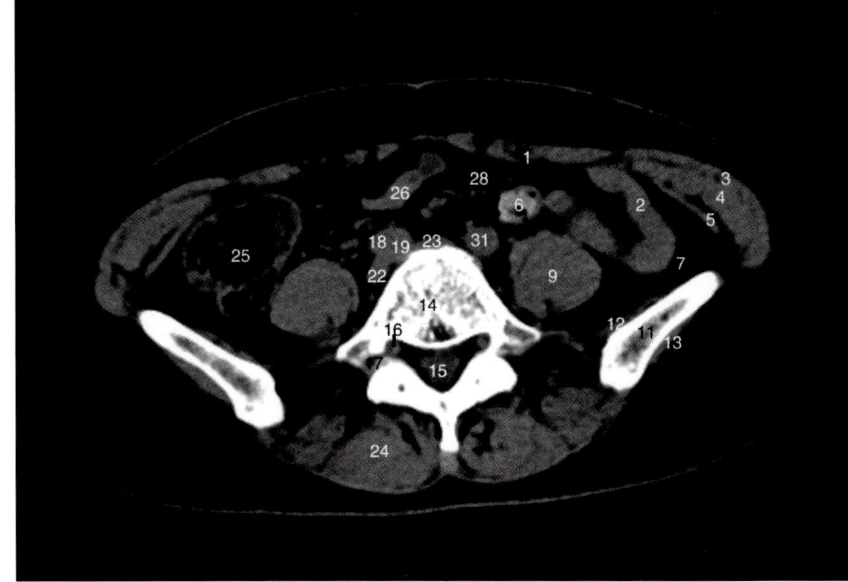

B. CT 平扫图像

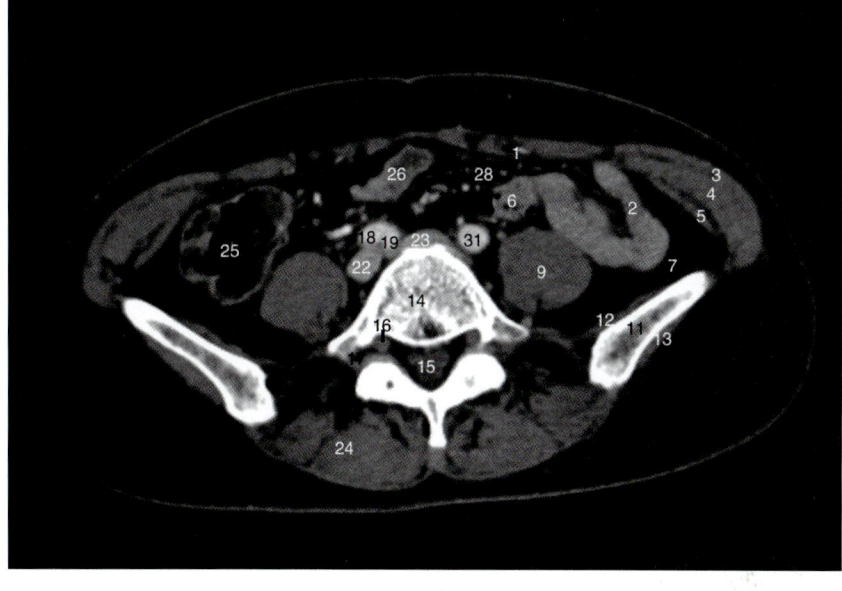

C. CT 增强图像

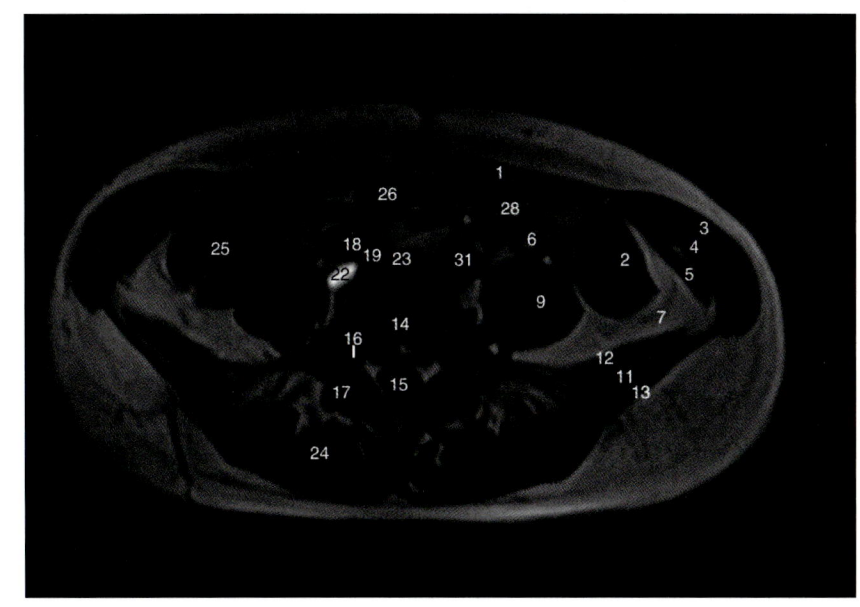

D. MR T1WI

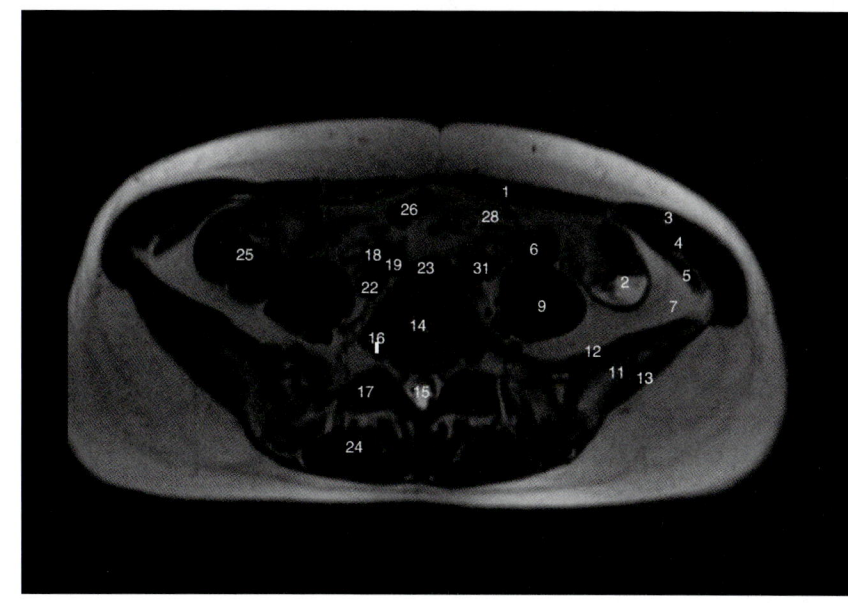

E. MR T2WI

关键结构：左髂外动脉，左髂内动脉，股神经。

此断面经过第 5 腰椎椎体。

左、右髂总静脉仍在椎体前方走行，右髂内、外动脉位于右髂总静脉前方。左髂总动脉在此断面分成左髂内动脉与左髂外动脉。腹腔右前份可见回肠和盲肠相交汇。在左髂窝中有乙状结肠下行，其系膜连于左腰大肌的内侧。右输尿管位于右髂外动脉右侧，左输尿管位于腰大肌与左髂外动脉之间。髂外动脉分支有腹壁下动脉和旋髂深动脉。腹壁下动脉是髂外动脉在穿越腹股沟韧带之前发出的分支，并于腹直肌深面与腹壁上动脉吻合。旋髂深动脉平腹壁下动脉起点自髂外动脉发出，分布于髂嵴及附近的腹肌。经皮动脉栓塞是治疗盆腔肿瘤的新兴治疗方式，但由于盆腔肿瘤患者常有膀胱和阴道出血等症状，若术中肿瘤供血血管栓塞不完全，不但无法抑制肿瘤生长，而且临床止血效果差。行盆腔肿瘤 TACE 时，常规做髂内动脉造影。近期研究发现在常规髂内动脉造影的基础上，进行双侧髂外动脉造影明确有无髂外动脉异常供血，栓塞全部肿瘤供血血管可保证介入栓塞效果[125]。

腹部连续横断层 123（FH.9470）

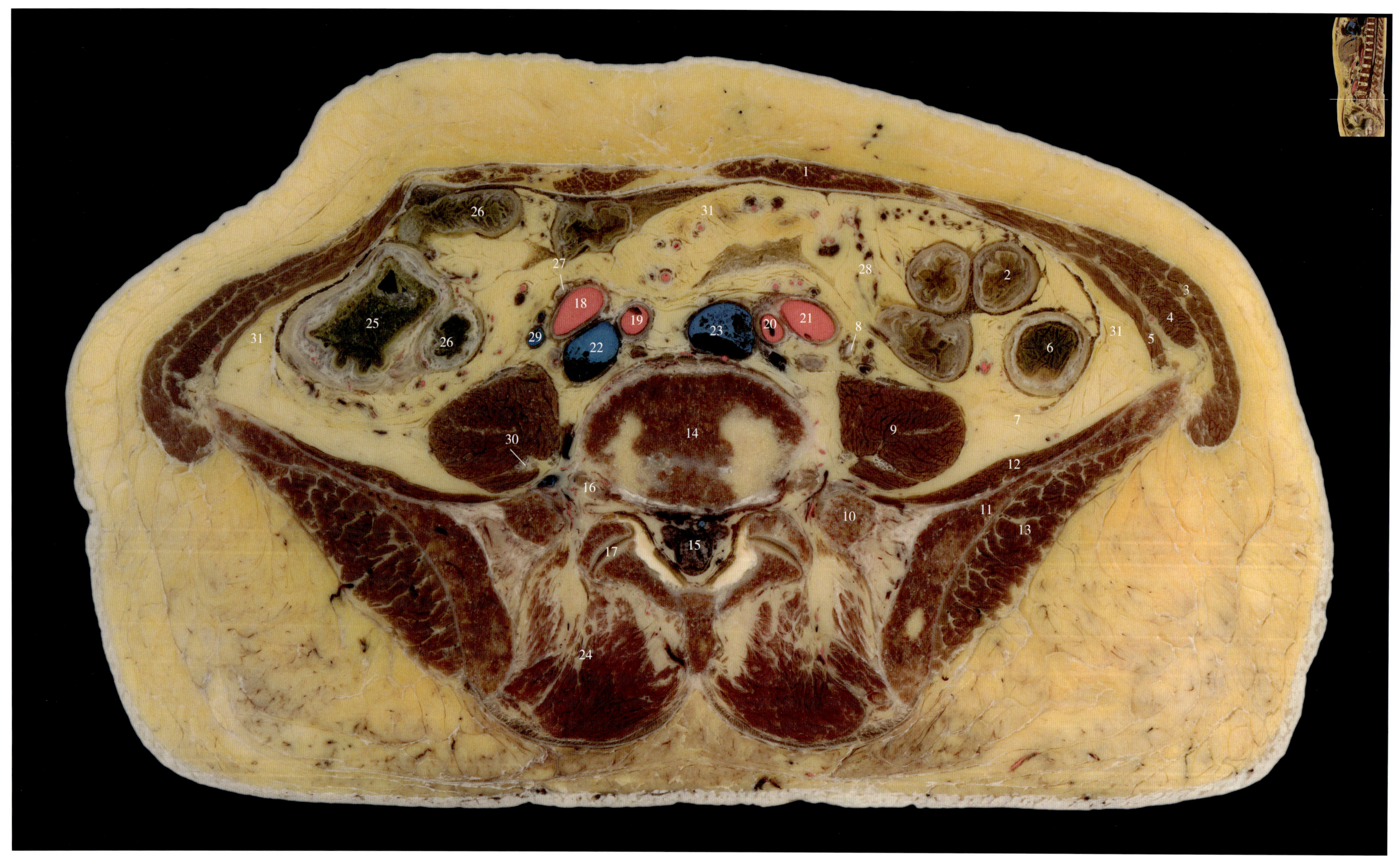

A. 断层标本图像

1. 腹直肌 rectus abdominis
2. 空肠 jejunum
3. 腹外斜肌 obliquus externus abdominis
4. 腹内斜肌 obliquus internus abdominis
5. 腹横肌 transverses abdominis
6. 乙状结肠 sigmoid colon
7. 腹膜外脂肪 extraperitoneal fat
8. 左输尿管 left ureter
9. 腰大肌 psoas majar
10. 骶翼 ala of sacrum
11. 髂骨翼 ala of ilium
12. 髂肌 iliacus
13. 臀中肌 gluteus medius
14. 第5腰椎椎体 body of 5th lumbar vertebra
15. 马尾 cauda equina
16. 第5腰神经 5th lumbar nerve
17. 关节突关节 zygapophysial joint
18. 右髂外动脉 right external iliac artery
19. 右髂内动脉 right internal iliac artery
20. 左髂内动脉 left internal iliac artery
21. 左髂外动脉 left external iliac artery
22. 右髂总静脉 right common iliac vein
23. 左髂总静脉 left common iliac vein
24. 竖脊肌 erector spinae
25. 盲肠 cecum
26. 回肠 ileum
27. 右输尿管 right ureter
28. 肠系膜 mesentery
29. 右卵巢静脉 right ovarian vein
30. 股神经 femoral nerve
31. 大网膜 greater omentum
32. 左髂总动脉 left common iliac artery

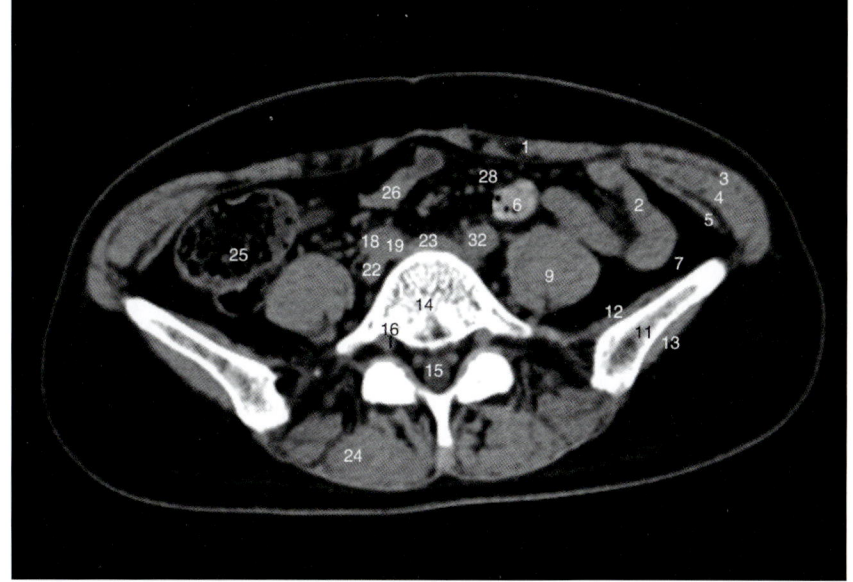

B. CT 平扫图像

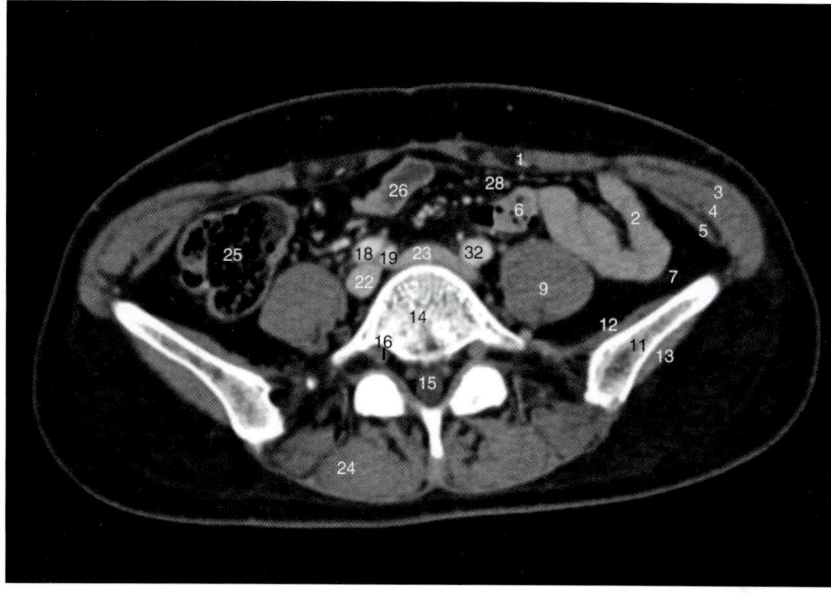

C. CT 增强图像

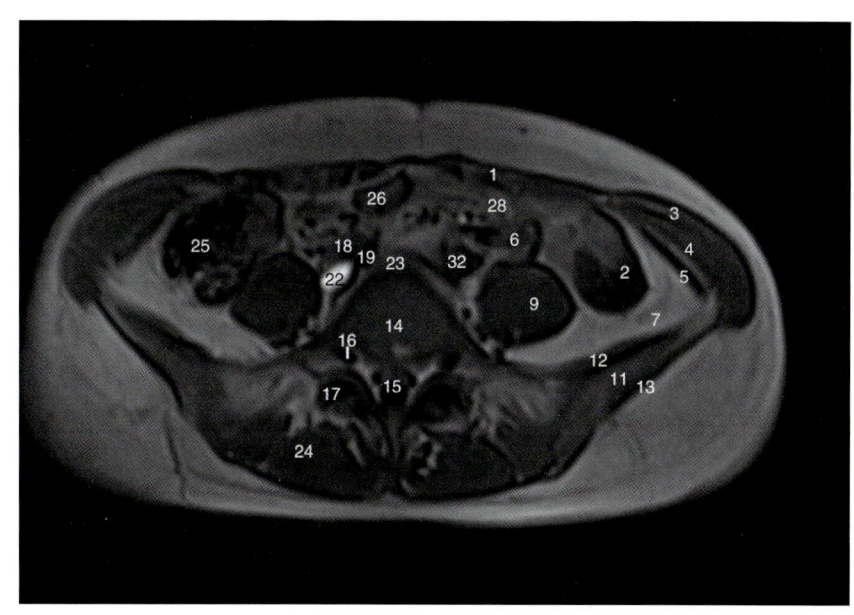

D. MR T1WI

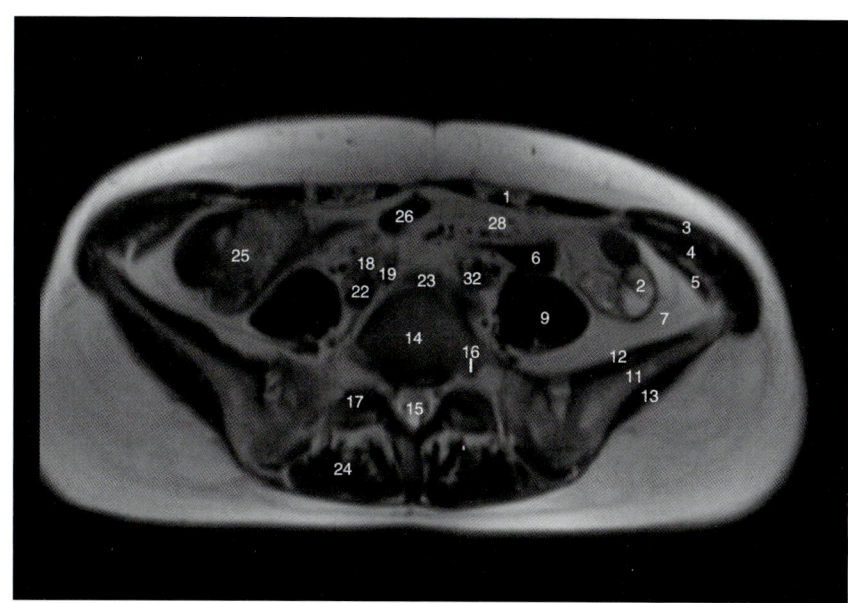

E. MR T2WI

关键结构：大网膜，肠系膜，右卵巢静脉。

此断面经过第5腰椎椎体。

大网膜位于腹腔前部，腹腔内结构同上一断面。大网膜是连接胃大弯和十二指肠起始部与横结肠之间的4层腹膜结构，呈围裙状下垂，遮盖于横结肠和小肠的前面，薄而透明，并含有大量脂肪。大网膜的长度是指从胃大弯中点到大网膜下缘之间的距离，宽度是指大网膜两侧缘中点之间的距离。大网膜的厚度以脂肪多少而定，根据大网膜血管周围和血管间区脂肪含量以及大网膜的透明程度分为薄、中、厚3型。薄型指大网膜的血管周围有脂肪，血管间区基本无脂肪，大网膜薄而透明；厚型指大网膜的血管周围及血管间区的脂肪均多，大网膜不透明；中型指大网摸的脂肪和透明度介于薄型与厚型之间。大网膜扭转是一种引起儿童急性腹痛的罕见疾病，以右下腹疼痛多见，分为原发性大网膜扭转和继发性大网膜扭转。大多情况下大网膜围绕其长轴顺时针扭转，继而出现大网膜水肿、缺血、坏死等病理改变。X线和超声对于大网膜扭转诊断的敏感性和特异性不高。大网膜扭转的CT图像表现为大网膜中存在模糊的同心线性脂肪块状结构，对诊断大网膜扭转具有较高的准确性，但手术探查仍是确诊的重要方法。大网膜扭转治疗方法主要是腹腔镜手术和保守治疗[126]。

腹部连续横断层 124（FH.9450）

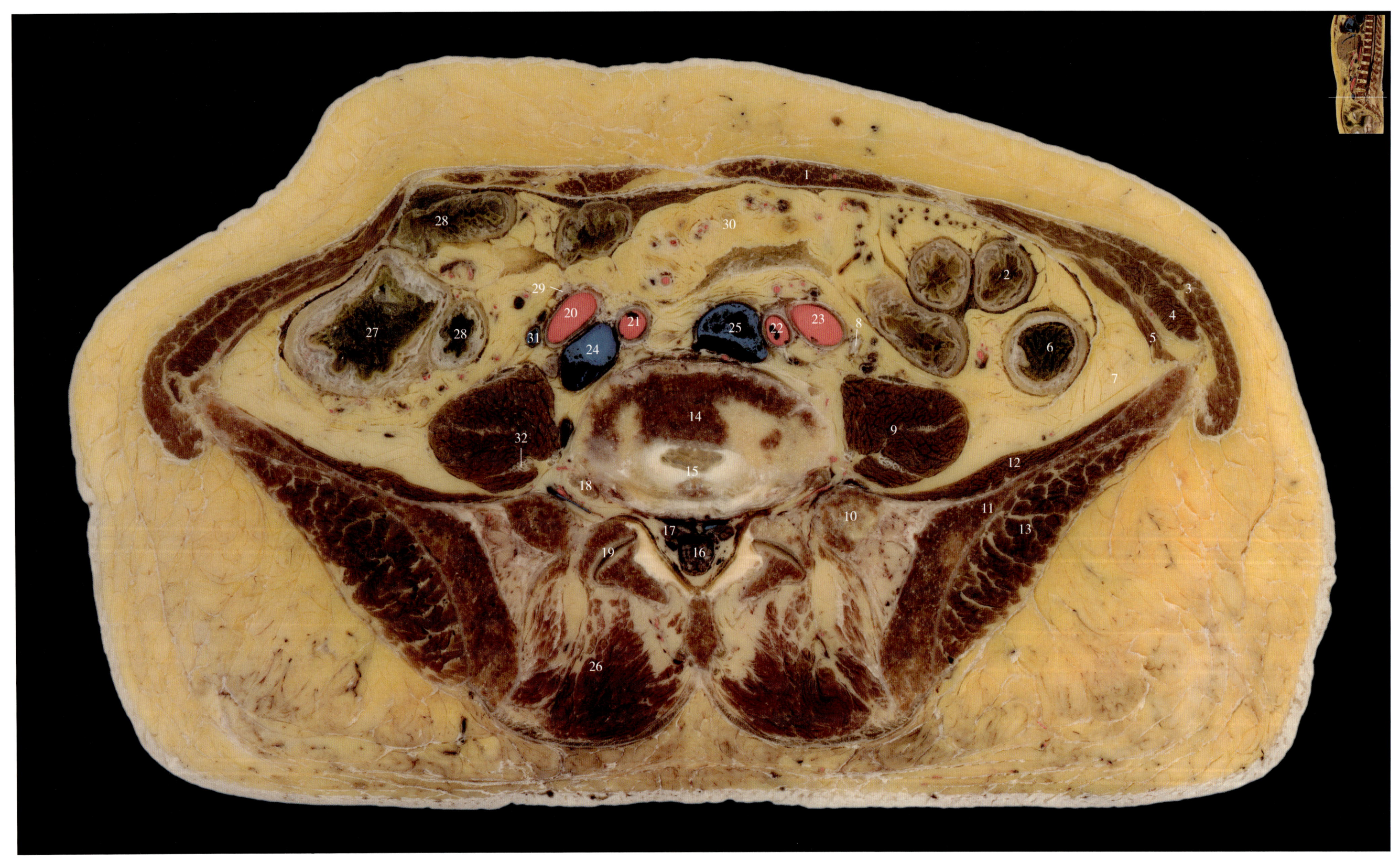

A. 断层标本图像

1. 腹直肌 rectus abdominis
2. 空肠 jejunum
3. 腹外斜肌 obliquus externus abdominis
4. 腹内斜肌 obliquus internus abdominis
5. 腹横肌 transverses abdominis
6. 乙状结肠 sigmoid colon
7. 腹膜外脂肪 extraperitoneal fat
8. 左输尿管 left ureter
9. 腰大肌 psoas major
10. 骶骨 sacrum
11. 髂骨翼 ala of ilium
12. 髂肌 iliacus
13. 臀中肌 gluteus medius
14. 第 5 腰椎椎体 body of 5th lumbar vertebra
15. L5-S1 椎间盘 L5-S1 intervertebral disc
16. 马尾 cauda equina
17. 第 1 骶神经 1st sacral nerve
18. 第 5 腰神经 5th lumbar nerve
19. 关节突关节 zygapophysial joint
20. 右髂外动脉 right external iliac artery
21. 右髂内动脉 right internal iliac artery
22. 左髂内动脉 left internal iliac artery
23. 左髂外动脉 left external iliac artery
24. 右髂总静脉 right common iliac vein
25. 左髂总静脉 left common iliac vein
26. 竖脊肌 erector spinae
27. 盲肠 cecum
28. 回肠 ileum
29. 右输尿管 right ureter
30. 肠系膜 mesentery
31. 右卵巢静脉 right ovarian vein
32. 股神经 femoral nerve

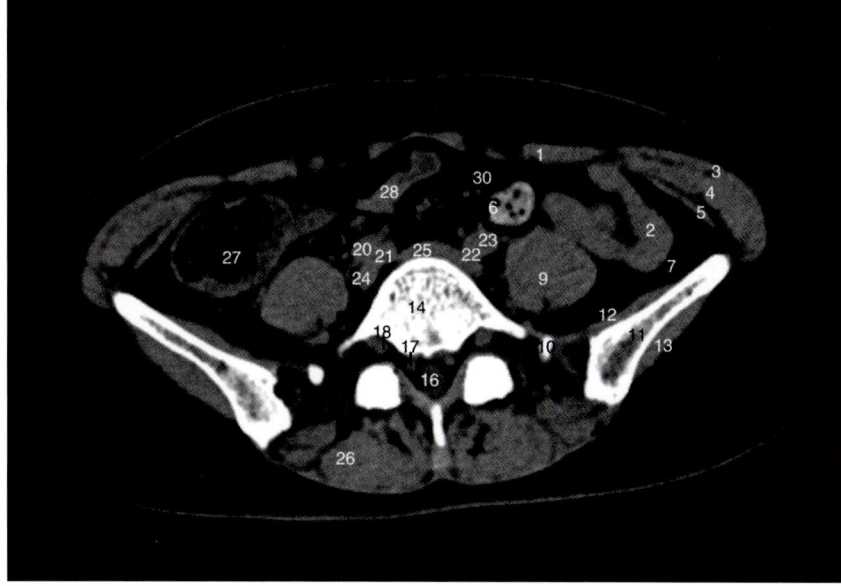

B. CT 平扫图像

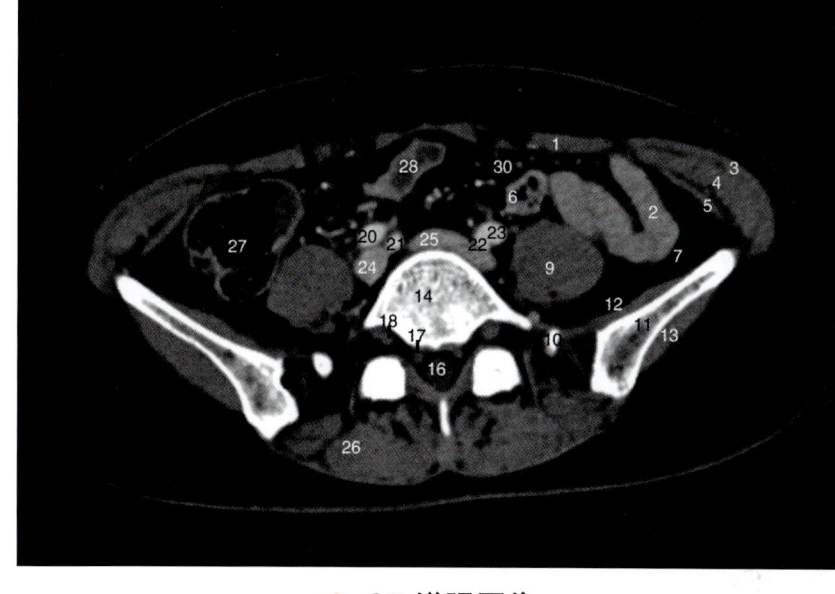

C. CT 增强图像

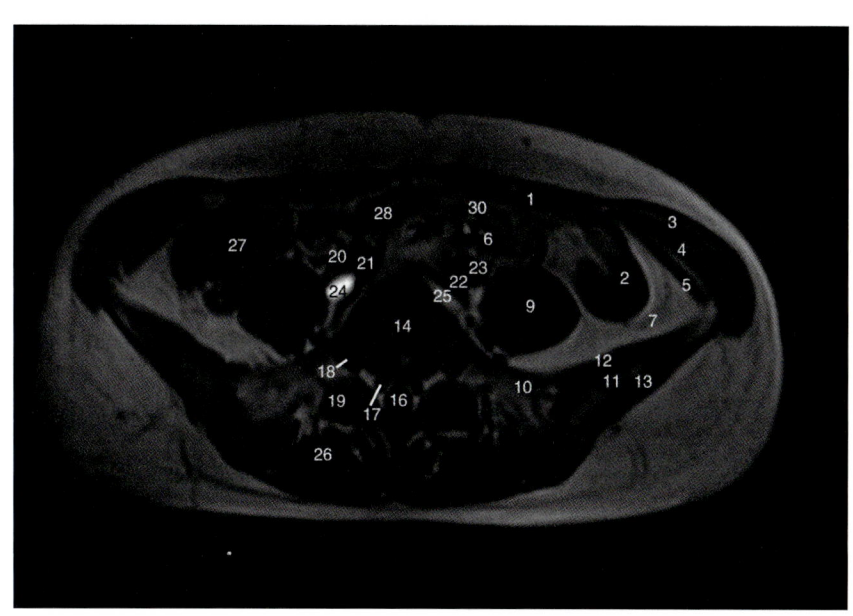

D. MR T1WI

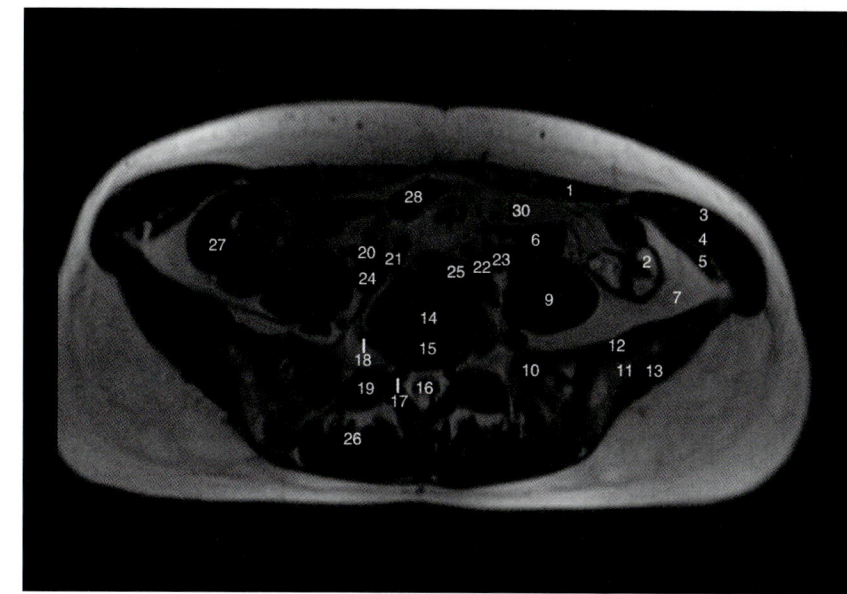

E. MR T2WI

关键结构：腹外斜肌，腹内斜肌，腹横肌，腹直肌。

此断面经过第 5 腰椎椎体。

腹直肌居腹前壁中线的两侧，腹直肌的两侧由浅至深分别有腹外斜肌、腹内斜肌和腹横肌，这 3 层肌肉在腹直肌的外侧缘延续为腱膜。腹内斜肌腱膜在腹直肌上 2/3 的外侧缘分为 2 层，前层与上方的腹外斜肌腱膜愈着构成腹直肌鞘的前层，后层与下方的腹横肌腱膜愈着构成腹直肌鞘的后层。但在腹直肌下 1/3、脐下 4~5 cm 处的下方，腹直肌鞘的后层完全转到腹直肌的前面与前层愈着，腹直肌鞘后层阙如，腹直肌后面直接与腹横筋膜相贴。梨状腹综合征是一种罕见的腹壁先天发育畸形，腹壁薄而松，因为缺少皮下组织而形成皱褶，像枯萎的梅干，也称梅干腹综合征。腹壁缺陷是其主要特点之一，患者腹直肌上部及腹外斜肌发育不良，腹壁下内侧腹肌阙如。产前 B 超可发现梨状腹综合征，胎儿 MRI 能够提供更多的诊断和评估信息[127]。

腹前外侧 3 层腹肌的腱膜向内包绕腹直肌形成腹直肌鞘后在两侧腹直肌内侧缘相互交织形成白线，如果在相互交织的结缔组织束之间留有裂隙，可发生白线疝。约在白线中点处有疏松的瘢痕组织区，称脐环，该处可发生脐疝[2]。

腹部连续横断层 125（FH.9430）

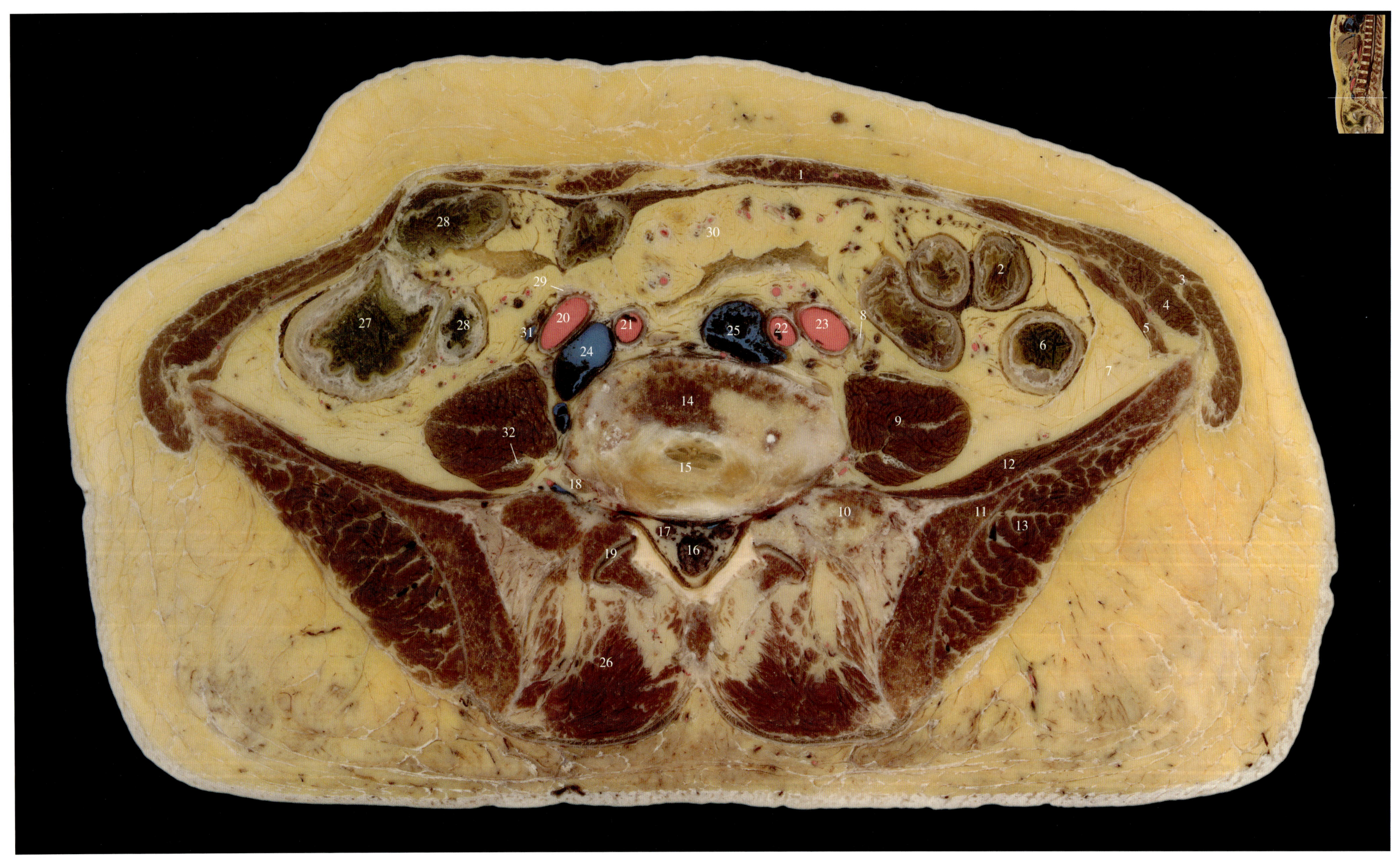

A. 断层标本图像

1. 腹直肌 rectus abdominis
2. 空肠 jejunum
3. 腹外斜肌 obliquus externus abdominis
4. 腹内斜肌 obliquus internus abdominis
5. 腹横肌 transverses abdominis
6. 乙状结肠 sigmoid colon
7. 腹膜外脂肪 extraperitoneal fat
8. 左输尿管 left ureter
9. 腰大肌 psoas major
10. 骶翼 ala of sacrum
11. 髂骨翼 ala of ilium
12. 髂肌 iliacus
13. 臀中肌 gluteus medius
14. 第5腰椎椎体 body of 5th lumbar vertebra
15. L5-S1 椎间盘 L5-S1 intervertebral disc
16. 马尾 cauda equina
17. 第1骶神经 1st sacral nerve
18. 第5腰神经 5th lumbar nerve
19. 关节突关节 zygapophysial joint
20. 右髂外动脉 right external iliac artery
21. 右髂内动脉 right internal iliac artery
22. 左髂内动脉 left internal iliac artery
23. 左髂外动脉 left external iliac artery
24. 右髂总静脉 right common iliac vein
25. 左髂总静脉 left common iliac vein
26. 竖脊肌 erector spinae
27. 盲肠 cecum
28. 回肠 ileum
29. 右输尿管 right ureter
30. 肠系膜 mesentery
31. 右卵巢静脉 right ovarian vein
32. 股神经 femoral nerve

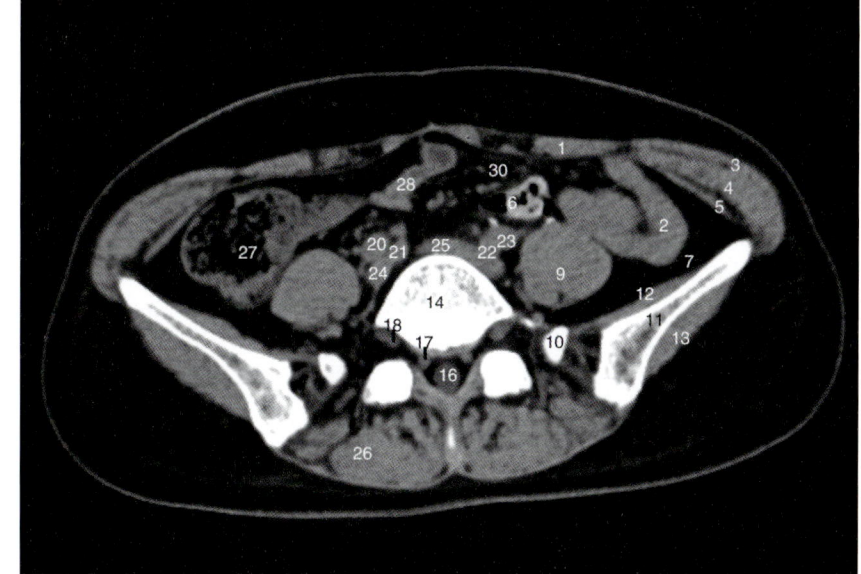

B. CT 平扫图像

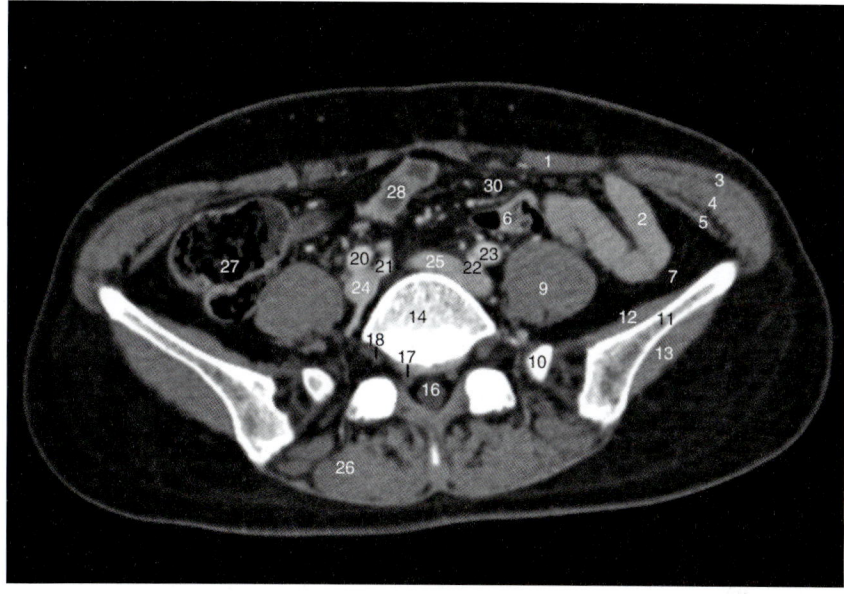

C. CT 增强图像

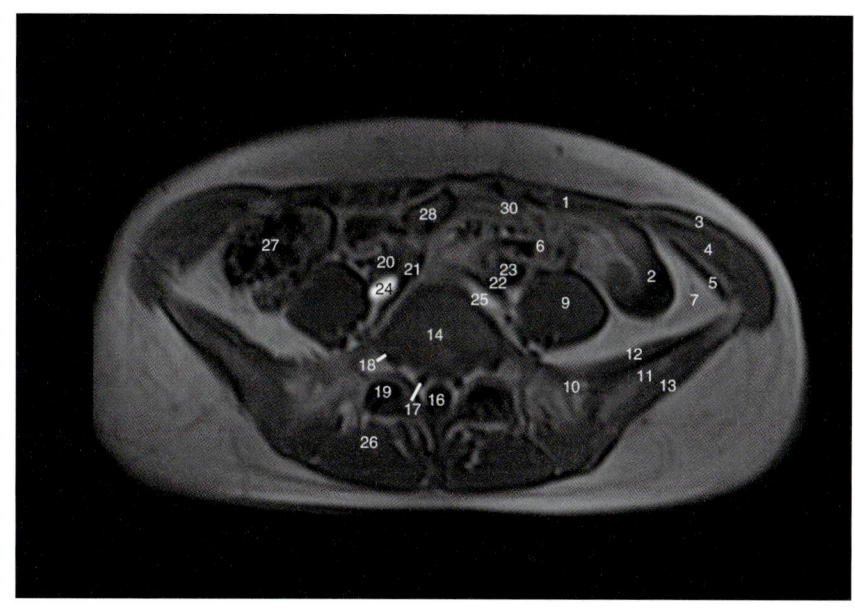

D. MR T1WI

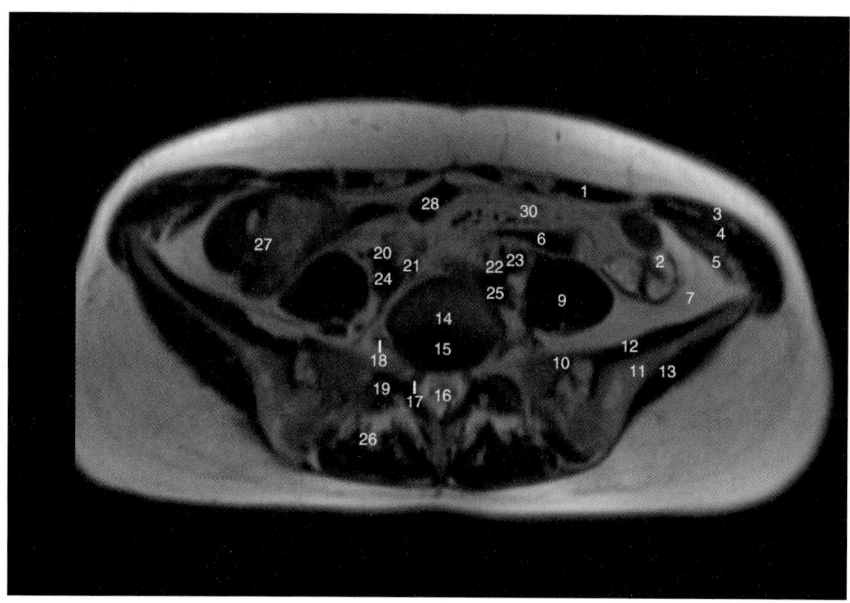

E. MR T2WI

关键结构：空肠，回肠，输尿管。

此断面经第5腰椎椎体下份。

空肠位于结肠下区左上方，接近十二指肠空肠曲，部分空肠肠袢可能向下落入盆腔内。从空肠到回肠的管腔直径和管壁厚度逐渐减小。空肠血管密度高，血液供应丰富，消化吸收功能强，表面呈肉红色，管腔大、管壁厚。间质瘤是独立起源于胃肠道间质干细胞的肿瘤，空肠是其好发部位之一。CT 显示空肠间质瘤的优势为：图像具有较高的组织对比，可清晰地显示肠管管腔、管壁及周围结构。间质瘤的肿块呈多种形态，以外生为主，大多数边界清晰，多不直接沿肠壁浸润蔓延，邻近管壁柔软无增厚。即使是巨大的恶性肿瘤，对周围浸润也相对轻微，与正常肠壁分界清晰，仅表现为边缘模糊。肿块密度可均匀或不均匀，内部出血、坏死显著。肿块多为富血供性，肿瘤实质中等以上强化，可有肝脏、腹膜转移，但周围淋巴结转移罕见。空肠和回肠的淋巴形成于肠绒毛中心的乳糜管，经肠壁的淋巴管丛汇集成淋巴管，伴血管走行，注入肠系淋巴结。肠结核不仅可以累及肠壁的淋巴小结，也可能累及肠系膜淋巴结，形成肿块或寒性脓肿。肠系膜淋巴结位于肠系膜内，约有160个，可分为3组：第1组位于肠的系膜缘处肠管壁附近，小肠动脉终末支之间；第2组位于空肠和回肠的各级动脉弓之间；第3组位于肠系膜根部，沿空肠动脉和回肠动脉起始部排列，淋巴结较大，其输出管注入肠系膜上淋巴结[26]。

腹部连续横断层 126（FH.9410）

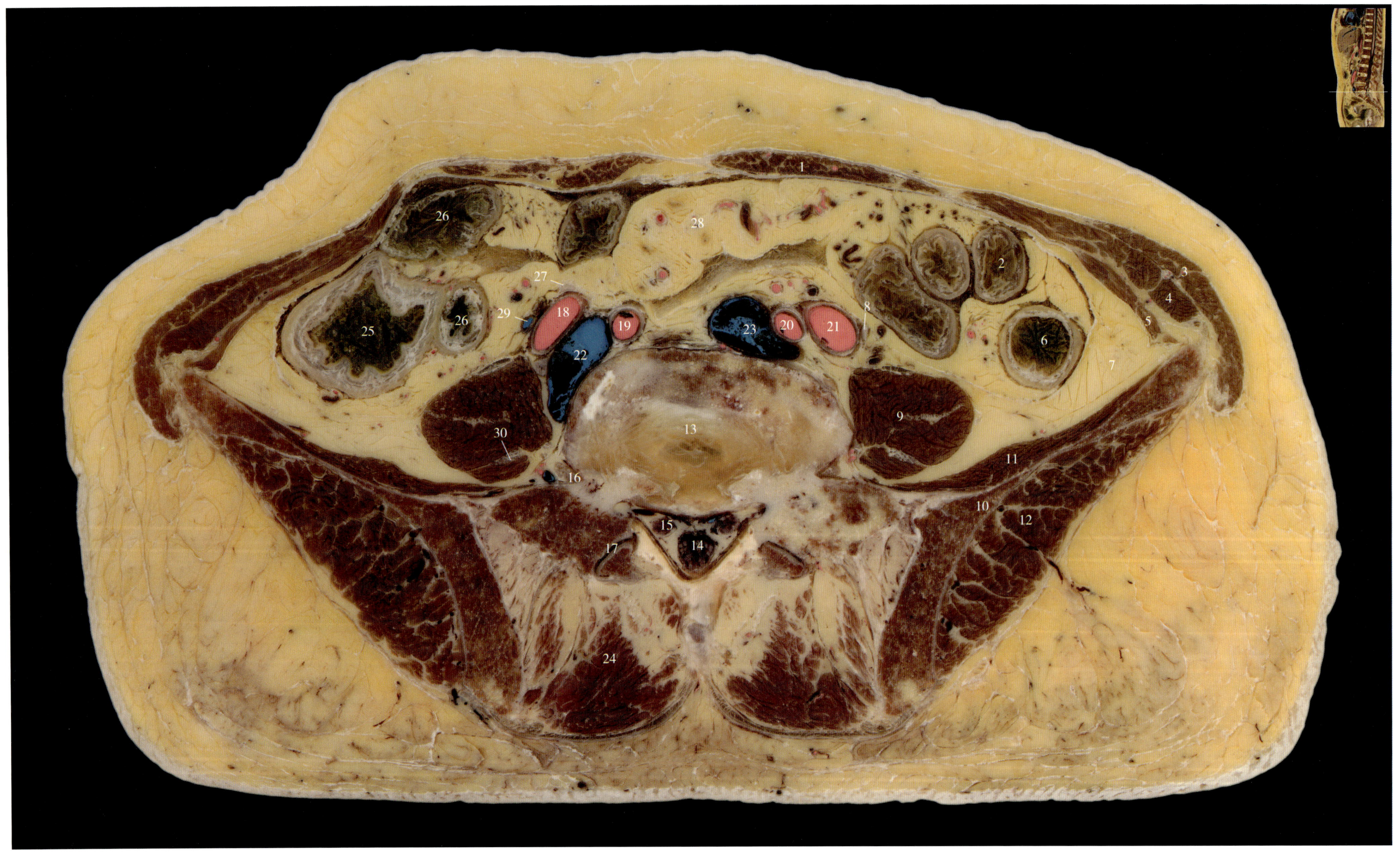

A. 断层标本图像

1. 腹直肌 rectus abdominis
2. 空肠 jejunum
3. 腹外斜肌 obliquus externus abdominis
4. 腹内斜肌 obliquus internus abdominis
5. 腹横肌 transverses abdominis
6. 乙状结肠 sigmoid colon
7. 腹膜外脂肪 extraperitoneal fat
8. 左输尿管 left ureter
9. 腰大肌 psoas major
10. 髂骨翼 ala of ilium
11. 髂肌 iliacus
12. 臀中肌 gluteus medius
13. L5-S1 椎间盘 L5-S1 intervertebral disc
14. 马尾 cauda equina
15. 第1骶神经 1st sacral nerve
16. 第5腰神经 5th lumbar nerve
17. 关节突关节 zygapophysial joint
18. 右髂外动脉 right external iliac artery
19. 右髂内动脉 right internal iliac artery
20. 左髂内动脉 left internal iliac artery
21. 左髂外动脉 left external iliac artery
22. 右髂总静脉 right common iliac vein
23. 左髂总静脉 left common iliac vein
24. 竖脊肌 erector spinae
25. 盲肠 cecum
26. 回肠 ileum
27. 右输尿管 right ureter
28. 肠系膜 mesentery
29. 右卵巢静脉 right ovarian vein
30. 股神经 femoral nerve

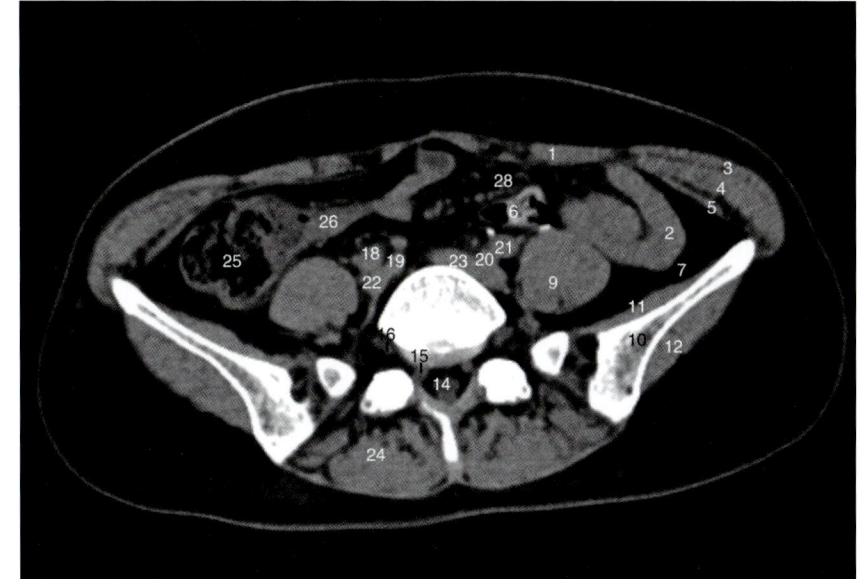

B. CT 平扫图像

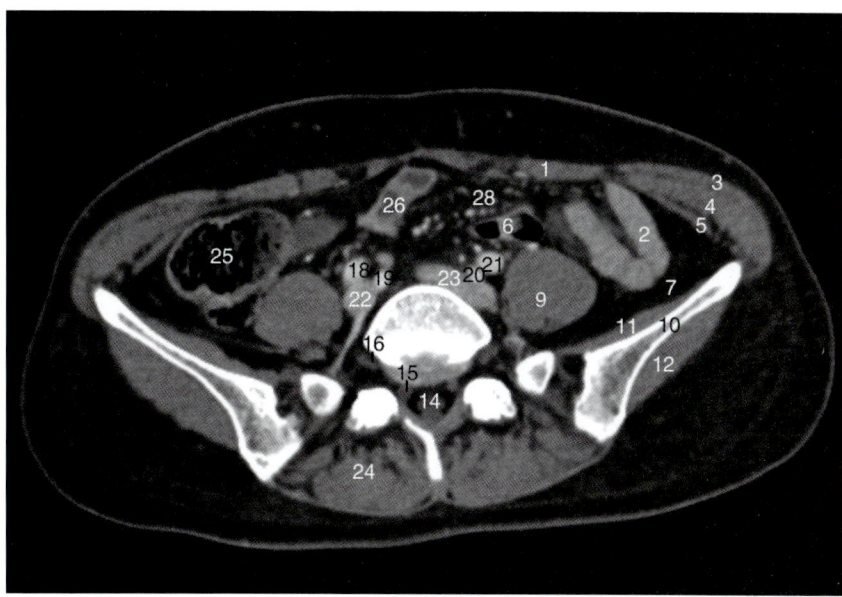

C. CT 增强图像

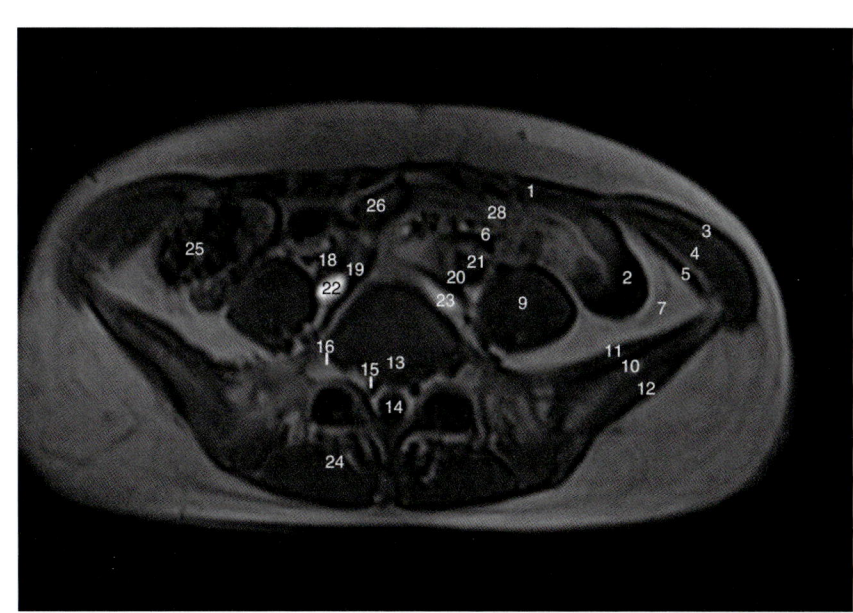

D. MR T1WI

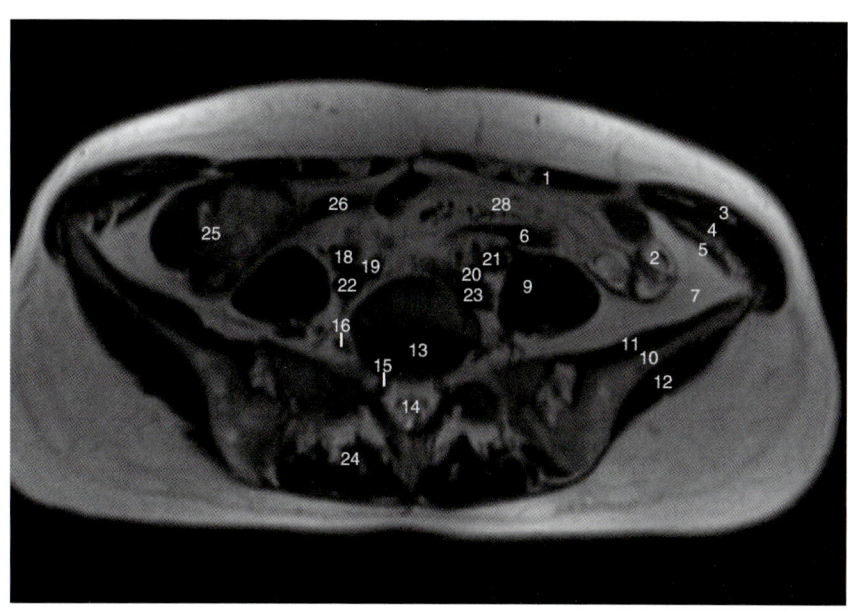

E. MR T2WI

关键结构：输尿管，股神经，髂血管。

此断面经过 L5–S1 椎间盘。

L5~S1 椎间盘前方的两侧分别有左、右髂总静脉和髂内、外动脉，左髂外动脉的左侧和右髂外动脉的前方有输尿管走行。输尿管结核是由于肾结核的结核菌下行至输尿管所引起的结核病变，患者多有肺结核或肾结核病史。输尿管狭窄、变硬、增粗和僵直，甚至完全梗阻。影像学表现为：①静脉尿路造影检查，早期输尿管结核主要表现为输尿管扩张，粗细不一，边缘不规则，失去自然形态，有时呈串珠状；晚期表现为挛缩而僵直，可有条索状钙化。重度输尿管狭窄可造成患侧肾脏及输尿管不显影。②CT 检查，只有大范围的连续扫描，才能显示输尿管中段和远端的狭窄，否则只能显示肾盂及输尿管的扩张。对近端输尿管狭窄，CT 在显示肾结核的同时，常能显示输尿管管壁增厚、管腔多发狭窄与扩张，以及管壁的钙化等，可与输尿管结石相鉴别[128]。此外，郑丽梅等通过 65 例女性盆腔 CTA 数据，观察输尿管腹盆段与周围结构的毗邻关系，发现输尿管跨越髂动脉后方的结构有以下几种：髂总动脉、髂总动脉分叉、髂外动脉。其中左侧输尿管后方结构为髂总动脉占 33.84%，髂总动脉分叉处占 13.85%，髂外动脉占 55.38%；右侧输尿管后方结构中，髂总动脉占 27.7%，髂总动脉分叉占 20.0%，髂外动脉占 52.3%。输尿管与血管间的水平距离为：①腹主动脉分叉处与输尿管的水平间距，左侧为 32.45 mm ± 6.24 mm，右侧为 39.3 mm ± 5.78 mm；②左、右髂总动脉分叉处与输尿管的水平间距，左侧为 10.55 mm ± 4.85 mm，右侧为 13.34 mm ± 5.49 mm；③左、右髂内动脉分叉处与输尿管的水平间距，左侧为 10.88 mm ± 5.55 mm，右侧为 9.97 mm ± 6.14 mm[129]。

腹部连续横断层 127（FH.9390）

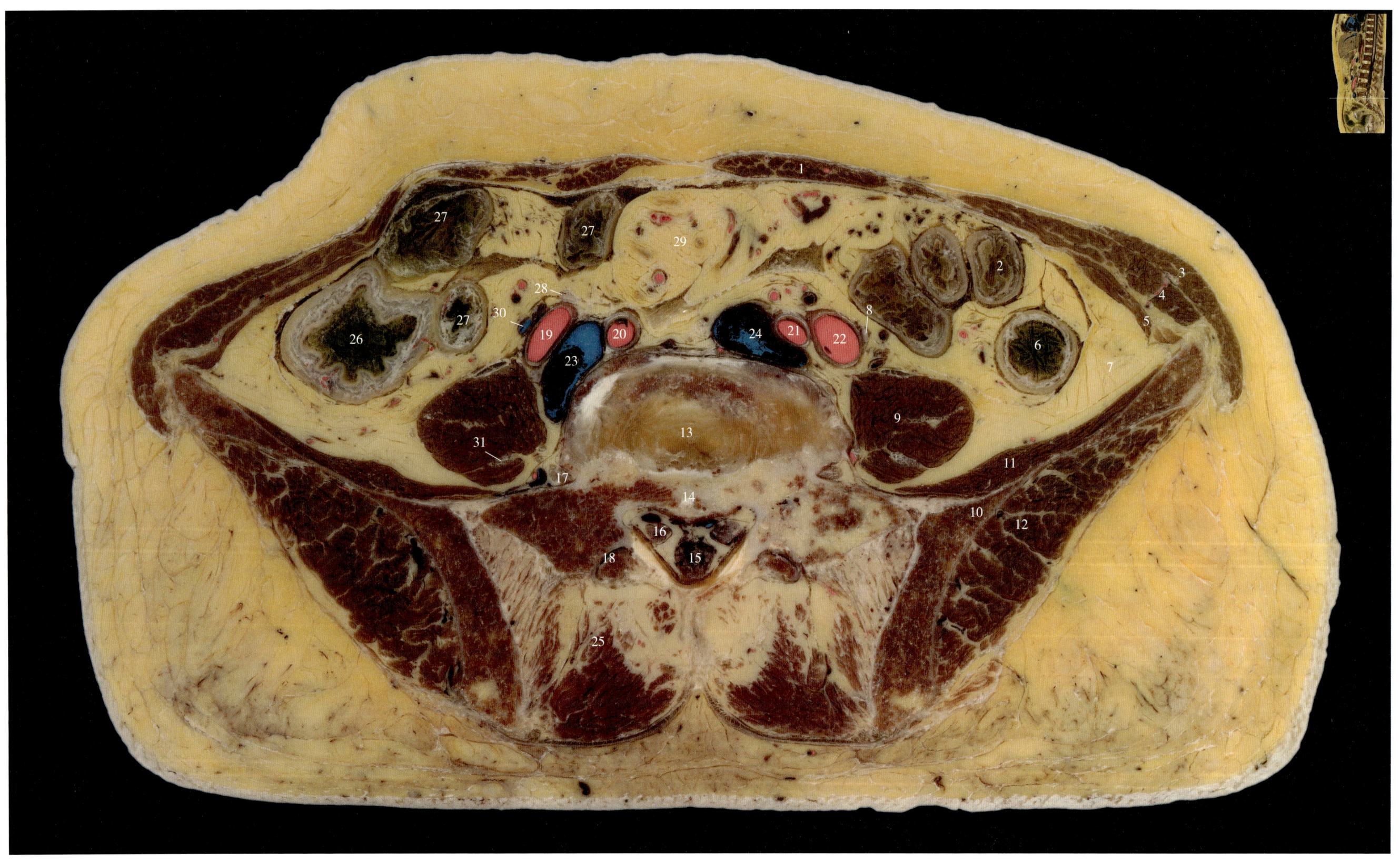

A. 断层标本图像

1. 腹直肌 rectus abdominis
2. 空肠 jejunum
3. 腹外斜肌 obliquus externus abdominis
4. 腹内斜肌 obliquus internus abdominis
5. 腹横肌 transverses abdominis
6. 乙状结肠 sigmoid colon
7. 腹膜外脂肪 extraperitoneal fat
8. 左输尿管 left ureter
9. 腰大肌 psoas majar
10. 髂骨翼 ala of ilium
11. 髂肌 iliacus
12. 臀中肌 gluteus medius
13. L5-S1 椎间盘 L5-S1 intervertebral disc
14. 第 1 骶椎 1st sacral vertebra
15. 马尾 cauda equina
16. 第 1 骶神经 1st sacral nerve
17. 第 5 腰神经 5th lumbar nerve
18. 关节突关节 zygapophysial joint
19. 右髂外动脉 right external iliac artery
20. 右髂内动脉 right internal iliac artery
21. 左髂内动脉 left internal iliac artery
22. 左髂外动脉 left external iliac artery
23. 右髂总静脉 right common iliac vein
24. 左髂总静脉 left common iliac vein
25. 竖脊肌 erector spinae
26. 盲肠 cecum
27. 回肠 ileum
28. 右输尿管 right ureter
29. 肠系膜 mesentery
30. 右卵巢静脉 right ovarian vein
31. 股神经 femoral nerve

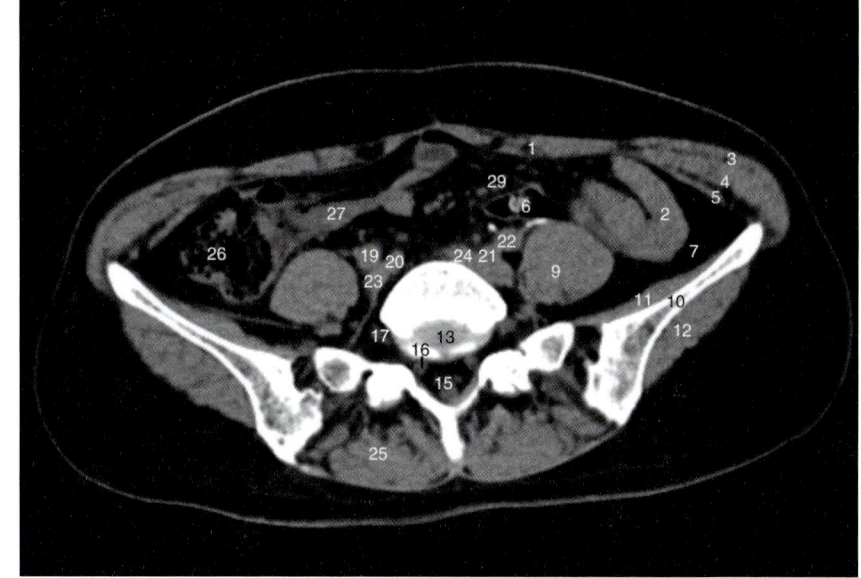

B. CT 平扫图像

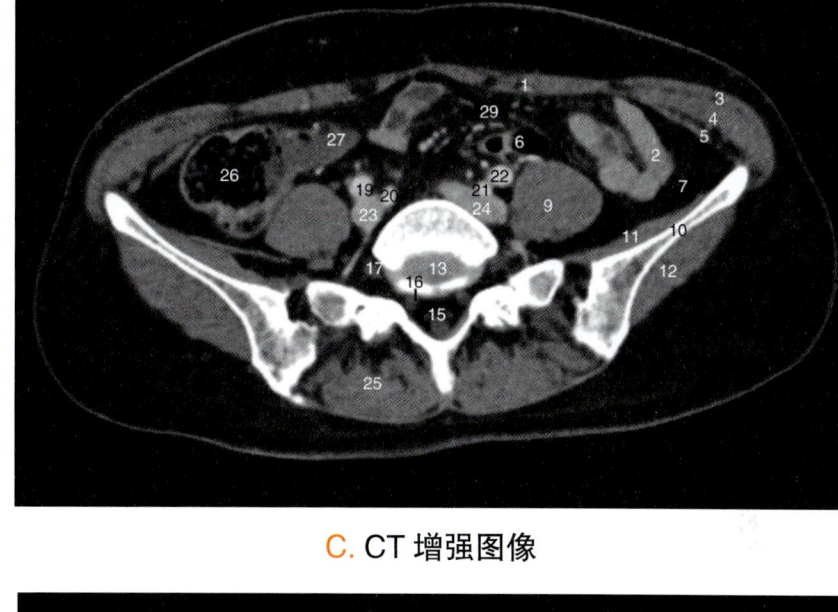

C. CT 增强图像

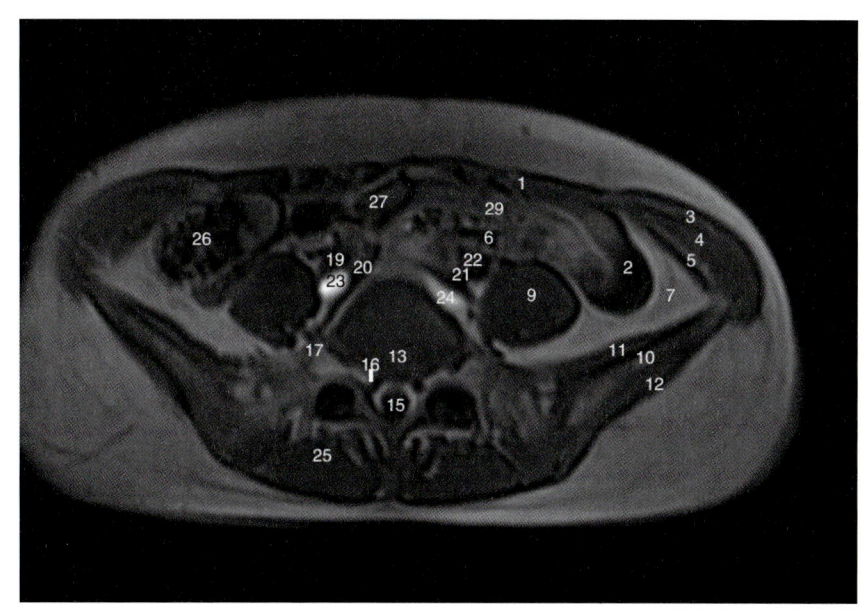

D. MR T1WI

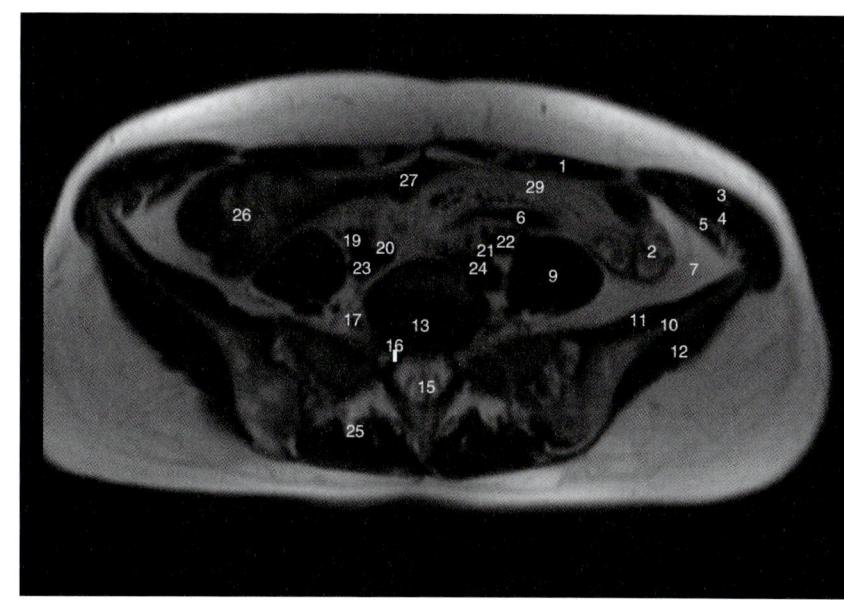

E. MR T2WI

关键结构：第 5 腰神经，马尾，第 1 骶神经。

此断面经过第 1 骶椎椎体。

第 1 骶椎的两侧可见第 5 腰神经走行，腰神经有 5 对，第 1~5 腰神经逐渐增大，第 5 腰神经是所有腰神经中最大的一对，但是第 5 腰椎椎间孔却比另外 4 个都要小，因此第 5 腰神经更易受到压迫。腰神经出椎间孔后分 4 支，较细的有脊膜支和交通支，较粗大的有前支和后支。第 5 腰神经后支比其他腰神经后支长，内侧支在第 1 骶椎上关节突根部呈拱形骑跨在骶骨翼上，在腰骶关节底部的后面发出 1 个分支进入腰最长肌最下部纤维，并以内侧支作为终末支钩绕腰骶关节周围，终止于多裂肌之前发出交通支汇入第 1 骶神经后支。第 5 腰神经前支与第 4 腰神经前支的一小部分合成腰骶干，与第 1、2 骶神经连接形成骶丛上干[27]。病因未明的腰背痛或伴有下肢痛称为"非特异性腰痛"，其中"腰神经后支综合征"约占非特异性腰痛的 80%。Bogduk 通过解剖学研究也证明了腰神经后支是产生腰痛的重要原因。目前临床治疗方法主要有：射频热凝神经毁损、体外冲击波、高频脉冲电针等，但各种方法均需要相对精确的腰神经后支的定位[130]。

腹部连续横断层 128（FH.9370）

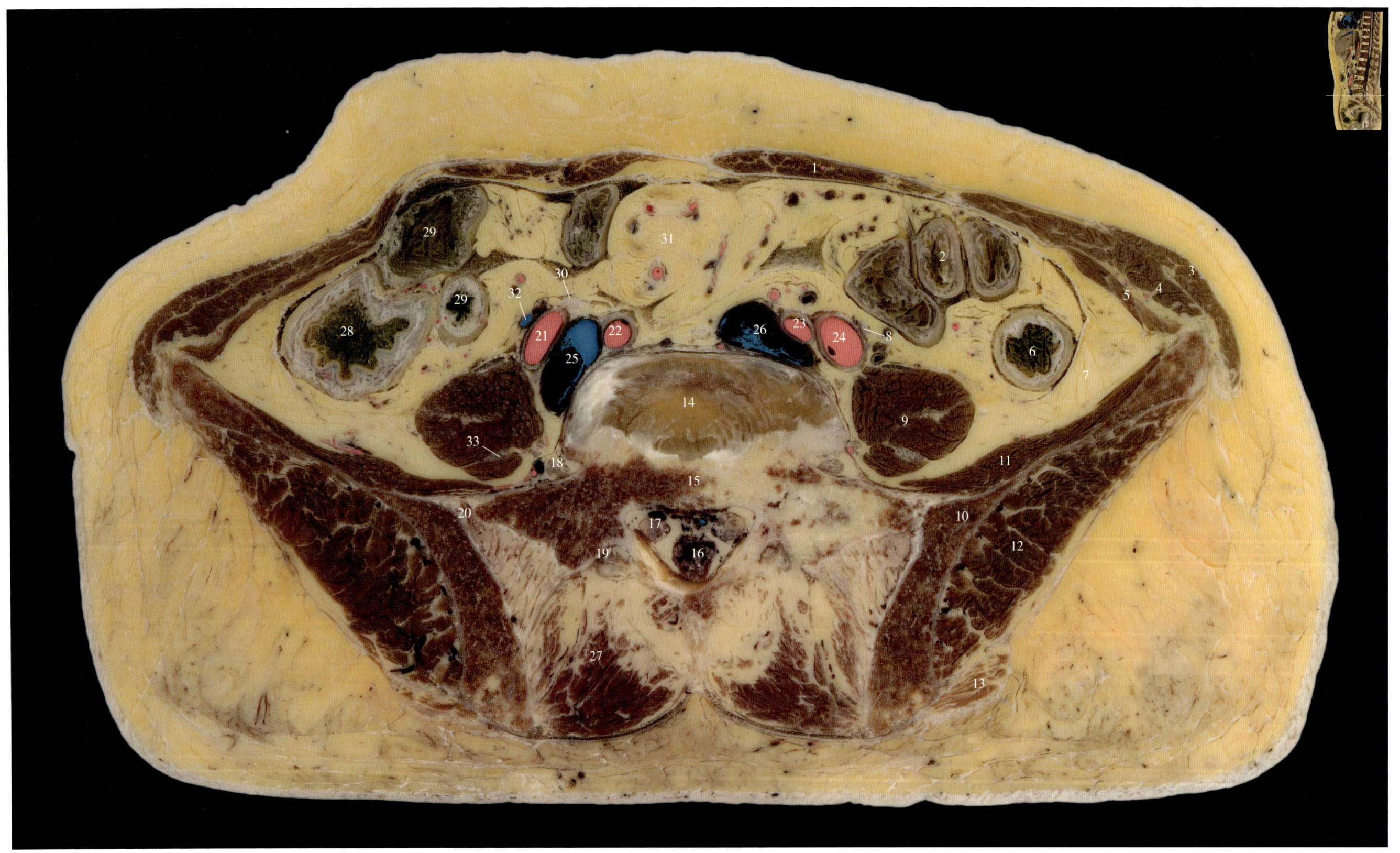

A. 断层标本图像

1. 腹直肌 rectus abdominis
2. 空肠 jejunum
3. 腹外斜肌 obliquus externus abdominis
4. 腹内斜肌 obliquus internus abdominis
5. 腹横肌 transverses abdominis
6. 乙状结肠 sigmoid colon
7. 腹膜外脂肪 extraperitoneal fat
8. 左输尿管 left ureter
9. 腰大肌 psoas major
10. 髂骨翼 ala of ilium
11. 髂肌 iliacus
12. 臀中肌 gluteus medius
13. 臀大肌 gluteus maximus
14. L5-S1椎间盘 L5-S1 intervertebral disc
15. 第1骶椎 1st sacral vertebra
16. 马尾 cauda equina
17. 第1骶神经 1st sacral nerve
18. 第5腰神经 5th lumbar nerve
19. 关节突关节 zygapophysial joint
20. 骶髂关节 sacroiliac joint
21. 右髂外动脉 right external iliac artery
22. 右髂内动脉 right internal iliac artery
23. 左髂内动脉 left internal iliac artery
24. 左髂外动脉 left external iliac artery
25. 右髂总静脉 right common iliac vein
26. 左髂总静脉 left common iliac vein
27. 竖脊肌 erector spinae
28. 盲肠 cecum
29. 回肠 ileum
30. 右输尿管 right ureter
31. 肠系膜 mesentery
32. 右卵巢静脉 right ovarian vein
33. 股神经 femoral nerve

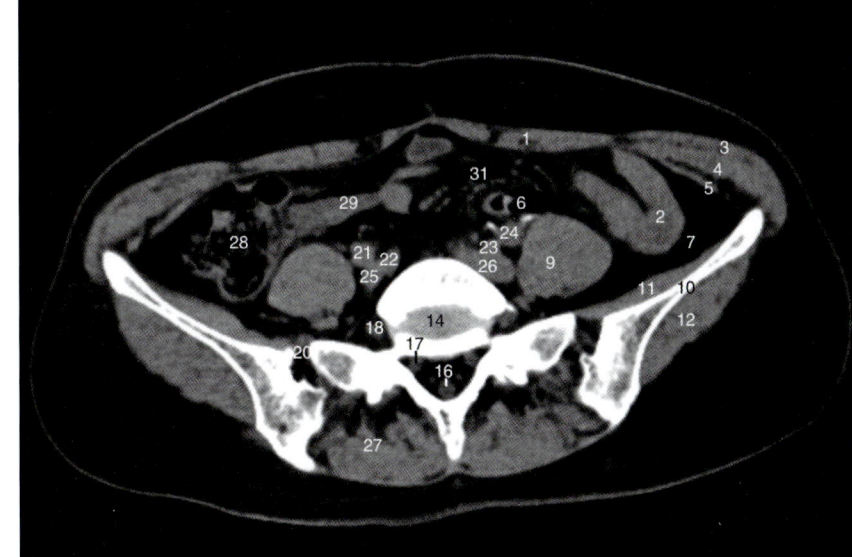

B. CT 平扫图像

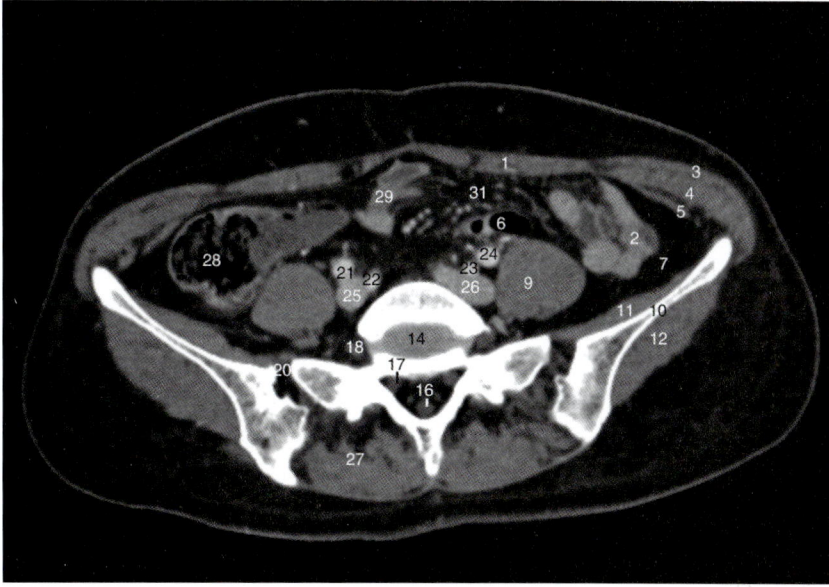

C. CT 增强图像

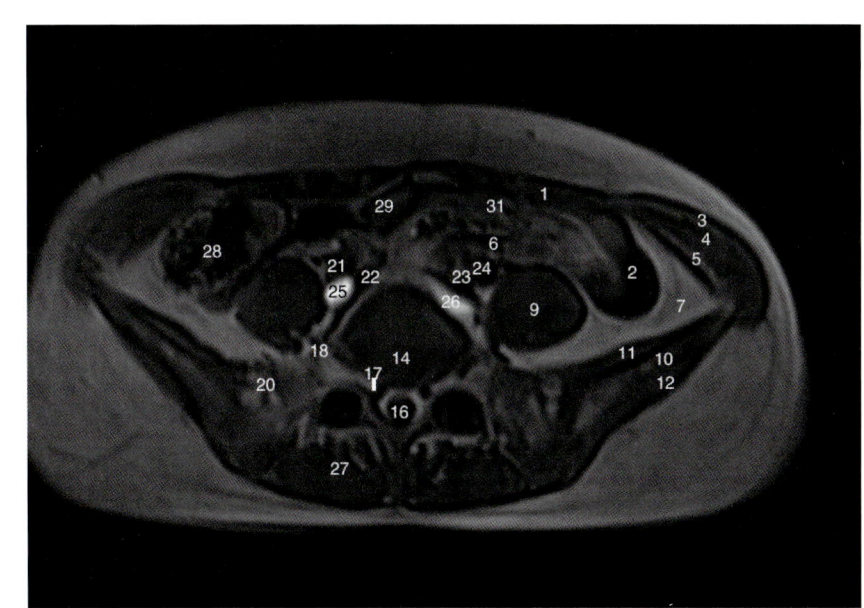

D. MR T1WI

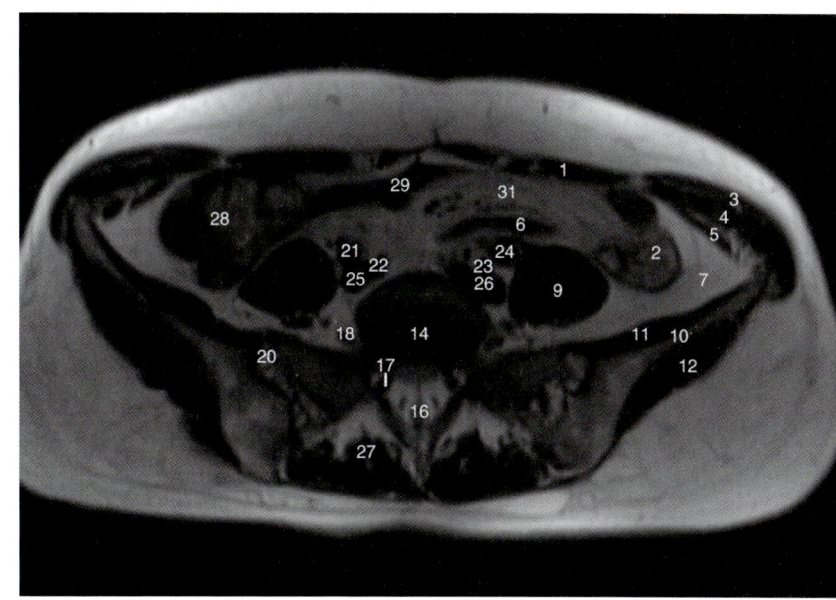

E. MR T2WI

关键结构：骶髂关节，左、右髂总静脉，髂外动脉，髂内动脉。

此断面经过第1骶椎椎体。

第1骶椎前方两侧为左、右髂总静脉及髂内、髂外动脉，后方骶管内有马尾和第1骶神经。第1骶神经向前外侧走行穿出骶管。断面后部两侧骨性部分为髂骨翼，髂骨翼内面覆盖有髂肌，外面被覆臀中肌。髂骨翼与内侧骶骨两侧之间形成骶髂关节。骶髂关节是全身最稳定的关节之一，关节由韧带连结部分和滑膜部分组成。随着年龄的增长，关节发生纤维粘连和逐渐闭塞。影像学调查显示，个别正常个体在50岁前骶髂关节就出现消失，而大多数是在50岁后消失，老年人此关节可完全纤维化，甚至偶尔出现骨化[27]。骶髂关节炎是骶髂关节最常见的病理改变，主要临床表现为疼痛、晨僵和黏着感。X线和CT的影像学表现为：关节面模糊、骨质破坏伴或不伴骨质增生硬化、关节间隙增宽及软组织肿胀。但是CT对于检测早期骶髂关节炎并不敏感；MRI可明确软组织和软骨的改变，对诊断早期活动性骶髂关节炎具有较好的敏感性。临床上多使用脂肪抑制的T2WI序列（FS-T2WI）来观察早期改变，其主要表现为双侧关节面下出现多发斑片状FS-T2WI高信号，提示骨髓炎性水肿[131]。

参考文献

[1] 刘树伟.人体断层解剖学.北京：高等教育出版社,2006.

[2] 张朝佑.人体解剖学(上).3版.北京：人民卫生出版社,2009.

[3] 赵洋,黄柱辉,付威,等.右心系统子宫静脉平滑肌瘤临床分析.中华医学杂志,2020,100(22):1741-1744.

[4] 刘树伟,李瑞锡.局部解剖学.8版.北京：人民卫生出版社,2013.

[5] 路福兴.肝硬化肝脏分叶体积变化研究.临床合理用药杂志,2015,8(11):18-21.

[6] Martakis K, Körber F, Dübbers M.Eventration of the diaphragm in a 4-year-old child diagnosed with dextrocardia.Klin Padiatr, 2016, 228(4):223-224.

[7] 刘树伟.断层解剖学.3版.北京：高等教育出版社,2017.

[8] 中华医学会放射学分会介入学组.布-加综合征介入诊疗规范的专家共识.中华放射杂志,2010,44(4):345-349.

[9] Fasel JH, Selle D, Evertsz CJ, et al.Segmental anatomy of the liver:poor correlation with CT.Radiology, 1998, 206(1):151-156.

[10] Fasel JH.Portal venous territories within the human liver:an anatomical reappraisal.Anat Rec (Hoboken), 2008, 291(6):636-642.

[11] Fasel JHD.Human liver territories:think beyond the 8-segments scheme.Clin Anat, 2017, 30(7):974-977.

[12] 钟世镇.临床应用解剖学.北京：人民军医出版社,1998.

[13] 周朋利,韩新巍.布-加综合征：副肝静脉解剖和介入治疗研究进展.临床放射学杂志,2009,28(10):1480-1482.

[14] 柏树令,应大君.系统解剖学.8版.北京：人民卫生出版社,2013.

[15] 中国临床肿瘤学会指南工作委员会.中国临床肿瘤学会(CSCO)胃癌诊疗指南2019.北京：人民卫生出版社,2019.

[16] 崔慧先,李瑞锡.局部解剖学.9版.北京：人民卫生出版社,2018.

[17] 沈柏用,施源.肝脏分段解剖的新认识.世界华人消化杂志,2008,16(9):913-918.

[18] 赵琪,姚冬雪,秦成勇.间位结肠综合征的临床特点与诊疗进展.中华消化杂志,2015,35(5):356-357.

[19] 徐鹏,刘丽,刘凤先,等.多层螺旋CT血管造影观察正常脾动脉解剖.中国医学影像技术,2011,27(9):1863-1866.

[20] 张彦,李振平,梁邦领,等.副肝静脉的影像解剖学研究.医学影像学杂志,2006,16(2):116-119.

[21] Kobayashi S, Matsui O, Gabata T.Pseudolesion in segment IV of the liver adjacent to the falciform ligament caused by drainage of the paraumbilical vein:demonstration by power Doppler ultrasound.Br J Radiol, 2001, 74(879):273-276.

[22] Kammen BF, Pacharn P, Thoeni RF, et al.Focal fatty infiltration of the liver:analysis of prevalence and CT findings in children and young adults.AJR Am J Roentgenol, 2001, 177(5):1035-1039.

[23] 王滔,陈梅鹃,尹阳,等.镰状韧带旁肝假性病灶的MRI诊断与鉴别诊断.医学影像学杂志,2019,29(5):794-797.

[24] Kollár D, Molnár FT, Zsoldos P, et al.Diagnosis and management of blunt pancreatic trauma.Orv Hetil, 2018, 159(2):43-52.

[25] Girard E, Abba J, Arvieux C, et al.Management of pancreatic trauma.J Visc Surg, 2016, 153(4):259-268.

[26] 张慧,周庭永,吕发金,等.64-MSCT重建肝门静脉左支的临床解剖学研究.解剖学杂志,2019,42(2):173-176.

[27] 刘树伟,邓雪飞,杨晓飞.临床解剖学腹盆部分册.2版.北京：人民卫生出版社,2014.

[28] 王云祥.实用淋巴系统解剖学.北京：人民卫生出版社,1984.

[29] 刘执玉.淋巴学.北京：中国医药科技出版社,1996.

[30] 蔡永辉,纪荣明,张成立,等.腹腔淋巴结群的应用解剖研究.解剖学杂志,1992,15(4):233-236.

[31] 蔡昌平,谢兴国,李成军,等.腹腔淋巴结影像断层解剖学的研究.局解手术学杂志,2010,19(4):261-262.

[32] 朱应礼,徐益民,金刚,等.胆囊癌的CT与MRI影像学表现及腹腔转移性淋巴结的分布特征探讨.中国临床医学影像杂志,2009,20(11):862-864.

[33] 孙伟英,袁建华,丁忠祥,等.腹部淋巴结核的CT诊断.放射学实践,2009,24(6):654-656.

[34] 杨志刚,杨开清,闵鹏秋,等.胰周区域淋巴结CT表现及其解剖病理基础.中国医学计算机成像杂志,2002,8(4):223-227.

[35] Michels NA.Newer anatomy of the liver and its variant blood supply and collateral circulation.Am J Surg, 1966, 112(3):337-347.

[36] Hitta JR, Gabbay J, Busuttil RW.Surgical anatomy of the hepatic arteries in 1000 cases.Ann Surg, 1994, 220(1):50-52.

[37] 侯燕红,崔爱玲,刘学敏,等.变异肝动脉的解剖学特点及其临床意义.中国临床解剖学杂志,2019,37(4):366-370.

[38] 中国解剖学会体质调查委员会.中国人解剖学数值.北京：人民卫生出版社,2002.

[39] 鲍光进,李树平,孙静,等.肝动脉解剖变异的640层容积CT血管成像研究.中国医学计算机成像杂志,2014,20(6):555-560.

[40] 李中辉,陈华,孙备.胰十二指肠切除术中变异肝动脉识别与处理.中国实用外科杂志,2017,37(9):1050-1053.

[41] Saeed M, Murshid KR, Rufai AA, et al.Coexistence of multiple anomalies in the celiac-mesenteric arterial system.Clin Anat, 2003, 16(1):30-36.

[42] 魏祯杰,晏玉洁,何璐,等.肝左动脉变异合并肝固有动脉、胃右动脉阙如一例.四川解剖学杂志,2016,24(3):65.

[43] Harold E, Vishy M.Clinical Anatomy:Applied Anatomy for Students and Junior Doctors.13th ed.Oxford, UK:Blackwell, 2006.

[44] Susan Standring.格氏解剖学.39版.徐群渊,译.北京：北京大学医学出版社,2008.

[45] Zirinsky K, Auh YH, Rubenstein WA, et al.The portacaval space:CT with MR correlation.Radiology, 1985, 156(2):453-460.

[46] Engels JT, Balfe DM, Lee JK.Biliary carcinoma:CT evaluation of

［46］ extrahepatic spread.Radiology, 1989, 172(1):35-40.

［47］ Dorfman RE, Alpern MB, Gross BH, et al.Upper abdominal lymph nodes:criteria for normal size determined with CT.Radiology, 1991, 180(2):319-322.

［48］ Araki T, Hihara T, Karikomi M, et al.Hepatocellular carcinoma: metastatic abdominal lymph nodes identified by computed tomography.Gastrointest Radiol, 1988, 13(3):247-252.

［49］ 钟世镇.血管外科临床解剖学.2版.济南：山东科学技术出版社，2020.

［50］ 张培华，蒋米尔.临床血管外科学.4版.北京：科学出版社，2014.

［51］ Jack L.Cronenwett K.Wayne Johnston.Rutherford's Vascular Surgery.8th ed.Philadelphia:Elsevier, 2014.

［52］ 刘昌伟，王深明.血管外科手术学.北京：人民军医出版社，2013.

［53］ 卢小刚，代远斌.腰交感干的局部解剖.解剖学杂志，2007(5):614-616.

［54］ Kim SH.Doppler US and CT diagnosis of nutcracker syndrome. Korean J Radiol, 2019, 20(12):1627-1637.

［55］ Ananthan K, Onida S, Davies AH.Nutcracker syndrome:an update on current diagnostic criteria and management guidelines.Eur J Vasc Endovasc Surg, 2017, 53(6):886-894.

［56］ Javier Casillas, Joe U Levi, Ruiz-Cordero Roberto, et al.Multidisciplinary teaching atlas of the pancreas.Berlin:Springer, 2016.

［57］ Zech, Christoph Johannes, MF Reiser.Multislice-CT of the abdomen.Berlin:Springer, 2012.

［58］ Liu Y, Song Q, Jin HT, et al.The value of multidetector-row CT in the preoperative detection of pancreatic insulinomas.Radiol Med, 2009, 114(8):1232-1238.

［59］ Fidler JL, Fletcher JG, Reading CC, et al.Preoperative detection of pancreatic insulinomas on multiphasic helical CT.AJR Am J Roentgenol, 2003, 181(3):775-780.

［60］ Zamboni GA, Kruskal JB, Vollmer CM, et al.Pancreatic adenocarcinoma:value of multidetector CT angiography in preoperative evaluation.Radiology, 2007, 245(3):770-778.

［61］ 谷涌泉，张建.全身血管影像解剖学图谱.北京：人民卫生出版社，2012.

［62］ Susan Standring.格氏解剖学.41版.丁自海，刘树伟，译.济南：山东科学技术出版社，2017.

［63］ Collins JT, Nguyen A, Badireddy M.Anatomy, abdomen and pelvis, small intestine.in:stat pearls.Treasure Island (FL):Stat Pearls Publishing, 2020.

［64］ Zhou ZM, Fang CH, Huang LW, et al.Three dimensional reconstruction of the pancreas based on the virtual Chinese human-female number 1.Postgrad Med J, 2006, 82(968):392-396.

［65］ O'Sullivan AW, Heaton N, Rela M.Cancer of the uncinate process of the pancreas:surgical anatomy and clinicopathological features. Hepatobiliary Pancreat Dis Int, 2009, 8(6):569-574.

［66］ Morrison TC, Wells M, Fidler JL, et al.Imaging workup of acute and occult lower gastrointestinal bleeding.Radiol Clin North Am, 2018, 56(5):791-804.

［67］ Surabhi VR, Menias C, Prasad SR, et al.Neoplastic and non-neoplastic proliferative disorders of the perirenal space:cross-sectional imaging findings.Radiographics, 2008, 28(4):1005-1017.

［68］ 金征宇.医学影像学.2版.北京：人民卫生出版社，2010.

［69］ Biasutto SN, Repetto E, Aliendo MM, et al.Inguinal canal development:the muscular wall and the role of the gubernaculum. Clin Anat, 2009, 22(5):614-618.

［70］ Acar HI, Comert A, Avsar A, et al.Dynamic article:surgical anatomical planes for complete mesocolic excision and applied vascular anatomy of the right colon.Dis Colon Rectum, 2014, 57(10):1169-1175.

［71］ 白人驹，张雪林.医学影像诊断学.2版.北京：人民卫生出版社，2010.

［72］ Srisajjakul S, Prapaisilp P, Bangchokdee S.Imaging spectrum of nonneoplastic duodenal diseases.Clin Imaging, 2016, 40(6):1173-1181.

［73］ Conley D, Hurst PR, Stringer MD.An investigation of human jejunal and ileal arteries.Anat Sci Int, 2010, 85(1):23-30.

［74］ Hamabe A, Park S, Morita S, et al.Analysis of the vascular interrelationships among the first jejunal vein, the superior mesenteric artery, and the middle colic artery.Ann Surg Oncol, 2018, 25(6):1661-1667.

［75］ Okahara M, Mori H, Kiyosue H, et al.Arterial supply to the pancreas; variations and cross-sectional anatomy.Abdom Imaging, 2010, 35(2):134-142.

［76］ Patel BN, Giacomini C, Jeffrey RB, et al.Three-dimensional volume-rendered multidetector CT imaging of the posterior inferior pancreaticoduodenal artery:its anatomy and role in diagnosing extrapancreatic perineural invasion.Cancer Imaging, 2013, 13(4):580-590.

［77］ Horiguchi S, Kamisawa T.Major duodenal papilla and its normal anatomy.Dig Surg, 2010, 27(2):90-93.

［78］ 柏树令.系统解剖学.2版.北京：人民卫生出版社，2010.

［79］ Sun CH, Li X, Chan T, et al.Multidetector computed tomography (MDCT) manifestations of the normal duodenal papilla.Eur J Radiol, 2013, 82(6):918-922.

［80］ Tang ZH, Qiang JW, Feng XY, et al.Acute mesenteric ischemia induced by ligation of porcine superior mesenteric vein:multidetector CT evaluations.Acad Radiol, 2010, 17(9):1146-1152.

［81］ Kopylov U, Amitai MM, Lubetsky A, et al.Clinical and radiographic presentation of superior mesenteric vein thrombosis in Crohn's disease:a single center experience.J Crohns Colitis, 2012, 6(5):543-549.

［82］ Grane P, Josephsson A, Seferlis A, et al.Septic and aseptic post-operative discitis in the lumbar spine-evaluation by MR imaging. Acta Radiol, 1998, 39(2):108-115.

［83］ Acosta S.Mesenteric ischemia.Curr Opin Crit Care, 2015, 21(2):171-178.

［84］ Eickhoff A, Pickhardt PJ, Hartmann D, et al.Colon anatomy based on CT colonography and fluoroscopy:impact on looping, straightening and ancillary manoeuvres in colonoscopy.Dig Liver Dis, 2010, 42(4):291-296.

［85］ Grubnic S, Vinnicombe SJ, Norman AR, et al.MR evaluation of normal retroperitoneal and pelvic lymph nodes.Clin Radiol, 2002, 57(3):193-204.

［86］ Sakala MD, Dyer RB.The horseshoe kidney.Abdom Imaging, 2015, 40(7):2910-2911.

［87］ D'Andrea G, Trillo G, Roperto R, et al.Intradural lumbar disc herniations:the role of MRI in preoperative diagnosis and review of the literature.Neurosurg Rev, 2004, 27(2):75-82.

［88］ Yussen PS, Swartz JD.The acute lumbar disc herniation:imaging diagnosis.Semin Ultrasound CT MR, 1993, 14(6):389-398.

［89］ 张启龙，代文杰.硬化性肠系膜炎.中华普通外科杂志，2008, 23(1):74-76.

［90］ 朱风尚，鲁星燧，杨长青.Lemmel综合征的临床特征和诊治进展.中华消化杂志，2018, 38(6):430-432.

［91］ 崔慧先，刘学政.系统解剖学.7版.北京：人民卫生出版社，2014.

［92］ 蒋宏毅，赵洪青，吴洪涛，等.后腹腔镜下输尿管切开取石治疗输尿管上段结石69例报告.中南大学学报(医学版)，2011, 36(8):791-793.

［93］ 程志远，贾伟，田轩，等.下腔静脉滤器回收后血管形态改变的CT静脉造影研究.中华解剖与临床杂志，2020, 25(3):272-277.

［94］ 唐建巍，李宁，梁径山，等.原发性马尾副神经节瘤35例临床

分析. 疑难病杂志, 2018, 17(4):408-411.

[95] Coughlan CH, Priest J, Rafique A, et al.Spinal tuberculosis and tuberculous psoas abscess.BMJ Case Rep, 2019, 12(12):e233619.

[96] Torres J, Mehandru S, Colombel JF, et al.Crohn's disease.Lancet, 2017, 389(10080):1741-1755.

[97] 黄志, 夏维, 彭晓红. 超声引导竖脊肌平面阻滞用于经皮穿刺球囊扩张椎体成形术老年患者镇痛的效果. 中华麻醉学杂志, 2020, 40(6):763-764.

[98] 丁文龙. 系统解剖学.9 版. 北京: 人民卫生出版社, 2018.

[99] Ordás I, Eckmann L, Talamini M, et al.Ulcerative colitis.Lanc-et, 2012, 380(9853):1606-1619.

[100] Gupta R, Farhat W, Ammar H, et al.Idiopathic segmental infarction of the omentum mimicking acute appendicitis:A case report.Int J Surg Case Rep, 2019, 60:66-68.

[101] Morimoto M, Higashino K, Manabe H, et al.Age-related changes in axial and sagittal orientation of the facet joints:Comparison with changes in degenerative spondylolisthesis.J Orthop Sci, 2019, 24(1):50-56.

[102] Vernon H, Wehrle CJ, Kasi A.Anatomy, Abdomen and pelvis, liver.In:StatPearls.Treasure Island (FL):StatPearls Publishing, 2020.

[103] Shimohira M, Ogino H, Sasaki S, et al.Transcatheter Arterial Embolization for Segmental Arterial Mediolysis.J Endovasc Ther, 2008, 15(4):493-497.

[104] Plowman RS, Javidan-Nejad C, Raptis CA, et al.Imaging of pregnancy-related vascular complications.Radiographics, 2017, 37(4):1270-1289.

[105] 陈水兵, 虞希祥. 腰动脉栓塞治疗经皮椎间孔镜引起的大出血 4 例. 介入放射学杂志, 2017, 26(11):1033-1037.

[106] Goodman BP.Disorders of the cauda equina.Continuum (Minneap Minn), 2018, 24(2):584-602.

[107] Sakalihasan N, Limet R, Defawe OD.Abdominal aortic aneurysm.Lancet, 2005, 365(9470):1577-1589.

[108] Nienaber CA, Clough RE.Management of acute aortic dissection. Lancet, 2015, 385(9970):800-811.

[109] Youn GJ, Chung WC.Micrometastasis in gastric cancer.Korean J Gastroenterol, 2017, 69(5):270-277.

[110] 龙茜, 柳曦, 刘定西, 等. MRN 在脊神经病变中的临床应用进展. 临床放射学杂志, 2012, 31(11):1666-1669.

[111] 韩华, 韩佳栩, 项燕, 等. 腰骶段脊柱前方大血管的解剖学研究. 局解手术学杂志, 2019, 28(2):91-95.

[112] 陈卫, 倪才方. 骶正中动脉造影及栓塞在骶骨肿瘤切除术中的价值. 中国介入影像与治疗学, 2008(3):215-217.

[113] 阮全丰. 多层螺旋 CT 对消化道穿孔不同穿孔部位腹腔游离气体、腹腔积液或炎性病变的分布特点分析. 影像研究与医学应用, 2020, 4(13):196-198.

[114] Brinegar KN, Sheth RA, Khademhosseini A, et al.Iliac vein compression syndrome:Clinical, imaging and pathologic findings.World J Radiol, 2015, 7(11):375-381.

[115] Cappell MS.Pathophysiology, clinical presentation, and management of colon cancer.Gastroenterol Clin North Am, 2008, 37(1):1-24.

[116] Kler A, Wilson P.Total endoscopic-assisted linea alba reconstruction (TESLAR) for treatment of umbilical/paraumbilical hernia and rectus abdominus diastasis is associated with unacceptable persistent seroma formation:a single centre experience.Hernia, 2020, 24(6):1379-1385.

[117] Kedia S, Das P, Madhusudhan KS, et al.Differentiating Crohn's disease from intestinal tuberculosis.World J Gastroenterol, 2019, 25(4):418-432.

[118] Olszewska-Szopa M, Wróbel T.Gastrointestinal non-Hodgkin lymphomas.Adv Clin Exp Med, 2019, 28(8):1119-1124.

[119] Reed LJ, Attarian S, Olson TR, et al.Feasibility and safety of targeting the anterior superior iliac spine to perform a bone marrow procedure:a prospective, clinical study.J Clin Patho, 2018, 71(12):1116-1119.

[120] Hagiwara A, Minakawa K, Fukushima H, et al.Predictors of death in patients with life-threatening pelvic hemorrhage after successful transcatheter arterial embolization.J Trauma, 2003, 55(4):696-703.

[121] Hansen LW, Dolgin SE.Trends in the Diagnosis and Management of Pediatric Appendicitis.Pediatr Rev, 2016, 37(2):52-58.

[122] Wende Nocton Gibbs, Amish Doshi.Sacral fractures and sacroplasty.Neuroimaging Clin N Am, 2019, 29(4):515-527.

[123] 卢小刚, 代远斌. 腰交感干的局部解剖. 解剖学杂志, 2007(05):614-616.

[124] 林维韶. 髂腰肌筋膜间隔区综合征 (附 6 例报告). 中国骨与关节损伤杂志, 1995(4):248-249.

[125] 闫磊, 梁昊, 张建好, 等. 髂外动脉造影在盆腔肿瘤介入栓塞中的应用价值. 介入放射学杂志, 2019, 28(6):571-573.

[126] 陈佳男, 季铃华, 葛文亮, 等. 儿童大网膜扭转的诊治进展. 中华小儿外科杂志, 2020(2):187-189.

[127] 梁化东, 倪宏彬, 王英, 等. 女性梨状腹综合征伴不完全重复膀胱等多器官畸型一例报告. 中华泌尿外科杂志, 2007(6):392.

[128] Muneer A, Macrae B, Krishnamoorthy S, et al.Urogenital tuberculosis-epidemiology, pathogenesis and clinical features. Nat Rev Urol, 2019, 16(10):573-598.

[129] 郑丽梅, 玉洪荣, 徐晓武, 等. 腹盆腔段输尿管及其周围结构的数字化解剖研究. 中国临床解剖学杂志, 2019, 37(4):386-389.

[130] Bogduk N.A narrative review of intra-articular corticosteroid injections for low back pain.Pain Med, 2005, 6(4):287-296.

[131] Antonelli MJ, Magrey M.Sacroiliitis mimics:a case report and review of the literature.BMC Musculoskelet Disord, 2017, 18(1):170.

索 引

B

白线 linea alba　139,141,151,161,227~239
白线疝 hernia of linea alba　227,249
半奇静脉 hemiazygos vein　5~47
背阔肌 latissimus dorsi　3~151
贲门癌 cardiac carcinoma　39
布加综合征 Budd-Chiari syndrome　25,33,103

C

Chilaiditi 综合征 Chilaiditi syndrome　49
Conn 综合征 Conn's syndrome　73
Cushing（库欣）综合征 Cushing syndrome　73
肠结核 intestinal tuberculosis　229,251
肠切除吻合术 enterectomy and anastomosis　133
肠系膜 mesentery　159~257
肠系膜动脉栓塞 mesenteric artery embolization　161
肠系膜静脉血栓 mesenteric venous thrombosis　155
肠系膜上动脉 superior mesenteric artery　97~237
肠系膜上静脉 superior mesenteric vein　109~235
肠系膜上静脉血栓 superior mesenteric venous thrombosis　177
肠系膜下动脉 inferior mesenteric artery　175~225
肠系膜下静脉 inferior mesenteric vein　119~225
超声引导下竖脊肌平面阻滞 ultrasound-guided erector spinae plane block (ESPB)　193
充血性脾肿大及脾功能亢进 congestive splenomegaly and hypersplenism　109

D

大动脉炎 aorto-arteritis　101
大网膜 greater omentum　37~205,247
大网膜扭转 torsion of greater omentum　247
胆囊 gallbladder　93~119
胆囊底 fundus of gallbladder　89~91
胆囊管 cystic duct　91~93
胆囊结石 cholecystolithiasis 97
胆总管 common bile duct　95~147
胆总管扩张 common bile duct dilation　105,135
低位胆道梗阻 low level biliary obstruction　135
骶骨 sacrum　249
骶髂关节 sacroiliac joint　257
骶髂关节炎 sacroiliitis　257
骶翼 ala of sacrum　247,251
骶正中动脉栓塞 median sacral artery embolization　217
第 10 肋骨 10th costal bone　69,103~127
第 10 肋软骨 10th costal cartilage　113,115,129
第 10 胸椎横突 transverse process of 10th thoracic vertebra　39~45
第 10 胸椎椎体 body of 10th thoracic vertebra　21~39
第 11 肋骨 11th costal bone　63~67
第 11 胸椎横突 transverse process of 11th thoracic vertebra　47~57
第 11 胸椎椎体 body of 11th thoracic vertebra　47~65
第 12 胸神经 12th thoracic nerve　95~97
第 12 胸椎横突 transverse process of 12th thoracic vertebra　69
第 12 胸椎棘突 spinous process of 12th thoracic vertebra　69
第 12 胸椎椎体 body of 12th thoracic vertebra　71~91
第 1 骶神经 1st sacral nerve　249~257
第 1 骶椎 1st sacral vertebra　255,257
第 1 腰椎椎体 body of 1nd lumbar vertebra　99~123
第 2 腰神经 2nd lumbar nerve　153~157
第 2 腰椎椎体 body of the 2nd lumbar vertebra　131~155
第 3 腰神经 3rd lumbar nerve　185~197,207~215
第 3 腰椎椎体 body of 3rd lumbar vertebra　163~191
第 4 腰神经 4th lumbar nerve　207~217,223~233
第 4 腰椎椎体 body of 4th lumbar vertebra　199~221
第 5 肋骨 5th costal bone　3
第 5 肋软骨 5th costal cartilage　3~45
第 5 腰神经 5th lumbar nerve　231~257
第 5 腰椎椎体 body of 5th lumbar vertebra　231~251
第 6 肋软骨 6th costal cartilage　47~51
第 7 肋骨 7th costal bone　3,21
第 7 肋软骨 7th costal cartilage　71~81
第 8 肋骨 8th costal bone　3,69,83~89
第 9 肋骨 9th costal bone　3~67,71~81,91~105
第 9 肋软骨 9th costal cartilage　107,109,111
第 9 胸椎椎体 body of 9th thoracic vertebra　3~13
第二肝门 the second porta hepatis　21,25,75,85
第三肝门 the third porta hepatis　67,75,85
第一肝门 the first porta hepatis　75,85

F

方向盘伤 chest steering wheel trauma　79
副肝静脉 accessory hepatic veins　29~37,65~77
副肝中静脉 accessory middle hepatic vein　35
副肝左动脉 accessory left hepatic artery　47
副神经节瘤 paraganglioma　187
腹白线 linea alba　41~71,75
腹壁上动脉 superior epigastric artery　3~15
腹部结核 abdominal tuberculosis　123
腹横肌 transverses abdominis　117~129,143~257
腹横肌腱膜 aponeurosis of transversus abdominis　139~141,151,161
腹膜外脂肪 extraperitoneal fat　153~257
腹内斜肌 obliquus internus abdominis　105~123,131~257
腹内斜肌腱膜 aponeurosis of obliquus internus abdominis　139~141,151,161
腹腔干 celiac trunk　83~93

腹腔积液 ascites　29,107,127,143
腹外斜肌 obliquus externus abdominis　3,11~25,27~69,87~257
腹外斜肌腱膜 aponeurosis of obliquus externus abdominis　139~141,151,161
腹直肌 rectus abdominis　11~61,71~257
腹主动脉 abdominal aorta　77~213
腹主动脉瘤 abdominal aortic aneurysm　211

G

GEJ 癌 gastro esophageal junction cancer　39
Gllisson 管道系统　Gllisson system　67
肝岛 hepatic island　61
肝段 hepatic segment　31,75,87
肝固有动脉 proper hepatic artery　91~99
肝固有动脉左支 left branch of proper hepatic artery　47
肝镰状韧带 falciform ligament of liver　25~61,65~97
肝镰状韧带旁假病灶 pseudo-lesion of liver sickle ligament　77
肝裸区 bare area of liver　19~99,101~109
肝门静脉 hepatic portal vein　81~107
肝门静脉高压症 portal hypertension　83
肝门静脉尾状叶支 caudate branch of hepatic portal vein　71,73
肝门静脉右后上支 right posterosuperior branch of hepatic portal vein　33~49,75~79
肝门静脉右后上支及肝动脉 right posterosuperior branch of hepatic portal vein and corresponding hepatic artery　45~73
肝门静脉右后下支 right posteroinferior branch of hepatic portal vein　99~129
肝门静脉右后下支及肝动脉、肝管 right posteroinferior branch of hepatic portal vein and corresponding hepatic artery and hepatic duct　77~85
肝门静脉右后支 right posterior branch of hepatic portal vein　51~73,89~97
肝门静脉右前下支 right anteroinferior branch of hepatic portal vein　11~61,99~129
肝门静脉右前下支及肝动脉、肝管 right anteroinferior branch of hepatic portal vein and corresponding hepatic artery and hepatic duct　79~97
肝门静脉右前支 right anterior branch of hepatic portal vein　31,63~77,89~97
肝门静脉右前支及动脉 right anterior branch of hepatic portal vein and correspondingartery　69~85
肝门静脉右支 right hepatic portal vein　73~89
肝门静脉左内叶支 left medial branch of hepatic portal vein　69~83,89
肝门静脉左内支 left medial branch of hepatic portal vein　31~57
肝门静脉左外上支 left laterosuperior branch of hepatic portal vein　17~25,39~45,51~61
肝门静脉左外上支及动脉、肝管 left laterosuperior branch of hepatic portal vein and corresponding artery and hepatic duct　65
肝门静脉左外上支及肝动脉 left laterosuperior branch of hepatic portal vein and corresponding hepatic artery　47~49,69~73
肝门静脉左外下支 left lateroinferior branch of hepatic portal vein　27~53,57~67
肝门静脉左外下支及动脉、肝管 left lateroinferior branch of hepatic portal vein and corresponding artery and hepatic duct　63,67~73
肝门静脉左外下支及肝动脉 left lateroinferior branch of hepatic portal vein and corresponding hepatic artery　75~81,85~97
肝门静脉左支横部 transverse part of left hepatic portal vein　59~73
肝门静脉左支角部 angular part of left hepatic portal vein　55,57
肝门静脉左支矢状部 sagittal part of left hepatic portal vein　59~71,91~109
肝内胆管细胞癌 intrahepatic cholangiocarcinoma　69
肝肾隐窝 hepatorenal recess　97~127
肝特异性对比剂 liver specific contrast agent　61
肝尾状叶 caudate lobe of liver　29~73,87~95
肝胃韧带 hepatogastric ligament　73~97
肝细胞肝癌 hepatocellular carcinoma　69
肝血管瘤 hepatic hemangioma　61
肝硬化 liver cirrhosis　11,49,51,77,83,115
肝右动脉 right hepatic artery　79~89,103~119
肝右管 right hepatic duct　53~73
肝右后上缘静脉 right posterosuperior marginal vein of liver　13~41
肝右后叶上段 superior segment of right posterior lobe of liver　5~81
肝右后叶下段 inferior segment of right posterior lobe of liver　83~137
肝右静脉 right hepatic vein　11~77
肝右静脉后根 posterior root of right hepatic vein　79~89
肝右静脉前根 anterior root of right hepatic vein　79~89
肝右静脉属支 tributary of right hepatic vein　91~115
肝右前叶上段 superior segment of right anterior lobe of liver　5~81
肝右前叶下段 inferior segment of right anterior lobe of liver　83~137
肝右叶 right lobe of liver　3,139~145
肝圆韧带 ligamentum teres hepatis　75~211
肝圆韧带裂 fissure for ligamentum teres hepatis　75~111
肝中静脉 middle hepatic vein　21~59
肝中静脉属支 tributary of middle hepatic vein　23,61~85,91~97
肝总动脉 common hepatic artery　89~119
肝总管 common hepatic duct　75~93
肝左动脉 left hepatic artery　77,81,87~97
肝左管 left hepatic duct　57~73
肝左后上缘静脉 left posterosuperior marginal vein of liver　29
肝左静脉 left hepatic vein　21~73
肝左静脉属支 tributary of left hepatic vein　75
肝左静脉下根 inferior root of left hepatic vein　77~87
肝左静脉下根属支 tributary of inferior root of left hepatic vein　89~97
肝左内叶 left medial lobe of liver　23~103
肝左内叶段 left medial lobe of liver　19,21
肝左外叶上段 superior segment of left lateral lobe of liver　19~73
肝左外叶下段 inferior segment of left lateral lobe of liver　21~111
膈 diaphragm　3~7,15~89
膈脚移位征 displaced crus sign　43,55
膈膨升 diaphragmatic eventration　15
膈脾韧带 phrenicosplenic ligament　63,65
梗阻性黄疸 obstructive jaundice　69,85
弓状切迹 arcuate notch　81~85
股神经 femoral nerve　243~257
关节突关节 zygapophysial joint　17,19,41~47,75,103~111,159~177,195~209,219~233,243~257
冠状窦 coronary sinus　3~19
冠状窦瓣 valve of coronary sinus　9
冠状韧带上层 superior layer of coronary ligament　3
冠状韧带下层 inferior layer of coronary ligament　3
横膈征 diaphragmatic sign　7

H

横结肠 transverse colon　49~211
后锯肌 serratus posterior　5~21
黄韧带 ligamenta flava　3,81~85
胡桃夹综合征 nutcracker syndrome　111
回肠 ileum　229~257
回肠动、静脉 ileal artery and vein　147
回盲瓣 ileocecal valve　227~235

J

急性阑尾炎 acute appendicitis　237
急性输尿管结石 acute ureterolithiasis　181
急性胰腺炎 acute pancreatitis　153
棘间韧带 interspinous ligament　67
脊神经根 root of spinal nerve　65~93
脊神经前根 anterior root of spinal nerve　59
脊髓 spinal cord　3~135
间位结肠综合征 chilaiditi syndrome　49
剑突 xiphoid process　35~39
降结肠 descending colon　65~221
交感干 sympathetic trunk　93~95,105
节段性动脉中膜溶解症 segmental arterial mediolysis (SAM)　203

结肠癌 colon cancer 225
结肠动脉 colic artery 201~203,219
结肠静脉 colic vein 157,159
结肠右曲 right colic flexure 139~145
结肠左曲 left colic flexure 67~73
结肠左曲综合征 syndrome of splenic flexure of colon 71
静脉韧带裂 fissure for ligamentum venosum 49~87
静脉韧带裂和肝胃韧带 fissure for ligamentum venosum and hepatogastric ligament 31~47,55
巨脾切除术 splenectomy for massive splenomegaly 109

K

克罗恩病 Crohn's disease 155,191
空肠 jejunum 91~257
空肠动、静脉 jejunal artery and vein 107~127,147
空肠动脉 jejunal artery 129~135,169
空肠梗阻 jejunal obstruction 133
空肠静脉 jejunal vein 99~105,151~157,171,177~197
溃疡性结肠炎 ulcerative colitis 195

L

L1-2 椎间盘 L1-2 intervertebral disc 121~133
L2-3 椎间盘 L2-3 intervertebral disc 153~163
L3-4 椎间盘 L3-4 intervertebral disc 185~199
L4-5 椎间盘 L4-5 intervertebral disc 219~231
L5-S1 椎间盘 L5-S1 intervertebral disc 249~257
肋膈隐窝 costodiaphragmatic recess 31~67
肋弓 costal arch 63
肋横突关节 costal transverse process joint 59,61
肋间后动脉 posterior intercostal artery 3~15,57,59,
肋间后静脉 posterior intercostal vein 49~63
肋间内肌 intercostale interni 5~31,51~61
肋间外肌 intercostale externi 5~49,57,63~89
肋头关节 joint of costal head 21~27,49~55
肋纵隔隐窝 costomediastinal recess 3
梨状腹综合征 prune belly syndrome 249
淋巴结 lymph nodes 89,135~149,213,215
淋巴结转移 lymph node metastasis 27,47,101,225,251
卵巢静脉血栓性静脉炎 ovarian vein thrombophlebitis 205

M

马尾 cauda equina 137~257
马蹄肾 horseshoe kidney 169
盲肠 cecum 237~257
门腔淋巴结 portocaval lymph node 95~111
门静脉高压 portal hypertension 25,77,83,103,109,201
迷走肝左动脉 aberrant left hepatic artery 41,47,87

P

盆腔肿瘤 transcatheter arterial chemoembolization of pelvic tumor (TACE) 245
脾 spleen 23~101
脾动脉 splenic artery 49~103
脾静脉 splenic vein 49~117
脾门 hilum of spleen 71,73
脾肾韧带 lienorenal ligament 75~101
脾肾隐窝 splenorenal recess 67,69

Q

奇静脉 azygos vein 3~63
脐 umbilicus 215~227
髂骨翼 ala of ilium 235~257
髂肌筋膜间隔综合征 iliacus compartment syndrome 243
髂肌 iliacus 235~257
髂嵴 iliac crest 229~233,241~245
髂静脉压迫综合征 iliac vein compression syndrome 223
髂内动脉栓塞 internal iliac artery embolization 217,235
前锯肌 serratus anterior 3,17~33
腔静脉过滤器 vena cava filter 185

R

韧带样瘤 desmoid tumor 183
乳头突 papillary process 75~85

S

肾癌 renal carcinoma 139
肾大盏 major renal calices 99,101,129
肾动脉 renal artery 85,103~107
肾动脉栓塞 renal artery embolization 127
肾动脉狭窄 renal artery stenosis 119
肾后筋膜 retrorenal fascia 139,141,167
肾结石 renal calculus 109
肾静脉 renal vein 85,103~107
肾前筋膜 prerenal fascia 139,141,167
肾上腺静脉 adrenal vein 85~91
肾小盏 minor renal calices 91~97,113~119
肾盂肾炎 pyelonephritis 109
肾锥体 renal pyramid 91~107,125~151,155~167
升结肠 ascending colon 133~235
升结肠癌 ascending colon cancer 143
十二指肠大乳头 major duodenal papilla 149~157
十二指肠降部 descending part of duodenum 111~181
十二指肠溃疡 duodenal ulcer 97
十二指肠旁疝 paraduodenal hernia 137
十二指肠憩室 duodenal diverticulum 145,175
十二指肠上部 superior part of duodenum 93~121
十二指肠升部 ascending part of duodenum 137~151
十二指肠水平部 horizontal part of duodenum 153~201
食管 esophagus 3~23
食管癌 esophageal cancer 17,39
食管腹部 abdominal part of esophagus 25~37
食管裂孔疝 esophageal hiatal hernia 23
室间隔 interventricular septum 5~19
输尿管结核 tuberculosis of ureter 253
竖脊肌 erector spinae 5~257
髓核 nucleus pulposus 157~163

T

T10-11 椎间盘 T10-11 intervertebral disc 39~47
T11-12 椎间盘 T11-12 intervertebral disc 65~73
T12-L1 椎间盘 T12-L1 intervertebral disc 93~101
T9-10 椎间盘 T9-10 intervertebral disc 15~21
特发性大网膜节段性梗死 idiopathic segmental infarction of the greater omentum 197
臀大肌 gluteus maximus 257
臀中肌 gluteus medius 233~257

W

网膜囊脾隐窝 splenic recess omental bursa　49~61
网膜囊上隐窝 superior omental recess　31~51
尾状突 caudate process　75~85
胃 stomach　39~77,121~123
胃癌 gastric cancer　27,39,47
胃癌区域淋巴结分组 regional lymph node grouping of gastric cancer　47
胃贲门 cardia of stomach　29~43
胃肠道间质瘤 gastrointestinal stromal tumor　251
胃底 fundus of stomach　15~37
胃动、静脉 gastric artery and vein　63~87
胃冠状静脉 gastric coronary vein　47
胃裸区 bara area of stomach　23~51
胃体 body of stomach　79~119
胃幽门部 pyloric part of stomach　87~123
胃潴留 gastric retention　93
胃左动脉 left gastric artery　27~85
胃左静脉 left gastric vein　47~89

X

下后锯肌 serratus posterior inferior　23~43
下腔静脉 inferior vena cava　3~217
先天性胆总管囊肿 congenital choledochus cyst　105
先天性巨结肠 hirschsprung's disease　71
消化道穿孔 gastrointestinal perforation　219
小肠梗 small bowel obstruction　129
小网膜 lesser omentum　49~55,61~71
心包前下窦 anterior inferior sinus of pericardium　5~25
心包腔 pericardial cavity　3~15
心包脂肪垫 pericardial fat pad　27~35
心大静脉 great cardiac vein　9~19
心小静脉 small cardiac vein　17,19
心中静脉 middle cardiac vein　21
胸导管 thoracic duct　3,29~69
胸骨体 body of sternum　3~33
胸廓内静脉 internal thoracic vein　3~11
胸膜腔 pleural cavity　5~39
胸主动脉 thoracic aorta　3~75

Y

腰椎间盘突出症 lumbar disc herniation　97,157,171,207,221,239
腰椎结核 tuberculosis of lumbar spine　189,207,215
胰岛素瘤 insulinoma　113
胰钩突 uncinate process of pancreas　113~165
胰颈 neck of pancreas　83~141
胰十二指肠下动脉 inferior pancreaticoduodenal artery　143~151
胰体 body of pancreas　75~129
胰头 head of pancreas　105~173
胰头钩突部癌 cancer of uncinate process of pancreatic head　135
胰头肿瘤 pancreatic head tumor　151
胰尾 tail of pancreas　83~101
胰腺导管腺癌 pancreatic ductal carcinoma　117
乙状结肠 sigmoid colon　223~257
硬化性肠系膜炎 sclerosing mesenteritis　173
硬脊膜 spinal dura mater　5~31,41~51,61~65
硬膜外隙 epidural space　41~47
右肺下叶 inferior lobe of right lung　3~37
右肺斜裂 oblique fissure of right lung　3~9
右肺中叶 middle lobe of right lung　3~23
右肝上间隙 right suprahepatic space　3,17~67,83~97
右膈脚 right crus of diaphragm　29~47,53,55,69~129
右冠状动脉 right coronary artery　5~19
右交感干 right sympathetic trunk　107~111,241
右卵巢静脉 right ovarian vein　203~257
右髂内动脉 right internal iliac artery　235~257
右髂外动脉 right external iliac artery　235~257
右髂总动脉 right common iliac artery　215~241
右髂总静脉 right common iliac vein　219~257
右肾 right kidney　89~187
右肾动脉 right renal artery　111~153
右肾静脉 right renal vein　117~153
右肾上极 the upper pole of right kidney　83~87
右肾上腺 right suprarenal gland　53~95
右肾盂 right renal pelvis　121~151
右输尿管 right ureter　153~257
右心房 right atrium　3~15
右心室 right ventricle　3~31
原发性小肠淋巴瘤 primary small intestinal lymphoma　231

Z

中间腰淋巴结 intermediate lumbar lymph node　155~167
终丝脂肪变性 filum terminalis steatosis　209
主动脉 abdominal aorta　173
主动脉瘤 aortic aneurysm　101,211
椎弓峡部 isthmus of vertebral arch　57
椎内静脉丛 internal vertebral venous plexus　41~59,65,67,75~89
椎外静脉丛 external vertebral venous plexus　33~39
左肺韧带 left pulmonary ligament　5~9
左肺上叶 superior lobe of left lung　3~23
左肺下叶 inferior lobe of left lung　3~39
左肺斜裂 oblique fissure of left lung　3~19
左肝上前间隙 anterior left suprahepatic space　31~69
左肝下前间隙 anterior left subrahepatic space　31~67,77
左膈脚 left crus of diaphragm　25,27,35,37,45,47,57~61,69~81,85~97,103~107
左冠状动脉 left coronary artery　13,15
左冠状动脉前室间支 anterior interventricular branch of left coronary artery　5~27
左冠状动脉左缘支 left marginal branch of left coronary artery　3
左交感干 left sympathetic trunk　109~123,153~175,241
左髂内动脉 left internal iliac artery　245~257
左髂外动脉 left external iliac artery　245~257
左髂总动脉 left common iliac artery　215~247
左髂总静脉 left common iliac vein　219~257
左肾 left kidney　61~169
左肾动脉 left renal artery　109~151
左肾静脉 left renal vein　109~141
左肾上腺 left suprarenal gland　53~103
左肾上腺三角 left adrenal triangle　71,73
左肾盂 left renal pelvis　109~133
左输尿管 left ureter　135~257
左心室 left ventricle　3~25
左叶间静脉 left interlobar vein　35~39